Handbook of
In Vivo Toxicity Testing

Handbook of
In Vivo Toxicity Testing

Douglas L. Arnold
Toxicology Research Division
Bureau of Chemical Safety
Food Directorate
Health Protection Branch
Health and Welfare Canada
Ottawa, Ontario

Harold C. Grice
CANTOX, Inc.
Nepean, Ontario

Daniel R. Krewski
Biostatistics and Computer Applications Division
Environmental Health Directorate
Health Protection Branch
Health and Welfare Canada
Ottawa, Ontario

ACADEMIC PRESS, INC.
Harcourt Brace Jovanovich, Publishers

San Diego New York Berkeley Boston London Sydney Tokyo Toronto

Academic Press, Inc.
San Diego, California 92101

United Kingdom Edition published by
Academic Press Limited
24–28 Oval Road, London NW1 7DX

Library of Congress Cataloging-in-Publication Data

Handbook of in vivo toxicity testing /
    edited by Douglas L. Arnold, Harold C. Grice, Daniel Krewski.
        p. cm.
    ISBN 0-12-063380-9 (alk. paper)
    1. Toxicity testing--in vivo. I. Arnold, Douglas L. II. Grice,
H. C. III. Krewski, D.
RA1199.4.I53I5 1990
615.9'07--dc20   89-37193
                                                           CIP

Printed in the United States of America
90 91 92 93   9 8 7 6 5 4 3 2 1

Contents

Part III
Hygiene

Part IV
Experimental Protocol

Part V
Conducting a Study

12. Developmental Toxicity Studies
Carole A. Kimmel and Catherine J. Price

13. Pharmacokinetics: Principles, Mechanisms, and Methods
James R. Withey

14. Pharmacokinetic Models
B. T. Collins

15. Principles and Procedures in Behavioral Toxicity Testing
Deborah C. Rice

16. Assessment of Immunotoxicity
Kenneth C. Norbury and Peter T. Thomas

Part VI
Monitoring the Study

17. Health Monitoring and Clinical Examination
Douglas L. Arnold and Harold C. Grice

18. Hematological Evaluation
Zofia Z. Zawidzka

19. Clinical Chemistry
D. L. Basel, D. C. Villeneuve, and A. P. Yagminas

Part VII
Data Analysis and Evaluation

Contributors

Numbers in parentheses indicate the pages on which the author's contributions begin.

R. Anderson (555), Health Protection Branch, Health and Welfare Canada, Ottawa, Ontario K1A OL2, Canada

Douglas L. Arnold (21, 149, 167, 449, 581, 589), Toxicology Research Division, Bureau of Chemical Safety, Food Directorate, Health Protection Branch, Health and Welfare Canada, Ottawa, Ontario K1A OL2, Canada

D. L. Basel (509), Staff Consultant, Southwest Veterinary Diagnostic Laboratory, Phoenix, Arizona 85022

Mikelis G. Bickis (113), Department of Mathematics, University of Saskatchewan, Saskatoon, Saskatchewan S7N OWO, Canada

R. T. Burnett (611), Environmental Health Center, Health Protection Branch, Health and Welfare Canada, Ottawa, Ontario K1A OL2, Canada

P. L. Carr (555), Health Protection Branch, Health and Welfare Canada, Ottawa, Ontario K1A OL2, Canada

M. D. Clarke (535), Toxicology Evaluation Division, Bureau of Chemical Safety, Food Directorate, Health Protection Branch, Health and Welfare Canada, Ottawa, Ontario K1A OL2, Canada

David B. Clayson (3, 643), Toxicology Research Division, Bureau of Chemical Safety, Food Directorate, Health Protection Branch, Health and Welfare Canada, Ottawa, Ontario K1A OL2, Canada

B. T. Collins (339, 611), Canadian Wildlife Service, Environment Canada, Ottawa, Ontario K1A 0L2, Canada

Darol E. Dodd (189), Bushy Run Research Center, Export, Pennsylvania 15632

James G. Fox (71), Division of Comparative Medicine, Massachusetts Institute of Technology, Cambridge, Massachusetts 02139

Claire A. Franklin (247), Environmental Health Directorate, Health Protection Branch, Health and Welfare Canada, Ottawa, Ontario K1A OL2, Canada

S. G. Gilbert (555), Health Protection Branch, Health and Welfare Canada, Ottawa, Ontario K1A OL2, Canada

M. J. Goddard (611), Environmental Health Directorate, Health Protection Branch, Health and Welfare Canada, Ottawa, Ontario K1A OL2, Canada

Harold C. Grice (149, 449, 535), CANTOX, Inc., Nepean, Ontario K2G 2X7, Canada

Carole A. Kimmel (271), Reproductive and Developmental Toxicology Branch/OHEA, U.S. Environmental Protection Agency, Washington, D.C. 20460

Daniel R. Krewski (3, 555, 643), Biostatistics and Computer Applications Division, Environmental Health Directorate, Health Protection Branch, Health and Welfare Canada, Ottawa, Ontario K1A OL2, Canada

Peter F. McGuire (589), Toxicology Research Division, Bureau of Chemical Safety, Food Directorate, Health Protection Branch, Health and Welfare Canada, Ottawa, Ontario K1A OL2, Canada

Sarah McLaughlin (31), Department of Mathematics and Science, ST. LAWRENCE COLLEGE, SAINT-LAURENT, Kingston, Ontario K7L 5A6, Canada

Jos Mes (45), Bureau of Chemical Safety, Health Protection Branch, Health and Welfare Canada, Ottawa, Ontario K1A OL2, Canada

D. J. Murdoch (611), Environmental Health Directorate, Health Protection Branch, Health and Welfare Canada, Ottawa, Ontario K1A OL2, Canada

Eduardo A. Nera (589), Toxicology Research Division, Bureau of Chemical Safety, Food Directorate, Health Protection Branch, Health and Welfare Canada, Ottawa, Ontario K1A OL2, Canada

Christian E. Newcomer (71), Department of Comparative Medicine, Tufts University School of Veterinary Medicine, Boston, Massachusetts 02111

Kenneth C. Norbury (409), Johnson & Johnson Patient Care, North Brunswick, New Jersey 08902

Catherine J. Price (271), Chemistry and Life Sciences, Center for Life Sciences and Toxicology, Research Triangle Institute, Research Triangle Park, North Carolina 27709

K. R. Reuhl (535), Neurotoxicology Laboratories, Department of Pharmacology and Toxicology, College of Pharmacy, Rutgers University, Piscataway, New Jersey 08854

Deborah C. Rice (383), Toxicology Research Division, Food Directorate, Health Protection Branch, Health and Welfare Canada, Ottawa, Ontario K1A OL2, Canada

Leonard Ritter (247), Environmental Health Directorate, Health Protection Branch, Health and Welfare Canada, Ottawa, Ontario K1A OL2, Canada

Harry C. Rowsell (59), Canadian Council on Animal Care and International Council for Laboratory Animal Science, Ottawa, Ontario K1P 5H3, Canada

William M. Snellings (189), Union Carbide Corporation, Danbury, Connecticut 06817

Peter T. Thomas (409), IIT Research Institute, Chicago, Illinois 60616

D. C. Villeneuve (509), Environmental Health Directorate, Health Protection Branch, Health and Welfare Canada, Ottawa, Ontario K1A OL2, Canada

James R. Withey (303), Bureau of Chemical Hazards, Environmental Health Directorate, Health and Welfare Canada, Ottawa, Ontario K1A OL2, Canada

A. P. Yagminas (509), Environmental Health Directorate, Health Protection Branch, Health and Welfare Canada, Ottawa, Ontario K1A OL2, Canada

Zofia Z. Zawidzka (463), Toxicology Research Division, Bureau of Chemical Safety, Food Directorate, Health Protection Branch, Health and Welfare Canada, Ottawa, Ontario K1A OL2, Canada

Preface

This book addresses, in a practical way, the design and conduct of *in vivo* toxicity studies used for purposes of safety assessment. In the course of our own laboratory work, it became evident that no single book provided a comprehensive treatment of all of the relevant considerations involved in *in vivo* toxicity testing. In response to this need, it was decided that a book on this topic would be of great value. All the contributors to this volume were selected on the basis of many years of practical experience in their respective areas of authorship. This will be evident in the thoroughness of their presentations and the guidance and recommendations provided on the specific topics addressed.

In general terms, the discipline of toxicology concerns itself with the detrimental effects of chemical and physical agents upon biological systems. Consequently, a wide range of knowledge and experience can and often must be brought to bear in the design, conduct, and interpretation of toxicological studies. This requires a depth of knowledge in such specialized areas as animal husbandry, hematology, clinical chemistry, pathology, biostatistics, and computer science as well as a global appreciation of the broader considerations involved in safety assessment based on toxicological data.

This book will be particularly useful to both graduate students and novice toxicologists as a practical guide to the conduct of toxicological research. It will be of value to more experienced practitioners interested in safety assessment practices outside their own area of expertise. Readers will find the book useful for appreciating the kinds of studies used by toxicologists today. The text describes the spectrum of *in vivo* protocols currently used in modern toxicology research laboratories and offers guidance on the detailed design and conduct of individual studies.

The text has been systematically organized to reflect the sequence of events involved in *in vivo* toxicity testing. After outlining the broad objectives of toxicity testing, the personnel requirements for the study team are described. The importance of good hygienic practices and techniques in the management of animal husbandry are discussed. General considerations in protocol development are delineated, including statistical principles. Because of the critical importance of the test animal in experimental studies, particular attention is paid to the selection and quality-control aspects of the test species. General principles are outlined for the conduct of particular studies, including acute, subchronic, and chronic studies in which the test agent is administered orally, by inhalation, or dermally. Criteria are included for the conduct of studies to examine developmental toxicity and pharmacokinetic disposition of test chemicals. Also featured are chapters covering the relatively new fields of behavioral toxicity and immunotoxicity.

During the course of a study, careful monitoring and follow-up is essential; attention needs to be given to animal health monitoring and clinical status. For large-scale studies, this requires computerized data acquisition, management techniques, and compliance with good laboratory practice regulations. After the completion of the study, data must be subjected to careful statistical analysis in order to ascertain the significance of any observed differences between exposed and unexposed animals. These results subsequently require careful interpretation to determine toxicological/biological significance. This book provides practical guidelines for carrying out these and other aspects of *in vivo* toxicity testing.

D. L. Arnold
H. C. Grice
D. R. Krewski

Part I
Objectives

1
Objectives of Toxicity Testing

David B. Clayson
Toxicology Research Division
Bureau of Chemical Safety
Food Directorate
Health Protection Branch
Health and Welfare Canada
Ottawa, Ontario

Daniel R. Krewski
Biostatistics and Computer Applications Division
Environmental Health Directorate
Health Protection Branch
Health and Welfare Canada
Ottawa, Ontario

I. INTRODUCTION: OCCUPATIONAL AND ENVIRONMENTAL CARCINOGENESIS

The Industrial Revolution that began in the late 18th century, and still continues today, has given humankind the opportunity to produce efficiently a large range of commercial and consumer products. Until recently, this was often achieved in very unhygienic surroundings with adverse health consequences for those workers engaged in the production or use of these products and with devastating consequences for the surrounding environment (Carson, 1962; Ashford, 1982). The Industrial

Revolution provided the financial strength necessary for the community to develop a strong scientific base, particularly in understanding why there was so much occupational ill-health and environmental destruction. This introductory chapter presents the major events and considerations that have led to the perception of modern toxicological science and its accompanying legislative framework as necessary parts of modern society. An attempt will be made to indicate when valid scientific conclusions can be drawn and how the residues of faith and superstition are still allowed to cloud attempts to develop a safer society.

In this chapter, the development of chemical carcinogenesis is traced in its relationship to the science of toxicology. Many other aspects of toxicology, such as teratogenicity, neurotoxicity, or behavioral toxicology, have grown in a similar way but at various rates and with differing starting times. Each aspect of toxicology is now generally investigated in living animals that are believed to reflect the probable results of human exposure to particular chemicals.

The earliest observations to connect life-style and cancer in humans were made by Ramazzini (1700) and Pott (1775). In *De Morbis Artificium* Ramazzini (1700) reported that nuns living in Appenine monasteries appeared more prone to breast cancer than did women in the general population. This occurrence was attributed to their celibacy, a prediction in keeping with modern epidemiological observations on parity and breast cancer (Wynder *et al.,* 1960). Pott (1775) observed that young children who had to sweep soot by hand from large old fashioned chimneys were peculiarly liable to scrotal skin cancer. He attributed this to soot particles lodged in the folds of the scrotal skin. It is noteworthy that a survey conducted in the 20th century demonstrated English chimney sweeps still to be liable to scrotal skin cancer (Henry, 1946). Subsequently, other astute clinicians have linked clusters of cancer cases to possible chemical exposures: Volkmann (1874) identified skin cancer in road repairmen; Bell (1976) noted skin cancer in shale oil workers; Rehn (1895) studied bladder cancer in dyestuff manufacturers; Barnett (1947) reported lung cancer in asbestos workers; and, most recently, Creech and Johnson (1974) associated occupational exposure to vinyl chloride with angiosarcoma of the liver.

The association of an industrial or environmental cancer with a cluster of cases is not sufficient evidence to establish the process or agent as carcinogenic. Two other types of observation are needed: epidemiological studies, in which populations of exposed and nonexposed individuals may be compared and possible confounding factors eliminated, and studies in surrogate species to reproduce the supposed human response under strictly controlled conditions. Both epidemiological and animal studies have been performed to confirm the carcinogenicity of each agent outlined in the previous paragraph, including soot (Henry, 1946), tars and oils (Henry, 1947), aromatic amines (Case and Hosker, 1954; Case et al., 1954; Melick et al., 1955, 1971; International Agency for Research on Cancer, 1977), asbestos, and vinyl chloride (International Agency for Research on Cancer, 1979).

Animal studies were developed in response to these cluster observations. Progress was delayed when researchers failed to realize that cancer induction generally required long periods of exposure and adequate doses of test agent to obtain meaningful results. In 1918 Yamagiwa and Ichikawa demonstrated that the continuous painting of coal tar on rabbits' ears led to the induction of carcinoma. Their critical observation was followed in 1921 by Bloch and Dreifuss' report of a similar effect in mice. Animals and humans suffered similar consequences from repeated exposure to coal tar.

Kennaway and his colleagues (Cook et al., 1932, 1933) synthesized dibenz (a,h) anthracene and showed it to be carcinogenic to mouse skin. They subsequently isolated benzo (a) pyrene from coal tar and showed it to be similarly carcinogenic. This first evidence that single chemicals could induce cancer was followed by Yoshida's (1932) report that ortho-aminoazotoluene induced tumors of the liver in rats. Since that time, it has been demonstrated that many hundreds of individual chemicals induce cancer in one or more animal tissues. Many of these chemicals belong to certain classes (Searle, 1976) — such as alkylating and arylating agents, polycyclic aromatic hydrocarbons, aromatic amines, nitro- and azo- compounds, N-nitroso compounds, aflatoxins, and metals — but a significant number, such as ethyl carbamate (Nettleship and Henshaw, 1943), do not. The existence of these outliers, and the fact that not all chemicals falling into the major classes of carcinogen demonstrate this activity, indicates that each chemical intended for use in the environment should, in theory, be tested for its potential to induce tumors. The economic and logistic requirements for properly conducted carcinogenicity bioassays are so great that only a small proportion of the total population of environmental chemicals can be adequately tested in this way. Current attempts to develop in vitro genotoxicity tests (DeSerres and Ashby, 1981), such as the Ames Salmonella/microsome assay and others (Ames et al., 1973a, 1973b; Ames, 1977; Langenbach et al., 1978; Brookes, 1981), constitute an effort to overcome the logistic problems. In general, this area is promising but still needs much scientific development before it can adequately replace animal bioassays (International Commission for Protection against Environmental Mutagens and Carcinogens, 1982).

II. THE SEARCH FOR SAFETY

Many new chemicals were introduced into western society as a result of technological innovations following World War II. Public concern about the safety of these and previously introduced chemicals escalated in the 1950s and 1960s. This anxiety was fueled by a growing realization, once infective diseases had been controlled with antibiotics and other pharmaceuticals, that chronic diseases, such as cancer and various heart diseases, were major causes of death. Public concern was further increased by the thalidomide disaster that resulted in the birth of several thousand badly deformed babies to mothers who used the drug to control morning sickness in early pregnancy (Wilson, 1973). The public responded in at least three ways: concern about cancer increased, leading to the passage of the Delaney clause of the U.S. Food and Drug Act in 1958; the consumer movement emerged as an unofficial watchdog over the regulatory machine; and emphasis in toxicology shifted from attempting to identify possibly toxic chemicals to trying to establish safety.

The Delaney clause of the U.S. Food and Drug Act (1958) states that "no [food] additive shall be deemed to be safe if it is found to induce cancer when ingested by man or animal, or if it is found after tests which are appropriate for evaluation of safety of food additives to induce cancer in man or animal". This clause has had a profound effect on regulatory thinking about food additives in many countries other than the United States and has also influenced thinking about the use of potential human carcinogens in other regulated areas of our environment. However, when the clause was enacted, only a few hundred chemicals were known to be carcinogenic and little was known about their mechanism of action. Also, analytical sensitivity was many orders of magnitude less than it is now. Because many critically important chemicals in the general environment, as well as some present in or added to the food supply, were discovered to be animal carcinogens (Searle, 1976), the Delaney clause appears somewhat less desirable now than formerly. Furthermore, increasing knowledge of the way in which chemicals may lead to cancer (Miller and Miller, 1976; Clayson, 1981; Squire, 1981; Weisburger and Williams, 1981; Clayson et al., 1983) indicates that some chemical carcinogens are less likely than others to induce human cancer. Mechanistic considerations may play an increasingly important role in carcinogen regulation and control in the years ahead. The success of such an approach will be apparent when it is no longer implicitly believed that animal bioassays for carcinogenicity can predict accurately for humans in every case (as is enshrined in the Delaney clause). However, evaluation of animal carcinogens with emphasis on their probable effectiveness in humans will become much more complex.

The emergence of consumer groups as unofficial watchdogs over regulatory toxicology has had a number of significant, but not always desirable, influences on the development of toxicology testing. There is little room for objection to one or more groups representing the public view on the outcome of toxicity testing and regulation. However, the dependence of these consumer groups on public funding means that they must retain public interest, a process which often leads to exaggeration of adverse findings and an apparent lack of judgment concerning what is optimal for society as a whole.

The objective of toxicological testing and ensuing regulation is to establish a "safe" environment and a correspondingly high level of public health. Absolute proof of safety is not possible since it would require an unequivocal demonstration that under no circumstances would a particular test agent produce an adverse effect. Thus, toxicological testing establishes an acceptable level of safety for each perceived adverse effect. This has led to an immense increase in toxicological testing requirements since World War II, which includes the enlargement of protocol size and complexity in established areas such as carcinogenesis and teratology and the introduction of new areas of concern such as immunotoxicology and behavioral toxicology. (Current protocol requirements for a variety of *in vivo* toxicological tests are discussed in Part IV of this book.) The large effort required in establishing the safety of a chemical to present-day standards is very costly and may be perceived to delay the introduction of new and extremely valuable chemicals into our environment. Overall, there is presently a clear necessity for the body politic through its political representatives to decide on the optimal level of toxicological testing necessary to provide adequate protection to public health without, at the same time, making innovation prohibitively expensive. In arriving at such a decision, it must be remembered that no action is ever free from risk. The wise person balances risk with achievement.

III. ERRORS AND THEIR ELIMINATION

The adage "to err is human, to forgive divine" (Pope, 1711) is admirable for the conduct of human relationships but totally inept as an approach to toxicity testing. Serious imperfections in the conduct of toxicological tests may lead to a dangerous chemical being introduced, with serious consequences to human health, or to a "safe" chemical being proscribed, with an economic loss to the developer and, ultimately, to the community. It is of little consequence to the public whether errors are accidental or deliberate.

The Industrial Bio-Test scandal, the most extensive example of toxicological testing error, led to many chemicals, particularly pesticides, being wrongly registered. Many person-years of effort auditing records were required to establish the details of which chemicals required retesting (Health and Welfare Canada, 1977, 1983). This incident provided one reason for the U.S. Food and Drug Administration (1976) to introduce "Good Laboratory Practices" (GLPs), a code designed to minimize the opportunity for significant error in toxicity testing. This code of practice is mandatory for all data to be submitted in support of regulatory submissions to the U.S. Food and Drug Administration. It has been recommended to member states by the Organization for Economic Co-operation and Development (OECD; 1982) and is the subject of several memoranda of agreement between the United States and other countries. Subsequently, the U.S. Environmental Protection Agency (1983a, 1983b) has adopted similar legislation on good laboratory practices.

The good laboratory practices code requires the preparation of a protocol before the experiment is started. Detailed operating instructions (called standard operating procedures or SOPs) must be written for each facet of the study and be readily available to the scientists or assistants responsible for the procedure. Data derived from the study must be signed by the person recording it. Modifications to the protocol, SOPs, and data are permissible provided they are recorded and signed by the appropriate person with a written explanation for the change. Once the experiment is complete, records of data and specimens must be collected and stored in a secured archive. The rigor of the requirements is established through an internal audit by the quality assurance unit and an external audit by the GLP inspectorate. GLP requirements will increase the manpower required for regulatory toxicological tests by up to 30% over the previous level. This will increase cost but may lead to economies overall, insofar as more manpower will largely eliminate the necessity to repeat studies on the grounds that they were flawed. From the scientific viewpoint, GLP adds little to what is considered prudent scientific practice.

IV. RELEVANCE OF ANIMAL STUDIES TO HUMANS

It is generally assumed that the results of animal tests on chemical toxicity are relevant to humans. In many cases, humans are considered at least as sensitive to the effects of the test agent as is the most sensitive species used in these tests. Such assumptions are necessitated by a current lack of knowledge of more appropriate methodology and reflect other assumptions made by our distant ancestors on the relevance of observations in animals to the human situation. Two series of questions arise from these assumptions. At the qualitative level, it should first be asked whether any specific animal tests are more likely than others to lead to results of questionable significance to humans. Second, it may be asked whether the risk to humans can be assessed quantitatively from animal data. The first series of assumptions are analyzed in this section, leaving the problems of more quantitative risk assessment to be discussed in the concluding chapter of this volume.

Some test protocols are particularly liable to produce misleading results. Khera (1985, 1987) has recently drawn attention to the fact that maternal toxicity induced by test agents, rather than the direct action of the test agent itself, may be responsible for the induction of certain patterns of teratogenic effects. Several examples of possibly confusing results obtained in carcinogenesis bioassays are presented here. Perhaps the first to be recognized concerned the induction of sarcomas following the local injection of chemicals subcutaneously in rats (Grasso and Golberg, 1966). Although there can be little doubt that the injection of small quantities of chemicals such as 7,12-dimethylbenz(a)anthracene actually induces these tumors, overloading the tissues with dyestuffs may well lead to cancer because of a mechanism dependent on factors other than the specific interactions of the test chemical. Similarly, bladder stone formation can lead to bladder cancer in rats and mice, thus making it difficult to be certain whether a chemical that leads to bladder stone formation and tumorigenesis is or is not a true carcinogen (Clayson, 1979).

Perhaps the greatest cause of confusion in the interpretation of carcinogenicity bioassays occurs when a substantial background incidence of tumors is enhanced (Clayson et al., 1983). It should be asked whether the test chemical is inducing such tumors or merely enhancing their incidence. Although this problem is clearly recognized with chemicals that enhance the already high incidence of pulmonary tumors in strain A mice (Shimkin and Stoner, 1975), there has been little discussion of the confounding effects of naturally occurring tumors that demonstrate a lower but still appreciable incidence (Tarone et al., 1981). The B6C3F1 male mouse used in the NCI/NTP Bioassay Program in the United States demonstrates a 15–60% incidence of hepatic cell tumors by two years of age (Sontag et al., 1976). Yet, whether this confounds the interpretation of a bioassay or whether enhancement of the yield of such tumors, as opposed to their direct induction, is relevant to the effects of the chemical in humans is not asked; instead, these chemicals are usually uncritically accepted as carcinogens and generally regulated as such.

There are many other tumors that have a naturally high incidence, such as tumors of the endocrine tissues in certain strains of rats. In each case, there is a need to consider the overall evidence that agents increasing the yield of such tumors may or may not induce cancer in humans. Such considerations require in-depth knowledge of biological and biochemical mechanisms of carcinogenesis and development of new and testable ideas. Increased emphasis on *how* agents exert their effect, rather than on *which* agents exert an effect, will move toxicology to the forefront of integrated biological science.

One further problem needs to be addressed regarding human and animal reactions to toxic agents. Although it is possible to control the exposure of a test animal quite precisely in a well-run experiment, humans are exposed to an ever changing multitude of chemicals as a result of the food they eat, the drugs they take, or the life-styles they have chosen. Therefore, single-substance toxicological tests may either over- or underemphasize the significance of the potential hazard to humans, except possibly in the case of massive exposures. There is very limited laboratory evidence on the effects of chemical mixtures because a single chemical assay is so expensive that the assay of mixtures becomes prohibitively costly. Yet the co-administration of a carcinogen and a promoting agent may lead to far more tumors than either agent alone (Berenblum and Shubik, 1947a, 1947b; 1949; Pitot and Sirica, 1980; Slaga, 1983); whereas two carcinogens, such as 4-dimethylaminoazobenzene and 3-methylcholanthrene, may fail to produce tumors when given together, they do so when given separately (Pitot and Sirica, 1980; Richardson *et al.*, 1952; Conney *et al.*, 1956). More information on chemical interactions is desperately needed if we are to extrapolate animal tests to humans even with qualitative accuracy.

V. SAFETY EVALUATION AND UNCERTAINTY

The fundamental objective of toxicology is the determination of safe levels at which humans can be exposed to toxicants present in the environment. Unfortunately, uncertainties prevail in many aspects of the safety evaluation process (Miller *et al.*, 1983). Scientifically, there still exists much uncertainty about the mechanisms of action underlying the induction of most toxic phenomena. This obscurity surrounding etiology presents researchers with serious difficulties in ascertaining dose–response relationships, particularly at low levels of exposure. The concept of safety *per se* is fraught with uncertainty. Because the absence of adverse effects in a sample of test animals does not guarantee that the entire population will be insensitive to the agent under study, negative experiments can provide only upper limits on potential risk (Schneiderman and Mantel, 1973). With the recognition that we do not and cannot live in a risk-free environment, there has been an increasing trend toward defining safety in terms of negligible or *de minimis* risks rather than zero risk (Wilson, 1979; Office of Technology Assessment, 1981). Finally, the increasing frequency with which safety decisions are being challenged in U.S. courts suggests that some degree of uncertainty exists in the legal statutes under which safety evaluation is mandated.

VI. CURRENT APPROACHES TO TOXICOLOGICAL TESTING

Today's toxicologist is faced with a large and expanding armamentarium of tests for determining the adverse effects of chemicals in living organisms and needs to select the most appropriate for the purpose in hand. Procedures are available for use with intact animals, single-cell organisms, or mammalian cell lines cultured in the laboratory. The toxic effects measured in these systems vary in terms of their nature, severity, time of onset, and reversibility. Although traditional endpoints such as acute lethality, weight loss, and carcinogenesis have been studied for many years, recent developments have emerged with exciting new tests for effects such as immunosuppression, behavioral abnormalities, and genetic damage.

Given this spectrum of different procedures, the need for an orderly and systematic approach to toxicological testing is evident. One of the most notable proposals in this regard is the so-called decision tree approach of the Food Safety Council Scientific Committee (1980). After the physical and chemical properties of the test material are carefully defined, a preliminary assessment of probable human exposure is made. Toxicological testing then follows in a systematic manner. Weisburger and Williams (1981) have proposed a formal decision point approach designed to divide chemical carcinogens into two broad categories, depending on whether their mechanism of action involves genotoxic effects or epigenetic effects such as hormonal imbalance, immunosuppression, chronic tissue injury, and promotion of previously altered cells. The Weisburger–Williams decision point approach to carcinogenicity testing involves five steps conducted in sequence, beginning with an assessment of chemical structure. Chemicals suspected of having genotoxic potential following the application of a battery of tests for genetic damage might be further evaluated in this context with a second battery of limited *in vivo* bioassays. These relatively short-term bioassays are less costly than the chronic bioassay, which may be required only when equivocal results have been obtained in the more limited test, when human exposure is high or is maintained for long periods, or when data on epigenetic effects are of interest. Unfortunately, however, there is considerable discordance at present among individual tests for genotoxicity and between results obtained in these tests and in whole animal bioassays (Upton *et al.,* 1984).

A structured approach to the identification of genotoxic carcinogens based solely on a battery of seven short-term tests has been proposed by Brusick (1981). A more general categorization scheme, in which information on the nature of the neoplastic events induced in the chronic bioassay is considered along with evidence of genotoxicity, has been proposed by Squire (1981). With this procedure, the most relevant toxicological data is used to construct five different categories of animal carcinogens, thereby providing a possible basis for prioritizing regulatory concerns.

VII. *IN VIVO* TOXICITY TESTING

This text is limited to *in vivo* toxicity testing procedures conducted in experimental animals. This by no means implies that the host of recently developed short-term *in vitro* tests for genotoxic effects in microorganisms and cultured cell lines (Hollstein *et al.,* 1979) is necessarily less relevant. Rather, it is felt that a discussion of both *in vivo* and *in vitro* procedures, which are in a state of vigorous development and validation and entail the application of a variety of unique laboratory procedures, cannot be adequately presented in a single volume. Individual *in vivo* testing areas are addressed in a practical fashion to provide a useful reference for those actively engaged in laboratory research.

The remainder of this book is organized in six parts. Part II outlines the personnel and areas of expertise required for the successful conduct of *in vivo* studies. Particular attention is paid to the roles of the principal investigator, often a board-certified toxicologist, and associates trained in disciplines such as animal care, pathology, analytical chemistry, nutrition, hematology, immunology, statistics, and computing. The functions of technical personnel involved in the conduct of the study as well as current training requirements are also considered. In Part III, laboratory hygiene and safety procedures that should be adhered to by all personnel involved in the study are described.

Part IV focuses on one of the most critical phases of the study, namely, protocol preparation. Unless the experimental protocol is well thought out and all anticipated difficulties discussed in advance, the success of the study is in jeopardy from the start. Thus, the selection of the most suitable animal model is considered, as are fundamental aspects of experimental design such as dose selection, duration of exposure, sample size, randomization, and analytical measurements. Several possible problems may arise if the appropriate statistical analysis is not considered as part of the protocol development. Failure to consider and control for sources of experimental error may yield a study of low statistical power, thereby sacrificing increased experimental sensitivity that could have been available with similar resources. Subsequent statistical analysis is often directly linked to the specific experimental randomization scheme, which must be organized before the study starts. Incorrect randomization may lead to biased results or to a situation in which no valid test is possible for an important hypothesis. It is best to anticipate criticisms of the experimental methodology and statistical analysis and to develop carefully a sound protocol that minimizes potential weaknesses prior to commencement of the study.

The detailed procedures involved in the conduct of a toxicological study are discussed in Part V. The execution of acute, subchronic, or chronic toxicity tests is presented, with separate chapters focusing on the particular requirements for oral or inhalation exposure. Conventional approaches to dermatological testing in mammalian species are also discussed along with recently developed combined *in vivo/in vitro* procedures. The conduct of pharmacokinetic studies designed to measure the distribution and fate of xenobiotic toxicants taken up by the body is then considered in tandem with pharmacokinetic models to describe in quantitative terms the rates of absorption, distribution, metabolism, and elimination of the test agent. The section concludes with a discussion of behavioral and immunological toxicology.

In Part VI, conditions necessary for the conduct of a study are described. Environmental factors such as lighting, temperature, humidity, and diet need to be monitored throughout the study in order to determine their constancy. Regular animal health examinations by qualified technical personnel are essential to an animal study because accurate records of animal health must be available for subsequent use in the interpretation of any toxicological findings. Periodic hematological and biochemical tests are also useful in support of clinical data because they indicate both health status and toxicity. More clinical chemistry assessments of blood and other tissue samples may also provide useful information on such specific indices as alteration in enzyme function.

The procedures to be followed in determining the nature of pathological lesions are described in detail, including both gross examinations during necropsy and subsequent evaluation of histologically prepared tissue samples. The pathological interpretation of an *in vivo* study is often considered to be a final and independent part of the study. This is not desirable. The pathologist should be a member of the study team from the start and should play an important role in the conduct of the experiment, particularly insofar as extensive clinical, hematological, and biological data are concerned.

Because of the large volume of data acquired during the course of most toxicological studies, the use of modern computing techniques for data acquisition, storage, and processing is discussed, including the use of microcomputers for statistical analysis of experimental data. The final chapter in Part VI relates to the need and mechanisms for compliance with current codes of good laboratory practice. As noted previously, such compliance is mandatory for studies intended to serve as the basis for regulatory decisions.

The statistical analysis of toxicological data is discussed in Part VII. Although many different statistical procedures are required to accommodate the spectrum of data generated, all are directed toward identifying significant findings (i.e., those that are unlikely to be attributable to chance alone) and estimating the magnitude of the effects induced. Consideration is also given to interpreting the biological significance of these findings and to evaluating their relevance to the human situation.

VIII. CONCLUSIONS

Competent conduct and adequacy of toxicological testing as expressed in this volume are essential if human risk factors posed by exposure to xenobiotics are to be identified. Despite the progress that has been made, especially during the past two decades, it is still necessary to scrutinize current toxicological science closely to ascertain how many of the age-old superstitions about results of animal tests predicting a product's effect on humans remain to cloud our current thinking. It is only by understanding and applying modern scientific philosophy to the interpretation of animal tests in terms of human risk assessment that we may hope to advance to an era of increased safety achieved more economically both in terms of tests done and chemicals wrongly identified as potentially dangerous.

Burns (1785) pointed out that "the best laid schemes of mice and men gang aft-a-gley". In all probability, we must guard against a potentiation of these undesirable consequences when mice and men become involved in the same schemes.

References

Ames, B. N. (1977). Environmental chemicals causing cancer and genetic birth defects: Developing a strategy for minimizing human exposure. In "California Policy Seminar, Dec. 14, 1977", pp. 1–37. Berkeley: Institute of Environmental Studies, University of California.

Ames, B. N., Burston, W. E., Yamasaki, E., and Lee, F. D. (1973a). Carcinogens are mutagens: A simple test system combining liver homogenates for activation and bacteria for detection. *Proc. Natl. Acad. Sci. USA* **70,** 2281–2285.

Ames, B. N., Lee, F. D., and Durston, W. E. (1973b). An improved bacterial test system for the detection and classification of mutagens and carcinogens. *Proc. Natl. Acad. Sci. USA* **70**, 782–786.

Ashford, N. A. (1982). "Crisis in the Workplace: Occupational Disease and Injury". Cambridge, Massachusetts: MIT Press.

Barnett, G. P. (1947). "Annual Report of the Chief Inspector of Factories for the year 1947", p. 79. London: H.M.S.O.

Bell, J. (1876). Paraffin epithelioma of the scrotum. *Edinburgh Med. J.* **22**, 135–138.

Berenblum, I., and Shubik, P. (1947a). The role of croton oil applications, associated with a single painting of a carcinogen, in tumor induction of the mouse's skin. *Br. J. Cancer* **1**, 379–382.

Berenblum, I., and Shubik, P. (1947b). A new, quantitative approach to the study of the stages of chemical carcinogenesis in the mouse's skin. *Br. J. Cancer* **1**, 383–391.

Berenblum, I., and Shubik, P. (1949). The persistence of latent tumor cells induced in the mouse's skin by a single application of 9:10-dimethyl-1:2-benzanthracene. *Br. J. Cancer* **3**, 384–386.

Bloch, B., and Dreifuss, W. (1921). Ueber die experimentelle Erzeugung von Carcinomen mit Lymphdrüsen- und Lungen Metastasen durch Teerbestandteile. *Schweiz. Med. Wochenschr.* **51**, 1033–1037.

Brookes, P. (1981). Critical assessment of the value of in vitro cell transformation for predicting in vivo carcinogenicity of chemicals. *Mutat. Res.* **86**, 233–242.

Brusick, D. (1981). Unified scoring system and activity definitions for results from *in vitro* and submammalian mutagenesis test batteries. *In* "Health Risk Analysis" (C. R. Richmond, P. J. Wash, and E. D. Copenhaver, eds.), pp. 273–278. Philadelphia: Franklin Institute Press.

Burns, R. (1785). *To a mouse,* stanza 7.

Carson, R. (1962). "Silent Spring". Boston: Houghton Mifflin.

Case, R. A. M., and Hosker, M. E. (1954). Tumour of the urinary bladder as an occupational disease in the rubber industry in England and Wales. *Br. J. Prev. Soc. Med.* **8**, 39–50.

Case, R. A. M., Hosker, M. E., McDonald, D. B., and Pearson, J. T. (1954). Tumours of the urinary bladder in workmen engaged in the manufacture and use of certain dyestuff intermediates in the British chemical industry. Part I. The role of aniline, benzidine, alpha-naphthylamine, and beta-naphthylamine. *Br. J. Ind. Med.* **11**, 75–104.

Clayson, D. B. (1979). Bladder carcinogenesis in rats and mice: Possibility of artifacts. *Natl. Cancer Inst. Monogr.* **52**, 519–524.

Clayson, D. B. (1981). I.C.P.E.M.C. working paper 2/3: Carcinogens and carcinogenesis enhancers. *Mutat. Res.* **86**, 217–229.

Clayson, D. B., Krewski, D., and Munro, I. C. (1983). The power and interpretation of the carcinogenicity bioassay. *Regul. Toxicol. Pharmacol.* **3**, 329–348.

Conney, A. H., Miller, E. C., and Miller, J. A. (1956). The metabolism of methylated aminoazo dyes. V. Evidence for induction of enzyme synthesis in the rat by 3-methylcholanthrene. *Cancer Res.* **16**, 450–459.

Cook, J. W., Hieger, I., Kennaway, E. L., and Mayneord, W. V. (1932). Production of cancer by pure hydrocarbons. Part I. *Proc. R. Soc. London Ser. B* **111**, 455–484.

Cook, J. W., Hewett, C. L., and Hieger, I. (1933). The isolation of a cancer-producing hydrocarbon from coal tar. Parts I, II, and III. *J. Chem. Soc.,* 395–405.

Creech, J. L., and Johnson, M. N. (1974). Angiosarcoma of liver in the manufacture of polyvinyl chloride. *J. Occup. Med.* **16,** 150–151.

DeSerres, F., and Ashby, J. (1981). "Evaluation of Short-term Tests for Carcinogens". Amsterdam: Elsevier–North Holland.

Food Safety Council Scientific Committee (1980). "Proposed System for Food Safety Assessment: Final report of the Scientific Committee of the Food Safety Council". Washington, DC: Food Safety Council.

Grasso, P., and Golberg, L. (1966). Subcutaneous sarcoma as an index of carcinogenic potency. *Food Cosmet. Toxicol.* **4,** 297–320.

Health and Welfare Canada (1977). "Validity of Data on the Safety of Numerous Chemicals Is Being Investigated". Ottawa: Health and Welfare Canada.

Health and Welfare Canada (1983). "Update on IBT Pesticides". Ottawa: Health and Welfare Canada.

Henry, S. A. (1946). "Cancer of the Scrotum in Relation to Occupation". London: Oxford University Press.

Henry, S. A. (1947). Occupational cutaneous cancer attributable to certain chemicals in industry. *Br. Med. Bull.* **4,** 389–401.

Hollstein, M., McCann, J., Angelosanto, F. A., and Nichols, W. W. (1979). Short-term tests for carcinogens and mutagens. *Mutat. Res.* **65,** 133–226.

International Agency for Research on Cancer (1977). Asbestos. *IARC Monogr. Eval. Carcinogen. Risk Chem. Man* **14,** 1–106.

International Agency for Research on Cancer (1979). Vinyl chloride, polyvinyl chloride and vinyl chloride–vinyl acetate copolymers. *IARC Monogr. Eval. Carcinogen. Risk Chem. Humans* **19,** 377–438.

International Commission for Protection against Environmental Mutagens and Carcinogens (1982). Committee 2, Final Report: Mutagenesis testing as an approach to carcinogenesis. *Mutat. Res.* **99,** 71–91.

Khera, K. S. (1985). Maternal toxicity—A possible etiological factor in embryo-fatal deaths and malformations of rodent–rabbit species. *Teratology* **31,** 129–153.

Khera, K. S. (1987). Maternal toxicity in human and animals: Effects on fetal development and criteria for detection. *Teratog. Carcinog. Mutagen.* **7,** 287–295.

Langenbach, R., Freed, H. J., and Huberman, E. (1978). Liver cell-mediated mutagenesis of mammalian cells by liver carcinogens. *Proc. Natl. Acad. Sci. USA* **75,** 2864–2867.

Melick, W. F., Escue, H. M., Naryka, J. J., Mezera, R. A., and Wheeler, E. P. (1955). The first reported cases of human bladder tumors due to a new carcinogen—xenylamine. *J. Urol. (Baltimore)* **74,** 760–766.

Melick, W. F., Naryka, J. J., and Kelly, R. E. (1971). Bladder cancer due to exposure to para-aminobiphenyl: A 17-year followup. *J. Urol. (Baltimore)* **106,** 220–226.

Miller, E. C., and Miller, J. A. (1976). The metabolism of chemical carcinogens to reactive electrophiles and their possible mechanisms of action in carcinogenesis. *In* "Chemical Carcinogens" (C. E. Searle, ed.), ACS monograph 173, pp. 737–762. Washington, DC: American Chemical Society.

Miller, C. T., Krewski, D., and Munro, I. C. (1983). Conventional approaches to safety evaluation. *In* "Safety Evaluation and Regulation of Chemicals" (F. Homburger, ed.), pp. 66–76. Basel: S. Karger.

Nettleship, A., and Henshaw, P. S. (1943). Induction of pulmonary tumors in mice with ethyl carbamate (urethane). *J. Natl. Cancer Inst. US* **4,** 309–319.

Office of Technology Assessment (1981). "Assessment of Technologies for Determining Cancer Risks from the Environment". Washington, DC: Congress of the United States/ Office of Technology Assessment.

Organization for Economic Co-operation and Development (1982). "Good Laboratory Practice in the Testing of Chemicals: Final Report of the Group of Experts on Good Laboratory Practice". Paris: Organization for Economic Co-operation and Development.

Pitot, H., and Sirica, A. E. (1980). The stages of initiation and promotion in hepatocarcinogenesis. *Biochim. Biophys. Acta* **605**, 191–216.

Pope, A. (1711). *An Essay on Criticism*, Part 2, line 325.

Pott, P. (1775). "Chirurgical Observations Relative to the Cataract, the Polypus of the Nose, the Cancer of the Scrotum, the Different Kinds of Ruptures, and the Mortification of the Toes and Feet". London: James, Clarke and Gillins.

Ramazzini, B. (1700). "De Morbis Artificum". Chapter XX. Capponi, Italy.

Rehn, L. (1895). Ueber Blasentumoren bei Fuchsinarbeitern. *Arch. Klin. Chir.* **50**, 588.

Richardson, H. L., Stier, A. R., and Borsos-Nachtnebel, E. (1952). Liver tumor inhibition and adrenal histologic responses in rats to which 3'-methyl-4-dimethylaminoazobenzene and 20-methylcholanthrene were simultaneously administered. *Cancer Res.* **12**, 356–361.

Schneiderman, M., and Mantel, N. (1973). The Delaney Clause and a scheme for rewarding good experimentation. *Prev. Med.* **2**, 165–170.

Searle, C. E., ed. (1976). "Chemical Carcinogens". (ACS monograph 173). Washington, DC: American Chemical Society.

Shimkin, M. B., and Stoner, G. D. (1975). Lung tumors in mice: Application to carcinogenesis bioassay. *Adv. Cancer Res.* **21**, 1–58.

Slaga, T. J. (1983). Overview of tumor promotion in animals. *Environ. Health Perspect.* **50**, 3–14.

Sontag, J. M., Page, N. P., and Saffiotti, U. (1976). "Guidelines for Carcinogen Bioassay in Small Rodents (NCI-CG-TR-1)". Washington, DC: U.S. Department of Health, Education, and Welfare, Public Health Service, National Institutes of Health.

Squire, R. A. (1981). Ranking animal carcinogens: A proposed regulatory approach. *Science* **214**, 877–880.

Tarone, R. E., Chu, K. C., and Ward, J. M. (1981). Variability in the rates of some common naturally occurring tumors in Fischer 344 rats and (C57BL/6N × C3H/HeN)F$_1$(B6C3F$_1$) mice. *J. Natl. Cancer Inst. US* **66**, 1175–1181.

U.S. Environmental Protection Agency (1983a). Pesticide programs; Good laboratory practice standards; Final rule. *Fed. Regist.* **48**, 53946–53969.

U.S. Environmental Protection Agency (1983b). Toxic substances control; Good laboratory practice standards; Final rule. *Fed. Regist.* **48**, 53922–53944.

U.S. Food and Drug Act (1958). Public Law 85–929. 85th Congress H.R. 13254, September 6.

U.S. Food and Drug Administration (1976). Nonclinical laboratories studies: Proposed regulations for good laboratory practice. *Fed. Regist.* **41**, 51206–51228.

Upton, A. C., Clayson, D. B., Jansen, J. D., Rosenkranz, H. S., and Williams, G. M. (1984). I.C.P.E.M.C. Publication No. 9: Report of I.C.P.E.M.C. task group 5 on the differentiation between genotoxic and non-genotoxic carcinogens. *Mutat. Res.* **133**, 1–49.

von Volkmann, R. (1874). Ueber Theer- und Russkrebs. *Klin. Wochenschr.* **11**, 218.

von Yoshida, T. (1932). Ueber die experimentelle Erzeugung von Hepatom durch die Fütterung mit o-Amido-azotoluol. *Proc. Imp. Acad. (Tokyo)* **8**, 464–467.

Weisburger, J. H., and Williams, G. M. (1981). Carcinogen testing: Current problems and new approaches. *Science* **214**, 401–407.

Wilson, J. G. (1973). Present status of drugs as teratogens in man. *Teratology* **7**, 3–15.

Wilson, R. (1979). Analyzing the daily risks of life. *Technol. Rev.* **81**, 40–46.

Wynder, E. L., Bross, I. J., and Hirayama, T. (1960). A study of the epidemiology of cancer of the breast. *Cancer* **13**, 559–600.

Yamagiwa, K., and Ichikawa, K. (1918). Experimental study of the pathogenesis of carcinoma. *J. Cancer Res.* **3**, 1–29.

Part II
Personnel

2
Principal and Associate Investigators

Douglas L. Arnold
Toxicology Research Division
Bureau of Chemical Safety
Food Directorate
Health Protection Branch
Health and Welfare Canada
Ottawa, Ontario

I. INTRODUCTION

Until recent times, a toxicological study was often designed by a toxicologist and conducted with the assistance of a small staff. Monitoring the test animal's well-being often consisted of determining its body weight and feed consumption on a weekly or biweekly basis, coupled with a very superficial assessment of the animal's general health status (see Chapter 17). Concern for the animal's environment and nutritional status was minimal. Currently, toxicology is a multifaceted discipline encompassing a spectrum of specialists including food toxicologists, behavioral toxicologists, analytical toxicologists, biochemical toxicologists, and veterinary toxicologists. These individuals collaborate with other medical and biological scientists as well as with statisticians and animal care professionals in the design, conduct, and interpretation of study results (see Parts IV, V, VI, and VII). In this introductory overview on personnel, the study team approach is discussed. Two detailed examples are presented in Chapters 3 and 4.

Handbook of
In Vivo Toxicity Testing

II. A TOXICOLOGY TESTING PROGRAM

The marketing of a chemical (e.g., food additive) or a mixture of chemicals (e.g., pesticide formulations, cleaning agents) as a consumer product cannot be accomplished solely on entrepreneurial whim. Regulatory agencies require nonclinical laboratory or toxicological data regarding the product. The amount of toxicological data is more extensive for a food additive or a pesticide intended for use with food products than for chemicals that have small sales volume and/or limited contact with humans and the environment. In addition, some evidence of efficacy is also required for drugs. Efficacy data, which are usually generated in a clinical setting, are not dealt with in this chapter.

The types of toxicological data required by regulatory agencies may include oral ingestion studies of various durations; reproduction, mutagenicity, teratogenicity, and/or pharmacokinetic/metabolic studies; and possibly inhalation and/or dermal studies. In view of the economic and practical restraints, as well as the ethical concerns about the use of animals, it is imperative that as much meaningful information as possible be obtained from each test and test animal.

III. THE STUDY TEAM

The team concept was used in our laboratory (Arnold *et al.*, 1978) prior to the introduction of good laboratory practice (GLP) legislation in the United States by the U.S. Food and Drug Administration (1978). The GLP regulations specifically require that a study director be appointed by management for each nonclinical laboratory study. Among other responsibilities, the study director "has overall responsibility for the technical conduct of the study" (U.S. Food and Drug Administration, 1978), which implies the use of a research team. Depending on the type of laboratory (contract, academic, or in house), the appointment procedure for the study director varies, but the appointment of a study director is the first "formal" step in the process of developing a study protocol. In the GLP context (see Chapter 22), the study protocol is prepared by the study director in collaboration with the cooperating scientists who comprise the study team.

The "tools of the trade" available to the toxicologist have improved dramatically in recent years. The most significant improvement is in the quality of laboratory animals available for research. For example, it was not much more than a decade ago that well over half the control animals in a two-year rat study or an 18-month mouse study would die or require euthanasia before completion of the study due to intercurrent and/or latent diseases. In this regard, the International Agency for Research on Cancer (1980) suggested that "an experiment is not really a satisfactory long-term carcinogenicity study if the mortality in the control or low dose group is higher than 50% before the end of week 104 of age for rats, week 96 for mice and week 80 for hamsters". In addition, improvements in transportation containers and sensitization of transportation personnel to the special requirements of laboratory animals reduced the probability of compromising an animal's health during transit (Fox *et al.,* 1979). Improvements in the investigator's laboratory facilities (controlled temperature, humidity, and lighting; vermin control procedures; caging that minimizes the spread of communicable diseases; improved hygienic practices; etc.) coupled with formal training of animal care personnel (see Chapter 3) have all enhanced control of extraneous factors that can artifactually affect experimental results.

Technological advances made during the last decade have opened up new research vistas for the toxicologist. The greater availability of radioisotopes has facilitated metabolic and pharmacokinetic studies. The development of radioimmunoassays and the use of immunological (see Chapter 16) and behavioral (see Chapter 15) tests have facilitated the monitoring of more subtle toxicological manifestations. The development of chromatographic equipment with greater resolution coupled with the introduction of bench-top mass spectrometers has enhanced the identity of toxic chemical entities. The availability of microscopes interfaced with microprocessors that allow for the morphometric measurement of cells has greatly extended the toxicologist's ability to quantitate effects at the cellular and subcellular levels.

Experience has shown that the core team needed for the design, conduct, and evaluation of toxicological tests consists of a toxicologist, pathologist, statistician, and laboratory animal specialist. However, it must be emphasized that these four disciplines represent only the core team, and requirements for additional personnel from other disciplines vary with each experiment.

A. The Study Director

The study director is often a toxicologist whose primary responsibilities are:

1. delineating the objectives of the study;
2. assembling the multidisciplinary study team;
3. developing the study protocol for approval by management (in the GLP context);

4. ascertaining that all routine procedures are delineated in the standard operating procedures (SOPs);
5. ensuring, in conjunction with management, that all staff are aware of the study objectives and the importance of their contribution in its attainment;
6. coordinating all facets of the study;
7. monitoring study progress and initiating corrective action for unanticipated problems;
8. preparing the study reports and summaries in conjunction with the participating scientists.

As the duration of a toxicity test increases, the number of things that can go awry often increases in a geometric manner. Indeed, the study director often has to use the wisdom of Solomon and the patience of Job to bring a chronic study to a successful conclusion.

B. The Pathologist

The pathologist's major responsibilities include determining the full extent of a test substance's manifestations upon the test animals' tissues and organs and assisting in any attempt to elucidate the toxicological mechanism involved. To achieve these objectives, the pathologist should be familiar with findings from previous toxicological studies to aid in the selection of tissues and organs to be examined and the methods to be utilized in the evaluation of lesions. In addition, the pathologist may be required to respond to unanticipated observations during the conduct of the study by changing the protocol's list of tissues and organs to be examined, clinical chemistry tests (see Chapter 19) to be performed, and/or hematological evaluations (see Chapter 18) to be conducted.

To accomplish these responsibilities, the pathologist should develop standard operating procedures in collaboration with the following staff:

1. a clinical chemist to analyze various enzymes and electrolytes in blood and/or urine in order to monitor organ "status";
2. a hematologist to detect occult "disease" and/or monitor the test animal's health status;
3. a toxicologist and animal care specialist for disease surveillance (see Chapter 17);
4. safety and medical personnel regarding precautions to be taken by staff members during necropsy, tissue processing, and tissue disposal;
5. pathology technicians for necropsy procedures, specimen preparation, fixation, and mounting, data handling, and storage of all study records and specimens;

6. a statistician regarding evaluation procedures to ascertain treatment effects (Fears and Tarone, 1977; Salsburg, 1977).

It may be desirable to develop procedures for the pathologist when specimens are to be evaluated without prior knowledge about the test group from which a particular animal came, commonly referred to as the "blind" evaluation technique (Arnold *et al.*, 1988).

C. The Statistician

It was not too many years ago that toxicologists designed and conducted their own tests and performed their own statistical analyses, consisting primarily of the student "t" or Chi square tests. However, statistical considerations in the design and evaluation of toxicological studies are currently of sufficient complexity that a trained statistician is required (Lagakos and Mosteller, 1981). The statistician (see Chapters 7, 14, 24) can enhance the evaluation and interpretation of a study, but an elaborate statistical analysis is not a panacea for poorly designed and conducted studies (Fox *et al.*, 1979). Some subjects considered by the toxicologist and statistician in the design of studies are described here.

1. The Number of Dose Groups

Three treated groups and a control group are standard in most studies. Some exceptions are the yes/no cancer bioassay (National Toxicology Program, Board of Scientific Counsellors, 1984), the low dose extrapolation study, and the effective/lethal dose (ED_{50}/LD_{50}) study. A yes/no cancer bioassay screen may contain one or possibly two treated groups and a control group. Subacute or chronic low dose extrapolation studies and acute ED_{50}/LD_{50} studies require at least four dose groups. Depending on the amount of toxicological data available for the chemical that is to undergo testing, the statistician may be of assistance in the actual selection of dose levels (Bickis and Krewski, 1985).

2. The Number of Animals per Test Group

Depending on the objectives of the study, 30 to 50 rodents of each sex constitute an acceptable group size for subchronic and chronic feeding studies. With larger species, groups of 10 or less are common. For studies in which the primary objective is to assess low-dose effects, as with saccharin (Arnold *et al.*, 1983a), it may be beneficial to assign more animals to the low-dose groups than to the high-dose groups. Decisions regarding group size should include consideration of the power of the statistical tests and the precision of the parameter estimates.

3. The Distribution of Test Animals

Multiple caging of animals is more economical but may not be consistent with study objectives (see Chapter 7). All studies require some form of randomization or random assignment of animals to cages and treatment groups. The relative merits of a simple design, such as a completely randomized design, should be compared with designs involving the grouping of animals into more homogeneous subgroups, the use of restricted randomizations, and/or the use of more complex sample structures. For example, blocking by body weight, litter, or extraneous environmental factors may result in a more efficient design.

4. The Scheduling of Tests and Serial Kills

Periodic tests (e.g., hematology, clinical chemistry) and interim kills are used when the progression of toxicological effects is followed.

5. Reduction of Potential Bias

Qualitative or judgmental observations (e.g., clinical evaluation; see Chapter 17) may be inadvertently biased by the technical staff's knowledge of the animal's treatment group. The use of "blinding" techniques (Weinberger, 1973; Fears and Schneiderman, 1974) have been recommended for pathologists, but this continues to be a highly controversial issue (Prasse *et al.*, 1986; Arnold *et al.*, 1988).

Some of the more complex statistical analyses now routinely undertaken for toxicological studies involve time-to-tumor analysis, longitudinal analyses of periodic specimen samples (e.g., blood, serum, tissues for test chemical or metabolite analysis), and quantitative risk assessment. A tendency for some toxicological manuscripts to contain separate sections exclusively for a trained statistician (Peto *et al.*, 1980; Arnold *et al.*, 1983b) is an indication of how complex some statistical analyses have become. Also note that all statistical tests are based on laws of probability, and there is no absolute guarantee that a probability *(p)* value of less than a generally accepted limit of 5% ($p \leq .05$) can be "translated" into a real or biologically significant difference. Indeed, the more statistical tests performed on any given set of data, the greater the probability that a false statistically significant difference will be found for some comparisons. Subsequently, a decision is required on whether the statistical difference can be translated into a biologically meaningful difference. In addition, not all statistical tests are "created" equal. For example, depending on the assumptions that an investigator is prepared to make and the types of alternative hypothesis being entertained, one statistical test may result in a significant difference whereas another test may not. Tests based on fewer assumptions are said to be "more robust" but may not be as powerful in detecting treatment differences. If the underlying assumptions are not satisfied, then the results of the statistical analysis may not be valid. Usually, professional statistical advice is required to appreciate the nuances in such situations. In this regard, statistical methods are often used to establish significant differences or relationships. Whether or not a particular level of significance is attained can depend on the magnitude of the underlying difference, the sample size, and the efficiency of the test used. Although the reporting of a p value is frequently an endpoint in the statistical analysis, further attention is often beneficial. For example, a nonsignificant result does not necessarily indicate the absence of a biological effect. A study with a small sample size or inefficient design may show only very large effects. Such "statistical power" considerations can involve specialized statistical arguments.

D. The Animal Care Specialist

The value of the animal care specialist who is charged with the responsibility for obtaining a quality research animal and maintaining its health during the study cannot be overestimated (Arnold et al., 1977; Fox et al., 1979). In most institutions, this individual is a laboratory animal veterinarian; however, senior personnel of the type described in Chapter 3 can fulfill many of the requirements.

The cost of a conventional chronic toxicity test increased from $155,300 (U.S.) in 1973 (Gehring et al., 1973) to $250,000 in 1981 (Grice et al., 1981). The latter figure does not include those costs associated with GLP regulations and probably does not cover all costs inherent in the maintenance and upkeep of the physical plant. Consequently, the longer the duration of a toxicological study and the more extensive its objectives, the greater is the requirement for a qualified, experienced, and certified animal care staff. The animal care personnel consist of individuals who are most familiar with each test animal and its particular personality. They are the first to notice any change in an animal's demeanor, which can be the first indication of a toxicological effect or disease. Their understanding of their role in a toxicological study is imperative to its successful conduct and is dealt with in more detail in Chapter 3.

E. Other Members

Depending on the objectives of the study and what is known about the test substance's toxicity, one or more additional disciplines may need to be represented on the study team. The following examples illustrate additional resources that the study director may need to achieve the study's objectives.

Epidemiology is the branch of medical science that deals with the incidence, distribution, and control of disease in a population. The major advantage of epidemiological studies over toxicological studies is that the results of the former are obtained from the ultimate research animal — the human. However, due to obvious ethical constraints, humans are not knowingly exposed to toxic agents for testing purposes. Occasionally, subpopulations are inadvertently exposed to various agents, and appropriate epidemiological investigative procedures often suggest causal relationships. Consequently, for studies with chemicals that might be considered environmental pollutants, such as halogenated hydrocarbons (New York Academy of Sciences, 1979), or food additives, such as saccharin (Arnold et al., 1983a), the addition of an epidemiologist to the study team provides insight and assistance to experimental procedures that might be more informative regarding hypotheses developed from the epidemiological studies.

The analytical chemist, whose role is described in more detail in Chapter 4, has a number of mandatory roles dictated by GLP and a number of additional capabilities that may be required by the research team (Burchfield et al., 1977). Regarding GLP, the purity and stability of the test substance must be determined for each batch of test substance. For example, toxicological testing of a pesticide's commercial formulation versus testing of its active ingredients only may reveal a toxicological problem due to an impurity in the formulation, not to the active ingredient(s) per se. A reformulation may reduce the toxicological hazard.

Additional requirements that may be placed on an analytical chemist in a GLP study relate to concerns about potential and/or known contaminants in feed, bedding, or drinking water. The amount of contamination present may need to be ascertained and found not to interfere with the objectives of the study. Conversely, it may be necessary to ensure that the concentration of a particular nutrient in the test animal's feed is above a specific concentration. Additionally, it may be necessary to ascertain the concentration of the test substance in the vehicle and whether it is uniformly distributed in the vehicle when the feed is the vehicle.

The acquisition of data in the animal laboratory via microprocessors, the use of microprocessors to direct the operation of various laboratory instruments, and the interfacing of such equipment to a larger computer for data handling have resulted in the addition of a computer hardware and software specialist and/or a data manager to the study team. Although there are software options available in the commercial sector for toxicological testing, such "packages" may not be ideal for every laboratory. Therefore, it is necessary to have personnel available with sufficient knowledge of computer software and hardware to maintain and interface various types of electronic equipment and develop *ad hoc* programs effectively and efficiently.

Ascertaining the mechanism by which a test substance elicits its toxicological response or dramatically affects one species as opposed to another may require a biochemist's knowledge and experience. A microbiologist may be required if the test substance results in changes to the alimentary tract flora or if the metabolism of the test substance is attributable solely to intestinal flora (e.g., cyclamate).

IV. CONCLUDING COMMENTS

The use of a team approach in the design, conduct, and evaluation of nonclinical laboratory studies is the most efficient and practical way to perform toxicological studies. The core team, which consists of a toxicologist, pathologist, statistician, and animal care specialist, should be augmented with whatever disciplines are needed to accomplish the objectives of the study. Depending on the setting in which the study is being conducted (i.e., academic, private, or commercial), there may be varying degrees of concern about subsequent publications. The resolution of authorship and related considerations should be addressed prior to initiation of a study.

References

Arnold, D. L., Charbonneau, S. M., Zawidzka, Z. Z., and Grice, H. C. (1977). Monitoring animal health during chronic toxicity studies. *J. Environ. Pathol. Toxicol.* **1,** 227–239.

Arnold, D. L., Farber, E., and Krewski, D. (1988). Carcinogenicity testing: Histopathology and the blind method. *Comments Toxicol.* **2,** 67–80.

Arnold, D. L., Fox, J. G., Thibert, P., and Grice, H. C. (1978). Toxicology studies. I. Support personnel. *Food Cosmet. Toxicol.* **16,** 479–484.

Arnold, D. L., Krewski, D., and Munro, I. C. (1983a). Saccharin: A toxicological and historical perspective. *Toxicology* **27,** 179–256.

Arnold, D. L., Krewski, D. R., Jenkins, D. B., McGuire, P. F., Moodie, C. A., and Munro, I. C. (1983b). Reversibility of ethylenethiourea-induced thyroid lesions. *Toxicol. Appl. Pharmacol.* **67**, 264–273.

Bickis, M., and Krewski, D. (1985). Statistical design and analysis of the long-term carcinogenicity bioassay. *In* "Toxicological Risk Assessment, Vol. I, Biological and Statistical Criteria" (D. B. Clayson, D. Krewski, and I. Munro, eds.), pp. 126–127. Boca Raton, Florida: CRC Press.

Burchfield, H. P., Storrs, E. E. and Green, E. E. (1977). Role of analytical chemistry in carcinogenesis studies. *In* "Advances in Modern Toxicology, Volume 3, Environmental Cancer" (H. F. Kraybill and M. A. Mehlman, eds.), pp. 173–207. New York: John Wiley & Sons.

Fears, T. R., and Tarone, R. E. (1977). Response to "use of statistics when examining lifetime studies in rodents to detect carcinogenicity". *J. Toxicol. Environ. Health* **3**, 629–632.

Fears, T. R., and Schneiderman, M. A. (1974). Pathologic evaluation and the blind technique. *Science* **183**, 1144–1145.

Fox, J. G., Thibert, P., Arnold, D. L., Krewski, D. R., and Grice, H. C. (1979). Toxicology studies. II. The laboratory animal. *Food Cosmet. Toxicol.* **17**, 661–675.

Gehring, P. J., Rowe, V. K. and McCollister, S. B. (1973). Toxicology: Cost/time. *Food Cosmet. Toxicol.* **11**, 1097–1110.

Grice, H. C., Munro, I. C., Krewski, D. R., and Blumenthal, H. (1981). *In utero* exposure in chronic toxicity/carcinogenicity studies. *Food Cosmet. Toxicol.* **19**, 373–379.

International Agency for Research on Cancer (1980). Long-term and short-term screening assays for carcinogens: A critical appraisal. *IARC Monogr. Suppl.* **2**, 21–83.

Lagakos, S., and Mosteller, F. (1981). A case study of statistics in the regulatory process: The PD+C red no. 40 experiments. *J. Natl. Cancer Inst. (US)* **66**, 197–212.

National Toxicology Program, Board of Scientific Counsellors (1984). "Report of the NTP Ad Hoc Panel on Chemical Carcinogenesis Testing and Evaluation". Washington, DC: U.S. Department of Health and Human Services.

New York Academy of Sciences (1979). Health effects of halogenated aromatic hydrocarbons. *Ann. N.Y. Acad. Sci.* **320**, 1–730.

Peto, R., Pike, M. C., Day, N. E., Gray, R. G., Lee, P. N., Parish, S., Peto, J., Richards, S., and Wahrendorf, J. (1980). Guidelines for simple, sensitive significance tests for carcinogenic effects in long-term animal experiments. *IARC Monogr. Suppl.* **2**, 311–426.

Prasse, K., Hilderbrandt, P., Dodd, D., Goodman, D., Leader, R., Ferrell, J., Squire, R., Hardisty, J., Newberne, J., Hilderbrandt, P., Burek, J., De Paoli, A., Boorman, G., Bendele, R., Payne, B., Ward, J., Todd, G., Webster, H., Piper, R., and Patterson, R. (1986). Letter to the editor. *Toxicol. Appl. Pharmacol.* **83**, 184–185.

Salsburg, D. S. (1977). Use of statistics when examining lifetime studies in rodents to detect carcinogenicity. *J. Toxicol. Environ. Health* **3**, 611–628.

U.S. Food and Drug Administration (1978). Nonclinical laboratory studies, good laboratory practice regulations. *Fed. Regist.* **43**, 59986–60020.

Weinberger, M. A. (1973). The blind technique. *Science* **181**, 219–220.

3
Animal Care Personnel

Sarah McLaughlin
Department of Mathematics and Science
ST. LAWRENCE COLLEGE SAINT-LAURENT
Kingston, Ontario

I. The Evolution of Animal Technician Training
II. Establishing Standards
   A. The Role of CALAS/ACTAL
   B. The Role of AALAS
III. Competencies of Animal Technicians
IV. The Role of the Laboratory Animal Technician in Toxicology
   A. Level of Training and Experience
   B. Orientation to the Project
   C. Importance of the Clinical Examination
V. Continuing Education for Animal Health Technicians

I. THE EVOLUTION OF ANIMAL TECHNICIAN TRAINING

Today it sounds obvious that toxicologists who use properly trained animal care technologists for their support personnel are likely to achieve better quality results as well as better standards of care than researchers who do not use this caliber of employee. Two decades ago, however, this was not so obvious and indeed at that time Canada had no formal training programs for animal care personnel. In the United States, some programs were in place by the early 1960s but most came on stream during the 1970s. In England, however, animal technician training is older, dating back to 1950. Before such graduates were available, the gap was filled by on-the-job training schemes run under the aegis of older technicians who, by virtue of their years of invaluable practical experience, taught the junior employees. Thus, most research institutes got along as well as they could with animal attendants chosen because they were "good with animals" and would put up with the low salaries and the generally menial nature of the work. Since then there has been a shift in attitude that has led to the increasing employment of personnel with

31

formal training. Giammattei and Anderson (1985) published the results of a 1983 survey identifying 78 schools in North America that offered some form of animal health technician (AHT) training. The current number of programs offered is unknown because some have started since the 1983 survey, whereas others have been phased out.

In Canada, the earliest official federal statement on the need for trained animal technicians to support the laboratory animal field came in the National Research Council's 1966 report of the Special Committee on the Care of Experimental Animals. In the section concerning the care of animals in teaching and research institutions, recommendation 5 advised "such institutions as technical and vocational schools in the several provinces [to] consider establishing courses for the training of animal technicians." The first Canadian animal health technician program (two years, four semesters) began the following year in Ridgetown, Ontario, and was moved to Huron Park, Ontario, in 1969. However, graduates of this program were intended primarily to support the veterinary profession in private practice. In 1969, Ontario Community College of Arts and Applied Technology, St. Lawrence, Kingston, registered its first students into a program of animal care technology (three years, six semesters),

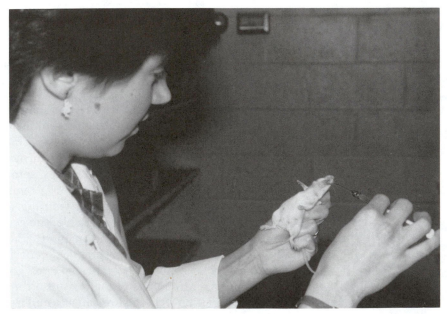

Fig. 1   Animal care technology student learning to oral dose a mouse, a skill taught in animal handling that is useful in toxicology.

with a curriculum geared specifically to training technologists to support the biomedical research field. Subsequently, animal technician/technology/husbandry/science care programs sprang up all across Canada, offering courses of study with different lengths and a bewildering variety of titles. In Ontario, the designation *technologist* tends to imply graduation from a three-year program, whereas a *technician* has received two years of training. This use of the terms *technologist* and *technician* has not been adopted uniformly by other provinces or by the United States. In addition, U.S. programs now favor the designation *veterinary technician* over *animal health technician.*

To make things even more confusing, the percentage of the curriculum devoted to laboratory animal technology varies widely among different programs. Toxicology as such is unlikely to appear as a specific course requirement in any of the programs; however, the subject is covered in portions of such courses as biology, physiology, gross and clinical pathology, pharmacology, large and small animal diseases, and animal handling (Fig. 1).

Table I

Formal Full-Time Programs in Animal Care and Health in Canada

Place	Type[a]	Semesters	Originated (year)	No. graduates/annum
Huron Park, Ont.	AHT (OMAF)	4	1967	30±
Kingston, Ont.	ACT (CAAT)	6	1969	30±
Windsor, Ont.	AHT (CAAT)	4	1970	20±
Edmonton, Alta.	Vet. assist. (IT)	2	1973[b]	20±
Toronto (1), Ont.	ACT (CAAT)	2	1973	20±
Saskatoon, Sask.	AHT (IT)	4	1973	20±
Montreal, Que.	AHT (CEGEP)	(6)2[c]	1973	15±
Sherbrooke, Que.	AHT (CEGEP)	(6)2[c]	1974	15±
St. Felicien, Que.	AHT (CEGEP)	(6)2[c]	1974	15±
St. Anne de la Pocatiere, Que.	AHT (CEGEP)	(6)2[c]	1974	15±
Toronto (2), Ont.	AHT (CAAT)	4	1975	20±
Olds, Alta.	AHT (Ag. Col.)	4	1976	20±
Fairview, Alta.	AHT (Ag. Col.)	4	1976	20±
Edmonton, Alta.	AHT (IT)	4	1976	20±
Vermilion, Alta.	AHT (Ag. Col.)	4	1976	20±
Kamloops, B.C.	AHT (Ag. Col.)	4	1981	20±
Red River, Man.	AHT (Ag. Col.)	4	1985	20±
Truro, N.S.	AHT (Ag. Col.)	6	1988	15±

Source: Modified from Greenwood (1981) with permission.

[a]CAAT, College of Arts and Applied Technology; CEGEP, College of General and Professional Education; Ag. Col., Agricultural College; OMAF, Ontario Ministry of Agriculture and Food; IT, Institute of Technology.

[b]This course was phased out in 1975.

[c]Indicates six semesters, two of which are in an animal health option.

In Canada, the number of graduates from provincially approved animal technician training programs is about 300 per year (Table I), but this number is increased by graduates from various other animal-related programs offered, for example, in vocational schools and universities. In the United States, animal technician graduates number over 2000 annually. Recently, however, some U.S. programs have closed because of declining enrollment. Several Canadian programs are also experiencing fewer applicants. At the same time throughout North America, there is a steady increase in employer demand for technicians. To some extent, this has sharpened competition between the veterinary clinics and the biomedical field for graduate AHTs. In general, the research facility has the advantage of offering better salaries and working conditions, but clearly these are not the sole criteria that determine choice of employment.

II. ESTABLISHING STANDARDS

A. The Role of CALAS/ACTAL

In 1969 when provincial education programs in animal care barely existed, the Canadian Association for Laboratory Animal Science/L'Association Canadienne pour la Téchnologie des Animaux de Laboratoire (CALAS/ACTAL) began a national certification scheme for laboratory animal technicians involving regionally organized extramural courses and examinations in written, oral, and practical form. With the growth of the formal provincial education programs, however, CALAS/ACTAL no longer felt the same pressing need to deliver education to technicians. The certification scheme was discarded, and in 1982 the association launched a voluntary registration scheme for laboratory animal technicians, designed to maintain and propagate national standards of competency. In order to write the registry board examinations, a candidate must have graduated from a formal training program in animal care of not less than two years' duration or the equivalent. In addition, candidates must have at least 12 months' full-time on-the-job experience in a laboratory animal facility accumulated within the two years prior to attempting the examinations. Success in the written examination qualifies the candidate to sit for an oral, which usually includes a practical component. Thereafter, the technician pays an annual fee to maintain registration.

The registry board of CALAS/ACTAL recognizes two categories of technicians working in the laboratory animal field. First, there is the technician who is involved in animal husbandry, that is, in maintaining animal colonies and facilities. This person is registered as an RLAT (registered laboratory animal technician). Second, the association also recognizes an animal technician who works in a research environment although this technician may not be involved with animals at the husbandry level. Such an individual is registered as an RLAT (Res) (registered laboratory animal technician in research).

In 1988 the registry board decided to allow the graduating class of AHTs in programs of two or more years' duration to sit for a written paper. Successful candidates are granted provisional registration, which is converted to full status upon their completion of the requisite work experience and the oral examination. Provisional registrants have two years in which to accomplish these requirements, otherwise the registration lapses.

The registry board also offers a higher level of registration, the master's. To qualify to write for this level, a candidate needs to have five years' experience in full-time relevant employment after attaining RLAT registration. Such a technician may be registered as an RMLAT or RMLAT (Res). These masters are few in number and usually are in a position of considerable seniority in which they carry supervisory responsibilities.

B. The Role of AALAS

The history of the American Association for Laboratory Animal Science (AALAS) dates back to 1950 when a group known as the Animal Care Panel formed to consider the educational needs of animal health technicians. The early 1960s saw the establishment of the Animal Technician Certification Board (ATCB) and later in that decade the Committee on Laboratory Animal Technicians (COLAT). The prime mission of COLAT is to give a voice to technicians within AALAS, including the opportunity to express their educational needs, whereas the mandate of the ATCB is to certify three levels of technicians: assistant laboratory animal technician (ALAT), laboratory animal technician (LAT), and laboratory animal technologist (LATG). These three levels reflect increasing levels of technical competence, knowledge, and ability to supervise more junior personnel.

Eligibility requirements for AALAS examination candidates stipulate a minimum educational background and length of relevant work experience for each level: ALATs must have a grammar school graduation plus one year's full-time employment in a laboratory animal facility; LATs must have a high school graduation or the equivalent plus three years' employment; LATGs must have a high school graduation or general education development certificate plus six years' employment. All candidates have to be recommended for examination by their immediate supervisor.

In some cases, education can be substituted for work experience. For example, a four-year degree in one of the life sciences qualifies the graduate for certification as an LAT after he or she has worked only one year in the field. Even without that one year's experience, such a graduate may apply for provisional certification as an LAT and have three years in which to acquire the twelve months' employment. Full status is granted after minimum work experience requirements are fulfilled, as documented in a letter from the applicant's supervisor.

The ATCB administers the AALAS examinations, which have a practical as well as a written component, through regional examining boards.

III. COMPETENCIES OF ANIMAL TECHNICIANS

One method that technical educators use to find an answer to the question "What must be learned?" is to summon a representative group of employees working together in the field to describe every technical procedure they actually perform in their work. These technical procedures are then grouped in categories of "competencies", and a chart eventually develops that is both a job description and a statement of curriculum objectives of a program geared toward servicing that field. This process of developing educational objectives is known as a DACUM (Design a Curriculum) study.

CALAS/ACTAL has done a DACUM study to define the competencies needed by laboratory animal technicians, including skills that are needed both by those working in animal husbandry and by those working on research protocols. Table II summarizes the competencies required by these two types of technician, and, for good measure, compares the skills these people require with those needed by technicians working in veterinary practice. One interesting feature is the greater array of skills needed by research technicians than by husbandry or veterinary technicians. Although there is no specific reference to toxicology in the competency chart, it is clear that a number of the skills listed are required for toxicological studies.

Because of variations in the individual training programs, all animal technician graduates cannot lay claim to the same competencies or even to the same degree of proficiency in each competency area. However, CALAS/ACTAL has supplied its DACUM study to all provincial educators across Canada involved in animal health technician training. The study advises them regarding the job skills needed in the field of labora-

Table II
Areas of Competence for Technicians

Skills	AHT[a] Vet. tech.	ACT An. man. RLAT	ACT An. res. RLAT (Res)
Perform animal management	+[b]	+	+
Perform animal health checks	+	+	+
Breed animals		+	+
Perform parasitic/mycotic examinations	+	±[c]	+
Collect/process blood samples	+	±	+
Perform microbiological techniques	+		+
Operate analytical equipment	+		+[d]
Perform necropsy	+		+
Perform histological techniques			+
Administer drugs, biologics, and reagents	+	+	+
Perform preventive medical techniques	+	+	+
Expose, develop, and store radiographs	+		
Administer anesthetics	+	±	+
Perform surgical techniques	+[e]		+
Perform postop care	+	+	+
Carry out tissue culture			+
Handle hazardous material		+	+
Process data			+
Perform business procedures	+		
Maintain supplies and equipment	+	+	+
Train other personnel	±	+	+

Source: Vet. tech. skills are derived from a DACUM study conducted by the Ministry of Colleges and Universities of Ontario. ACT skills are derived from a DACUM study performed by CALAS/ACTAL (1982).

[a]AHT, animal health technician; ACT, animal care technologist; Vet. tech., veterinary technician; An. man., animal management; An. res., animal research; RLAT, registered laboratory animal technician; RLAT (Res), registered laboratory animal technician in research.

[b]Indicates DACUM study showed competence needed in this area.

[c]Indicates may or may not need competence; in general becoming more commonplace.

[d]Higher level of sophistication.

[e]Veterinary technician skills limited to assisting in surgery.

tory animal technology. Programs that train graduates for this market are beginning to modify their curricula accordingly.

AALAS has also expressed interest in developing an occupational analysis similar to a DACUM study to define more closely the competencies of technicians. Meanwhile the association has outlined minimum job capabilities for each of its three certification levels. These capabilities range from relatively simple tasks, such as restraint required at the assistant technician level, through more complicated skills, such as injection administration at the technician level, to quite complex responsibilities, such as fiscal budgeting at the technologist level (*AALAS Bulletin,* 1978).

IV. THE ROLE OF THE LABORATORY ANIMAL TECHNICIAN IN TOXICOLOGY

A. Level of Training and Experience

Arnold and his colleagues (1978) have observed that toxicology research profits best from a multidisciplinary approach requiring as a minimal core a toxicologist, a pathologist, a statistician, and a laboratory animal specialist. Although there may be some argument about the exact makeup of such a "toxicology team", there is no doubt the people whose primary responsibility is the day-to-day handling of the animals must be represented on it. They are in closest proximity to the animals, and it is ultimately upon their competence and diligence in maintaining and monitoring the health of the animals that the success of a study depends. Indeed it has been said that "the wise investigator has as much respect for his animal technician as he has for his director, and it may be that his future as a scientist depends as much on the one as on the other" (Lane-Petter, 1967).

The level of training and experience needed for the "laboratory animal specialist" on the toxicology team varies for the individual project. Institutions are, of course, at liberty to hire whom they choose, and when economics dictate, institutions may choose to hire personnel who have no formal training in animal care. In this case, the institution itself usually offers some form of internal training program to teach at least the basic skills in animal care. At the same time, the employee may be offered a chance for eventual job promotion after a prescribed training period is completed. Examples are described in the literature (Arnold *et al.,* 1977). However, since the development of numerous formal educational programs (reviewed in Section I), there has been a tendency for institutions to discard in-house courses at this basic level because they can now hire personnel who already have these skills.

In Canada, it should also be noted that technicians without formal training are not eligible to write the CALAS/ACTAL registry board examinations (see Section II, A). Furthermore, at least eight university animal research facilities in Canada currently hire only personnel who already have or who are eligible for CALAS/ACTAL registration. Indeed, some projects are funded by grant monies that are conditional upon laboratory animal technicians having CALAS/ACTAL registration (personal communication, J. Kenyon, Director of Animal Care, Toronto General Hospital). This growing concern with the qualifications of support personnel involved in animal research is undoubtedly a response to the increasingly vocal animal rights activist groups that are demanding more accountability from animal researchers. The Medical Research Council of Canada requires exemplary care for animals in research projects. In its accreditation reports, the Canadian Council on Animal Care (CCAC) assesses the competence of personnel, and considers training an important indicator of competence. Under these circumstances, it is easy to understand the growing preference for formally trained animal care personnel.

Institutions usually decide upon job titles for their animal care employees that reflect a rising scale of seniority and pay, although the number of levels varies widely among institutions. For simplicity, a three-tier hierarchy that corresponds roughly to the three levels of AALAS certification is described next.

1. The Junior Technician

At the lowest level is the junior technician, or animal attendant, who is not expected to have any formal training. In some facilities, the tasks performed by this individual involve little animal contact: cleaning and/ or sanitizing rooms, cages, and water bottles; feeding and watering animals; and transporting bedding and feed. In other facilities, the junior technician who has received basic in-house training is expected to handle and restrain animals as well as to perform physical health checks. Careful observation of the animals can obviously be of great value in a toxicology study.

2. The Senior Technician

A technician working at the next level usually has a formal educational background (college or university) and is competent in the basic chores outlined for animal attendants. Through a study of the tasks that senior technicians perform at work, CALAS/ACTAL has found that they either engage in animal husbandry activities or directly assist the researcher with experimental protocols. Although some required skills are common to these two groups, as has been noted, the research technician needs additional skills (see Table II and Fig. 2). Table III lists the duties that can be assigned to a senior technician assisting in a toxicological study.

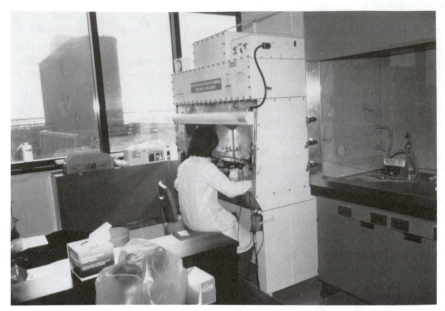

Fig. 2 Sophisticated skills are often needed by research technicians. An animal care technologist works at a Baker Class IIa biohazard containment work station. Model number #B40–112 "Biogard" (Baker Co. Ltd., Stanford, Maine).

3. The Master Technician

Technicians employed at the master's level will have prolonged experience in the laboratory animal field and a formal educational background which is at least equivalent to that of a senior technician. Master technicians, like seniors, work either in the field of animal husbandry or animal research and need the same competencies as their counterparts at the senior level; however, master technicians have more in-depth knowledge and experience. When engaged in a toxicological project, the master technician may assume some duties outlined for the senior technician (see Table III), but typically will have more supervisory duties, including fiscal and personnel responsibilities. The latter may extend to running in-house training programs for junior personnel.

B. Orientation to the Project

Once decisions have been made regarding the number and caliber of technicians to be employed in a particular study, the task of orienting and training these personnel on specific procedures and laboratory poli-

Table III
Duties Assigned a Senior/Master Technician for
a Toxicology Study

Animal identification
Health checking
Record keeping on individual animals and on
    environmental variables
Preparation of test diets
Administration of test chemicals
Collection and processing of tissue, blood, and
    other body fluids
Necropsy
Tissue culture
Histology
Surgical services (including pre/postoperative
    care, anesthesia)
Data entry on a computer system
Troubleshooting equipment
Assisting in the development of experimental
    protocol
Communicating with other members of the
    toxicology team

---

cies remains. If possible, all technicians working on a project, including temporary staff, should be oriented and trained by the same person so that all will be familiar with the same features of the experimental protocol and perform tasks in an identical manner. This maximizes the opportunity for reproducible results.

An orientation that proceeds from the general to the specific is logical. For example, technicians should be oriented to the department, then to the project, and then to specific policies and techniques. Orientation to the project allows technicians to understand the objectives and significance of the study, as well as their roles and responsibilities as members of the toxicology team. In this way, they are imbued with a sense of purpose in what they do so that they will never knowingly let the system down. Any safety precautions should be made clear at the outset (Arnold *et al.*, 1978).

Specific training in proper techniques involves demonstration. Some supervisors have found it useful to do a task analysis, breaking down a task into individual steps that have to be performed; key points of the task are highlighted and reasons for performing each step in a particular manner are explained (Thompson, 1979). For an animal health technician involved in a toxicological project, task analysis might be done on the following:

1. preparation of dosage forms
2. administration of dosage
3. observation of animal reactions
4. recording and summarizing observations
5. clinical pathology tests
6. necropsy examinations

For evaluation purposes, it may be useful to list the job skills across the top of a chart and write the technicians' names down the side. As each employee demonstrates mastery of a particular task, this can be indicated on the chart. The chart then verifies that qualified and trained people are involved in the study; it also indicates those technicians who need additional training (Thompson, 1979).

As Arnold *et al.* (1978) have pointed out, once the animal health technicians have been assigned to a study, it is important that they remain for the study's duration to avoid the undue stress that animals experience when handled by unfamiliar personnel. Using the same personnel avoids the introduction of another variable into the study. In a long-term study, this requires considerable forethought regarding vacation scheduling and possible sick leaves. The benefits, however, are worth it. For example, Scala (1983) has found that even in recording observations, more reproducible results are obtained with a constant staff of people. Moreover, when the same people are repeatedly in contact with the same animals, they are more likely to recognize behavioral changes that can signify impairment of an animal's health (Arnold *et al.,* 1978).

C. Importance of the Clinical Examination

The clinical examination plays a role of special importance in a toxicological study, especially in long-term studies. Protocols and procedures have to be established for daily and weekly monitoring of animals. Arnold and his colleagues (1977) have described a regime for thorough clinical monitoring involving extensive use of technicians. This monitoring includes a visual assessment of each animal on test twice daily for:

1. behavioral status
2. respiratory signs
3. skin condition
4. eye and mucous membrane condition
5. bleeding from orifices/surfaces

6. excretory products
7. food and water consumption

Abnormalities are recorded and brought to the attention of the senior technician who conducts a more detailed physical examination, which can be summarized as follows:

1. visual examination for signs of disease
2. palpation for nodules, lymph node enlargement, changes in abdominal viscera
3. observation of gait and postural changes
4. assessment of body temperature
5. observation of presence or absence of gross/occult blood in feces/urine
6. heart–lung ascultation
7. assessment of changes in body weight and food consumption
8. assessment of pain sensitivity (i.e., tail pinch)

Depending on the findings, the animal is returned to its original cage, admitted to an intensive care unit, or seen in consultation with the veterinarian or toxicologist. Animals in the intensive care unit are subjected to even more rigorous monitoring.

As well as performing these daily examinations, the senior technician also examines each animal weekly for tumors or other abnormalities. At this time, body weight and weekly feed consumption are recorded.

Arnold *et al.* (1977) noted that strict adherence to this monitoring system decreases the number of animals lost for histopathological examination due to autolysis, although it increases the technician's workload considerably.

V. CONTINUING EDUCATION FOR ANIMAL HEALTH TECHNICIANS

Most facilities acknowledge an obligation to foster interest in continuing education, especially for animal technicians who desire career development. There are various ways to accomplish this. Some institutions have had success with workshops and seminars that overlap part of the employer's time and part of the technician's off-hours. In some centers, regional chapters of CALAS/ACTAL or AALAS engage in promoting continuing-education activities. CALAS/ACTAL promotes lifelong learning through a Continuing Education Recognition Award that takes the form of a certificate and a congratulatory letter, a copy of which is sent to the individual's supervisor. The award is based on the self-reporting of 60 continuing-education credit hours accumulated over two years.

Some facilities send their technicians to conventions; others encourage enrollment in part-time courses that are job related. Some institutions even offer their senior technicians an in-house training program consisting of lectures, reading assignments, technical seminars, and small-group instruction on special clinical equipment. In the United States, AALAS provides a correspondence program to prepare candidates for higher certification. In Canada, independent study materials recognized by CALAS/ACTAL are available to enable technicians without access to a community college to complete the equivalent of a two-year college program.

The more successful endeavors are strengthened by the employer's willingness either to allow the employee time off to participate in such activities and/or to subsidize participation partially. It also helps if participation in continuing education demonstrably enhances the technician's career prospects. There is an obvious benefit to researchers who have well-trained and well-motivated technicians because this helps to ensure that studies will be properly conducted. Making the job sufficiently attractive helps to minimize turnover of personnel. For the sake of the animals, the study, and the technicians, the work of animal care personnel should be made dignified, rewarding, and agreeable.

References

AALAS Bulletin (1978). **17**, 6.

Arnold, D. L., Charbonneau, S. M., Zawidzka, Z. Z., and Grice, H. C. (1977). Monitoring animal health during chronic toxicity studies. *J. Environ. Pathol. Toxicol.* **1**, 227–238.

Arnold, D. L., Fox, J. G., Thibert, P., and Grice, H. C. (1978). Toxicology studies. I. Support personnel. *Food Cosmet. Toxicol.* **16**, 479–484.

Canadian Association for Laboratory Animal Science (1982). "DACUM Competency Study". Kingston: Canadian Association for Laboratory Animal Science.

Giammattei, V. M., and Anderson, J. G. (1985). "Training Programs & Careers in Animal Health Technology & Veterinary Nursing in North America". Napa, California: Dillon–Tyler.

Greenwood, R. (1981). The evolution of animal technologist training (1967 to 1981) in Canada. *20th Annual Convention, Canadian Association for Laboratory Animal Science, Montreal.*

Lane-Petter, W. (1967). Selection, training and control of staff. *In* "Husbandry of Laboratory Animals" (M. L. Conalty, ed.), p. 69. London: Academic Press.

National Research Council (1966). "Report of Special Committee on the Care of Experimental Animals, Ottawa, 1966", p. 15. Ottawa: National Research Council.

Scala, R. A. (1983). Comment in discussion following Part III. *Ann. N.Y. Acad. Sci.* **406**, 106–107.

Thompson, H. (1979). Personal elements of good laboratory practices. *Clin. Toxicol.* **15(5)**, 527–538.

4
Analytical Chemistry Aspects of Toxicity Studies

Jos Mes
Bureau of Chemical Safety
Health Protection Branch
Health and Welfare Canada
Ottawa, Ontario

I. INTRODUCTION

In the context of this chapter, only those aspects dealing with analytical organic chemistry are considered although they may have a broader application. The analytical function within a toxicological study is directly related to both the availability of capable support personnel and validated analytical technology. Although the following discussion of these two factors is not exhaustive, it conveys some basic considerations.

II. PERSONNEL ASPECTS

In the supporting analytical laboratory, both professional and technical staff are involved. Their educational requirements, experience, and duties are briefly outlined in the following two sections.

Handbook of
In Vivo Toxicity Testing

45

A. Professional Staff

Analytical laboratories associated with toxicological studies should be staffed by chemists with at least a bachelor of science degree or the equivalent level of education. In studies involving organic compounds, as is the case with many drugs or environmental chemicals, a major in organic chemistry may be desirable.

The head of the analytical laboratory should have extensive experience in analytical chemistry (5–10 years), with formal training in biochemistry and/or biology in order to participate knowledgeably in discussions regarding appropriate biological specimens and possible effects of metabolic processes on the test chemical.

The continuity and reliability of analytical services is very important, especially in toxicological investigations that span many years because they are costly, require a particular expertise, and are difficult to repeat. Consequently, it is wise to have another chemist available as part of a contingency plan. The duties of a chemist in charge of the analytical laboratory for a toxicological study include the following:

1. to evaluate and decide upon the methodology and equipment to be used;
2. to advise the study's project leader on analytical problems, such as the required specimen size;
3. to train and instruct technical personnel in the analysis of animal tissues and fluids;
4. to eliminate potential and on-the-spot analytical problems;
5. to interpret, evaluate, and present results;
6. to maintain laboratory performance and safety;
7. to prepare or assist in the preparation of standard operating procedures (SOPs);
8. to follow SOPs and collect and store data in accordance with good laboratory practice (GLP; see Chapters 5–8).

The chemist must possess tact in supervising technical staff and display good judgment in making decisions that may affect the efficiency of the analytical operation. Frequent communication with the study director is also essential.

B. Technical Staff

For technical staff, such as technicians or technologists, the current-day standards require a diploma from a technical college or institute of technology as a prerequisite for any job in a chemical laboratory.

For junior staff, one or two years' experience or on-the-job training is acceptable, depending on the type and complexity of the analysis. A technician having only minimal supervision while working with a capillary gas chromatograph would obviously require a longer apprenticeship than one using an analytical balance for gravimetric measurements. On-the-job training offers the advantage that the supervisor has an opportunity to prevent the technician from acquiring unsafe and dubious techniques.

Senior technologists, who frequently oversee general day-to-day activities in the laboratory, must have at least five years' experience in analytical laboratory practice and possess good supervisory qualities.

An efficient analytical laboratory with several technicians requires cooperation among all its members, especially when practical considerations require that equipment and fume hood space be shared. The duties of an analytical laboratory technician are summarized as follows:

1. analysis of biological specimens;
2. adherence to established analytical procedures as described in appropriate SOPs;
3. observation and reporting of any anomalies during analysis;
4. calculation of results and recording of procedures;
5. maintenance and simple modification of equipment;
6. procurement of laboratory supplies;
7. supervision of junior staff where applicable.

In many toxicological studies, a large number of samples have to be analyzed. It is important to keep up with the study in terms of analyses so that no appreciable backlog of samples accumulates. Decisions affecting the future conduct of a study may often depend on the results of previous analyses. For example, a study protocol may state that breeding of the test animal may be started only after the level of the test substance in the animal's blood has reached an "apparent" state of pharmacokinetic equilibrium. Consequently, coordinated teamwork is an important factor in the analytical laboratory.

Like many aspects of a chronic toxicological study, the analytical part is often routine; that is, one repeatedly analyzes for the same drug or xenobiotic chemical using the same basic technique and the same types of specimen. The managerial question arises as to how maximum productivity can be best achieved, especially when the boredom inherent in routine analysis and the necessity to avoid sloppy work due to familiarity with the procedure are taken into account. During a complex analysis of polychlorinated biphenyl (PCB) in animal specimens, for example, several distinct manipulations such as extraction, sample cleanup, separation of interfering substances, detection, and quantification have to be carried out. Thus, each technician can be assigned one step in the process. On first sight, this work division seems efficient, but two disadvantages cannot be overlooked. For the supervisor, this approach leaves no means of accountability for end results, whereas from the technician's point of view, exposure to potential health hazards for long periods of time is not desirable as, for example, in the handling of monkey feces that may contain potential pathogens.

The alternative, in which each technician carries out the entire analysis of a given specimen, not only gives more personal satisfaction in producing a good end result, but any suspected error can be traced more easily. This approach may provide an incentive for higher productivity and allows for rotating the analysis of different specimens among the technical staff, thus further diminishing boredom and long-term exposure to potential pathogens.

Increased productivity can also be obtained by the introduction of automation in the analytical laboratory. Many analyses for toxicological studies can be perceived as readily adaptable to automation (including robotics), either entirely or in part. The chemist should weigh the pros and cons of automation with regard to such factors as cost, manpower, downtime, reliability of results, and percentage of increase in productivity.

III. TECHNOLOGICAL ASPECTS

The analyst involved in a toxicological study should consider beforehand the entire analytical process, from sampling and analysis to data recording and storage, in order to correct, strengthen, or verify certain steps of the process when necessary. In the following examples, decisions have to be made that can affect not only the analytical results but also the final evaluation and extrapolation of data as well.

A. Sampling

Sampling is an important part of any analytical procedure, particularly when biological specimens are involved. Some sampling details that should be considered are discussed next.

1. Sample Size

The analyst is often asked to decide on sample size. This is not much of a problem at necropsy, unless large samples are required by the pathologist or other team members, but certainly is in the case of biopsies because sample size is necessarily restricted. In those toxicological studies in which the parameter to be measured concerns a rapid increase in the test chemical or its metabolite in the body tissues or fluids of the test animal, the residue concentration in even relatively small samples may be sufficient for its analytical determination. In those studies, however, in which the "disappearance" of the test chemical from the body is of paramount interest, the sample size may have to be increased as the study progresses. Relatively large samples will also be required from control or low dose animals in order to increase confidence in the analytical findings. If this is not possible, the analytical limitation due to sample size should clearly be stated. Sample size is also limited by the size of the animal and the frequency of sampling, which should not be excessive to the extent that it alters homeostasis.

The question of representative sampling must also receive special attention. Representative sampling of biological specimens, such as fat, present unique problems when the fat depot is small and can contain other types of tissues in the proximity of the sampling site. To minimize possible variation, it is preferable, but by no means always practical, to sample the same area in repeated biopsies. Although representative sampling is not an issue with blood, the analyst should determine whether it is whole blood, plasma, or serum that provides the best measure of residue level.

2. Sample Container

Sample containers should be properly cleaned prior to sample collection to avoid contamination of the specimen. This is of particular importance with control samples in which the absence of the test chemical has to be demonstrated or with test chemicals (e.g., PCBs) that contribute to the background level due to existing environmental contamination.

Glass containers can be cleaned by high temperature treatment (350°C) or rinsed with organic solvents free of interfering substances. This technique has been successfully applied to containers used for the collection of human milk to be analyzed for chlorinated hydrocarbons (Mes, 1981). If glass containers cannot be used because the chemical in question is adsorbed onto the glass surface, Teflon[1] may be an alternative. All caps for glass containers should have precleaned Teflon or aluminum foil liners.

In general, plastic containers should be avoided because some plasti-

---

[1] Teflon is a product made by Du Pont.

cizer may be absorbed by the specimen when it comes in contact with the plastic. However, preliminary experiments can be carried out to investigate the extent of sample contamination and its effect on the analysis.

3. Sample Labeling

The analyst may have little direct control over labeling but should have sufficient input to ensure that the system used by the toxicologist is compatible with that required by the analytical laboratory for processing and storing of samples. However, access to such information as dose groups and intervals of dosing are essential in the preparation of interim and final reports. The labeling procedures should be designed to minimize sample confusion or misidentification.

4. Sample Storage

The effect of storage on the chemical residue analysis of biological specimens should not be overlooked. Breakdown or disappearance of the analyte has been reported to occur, even when it is frozen (McCully, 1971). Although it is customary to store samples that cannot be immediately analyzed at $-20°C$, storage of sample extracts is often more preferable. Relatively small samples, such as biopsy tissues or breast milk, readily dehydrate when stored for short periods of time. If such specimens are not stored preweighed, chemical residue levels cannot be accurately calculated on a total wet weight basis. Tissue samples up to 1 g can be preweighed on cleaned aluminum foil and stored in the foil inside a sample container. Analyzing the entire preweighed sample is most efficient. The same efficiency can be achieved for small samples of body fluids if the sample vial or container is used as the extraction flask, thereby avoiding unnecessary losses due to sample transfer.

Thawing and refreezing of specimens should be kept to a minimum, especially with such body fluids as milk, because these changes can affect analysis of fat-soluble compounds due to changes in physical consistency.

5. Subsampling

Large tissue samples other than liquids may need some form of homogenization before subsampling. Subsampling of such biological samples as adipose tissue, liver, kidney, and brain from nonhuman primates is never ideal due to lack of uniformity. If at all possible, the entire sample should be used for analysis. In this respect, removing an aliquot from the total sample extract is preferable to subsampling of the tissue or organ.

In a recent study in our laboratory, five small ($\cong$ 300 mg) subsamples of homogenized subcutaneous fat were analysed for PCBs. The coefficient of variation (CV) was approximately 20 although the fat content of each specimen was close to 100% (Mes, 1984).

Generally, body fluids are more easily subsampled when fresh. Freezing and thawing may cause precipitation or conglomeration of particles, whereas an anticoagulant should be immediately added to avoid clotting in the case of blood. In contrast to the example of subcutaneous fat mentioned previously, when four subsamples of fresh human blood ($\cong$ 5 g) were analysed, a CV of only 7 was observed (Mes, 1984).

It is important for the chemist to have well-defined sampling procedures as part of the overall documentation for the toxicological study, especially in those cases in which the analyst has little control over the sampling process itself, including the weighing and storing of specimens.

B. Methodology

Many methods may be available to determine the test chemical, its metabolites, or its breakdown products, whether in the dosing vehicle (i.e., diet, solution, inhaled atmosphere) or in animal tissues or fluids. The choice of an analytical method is important from both a scientific and an economic point of view. The method chosen must be well documented, that is, established in the scientific literature or developed in house. In either case, accurate and precise data should be available not only for quality control but also for comparison with other methods. A comparison of several methods with regard to accuracy, precision, efficiency, and general applicability is a good investment, particularly when long-term and costly studies are considered.

Wallace *et al.* (1977) evaluated four methods for determining cocaine and its metabolite benzoylecgonine in urine based on different scientific approaches. Briefly, these investigators found gas–liquid chromatography (GLC) the most precise, thin-layer chromatography (TLC) the most applicable to simultaneous determination, enzyme immunoassay the least time-consuming for small numbers of samples, and radioimmunoassay (RIA) the most sensitive method. They also calculated that a single determination was approximately three times more expensive than samples analyzed by the dozen, and half again as expensive when one gross was analyzed at the time.

The foregoing example illustrates the need to evaluate all available methodology, not only for scientific reasons but also for economic and efficiency considerations. A considerable increase in analysis costs is seldom justified for a slight increase in precision and accuracy. On the other hand, the use of microtechniques should be promoted if they result in significant savings of materials and supplies and/or analysis time. Although chronic toxicological studies are expensive in general, the analyst making a choice of methodology must not neglect sound scientific principles for the sake of cutting costs. Inaccurate analytical results may adversely affect the evaluation and extrapolation of study results or, in the worst case, invalidate the whole study.

For the analyst to make an informed decision on the method to be chosen or developed, it may be helpful to examine in more detail some individual stages of the analytical methodology. The following outline presents some procedural steps encountered in the analysis of environmental chemicals. These steps can be directly or indirectly applicable to other areas of methodology.

1. Extraction

Extraction is one of the most important stages in the analysis of the test chemical because the quantity of chemical to be measured is released during this stage. Poor extraction efficiency inevitably leads to incorrect results no matter how good further cleanup, detection, or quantitation is. Extractions can be carried out with a great variety of solvents or solvent systems. The foremost guiding principle for extraction of the analyte from tissues, excluding blood, is its solubility in the solvent of choice. For body fluids, the same guiding principle is valid, but the solvent must be immiscible with the substrate. For example, it is a poor choice to select acetone as an extraction solvent for the determination of residues in body fluids, even if the residues are readily soluble, because acetone itself is soluble in water.

During the extraction process, compounds of similar polarity to the test chemical can be coextracted. Such coextractants can interfere with the analysis. In general, therefore, the least polar solvent that enables complete removal of the test chemical from the sample is the preferable one. In those cases in which the method calls for concentration of the solvent or for evaporation to dryness, the choice of extraction solvent may also be based on its boiling point and purity.

The selection of an extraction method largely depends on such test chemical characteristics as thermal lability, volatility, tendency to codistill, photodegradation, reactivity, or instability. A heat labile chemical should not be extracted in a Soxhlet apparatus or a volatile compound at an elevated temperature. Similarly, chemical treatment of the sample prior to extraction to destroy coextractants or break chemical bonds should be carefully evaluated in order not to destroy or alter the test chemical. For example, concentrated H_2SO_4 may not only destroy the easily coextracted fat from an adipose tissue sample containing the pesticide dieldrin, but the acid may destroy the dieldrin as well (Saxena and Siddiqui, 1981).

Sometimes an exhaustive extraction of the analyte from the specimen may be needed in order to get quantitative results. In most cases, however, a single extraction is sufficient if such extraction parameters as time, temperature, surface area contact, and, of course, choice of solvent are adjusted. If 98% of the dosing chemical is extracted initially, the remaining 2%, obtainable by successive reextraction of the substrate, may not add significantly to the accuracy of the results yet will considerably increase analysis time.

The choice of extraction apparatus depends also on the sample size. A small tissue sample, as from a biopsy, cannot be extracted in a Soxhlet apparatus but can be perfectly macerated in solvent with a microhomogenizer.

2. Cleanup and Separations

Most sample extracts need some form of coextractant cleanup before the toxic chemical(s) can be detected, identified, or quantified. The extent of cleanup depends largely on the concentration of the test chemical and/or metabolites present in the biological substrate to be analyzed. For example, during the extraction of chlorinated hydrocarbons, such as DDTs, from fatty tissues, large quantities of fat are coextracted which can seriously interfere with the detection and quantification of these residues if the chlorinated hydrocarbons are present in relatively small concentrations. If the concentration of the test chemical far exceeds that of the coextractants, however, detection may be possible by simple dilution without cleanup. Although the effect of some interferences on the determination of the analyte can be minimized by dilution, precipitation, or destruction, other interferences that are closely related chemically to the analyte need further separation by some selective physical–chemical process, such as adsorption chromatography, gel permeation, or ion exchange.

For highly toxic chemicals, the dosing levels in a toxicological study should be kept low; consequently, the small residue levels to be determined can lead to laborious workup of the extract. This is probably best illustrated in the analysis of the extremely toxic dioxins and dibenzofurans in body fluids and tissues. Several cleanup and separation steps, such as acid treatment and different column chromatographies are needed before these chemicals can be detected and identified (Tosine, 1981).

In addition to coextractants, note that impurities from solvents, adsorbents, or glassware can contribute considerably to background interference, especially when the test chemical, due to its ubiquitous nature, is already present in the tissues and fluids from control animals.

3. Detection, Identification, and Quantification

Methods available for the detection of test chemicals range from spectrophotometry to mass spectrometry. The most common approach has been the use of thin-layer, high pressure liquid, or gas–liquid chromatography. The latter in particular has been a useful analytical tool for the detection and separation of many compounds, especially with the appearance of capillary columns, which have been applied to routine toxicological analysis (Anderson and Stafford, 1983).

The analyst must consider the detection limit of the test chemical at the outset of the study. For toxicological experiments, this detection limit can be defined as the lowest possible test chemical concentration that can be measured as statistically different from a blank, and must relate to both method and instrument(s). The instrument is often the limiting factor in analyte detection and requires careful optimization. In toxicological studies, the animals are dosed with a chemical of known purity. Identification of the chemical should pose no problem if its concentration is detectable and if there is no interference. However, when unknown metabolites have to be analyzed and their identification confirmed, the use of a mass spectrometer will likely be required. Unfortunately, not every analyst has ready access to such expensive equipment; however, relatively inexpensive "bench-top" mass spectrometers have now been developed, which can be used for routine analysis in conjunction with capillary gas chromatography.

Confirmation of the test chemical should be carried out initially to establish that, indeed, the test chemical has been identified in body tissues or fluids. Gas chromatographic retention times can supplement, but not take the place of, proper identification techniques. For example, a predioxin can easily be misidentified as a dioxin by GLC when a high injection temperature is used, which will favor the conversion of predioxin into the corresponding dioxin.

The test chemical can be quantitated only within the linear range of the detector response. If this range is not known, the analyst should establish a range for each compound to be analyzed. The stability of the test compound in the extraction solvent can also affect quantification, as in the case of the antibiotic cefoperazone, which is unstable in methanol

(Kinniburgh *et al.*, 1982). Standards used for quantification should be of known purity and of the same source as the test chemical (if possible) in the toxicological study.

Interpretation of the analytical results should be carried out according to a specified limit of quantitation. The limit of quantitation is an expression of the degree of confidence in the analytical results. Keith *et al.* (1983) recommend a limit of quantitation equal to 10X the standard deviation. Since computers are becoming an integral part of analytical instrumentation, quantification has become less laborious but not necessarily more accurate. Quantification of the test chemicals, as represented by chromatographic peaks is only as good as their separation.

C. Evaluation

Good analytical practice requires that fortification experiments be carried out. These experiments involve the subdivision of a sample and the addition of a known quantity of test chemical (within the working range) to one or more subsamples. The test chemical is then determined in both the fortified and nonfortified subsamples and its recovery calculated. Nevertheless, even excellent fortification results do not necessarily give an accurate representation of the residue level in the sample, as was pointed out by Albro (1979). In some instances, the use of radioisotopes may be required. The chemist in charge of the analytical laboratory should examine all data and evaluate them regarding their analytical validity before reporting them to the project leader. In this process, gross anomalies are often easily recognized but not always easily corrected.

In toxicological studies, the analysis of body tissues and fluids often cannot be easily reproduced due to the limited amount of specimen available, as, for example, in biopsy cases. In the evaluation of single determinations, especially of low residue levels, caution should be exercised because variations anywhere from ± 20 to $\pm 200\%$ are not uncommon (Gunther, 1980). Therefore, a preliminary workup should include attempts to establish the repeatability of the entire analytical process. At the same time, the reliability of the method may be tested by another laboratory.

D. Data Handling

The data generated from a long-term and comprehensive toxicological study can be voluminous, and the analyst can be faced with enormous storage and retrieval problems. In many toxicological studies, proper storage and filing of all data, including laboratory notebooks, are carried out according to good laboratory practice (GLP) guidelines to ensure their safety and to avoid unauthorized retrieval. Raw data can be easily stored on computer tapes and/or disks but not always so easily retrieved from them; data printouts, chromatograms, and spectra have to be filed.

A coding system for hard-copy material should be devised to facilitate retrieval and transfer of data, especially when no long-term computer storage is available. In studies lasting several years, it is not unusual to reexamine a sample chromatogram one or two years later.

IV. CONCLUDING COMMENTS

It is evident that many aspects have to be considered in any routine analytical procedure. Therefore, the analyst has to decide before the start of any toxicological experiment how the various stages of the analytical process should be carried out and how results should be evaluated and confirmed.

The final decision will be influenced by such factors as available man- power and equipment, analysis time, dosing level, and required precision. In addition, a nonscientific judgment often has to be made based on priorities, costs, and safety. Within these realms the analyst must ensure that the practice of sound science is not jeopardized.

References

Albro, P. W. (1979). Problems in analytical methodology: Sample handling, extraction, and cleanup. *Ann. N.Y. Acad. Sci.* **320,** 19–27.

Anderson, W. M., and Stafford, D. T. (1983). Applications of capillary gas chromatography in routine toxicological analyses. *J. High Resolut. Chromatogr. Chromatogr. Commun.* **6,** 248–254.

Gunther, F. A. (1980). "Residue Reviews", pp. 155–171. New York: Springer-Verlag.

Keith, L. H., Crummett, W., Deegan, J. Jr., Libby, R. A., Taylor, J. K., and Wentler, G. (1983). Principles of environmental analysis. *Anal. Chem.* **55,** 2210–2218.

Kinniburgh, D. W., Jennison, T. A., and Matsen, J. M. (1982). Factors affecting the analysis of Cefoperazone in cerebral spinal fluid. *J. Anal. Toxicol.* **6,** 85–87.

McCully, K. A. (1971). "Methods in Residue Analysis/Pesticide Chemistry", pp. 315–356. New York: Gordon and Breach.

Mes, J. (1981). Experiences in human milk analysis for halogenated hydrocarbon residues. *Int. J. Environ. Anal. Chem.* **9,** 283–299.

Mes, J. (1984). Chlorinated hydrocarbon residues in primate tissues and fluids. *In* "Trace Analysis" (J. F. Lawrence, ed.), pp. 71–112. New York: Academic Press.

Saxena, M. C., and Siddiqui, M. K. J. (1981). Reduced recovery of dieldrin residues — A shortcoming of sulfuric acid cleanup of biological samples. *J. Anal. Toxicol.* **5,** 150–152.

Tosine, M. (1981). Report No. 18576. Ottawa: National Research Council of Canada.

Wallace, J. E., Hamilton, H. E., Christenson, J. G., Shimek, E. L. Jr., Hand, P., and Harris, S. C. (1977). An evaluation of selected methods for determining cocaine and benzoylec- gonine in urine. *J. Anal. Toxicol.* **1,** 20–26.

Part III
Hygiene

5
Hygiene Programs

Harry C. Rowsell
Canadian Council on Animal Care and
International Council for Laboratory Animal Science
Ottawa, Ontario

I. INTRODUCTION

Every facility employing personnel engaged in toxicological studies involving animals should institute a program that embraces injury, diseases transmitted from humans to animals and from animals to humans, allergies, and social and ethical implications that may impact on the psychological well-being of personnel (Bartosek *et al.,* 1982; Nethery, 1985; Hamm, 1986). Every institution should be familiar with any legislation concerning industrial health and safety (Government of Ontario, 1978), as well as with any procedures laid down by the institution that ensure adequate handling and hygiene practices.

Occupational safety and health issues are discussed by Penn (1977) and Jonas (1976). In *Guide to the Care and Use of Experimental Animals,* volume 1, the Canadian Council on Animal Care (CCAC; 1980) has discussed personnel safety.

> In addition to dangers from infectious diseases transmissible from animals to man, there are many personnel hazards inherent in the animal house including damage inflicted by animals, chemicals, machinery and equipment in the animal facility.

Like other laboratories, the animal care facility should have a safety program which includes fire drills, instruction in using equipment safely and first aid training. All persons using a facility should be familiar with the requirements of the institution and/or facility safety program in case of accidental injury. Responsibility must be designated to ensure that all personnel working with animals understand how to handle the species involved both for their own safety and health and for that of the animals.

II. HEALTH PROTECTION

It is important to recognize that the transmission of disease is a two-way street between humans and animals. Unfortunately, in most hygiene programs, the transmission of diseases from humans to animals is overlooked. However, it should be included in a monitoring program encompassing the pre-employment physical examination. Such health examinations should not be restricted only to those involved in the day-to-day handling of experimental animals, that is, to animal technicians, but should include any professionals who will be working with animals. Particular attention should be paid to the matter of allergy to laboratory animals. Dander, serum, urine, and other animal tissue products can be allergenic (Ohman, 1978; "Allergic reactions," 1980; Edwards et al., 1983; Dewdney, 1984).

It is especially important in any effective hygiene program to inform employees in contact with nonhuman primates of the "substantial zoonoses that pose a serious potential health hazard to personnel" (Canadian Council on Animal Care, 1984), and of animal susceptibility to human diseases. As well, employees should be instructed regarding the protective clothing they must wear and the devices they must use in handling these animals. They should be informed of the necessity for routine health examinations for diseases such as tuberculosis. Yearly medical attention should include X ray, fecal culture, and possibly prophylactic immunization with human immune globulin against hepatitis A (Canadian Council on Animal Care, 1984). Rabies is a danger (Charlton et al., 1986; Gardner, 1986; "Rabies Report," 1986), and DF-2 septicemia is a life-threatening infection that occurs after dog bites (Huminer, 1986).

Other chapters in this book describe the prevention of infection involving microbiological monitoring of the important laboratory animal diseases that must be controlled (U.S. Department of Health, Education, and Welfare, Public Health Service, 1976; Richardson and Barkley, 1984; Nomura and Held, 1986). Many of these may infect human beings, and some may spread from human subjects to animals. Thus, again, those responsible for the hygiene program must be aware of this two-way street.

One of the most devastating diseases that may be transmitted from humans to their animal subjects, particularly from humans to nonhuman primates, is tuberculosis. Evidence of such transfer is documented (Franklin *et al.,* 1986). Other human diseases that may be transmitted to laboratory animals, including nonhuman primates, are salmonellosis, streptococcal, staphylococcal, and *Escherichia coli* infections, and infections of newborn and juvenile animals. When initial infections are observed in laboratory animal species, the source of the disease must be investigated. If a specific animal source is not indicated, then the possibility of a human source must be considered (Schultz, 1982). Over 200 laboratory-associated diseases have been identified, with over 300 resultant deaths by 1979 (Wallbank, 1979).

Diseases Transmitted from Animals to Humans

Personnel health, monitoring programs, and prophylactic programs that may prevent the transmission of diseases from animals to humans should be instituted as directed by the CCAC Guide (1980, 1984) and *Syllabus of the Basic Principles of Laboratory Animal Science* (1985). The most valuable reference source for the myriad of diseases that can be transmitted between humans and animals is that of Schurrenberger and Hubbert, (1981). Schwabe (1984) should also be consulted.

Similarly, the *Diseases Transmitted from Animals to Man* by Hubbert *et al.* (1975) is all inclusive. Soulsby (1974) has discussed parasitic diseases and Fiennes (1978), the origins of diseases. However, there are some rarely-thought-of diseases that pose a danger to the animal technician including Q fever (Bernard *et al.,* 1985; Grant *et al.,* 1985; Ruppaner *et al.,* 1985), pasteurellosis (Weber *et al.,* 1984; Goldstein *et al.,* 1986), and lymphocytic choriomeningitis, which is carried by a number of laboratory rodents including hamsters. Parasites, for example, the ectoparasite *Sarcoptes scabie* that causes scabies, represent a hazard (Soulsby, 1974).

The numerous sources of information concerning the zoonoses and infectious disease hazards to personnel employed in the animal facility should be well known to the personnel safety officer and the veterinary director (Ganaway, 1974; Quist, 1974; Pyke, 1976, 1978; Fiennes, 1978; Wallbank, 1979; Boulter, 1981; Davies *et al.,* 1981; World Health Organization, 1983; Fox *et al.,* 1984; Elliot *et al.,* 1985; Povey, 1985; Sataline, 1986).

III. HYGIENIC HAZARDS

The major emphasis of many publications is related to the importance of health examinations and disease-related hazards that affect both the animal population and human personnel. However, any hygiene program must also recognize many other hazards associated with health and safety in the animal facility and laboratories in which animals are used.

A. Physical Hazards

There are numerous physical hazards caused by animals (Canadian Council on Animal Care, 1984; Kalb *et al.,* 1985). It is a historical truism that those handling or treating animals must realize that animals do not understand the reason for restraint or examination, nor do they recognize that, in cases of illness or trauma, handling is essential to diagnosis, treatment, and/or prophylactic measures. The necessary procedures must therefore be instituted to prevent animal-related injuries.

It is accepted that certain species of animals are more amenable to manipulation than others; even within species, certain strains may be more easily handled than others. Again, a predisposition to the acceptance of handling is related to the human – animal bonding between animals and technicians, investigators, and laboratory personnel (Bustad, 1985; Wolfle, 1985). However, there are certain species that will automatically resist handling and treatment for the prevention of pain and disease. Most nonhuman primates and domestic animals, including swine, are among these species. Thus, it is important to understand the animal with which one is dealing and to know its defense mechanisms.

An essential requirement of any hygiene program is the documentation of conditions under which injury has occurred: the description of the injury, the circumstances under which it occurred, and the species involved. Some non-animal-related physical injuries are due to negligence on the part of the animal technician or the investigator. For example, it is necessary that disposable syringes, needles, and scalpel blades be disposed of after use in order to eliminate the possibility of contamination and physical injury to personnel. Protective devices for disposing of sharp materials have been designed, and their use should be mandatory by institutional regulations.

Although more difficult to measure, dust and aerosols can be deleterious to the health of the personnel as well as to the animals within the facility. Therefore, biosafety and industrial health regulations to control such hazards are essential. Relevant recommendations are contained in both volumes of the Canadian Council on Animal Care guides (1980, 1984).

One of the most detrimental physical hazards, not only to animals but to humans, is smoke. Smoking should be banned in all animal rooms and limited to designated areas elsewhere in the building. Each institution should inform its personnel of the location of a "no smoking" area. The building as a whole may be considered a "no smoking" area. The potential ill effects from secondary smoke are well known; therefore, such a hazard to nonsmoking personnel and to animals should be recognized and methods instituted to preclude exposure to tobacco smoke. It has been demonstrated that nicotine on the hands of animal technicians significantly affects drug testing programs.

B. Biological Hazards

Biological hazards that may pose a danger for employees should be considered in all hygiene programs. Such hazards should be discussed with the biohazard committee, and guidelines of such committees should be adhered to by all personnel. Study programs should be designed in collaboration with the biohazard committee so that personnel can understand the proper handling of potentially dangerous biological materials such as animals, carcasses, waste, and bedding. The requirements of the *Guidelines for Handling Recombinant DNA and Animal Viruses* (Medical Research Council of Canada, 1980) should be made available to the animal care staff and technical assistants who come in contact with such material. Additional information as published by Wallbank (1979), Boulter (1981), Fox *et al.* (1984), and Wedum (1974) should be on hand as well.

Regulations and requirements of biohazard containment facilities should be available to personnel in order for them to understand entry restrictions and to be assured that the facilities in which they work are not inadvertently or deliberately used to contain biohazardous material. It is essential that the animal care staff work in cooperation and liaison with the biohazard committee and know who should be informed of any possible irregularities.

C. Chemical Hazards

Chemicals represent by far the most insidious hazard to the health and well-being of both animals and humans (Caldwell *et al.*, 1972). Most manufacturers of disinfectants and chemicals used by animal facilities (Prindle, 1983; Schiefer, personal communication) have been required to carry out safety and toxicity testing of their compounds before they are released to the market; however, such information is rarely made available to personnel using or handling the product. Therefore, a safety program should emphasize the toxic levels of all chemical compounds used, the dangers of absorption through the skin and by inhalation, as well as the dangers of inappropriate use or use beyond recommended strength.

The use of insecticides, particularly those containing organophosphates, as well as pesticides may be required in the animal house (Hayes, 1975; Rowsell *et al.,* 1979). Personnel handling such compounds should know the signs of toxicity (such as fatigue, weakness, or dizziness) particularly associated with the use of such compounds in closed and poorly ventilated areas.

It is also important that personnel know whether or not the compounds they are using are biodegradable. They should be aware of the risks when exposures to chemicals occur frequently, resulting in buildup of tissue residues in animals as well as in themselves. Knowledge is necessary in the use of compounds that may not only pose a danger to the health and well-being of personnel but also may affect the experimental results of animal studies.

D. Waste Disposal Hazards

Most animal waste and by-products, if handled and disposed of by acceptable methods, pose little risk to the handler. It is important, however, that the hygiene program address the potential dangers associated with *Toxocara canis* infection in dogs (Wilson *et al.,* 1980; Duwel, 1983) and the possible development of visceral larval migrans (Elliot *et al.,* 1985) in young children who may be brought into the animal facility. One cannot overemphasize the importance of educating and protecting female technicians of childbearing age regarding toxoplasmosis acquired from cats, which can result in fetal malformation (Frankel and Dupey, 1972; Wilson *et al.,* 1980; Hunter *et al.,* 1983; Carter and Frank, 1986). A waste disposal program is an inexpensive component of the overall hygiene strategy.

Additionally, waste disposal hazards may expose technicians and investigators to new diseases such as cryptosporidiosis, as yet untreatable (Elsser *et al.,* 1976), which appears to be associated with human exposure to fecal material of dogs and cats. It is of particular danger to those individuals who may be immunodeficient; such persons also risk infections with *Pasteurella multocida* organisms (Goldstein *et al.,* 1986).

Proper waste disposal systems should be addressed in a hygiene program; however, they are an integral part of any management program of sanitation in an animal facility. Their inclusion in this section is to reemphasize the dangers and to draw attention to specific known hazards.

IV. ETHICAL, SOCIAL, AND PSYCHOLOGICAL CONSIDERATIONS

Most hygiene programs tend to deal with the control and prevention of infectious diseases and other biological and chemical hazards. However, the psychological well-being of those involved in animal research is of extreme importance in view of the marked publicity given to animals in research by animal rights activists and those who vandalize animal facilities, such as members of the Animal Liberation Front (Jacobs, 1985; ALF, 1986). One must be aware of the words of Vicki Miller, founder and president of ARK II, and former president of the now activist Toronto Humane Society who wrote recently, "I believe that this decade will see the first acts of true violence. Some may be accidental—like a bystander killed in a bomb blast; some will be deliberate—like a vivisector shot in the street" (Miller, 1986).

Such threats necessarily cause anxiety and stress among those who are involved in the use of animals in research and often pose psychological stressors that may affect the work habits and the well-being of animal care personnel (Wolfle, 1985). Therefore, any hygiene program should include discussions with animal care personnel concerning the need for research involving animals (Gay, 1986; Fox, 1986), the contributions of biomedical research, and the need for adherence to ethical standards. This reinforcement provides psychological benefits to animal care personnel.

The concerns of the technician who becomes closely identified with the research animal and develops a bonding also should be understood by those responsible for the direction of animal-based research (Wolfle, 1985). Technicians should be allowed to express their concern for animals to which they have become bonded through association and tender loving care (Bustad, 1985).

In addressing the ethical psychological concerns of animal care technicians, programs should foster the proper methods of euthanasia to render an animal immediately unconscious and insensitive to pain (Rowsell, 1979). Technicians who find the killing of animals repugnant should not be forced to do so. In all likelihood, they will not carry out the technique well and may, because of their reluctance to do so and their abhorrence of killing animals, cause an animal unnecessary pain and suffering. Only those individuals who have the necessary stability and understanding should be selected for this task. Animals should have their total well-being addressed, including their behavioral needs (Fraser, 1984; Ellis, 1985), and those caring for the animals should have their sensitivities and concerns recognized. In this way, programs will develop to address these needs.

References

ALF Canada Front Line News (1986). U. of T. dentistry raid. Interview with the ALF. *ALF Canada Front Line News* **3**, 6–7.

Bartosek, I., Guaitani, A., and Pacei, E. (eds.) (1982). "Animals in Toxicological Research". New York: Raven.

Bernard, K. W., Parham, G. L., Winkler, W. F., and Helmick, C. G. (1985). Q fever control measures: Recommendations for research facilities using sheep. *In* "The Contribution of Laboratory Animal Science to the Welfare of Man and Animals" (J. Archibald, J. Ditchfield, and H. C. Rowsell, eds.), pp. 89–104. New York: Gustav Fischer Verlag.

Boulter, E. A. (1981). Infectious hazards. *In* "Safety in the Animal House," (J. H. Seamer and M. Wood, eds.), 2nd Rev. Ed., Laboratory Animal Handbooks 5, pp. 11–35. London: Laboratory Animals.

Bustad, L. K. (1985). Laboratory animal scientists and their new role in human–animal bonding. *In* "The Contribution of Laboratory Animal Science to the Welfare of Man and Animals" (J. Archibald, J. Ditchfield, and H. C. Rowsell, eds.), pp. 319–337. New York: Gustav Fischer Verlag.

Caldwell, R. S., Nakaue, H. S., and Buhler, D. R. (1972). Biochemical lesion in rat liver mytochondria induced by hexachlorophene. *Biochem. Pharmacol.* **21**, 2425–2441.

Campbell, J. S. (1979). Occupational health — the legal implications. *Proc. Can. Assoc. Lab. Anim. Sci. Guelph, Ont. 1979* 260–262.

Canadian Council on Animal Care (1980). Personnel safety. *In* "Guide to the Care and Use of Experimental Animals," Vol. 1, pp. 50–52. Ottawa, Canadian Council on Animal Care.

Canadian Council on Animal Care (1984). Non-human primates. *In* "Guide to the Care and Use of Experimental Animals," Vol. 2, pp. 164–173. Ottawa: Canadian Council on Animal Care.

Canadian Council on Animal Care (1985). Hazard control in animal facilities. *In* "Syllabus of the Basic Principles of Laboratory Animal Science," p. 23. Ottawa: Canadian Council on Animal Care.

Carter, A. O., and Frank, J. W. (1986). Congenital toxoplasmosis: Epidemiologic features and control. *Can. Med. Assoc. J.* **135**, 618–623.

Charlton, K. M., Webster, W. A., Casey, G. A., Rhodes, A. J., MacInnes, C. D., and Lawson, K. F. (1986). Recent advances in rabies diagnosis and research. *Can. Vet. J.* **27**, 85–89.

Davies, J. W., Karstad, L. H., and Trainer, D. O. (eds.) (1981). "Infectious Diseases of Wild Mammals." Ames, Iowa: Iowa State University Press.

Dewdney, J. M. (1984). Animals in the aetiology of asthma. *J. R. Soc. Med.* **77**, 629–631.

Duwel, D. (1983). Toxocariasis in human and veterinary medicine — And how to prevent it. *Helminthologia* **20**, 277–286.

Edwards, R. G., Beeson, M. F., and Dewdney, J. M. (1983). Laboratory animal allergy: The measurement of airborne urinary allergens and the effects of different environmental conditions. *Lab. Anim.* **17**, 235–239.

Elliot, D. L., Tolle, S. W., Goldberg, L., and Miller, J. B. (1985). Pet associated illness. *N. Eng. J. Med.* **313**, 985–995.

Ellis, D. V. (1985). "Animal Behaviour and Its Applications." Chelsea, Michigan: Lewis.

Elsser, K. A., Moricz, M., and Proctor, E. M. (1976). Cryptosporidium infections: A laboratory survey. *Can. Med. Assoc. J.* **135**, 211–213.

Fiennes, T. W. (1978). "Zoonosis and the Origins and Ecology of Human Disease." New York: Academic Press.

Fox, J. G., Cohen, B. J., and Loew, F. M. (eds). (1984). "Laboratory Animal Medicine." Orlando, Florida: Academic Press.

Fox, M. A. (1986). "The Case for Animal Experimentation: An Evolutionary and Ethical Perspective." Berkeley: University of California Press.

Frankel, J. K., and Dupey, J. P. (1972). Toxoplasmosis and its prevention in cats and man. *J. Infect. Dis.* **126,** 664–673.

Franklin, J. A., Austin, J. C., Kleeberg, G., and Knoetze, K. (1986). Monitoring of laboratory animal personnel for T.B. at the University of Witwatersrand. *5th Bienn. Congr. South Afr. Assoc. Lab. Anim. Sci. Cape Town,* 16.

Fraser, A. F. (1984). "The Behaviour of Self Maintenance in Laboratory Animals." St. John's: Memorial University of Newfoundland.

Gardner, S. D. (1986). In pursuit of the perfect rabies vaccine. *Br. Med. J.* **293,** 516.

Gay, W. I. (ed.) (1986). "Health Benefits of Animal Research." Washington, DC: Foundation for Biomedical Research.

Ganaway, J. R. (1974). Zoonoses of laboratory animals — Bacterial. *In* "CRC Handbook of Laboratory Animal Science," (E. C. Melby and N. H. Altman (eds.), Vol. 2, pp. 245–257. Cleveland: CRC Press.

Goldstein, R. W., Goodhart, G. L., and Moore, J. E. (1986). *Pasteurella multocida* infection after animal bites. *N. Eng. J. Med.* **315,** 460.

Government of Ontario (1978). Ontario Health and Occupational Safety of Workers, Bill 70.

Grant, C., Ascher, M. S., Bernard, K. W., Ruppaner, R., and Bellend, H. (1985). Factors to be considered in formulating guidelines for Q Fever and experimental sheep. *In* "The Contribution of Laboratory Animal Science to the Welfare of Man and Animals" (J. Archibald, J. Ditchfield, and H. C. Rowsell, eds.), pp. 81–84. New York: Gustav Fischer Verlag.

Hamm, T. E. (ed.) (1986). "Complications of Viral and Mycoplasmal Infections in Rodents to Toxicology Research and Testing." Washington, DC: Hemisphere Publishing.

Hayes, W. J. (1975). "Toxicology of Pesticides." Baltimore: Williams and Wilkins.

Hubbert, W. T., McCulloch, W. F., and Schnurrenberger, P. R. (1975). "Diseases Transmitted from Animals to Man." Springfield, Illinois: Charles C. Thomas.

Huminer, D. (1986). Pet-associated illness. *N. Eng. J. Med.* **314,** 1046.

Hunter, S., Stagno, S., Capps, E., and Smith, R. J. (1983). Prenatal screening of pregnant women for infections caused by cytomegalovirus, Epstein–Barr virus, herpes virus, rubella, and *Toxoplasma gondii. Am. J. Obstet. Gynecol.* **145,** 269–273.

Jacobs, D. (1985). A guerrilla war for animals. Why the ALF breaks the law. *The Sunday Sun, (Ottawa)* **Jan. 30,** p. 60.

Jonas, A. M. (1976). The research animal and the significance of a health monitoring program. *Lab. Anim. Sci.* **26,** 339.

Kalb, R., Kaplan, M. H., Tenenbaum, M. J., Joachim, G. R., and Samuels, S. (1985). Cutaneous infection at dog bite wounds associated with fulminant DF-2 septicemia. *Am. J. Med.* **78,** 687–690.

Medical Research Council of Canada (1980). "Guidelines for the Handling of Recombinant DNA Molecules and Animal Viruses and Cells" (Cat. No. MR 21-1/1980). Ottawa: Ministry of Supplies and Services Canada.

Miller, V. (1986) Forum. *Animals Agenda* Jan./Feb. p. 8.

Nethery, L. B. (1985). "Animals in Product Development and Safety Testing: A Survey." Washington, DC: Institute for the Study of Animal Problems.

Nomura, T., and Held, J. R. (eds.) (1986). "Manual of Microbiologic Monitoring of Laboratory Animals" (NIH Publication No. 86-2498). Bethesda, Maryland: U.S. Department of Health and Human Services, Public Health Services, National Institutes of Health.

Ohman, J. L., Jr. (1978). Allergy in man caused by exposure to mammals. *J. Am. Vet. Med. Assoc.* **172,** 1403.

Penn, A. C. (1977). How to work safely with laboratory animals. *In* "Job Safety and Health," pp. 29–39. Washington, DC: Occupational Safety and Health Administration.

Prindle, R. F. (1983). Phenolic compounds. *In* "Disinfection and Sterilization" (S. S. Block, ed.), pp. 197–224. Philadelphia: Lea and Febiger.

Povey, R. C. (1985). "Infectious Diseases of Cats: A Clinical Handbook." Guelph, Ontario: Centaur Press.

Pyke, R. M. (1976). Laboratory-associated infections: Summary analysis 3921 cases. *Health Lab. Sci.* **13,** 105–114.

Pyke, R. M. (1978). Past, present hazards of working with infectious agents. *Arch. Pathol. Lab. Med.* **102,** 333–336.

Quist, K. D. (1974). Zoonoses of laboratory animals — Viral and rickettsial. *In* "CRC Handbook of Laboratory Animal Science," (E. C. Melby and N. H. Altman, eds.) Vol. 2, pp. 259–269. Cleveland: CRC Press.

Richardson, J. H., and Barkley, W. E. (eds.) (1984). "Biosafety in Microbiological and Biomedical Laboratories" (Stock #0170230016). Washington, DC: U.S. Department of Health and Human Services, U.S. Government Printing Office.

Rowsell, H. C. (1979). Euthanasia: The final chapter. *Proc. 2nd Symp. Pets Soc. Vancouver* 125–139.

Rowsell, H. C., Ritcey, J., and Cox, F. (1979). Assessment of humaneness of vetebrate pesticides. *Proc. Can. Assoc. Lab. Anim. Sci. Guelph, Ont.* 236–249.

Ruppaner, R., Brooks, D. E., Behymer, D. E., and Ermel, R. W. (1985). *C. burnetii* infection in ewes: Will vaccination prevent shedding in exposed animals. *In* "The Contribution of Laboratory Animal Science to the Welfare of Man and Animals" (J. Archibald, J. Ditchfield, and H. C. Rowsell, eds.), pp. 85–88. New York: Gustav Fischer Verlag.

Sataline, L. (1986). Pet-associated illness. *N. Eng. J. Med.* **314,** 1046.

Schnurrenberger, P. R., and Hubbert, W. T. (1981). "An Outline of Zoonoses." Ames, Iowa: Iowa State University Press.

Schultz, R. D. (1982). Theoretical and practical aspects of an immunization program for dogs and cats. *J. Am. Vet. Med. Assoc.* **181,** 1142–1149.

Schwabe, C. W. (1984) Zoonoses. *In* "Veterinary Medicine and Human Health" (eds.), Vol. 3, pp. 194–242. Baltimore: Williams and Wilkins.

Soulsby, E. J. W. (ed.) (1974). "Parasitic Zoonoses." New York: Academic Press.

U.S. Department of Health, Education, and Welfare, Public Health Service (1976). "Classification of Etiologic Agents." Atlanta: Centers for Disease Control.

Veterinary Medicine Publishing Company (1986). "Rabies Report: Mounting a Strong Defense" (Special Issue). Lenexa, Kansas: Veterinary Medicine Publishing.

Veterinary Records (1980). Allergic reactions to laboratory animals. *Vet. Rec.* **Aug.9,** 122–123.

Wallbank, A. M. (1979). Biohazards in the animal facility and laboratory. *Proc. Can. Assoc. Lab. Anim. Sci. Guelph, Ont.* 263–287.

Weber, D. J., Wolfson, J. S., Schwartz, M. N., and Hooper, D. C. (1984). *Pasteurella multocida* infections: Report of 34 cases and review of the literature. *Medicine* **63,** 133–154.

Wedum, A. G. (1974). Biohazard control. *In* "CRC Handbook of Laboratory Animal Science," (E. C. Melby and N. H. Altman, eds.), Vol. 1. pp. 193–210. Cleveland: CRC Press.

Wolfle, T. (1985). Laboratory animal technicians. Their role in stress reduction and human–companion animal bonding. *Vet. Clin. North Am. Sm. Anim. Pract.* **15,** 449–454.

World Health Organization (1983). "Laboratory Biosafety Manual." Geneva: World Health Organization.

Wilson, C. B., Remington, J. S., Stagno, S., and Reynolds, D. W. (1980). Development of adverse sequelae in children born with subclinical congenital *Toxoplasma* infection. *Pediatrics* **66,** 767–774.

6
Rodent-Associated Zoonoses and Health Hazards

James G. Fox
Division of Comparative Medicine
Massachusetts Institute of Technology
Cambridge, Massachusetts

Christian E. Newcomer
Department of Comparative Medicine
Tufts University School of Veterinary Medicine
Boston, Massachusetts

I. Introduction
II. Viral Diseases
   A. Korean Hemorrhagic Fever
   B. Lymphocytic Choriomeningitis Virus
   C. Rabies
III. Rickettsial and Chlamydial Diseases
   A. Psittacosis
   B. Other Rickettsial Diseases
IV. Bacterial Diseases
   A. Leptospirosis
   B. Plague
   C. Ratbite Fever
   D. Salmonella
   E. Other Potential Bacterial Diseases
   F. Cutaneous Infections
V. Mycoses
VI. Protozoan Diseases
   A. *Entamoeba coli*
   B. Toxoplasmosis
   C. Cryptosporidiosis
   D. Other Protozoan Diseases
VII. Helminth Diseases
   A. Tapeworms
   B. Roundworms

Handbook of
In Vivo Toxicity Testing

71

I. INTRODUCTION

Zoonotic diseases and other health hazards are sometimes associated with laboratory species. This chapter focuses on rodents and their potential to transmit a number of diseases, since rodents are the most frequently used laboratory species. Some of the diseases discussed can be transmitted by other species as well. Relevant epidemiological factors, modes of transmission, clinical features, and prevention and control of rodent-associated diseases are reviewed. Other health hazards such as bites and allergies are briefly mentioned.

II. VIRAL DISEASES

A. Korean Hemorrhagic Fever

Korean hemorrhagic fever (KHF), also called epidemic hemorrhagic fever-Osaka, is a febrile disease with renal involvement caused by the RNA Hantaan virus that is transmitted by rodents (Johnson, 1982; Lee et al., 1978).

1. Reservoir and Incidence

KHF, first identified among troops in the Korean War, infected over 100 Japanese researchers and animal technicians working with rats in 15 institutions between 1975 and 1981 (Unemai et al., 1979; Kawamata et al., 1980). Serological evidence indicates that laboratory rats with enzootic KHF are the source of human KHF in Japan. Laboratory rats do not manifest clinical signs and lesions but do develop relatively high antibody titers to the agent.

Hantaan virus is enzootic in wild rodents. In Korea, Apodemus spp. carry the Hantaan virus, and it has been suggested that this virus — or one closely related to it—is present in wild *Rattus norvegicus* (Lee, 1982). The virus may also be present in *Microtus* spp. and *Clethriomys glareolus* in the United States.

2. Mode of Transmission

Transmission is by direct contact with the excreta of infected rodents. Experimental animals excrete the virus in urine for prolonged periods and should be handled with proper precautions.

3. Clinical Features

In humans, the clinical features of KHF include high fever, severe malaise, myalgia, headaches, diarrhea, nausea, vomiting, proteinuria, oliguria or polyuria, and hemorrhage.

4. Prevention and Control

When laboratory rats, *Apodemus* spp., other wild rodents, and possibly wild mice are transported from parts of the world where Hantaan virus may exist, such as Japan and Belgium, serological monitoring should be considered. Sera testing for KHF antibody can be done with immunofluorescent antibody technique (IFA) and should be performed either prior to shipping or at the recipient site while the animals are in quarantine. Such tests are not routinely performed in the United States, but IFA tests recently have become commercially available from Microbiological Associates.[1]

B. Lymphocytic Choriomeningitis Virus

Lymphocytic choriomeningitis virus (LCM) can be considered an arthropod-borne virus, often transmitted by various blood-sucking insects such as mosquitoes *(Aedes aegypti),* Rocky Mountain wood ticks *(Dermacentor andersoni),* and fleas. LCM is latent in mice but creates an influenzalike illness in humans.

1. Reservoir and Incidence

Three sources of LCM infection in humans have been identified: wild and laboratory mice, hamsters, and passage of transplantable tumors in

[1] Microbiological Associates, 5221 River Road, Bethesda, Maryland 20016.

laboratory mice, including experimentally induced leukemia. Wild mice represent the most important source. They are the ultimate reservoir of infection for laboratory mice and other hosts (Maurer, 1964). The LCM virus lives symbiotically in mice, and neither the virus nor the host significantly suppresses the other. The other species in which long-term, asymptomatic LCM infection exists to a lesser extent is the hamster.

LCM virus has been detected in wild mice throughout the United States, Asia, Africa, and Europe, and is probably present globally, although it has not been isolated from mice in Australia. A 1940 survey of wild mice in the Washington, D.C., area showed 21.5% of the sample to be infected with LCM virus (Armstrong et al., 1940).

A survey of 22 laboratory mouse colonies performed between 1967 and 1970 in the United States showed only 2 colonies containing the virus (Poiley, 1970). This survey was carried out in retired breeding stock in production and research colonies, and only nontolerant infections were detectable with the monitoring technique used. Other reports of LCM virus in mouse colonies have appeared in studies of research animals in the United States (Soave and Van Allen, 1958) and in selected English institutions (Skinner and Knight, 1971). LCM certainly persists in some colonies today, although rigorous controls have all but eradicated it (see Section II, B, A).

Laboratory hamsters also harbor the virus, and epizootics in this species during 1973 and 1974 were responsible for 236 human cases of LCM in the United States (Gregg, 1975). LCM viral infections have also developed in commercial hamster colonies in Germany, where it has been estimated that pet hamsters are responsible for about 1000 human cases each year (Parker et al., 1976). In the United States, the first infected commercial hamster colony was detected in 1974 (Gregg, 1975).

A third source of LCM infection in humans results from the presence of the virus as a contaminant in experimentally passaged mouse tumors, mycoplasmas, and murine poliovirus. Transplantable leukemia in C58 mice was the first recognized experimental tumor source. Inoculation of the tumor produced mild clinical illness in mice, at first attributed to leukemia-related toxin and later to LCM (Taylor and MacDowell, 1949; Lindorfer and Syverton, 1953). Since then, LCM has been found in other commonly used tumor lines (Collins and Parker, 1972).

Arthropods may transmit the virus to laboratory animals or receive it from them and transmit it directly to human beings. LCM has been transmitted experimentally by various blood-sucking insects, as described in Hotchin and Benson (1973). Lymphocytic choriomeningitis virus has also been recovered from cockroaches (Armstrong, 1963).

2. Mode of Transmission

LCM virus transmits easily from animals to humans either directly, through physical contact with host animals, their excreta, and tissues, or indirectly through aerosol transmission of the virus (see the literature review in Lehmann-Grube, 1971).

Congenitally infected mice are normal at birth and appear normal for most of their lives, although they are persistently viremic and viruric. Almost all mouse cells are susceptible to this viral infection. Improper handling of infected murine tissues has been associated with most cases of LCM in human laboratory workers (Baum *et al.,* 1966; Tobin, 1968). Contact with mouse feces and urine and inhalation of dried excreta carried on aerosolized dust can also result in LCM infections in humans. Handling LCM-infected mice and being bitten by them are also significant causes of human LCM.

The cage type and location of infected pet hamsters are associated with LCM acquired in households. Wire cages are associated with the highest infection rate and aquariums or deep boxes with lower infection rates, presumably because their poor ventilation does not facilitate transmission of the virus. Cages placed in common living areas are associated with a high infection rate in contrast to cages placed outside the usual human occupancy areas (i.e., basements) in which no household infections occurred (Biggar *et al.,* 1975). Biggar's study, along with one by Hinman *et al.* (1975), supported the notion of aerosol transmission of LCM virus. The Hinman study showed that LCM infection — most common among medical personnel who had physical contact with the animals — also occurred among people who denied having any physical contact with the animals. The rate of seroconversion in those without physical contact related to the frequency with which they entered rooms housing LCM-infected hamsters, providing further evidence of airborne LCM viral transmission.

3. Clinical Features

LCM viral infection most frequently manifests itself as a mild nervous system disorder (Duncan *et al.,* 1951). The disease cannot be regarded merely as a minor, flulike illness because its expression varies greatly, sometimes necessitating prolonged hospitalization (Biggar *et al.,* 1975). The wide variety of clinical signs and symptoms associated with LCM makes elevations in antibody titers the most definitive means of diagnosis (other than viral isolation).

4. Prevention and Control

Cesarean derivation, routine serological monitoring, culling, and prevention of wild mice entering the laboratory have eradicated LCM infection in almost all colonies in the United States. To prevent infection either through contact or airborne transmission, use these measures: screen all murine tumor lines for LCM virus before beginning manipulative procedures; wash hands thoroughly and use disposable gloves when touching animals, their tissues, or cages; restrict personnel movement in and out of enclosures of LCM-infected animals.

C. Rabies

Rabies, an acute, almost invariably fatal disease caused by a member of the rhabdovirus group, is worldwide in distribution with the exception of a few countries that have maintained rabies-free status because of strict importation and animal control regulations and because of geographic barriers (Gillespie and Timoney, 1981). Geographically varying primary reservoirs of rabies may involve many domestic and wild species, including rodents, but incidence of rabies in this species, especially in laboratory animals, is rare to nonexistent.

III. RICKETTSIAL AND CHLAMYDIAL DISEASES

A. Psittacosis

Psittacosis, also known as ornithosis, parrot fever, and chlamydiosis, is caused by *Chlamydia psittaci,* an obligate intracellular organism with a unique development cycle.

1. Reservoir and Incidence

Two species, *C. trachomatis* and *C. psittaci,* compose the genus *Chlamydia.* Mice and humans are the only natural hosts of *C. trachomatis;* mice can carry several strains causing pneumonitis. The zoonotic potential of mouse-adapted *C. trachomatis* has not been recorded. A broad range of species can host *C. psittaci,* including mice, guinea pigs, and other laboratory animal species (Storz, 1971; Newcomer *et al.,* 1982). Birds are the main reservoir of *C. psittaci* infection; the mammalian-derived strains are rarely implicated as a source of zoonotic infection (Schachter and Dawson, 1978). Approximately 25% of humans who contract psittacosis have no history of contact with birds, and the source of the organism has never been identified (Schachter and Dawson, 1978). Some of these outbreaks came from highly virulent strains of *C. psittaci.*

2. Mode of Transmission

The organism is shed enterically in gastrointestinal infection, making dried aerosolized fecal material highly infective. The organism can cause latent infection or fulminant disease in the same host species.

3. Clinical Features

Psittacosis may be either asymptomatic or clinically evident after a 1- to 2-week incubation period. Clinical onset may be acute or insidious. Symptoms include fever, chills, myalgia, anorexia, headache, and a nonproductive cough. The disorder frequently has a respiratory component.

Pneumonitis or atypical pneumonia displaying extensive pulmonary involvement may be indicated radiographically. Respiratory lesions are less prominent in some cases, and the disease presents itself as a toxic or septic condition. Characteristics of this form of the disease include hepatosplenomegaly with hepatitis, meningoencephalitis, and cardiac involvement. To ensure that relapses do not occur, antibiotic regimens for 21 days or longer are generally prescribed.

4. Prevention and Control

Because birds serve as the primary reservoir of this disease, only those free of psittacosis should be introduced into an animal facility. If birds from the wild or those of unknown disease status must be used, animal care and research personnel should implement chlortetracycline chemoprophylaxis, and use protective clothing, particularly masks. Rodents in toxicological studies should not be housed in rooms with birds because of potential interspecies transmission of diseases.

B. Other Rickettsial Diseases

Excepting their possible transmission of psittacosis, rodents do not ordinarily transmit other rickettsial infections in research animal facilities. Wild rodents — as well as other wild animals — do carry infectious rickettsial species that may be introduced into laboratory animal populations if such wild animals are required for investigative purposes. Rickettsial diseases transmitted by wild rodents and other animals are discussed in the following sections.

1. Rocky Mountain Spotted Fever

Rocky Mountain spotted fever is a serious disease of humans caused by *Rickettsia rickettsii.*

a. Mode of Transmission

Ixodid ticks (*Dermacentor andersonii* and *D. variabilis*) and their host species transmit *Rickettsia rickettsii* to humans. The mammalian hosts from which the organism has been isolated include numerous wild rodents and lagomorphs (Burgdorfer, 1979).

b. Clinical Features

The disease is characterized by fever, headache, myalgia, and a generalized maculopapular rash that frequently becomes hemorrhagic.

c. Prevention and Control

Controlling ectoparasites on newly arrived, wild-caught rodents and other animals helps prevent this disease from entering the laboratory.

2. Rickettsialpox

Rickettsialpox is caused by *R. akari,* a member of the spotted fever group of *Rickettsia.* In humans, rickettsialpox is a mild, self-limiting disease.

a. Reservoir and Incidence

Domestic mice, rats, and moles are the natural hosts of this organism. The disease is primarily transmitted to humans dwelling in rodent-infested urban buildings in which mice, mites, and rickettsia maintain a cycle of infection (Greenberg *et al.,* 1947; Nichols *et al.,* 1953). *Allodermanyssus sanguineus,* the natural vector of the disease, is present in many areas of the world but has not been documented in laboratory rodent colonies.

b. Mode of Transmission

Transmission via the respiratory route has been reported in laboratory-acquired infections in humans (Sulkin, 1961); however, laboratory infection from mite bites has not been reported.

c. Clinical Features

Rickettsialpox presents the following clinical features in humans: escharlike lesions, fever for several days, headache, myalgia, lymphadenopathy, leukopenia, and a generalized papulovesicular rash.

d. Prevention and Control

The elimination of wild mice and the mite vector is necessary for the control and prevention of this disease in both laboratory and human dwellings.

3. Murine Typhus

Rickettsia typhi is known to infect the mite *Ornithonyssus bacoti,* which experimentally can transmit the infection to guinea pigs (Dove and Shelmire, 1932). Rat fleas also harbor the organism, although natural laboratory rodent infections with *R. typhi* have not been observed. Outbreaks of the disease in humans living in rodent-infested dwellings continue to occur throughout the United States, particularly in Texas.

a. Mode of Transmission

The organism is known to be transmitted to humans by rat fleas (*Xenopsylla cheopsis* and *Nasopsyllus fasciatus*) or directly through laboratory animals experimentally infected with the disease. Laboratory-acquired infections in humans from experimentally inoculated mice have been reported (Fox and Brayton, 1982).

b. Clinical Features

The clinical signs and symptoms of murine typhus in humans are similar to those of rickettsialpox.

c. Prevention and Control

Prevention of ingress of wild rodents and insects will effectively limit introduction of this disease in laboratory rodents used in toxicological studies.

IV. BACTERIAL DISEASES

A. Leptospirosis

Leptospirosis is a potentially severe biphasic disease that may affect renal, pulmonary, and hepatic function. Gastrointestinal and conjunctival findings may also be abnormal (Barkin *et al.,* 1974).

1. Reservoir and Incidence

Rodent hosts of leptospirosis include rats, mice, field moles, gerbils, and hamsters. Most serotypes can be carried by several hosts. Leptospira adapt particularly well to wild animals and rodents. Chronic clinical manifestations are inconspicuous; organisms are shed in the urine for long periods of time. Active shedding of leptospira prototypes, including *L. australis, bataviae, grippotyphosa, hebdomidis icterohaemorrhagiae, pomona,* and *pyrogenes,* is found in the house mouse (Torten, 1979). *Leptospira ballum* has also been reported in mice and is most commonly associated with zoonotic outbreaks (Borst *et al.,* 1948; Stoenner and Maclean, 1958; Friedmann *et al.,* 1973).

Although rats and mice are common hosts for *L. ballum,* it exists in other wildlife as well. The infection in mice is inapparent and can persist for the animal's lifetime (Torten, 1979). Although earlier reports indicated that several colonies of laboratory mice harbor the organism (Wolf *et al.,* 1949; Yager *et al.,* 1953), no current estimates of carrier rats among laboratory rodents in the United States are available. Recently, a laboratory mouse colony used for biomedical research was diagnosed as having *L. ballum* infection (Barkin *et al.,* 1974). Several European laboratories have reported transmission of leptospira from laboratory rats to laboratory personnel (Geller, 1979). A Georgia study of 2673 feral rodents from 10 species isolated *L. ballum* (the only serotype cultured) in 22% of the house mice and 0.8% of the field mice *Peromyscus polionotus* (Brown and Gorman, 1960).

The difficulty in diagnosing leptospirosis in humans may mean that the low reported incidence of human *L. ballum* is misleading. Only 17 human cases of this disease were recorded in the United States between 1947 and 1973 (Stoenner and Maclean, 1958; Boak *et al.,* 1960; Centers for Disease Control, 1965, 1966; Friedmann *et al.,* 1973). Outbreaks in personnel working with laboratory mice in the United States have also been documented (Stoenner and Maclean, 1958; Boak *et al.,* 1960; Barkin *et al.,* 1974). In one study, 8 of 58 employees handling infected laboratory mice experienced leptospirosis; 80% of the breeding female mice were excreting *L. ballum* in their urine. Humans have also contracted leptospiral infection by handling infected pet mice (Friedmann *et al.,* 1973).

2. Mode of Transmission

Infection with *L. ballum* most frequently results from handling infected mice (contaminating the hands with urine) or from aerosol exposure during cage cleaning. Because *L. ballum* presumably does not penetrate intact skin, skin abrasions may serve as the portal of entry. In one instance, it was speculated that a father became infected when his daughter used his toothbrush to clean the contaminated pet mouse's cage after she had an argument with him (Friedmann *et al.,* 1973).

3. Clinical Features

Infected individuals experience a biphasic disease (Heath and Alexander, 1970). At first, they suddenly become ill and weak, with headache, myalgia, malaise, chills, and fever. Although usually associated with leptospirosis, leukocytosis is inconsistently presently in *L. ballum* infection.

Painful orchitis is often present during the second phase of this disorder but does not usually cause the enlarged testes seen in mumps (Friedmann *et al.*, 1973). Serological diagnosis, or actual isolation of leptospira, provides the means to identify this disease (Stoenner, 1954; Torten, 1979). Leptospira can sometimes be observed by examining or directly staining body fluids or fresh tissue suspensions. A definitive diagnosis in human or mouse is made by culturing the organisms from tissue or fluid samples or by inoculating animals (particularly 3- to 4-week-old hamsters) and subsequently culturing and isolating the organisms.

In a survey of trapped urban rats, diagnosis of leptospirosis was more accurate by urine or kidney culture rather than by indirect fluorescent antibody or macroscopic slide agglutination (Sulzer *et al.*, 1968; see also Higa and Fujinaka, 1976).

4. Prevention and Control

In mouse colonies infected with *L. ballum,* antibodies against *L. ballum* were detected in sera of mice of all ages, but leptospira could be recovered only from mature mice. Progeny of seropositive females had detectable serum antibodies at 51 days of age but not at 65 days. Progeny of seropositive female mice possessed antibodies at birth and acquired additional antibodies from colostrum; they remained free of leptospira when isolated from their mothers at 21 days of age, despite exposure during the nursing period (Stoenner, 1957).

Studies in mice experimentally infected with *L. grippotyphosa* demonstrated that maternal antibodies, whether passed through milk or placenta, conferred long-lasting protection against the carrier state and shedding of leptospira (Birnbaum *et al.*, 1972). Thus, serologically positive immune mothers do not transmit the disease to their offspring. However, mice born to nonimmune mothers — if infected at 1 day postpartum — become carriers with no trace of antibodies. A population of pregnant carrier mice without antibodies can precipitate outbreaks among susceptible mouse populations (Birnbaum *et al.*, 1972). The fact that many carrier mice do not have antibodies has led to a diagnostic approach in which both serological and isolation methods are used to determine the rate of leptospiral infection in rodents (Galton et al., 1962).

Leptospira ballum is frequently found in the common house mouse (*M. musculus;* Yager et al., 1953; Brown and Gorman, 1960), and *L. icterohae-morrhagiae* is found in wild rats (Higa and Fujinaka, 1976). Eradication of infected colonies, use of surgically derived and barrier-maintained rodents or of conventional laboratory rodents free of leptospiral infection, coupled with the prevention of ingress of wild rodents into laboratories should effectively preclude introduction of the organism into research and commercial laboratories (Loosli, 1967). Any laboratory or wild rodents to be used for primary kidney tissue cultures should first be examined to assure that they are free of leptospira (Turner, 1970).

Administering feed containing 1000 g chlortetracycline hydrochloride per ton to infected mice for 10 days eliminated *L. ballum* from one colony. On the seventh day of antibiotic therapy, the mice were transferred to clean containers and given clean water (both previously steam-sterilized). Mouse traps and DDT destroyed escaped mice and prevented house mice from reintroducing *L. ballum* (Stoenner et al., 1958).

B. Plague

Plague is a febrile zoonotic disease caused by the gram-negative bacteria *Yersinia pestis.* Human infections in the United States are sporadic and limited. Plague affects the lymphatic system and, if left untreated, may progress to severe pneumonic or systemic plague.

1. Reservoir and Incidence

Plague is endemic in scattered wild rodent populations in the western third of the United States. Incidence of human infection has been on the rise since 1965 (Poland and Barnes, 1979; Christie et al., 1980; Kaufman et al., 1981; Sanford, 1982). Human infection usually results from contact with infected fleas or rodents. In addition, animals such as dogs and cats may serve as passive transporters of infected rodent fleas into the home or laboratory.

2. Mode of Transmission

Infected fleas or rodents transmit plague through bites.

3. Clinical Features

Bubonic plague in humans is usually characterized by fever and large, tender, swollen lymph nodes or buboes, which may progress to severe pneumonic or systemic plague if untreated. Inhalation of infective particles may also result in pneumonic plague. Proper antibiotic therapy can significantly reduce the mortality rate, which may exceed 50% in untreated cases. The general population is widely susceptible, with relative immunity present only after recovery.

4. Prevention and Control

A presumptive diagnosis can be made through visualization of bipolar-staining, ovoid, gram-negative rods on microscopic examination of fluid from buboes, blood, sputum, or spinal fluid. Culturing confirms the diagnosis. Complement fixation, passive hemagglutination, and immunofluorescence staining of specimens provide serological confirmation.

Plague prevention is aimed at controlling wild rodents. Feral or random-source animals acquired in known endemic plague areas for use in laboratories should be carefully quarantined and treated with appropriate insecticides to kill fleas. Beyond rodent control, routine flea control should be carefully followed in animals housed outdoors in plague-endemic areas. A vaccine is available for high-risk personnel doing field work in endemic areas.

C. Ratbite Fever

Ratbite fever can be caused by either of two microorganisms: *Streptobacillus moniliformis (Actinomyces muris)* or *Spirillum minus (Spirillum minor; Spirillum morsus muris)*, synonym (sodoku). It is a serious human disease causing arthritis, pneumonia, hepatitis, enteritis, and endocarditis.

1. Reservoir and Incidence

These organisms are present in the oral cavity and upper respiratory passages of asymptomatic rodents. Mice are not asymptomatic carriers of either *S. moniliformis* or *Sp. minus,* but rats are (Strangeways, 1933). Paegle *et al.* (1976), in a more recent study of laboratory Sprague–Dawley rats, isolated *S. moniliformis* as the predominant microorganism from the upper trachea of control animals. The lack of reported carrier rates in mice is attributed partly to the usual asymptomatic carrier state and partly to the difficulty in isolating the organisms. *Spirillum minus* cannot be cultured *in vitro* and requires inoculation of culture specimens into laboratory animals and subsequent identification of the organism by dark-field microscopy. *Streptobacillus moniliformis* grows slowly on artificial media but only in the presence of sera, usually 10–20% rabbit or horse serum incubated at reduced partial pressures of oxygen (Holmgren and Tunevall, 1970; Rogosa, 1974).

Uncommon in man, the disease has nonetheless appeared among researchers working with laboratory rodents, particularly with rats (Holden and MacKay, 1964; Cole *et al.,* 1969; Arkless, 1970; Gilbert *et al.,* 1971; Anderson *et al.,* 1983). Historically, however, wild rat bites and subsequent illness relate to poor sanitation and overcrowding. Almost 50% of all cases have involved children under the age of 12 (Brown and Nunemaker, 1942; Richter, 1945; Roughgarden, 1965; Raffin and Freemark, 1979).

Ratbite fever is not a reportable disease, which makes its incidence, geographic location, racial data, and source of infection in humans difficult to assess. Because acute febrile diseases — especially those associated with animal bites — are routinely treated with penicillin or other antibiotics before culturing the bite wound, accurate recording of the disease is impossible.

2. Mode of Transmission

The bite of an infected rodent, usually a wild rat but occasionally a laboratory rat or mouse, is the usual source of infection. In some cases, other animal bites or rare traumatic injuries unassociated with animal contact cause the infection (Richter, 1945; Roughgarden, 1965). Occasional outbreaks have been associated with streptobacillus-contaminated milk or food (Place and Sutton, 1934).

3. Clinical Features

Streptobacillus moniliformis incubation varies from a few hours to 1–3 days, whereas *Sp. minus* incubation ranges from 1 to 6 weeks. Fever is present in either form. Inflammation and lymphadenopathy are frequently accompanied by headache, general malaise, myalgia, and chills (Raffin and Freemark, 1969; Gilbert *et al.,* 1971). The discrete macular rash that often appears on the extremities (e.g., palms and soles) may generalize into pustular or petechial sequelae. Arthritis occurs in 50% of all cases of *S. moniliformis* but is less common in *Sp. minus.* Serous to purulent effusion can be recovered from affected larger joints, and *S. moniliformis* cultured from this fluid.

If antibiotic treatment is not instituted early, complications such as pneumonia, hepatitis, pyelonephritis, enteritis, and endocarditis may develop (McGill *et al.*, 1966). Death has occurred in cases of *S. moniliformis* involving preexistent valvular disease.

D. Salmonella

Of the 1600 recognized serotypes, *Salmonella typhimurium* and *Salmonella enteritidis* represent those most associated with infection in laboratory rodent colonies (Habermann and Williams, 1958; Hoag and Rogers, 1961). *Salmonella typhimurium* was the most frequently isolated serotype in the United States from 1974 to 1978 (Centers for Disease Control, 1976; Morbidity and Mortality Weekly Report, 1980). Other frequently isolated serotypes include *S. newport, S. enteritidis,* and *S. heidelberg.*

1. Reservoir and Incidence

Salmonella infection in humans and animals, including mice and rats, occurs worldwide. The organism is an enteric bacterium inhabiting the intestinal tract of many animals. Salmonella routinely contaminates food, sewage, and many environmental water sources.

Despite the recent decreases in incidence of salmonella in laboratory rodents brought about by improved management practices, environmental contamination by these bacteria continues to threaten laboratory animals and personnel. Contaminated animal feed poses particular danger, especially if the diet consists of raw, unpelleted meal (Hoag *et al.*, 1964; Williams *et al.*, 1969; Stott *et al.*, 1975).

Salmonella-infected rodents have also caused food-borne outbreaks of salmonellosis. In an interesting epidemiological study performed in England, *S. enteritidis* (var. *danzy*) was isolated from two adults living four miles apart. The source of infection was contaminated cakes from a local bakery where mice had acquired the infection from living *S. danzy* cultures in rodenticide baits and had infected food in the bakery (Brown and Parker, 1957).

Although both humans and animals are carriers and periodic shedders of salmonella, they may have mild, unrecognized, asymptomatic cases. Asymptomatic, salmonella-shedding animals are particularly hazardous in biomedical research because they can infect other animals, animal technicians, and investigators (Fox and Beaucage, 1979). Incidence of asymptomatic carrier mice within a colony varies from 1–20% (Habermann and Williams, 1958); indeed, Margard *et al.* (1963) suggested that clinically apparent salmonellosis is rare in infected mice. A total of 227 isolates were recovered from rodents in a survey conducted in the United States from 1962 to 1965 of 19,137 salmonella isolations of nonhuman origin from pet animals (Kaufman, 1966). The incidence of salmonellosis transmission from humans to mice or vice versa is unknown.

2. Mode of Transmission

Salmonella is most commonly transmitted through human handling of infected animals or contaminated materials, such as animal feed.

3. Clinical Features

Clinical signs of salmonellosis in humans include acute sudden gastroenteritis, abdominal pain, diarrhea, nausea, and fever. Loose bowels and anorexia may persist for several days. Organisms invading the bowel wall may create febrile septicemia without severe intestinal involvement; most clinical signs are attributed to hematogenous spread of the organisms (Robbins, 1974). As with other microbial infections, the disease's severity relates to the organism's serotype, the number of bacteria ingested, and the host's susceptibility. Because infection is often inapparent, laboratories maintaining rodent colonies should consider screening animal technicians for subclinical salmonella infections.

E. Other Potential Bacterial Diseases

On rare occasions, rodents may transmit other bacteria, such as *Pasteurella,* to humans. *Yersinia pestis,* transmitted by flea bite, is endemic in wild rodent populations (Hudson *et al.,* 1964) but should not be found in established mouse colonies provided those mice have had no contact with wild rodents.

Another disease, campylobacteriosis, caused by *Campylobacter jejuni/ coli,* has occasionally been isolated in hamsters. It is not known, however, if this disease is routinely transmitted by rodents in the laboratory.

Migrating meadow mice and house mice in California (Wayson, 1972) suffer epizootic infection from *Erysipelothrix rhusiopathiae,* but handling of infected animals has not yet been shown to bring about human infection.

Evaluating the zoonotic potential of *Pseudomonas aeruginosa* is difficult because of its environmental ubiquity. Human-to-animal transmission, linked to infected animal caretakers, has been documented in two outbreaks within a mouse colony (Van der Waaij *et al.*, 1963), but animal-to-human transmission has not been documented. *Pseudomonas aeruginosa* is a virulent pathogen in immunosuppressed mice as well as a potential pathogen in conventional or SPF mice.

Finally, pathogenic *Staphylococcus aureus* of human phage type can cause clinical disease in mice and rats. This organism has been introduced into SPF barrier-maintained mouse colonies and SPF rats and guinea pigs; the same phage type was isolated from their animal caretakers (Davey, 1962; Blackmore and Francis, 1970; Shults *et al.*, 1973). Nasopharyngeal colonization by normal *S. aureus* strains in humans presumably minimizes zoonotic potential of animal-originated *S. aureus* in humans.

Streptococci of Lancefield groups A, B, C, and D have been isolated from disease outbreaks in mice (Besch-Williford and Wagner, 1982), but there is no documented evidence that streptococci isolated from mice are transmitted to or acquired from humans.

F. Cutaneous Infections

Numerous bacterial species can cause cutaneous infections, but the danger of such transmissions is minor when compared with other diseases. For example, wild and laboratory mice can transmit dermatophilosis and erysipeloid; and guinea pigs may, under certain circumstances, transmit dermatophilosis or listeriosis.

V. MYCOSES

Ringworm (favus) in the mouse was first recorded in England in 1850. In almost all mouse-associated ringworm infections in humans, *Trichophyton mentagrophytes* has been isolated as the etiological agent (see Table I). Many other zoophilic dermatophytes associated with infections of mice can cause ringworm in humans, including *Epidermophyton floccosum, Microsporum gallinae, M. gypseum, T. erinacai, T. schoenleini,* and *T. (Keratinomyces) ajelloi* (Dvorak and Otechenasek, 1964; Krempl-Lamprecht and Bosse, 1964; Marples, 1967; Refai and Ali, 1970). Classical murine ringworm, reportedly caused by *Trichophyton quinckeanum,* is usually restricted to feral rodents, but successful crossing of cultures of this strain with tester strains of perfect-state *T. mentagrophytes (Arthroderma benhamiae)* proves that *T. quinckeanum* is not a distinct species and is indistinguishable from *T. mentagrophytes* (Ajello *et al.*, 1968).

Table I

Trichophyton mentagrophytes Infections Associated with Laboratory Mice, Rats, or Pet Mice

Probable source of infection	Number of persons infected	Lesions appearing on infected mice or rats	References
Pet white mice; inbred albino laboratory mice (VSBS, A2G)	7 children; 2 laboratory technicians	2 of 104, diffuse alopecia	MacKenzie (1961)
Laboratory mice	6 laboratory technicians		Alteras (1965)
Laboratory mice	2 laboratory technicians	0 of 96 (222 cultured), survey of commercial stock	Dolan *et al.* (1958)
BALB/c C3H/Bi mice	6 laboratory technicians	<1% of all mice, carrier rate 90%	Davies and Shewell (1964)
White mice	1 laboratory worker	% ND[a], alopecia, increased scaling on head and back, 10 mice	Booth (1952)
White mice	1 bacteriologist	60 of 400, crusted or crustless plaques, circular with prominent periphery; general alopecia; mortality in some mice	Cetin *et al.* (1965)
Wistar rats	1 technician	20% colony with alopecia and scaly skin	Dolan *et al.* (1958)
Rats	1 technician	Alopecia with crusting and erythema	Povar (1965)

[a]ND, not determined.

1. Reservoir and Incidence

Dermatophytes are distributed worldwide, with some species reportedly more common in certain geographic locations. From a study of 1288 animals from 15 different species of small mammals in their natural habitats, 57 *T. mentagrophytes* were isolated most commonly from the bank vole *(Clethriomys glareolus),* followed by the common shrew *(Sorex araneum)* and house mouse (*M. musculus;* Chmel *et al.,* 1975). Agricultural workers exposed to these mammals in granaries and barns risked contracting *T. mentagrophytes* infections; indeed, 77% of 137 agricultural workers were infected with ringworm. Only 23% of the workers showed signs of *T. verrucosum* infection.

In laboratory mice and rats, ringworm infection is often asymptomatic, going unrecognized until laboratory personnel become infected (see Table I). The prevalence of *T. mentagrophytes* among laboratory mouse stocks has been recorded as high as 80–90% (Davies and Shewell, 1964). For the 8-month period before these infected mice were treated, almost half the people handling the mice developed ringworm, although less than 1% of the mice showed any signs of the disease. Fungicide treatment reduced the level of carriers from 90 to 21% of the mice.

2. Mode of Transmission

Transmission occurs via direct or indirect contact with asymptomatic carrier animals, skin lesions of infected mice, contaminated grain, or animal bedding. Causal fungi present in air, dust, or on surfaces of animal holding rooms are also transmittal sources. (MacKenzie, 1961). Transmission often goes unsuspected until symptoms appear because laboratory animals have few visible skin lesions (Dolan *et al.*, 1958; Cotchin and Roe, 1967).

3. Clinical Features

Ringworm is in many cases nonfatal, usually self-limiting, and, because it is sometimes asymptomatic, often ignored by the affected person. The dermatophytes cause scaling, erythema, and occasionally vesicles and fissures; the fungi cause thickening and discoloration of the nails. On the skin of the trunk and extremities, lesions may be circular with a central clearing (Mescon and Grots, 1974). Fungal locations create clinical categories, for example, tinea capitis or tinea ungium. When humans are infected by one of the dermatophytes recovered from mice, the fungus appears on the body and/or extremities, most commonly on the arms and hands.

Zoophilic *T. mentagrophytes* is highly inflammatory and often undergoes rapid resolution; the infection may produce furunculosis, widespread tinea corporis, and deep involvement of the hair follicles (also seen in infections of *E. floccosum*). A technician who acquired *T. (Keratinomyces) ajelloi* while working with mice developed small, grayish-white scaly lesions on both hands. The organism isolated from the hand lesions appeared in 2 of 250 apparently healthy mice (Refai and Ali, 1970).

4. Prevention and Control

Strict environmental and personal hygiene help lower the incidence of ringworm. Animal handlers should wear rubber gloves when touching infected animals.

VI. PROTOZOAN DISEASES

A. *Entamoeba coli*

A nonpathogenic protozoan in humans, *Entamoeba coli* morphologically resembles *E. muris,* seen in mice and rats. Whether transmission between humans and rodents is possible is unknown. *E. coli* infection has been established in rats, but little attempt has been made to reduce possible cross-infection with *E. muris* (Kessel, 1923). A 1950 study neither transmitted nor established *E. coli* in either mice or rats (Neal, 1950).

More recently, researchers have attempted to establish *E. coli* in laboratory rodents by passaging cysts of *E. coli* from 15 human and 4 primate stools in SPF guinea pigs, rats, and mice. In only one instance were cysts established in mice and eventually in rats (Owen, 1978). The morphological similarity between *E. coli* and *E. muris* prevented Owen from determining whether the *Entamoeba* (originally isolated from an Ethiopian) was a true transmission of *E. coli* in the rodent or a contaminant of the human feces with *E. muris.* The author concluded that human–rodent contact is not responsible for the introduction of *Entamoeba* spp. (most likely *E. muris*) in SPF-barrier-maintained rodent colonies. No evidence in the literature lists humans as *E. muris* carriers.

The mouse can also be infected experimentally with *E. histolytica,* but natural infections with this parasite have not been reported (Flynn, 1973).

B. Toxoplasmosis

Infection due to *Toxoplasma gondii* is widespread in humans and lower animals (Frenkel, 1973; Levine, 1973). Approximately 500 million humans have been infected with this organism, primarily through the ingestion of contaminated food (Kean, 1972).

The life cycle of *T. gondii* consists of definitive and intermediate hosts. Mice, rats, hamsters, guinea pigs, and other rodents are some laboratory animals that might serve as intermediate hosts. These hosts have not proved to be important in zoonotic infection by *T. gondii* in the laboratory because the organism is replicating asexually in extraintestinal sites only.

C. Cryptosporidiosis

Cryptosporidiosis was first described in the mouse (Tyzzer, 1907). The genus *Cryptosporidium* now contains approximately 11 named species

(Levine, 1980), many of which have been incriminated as opportunistic pathogenic parasites.

1. Reservoir and Incidence

Although cryptosporidial infection most commonly occurs in the intestinal epithelium, it has been observed in the stomach of mice and other animals. Guinea pigs have sometimes been infected with enteric cryptosporidial infection or bovine cryptosporidia from calves.

2. Mode of Transmission

Recent studies suggest infectivity across species lines.

3. Clinical Features

Most cases of human cryptosporidiosis have occurred in immunodeficient individuals and are regarded as opportunistic endogenous infections (Messel *et al.*, 1976; Lasser *et al.*, 1979; Stemmermann *et al.*, 1980). The disease produced low grade fever, malaise, anorexia, nausea, abdominal cramps, and protracted water diarrhea. Endogenous cryptosporidial stages and clinical signs have persisted in some cases for over a year.

In one case, experimental transmission studies were conducted in mice and rats in which human and calf isolates were compared. Indistinguishable infections were produced (Reese *et al.*, 1982), adding support to the theory that cryptosporidiosis may be zoonotic and that some species of *Cryptosporidium* may not be host specific.

4. Prevention and Control

There is no established therapeutic regimen for this disease.

D. Other Protozoan Diseases

Laboratory rodents can transmit *Pneumocystis carinii,* but zoonotic transmission has not been confirmed. In humans and animals, clinical disease is usually seen in individuals with intercurrent debility, poor nutrition, neoplasia, or immunodeficiency. In humans, the disease is frequently characterized by diffuse desquamative alveolitis (Hughes, 1981).

VII. HELMINTH DISEASES

A. Tapeworms

1. The Rat Tapeworm (*Hymenolepis diminuta*)

a. Reservoir and Incidence

This parasite is most commonly associated with rats, especially wild Norway *(Rattus norvegicus)* and black *(Rattus rattus)* rats throughout the world (Wardle and McLeod, 1952). It can also be found in the mouse intestine but is rarely encountered in humans (Stone and Manwell, 1966; Faust and Russell, 1970).

b. Mode of Transmission

Like other tapeworms, *H. diminuta* requires an intermediate host, usually a flour beetle *(Tribolium* spp.), moth, or flea (Voge and Heyneman, 1957). *Tribolium* larval development requires 8 days at 30°C. Humans become infected only through ingesting infected insects, which may infest rodent food or cereal marketed for human consumption.

c. Clinical Features

Usually asymptomatic, moderate to heavy infections may cause headache, dizziness, and abdominal discomfort.

d. Prevention and Control

Elimination of feral rodents in animal facilities will effectively preclude introduction of this parasite. Routine health monitoring of newly introduced rodents for use in research is also warranted.

2. The Dwarf Tapeworm of Humans (*Hymenolepis*)

a. Reservoir and Incidence

Although the dwarf tapeworm is a common parasite of both the wild house mouse and the laboratory mouse, its incidence is low in most well-managed mouse colonies (Wescott, 1982).

In 1947 Stoll listed *H. nana* infections in 100,000 North Americans and in 20 million people worldwide. Central European surveys find this tapeworm more prevalent in warmer regions. Some South American countries suffer 10% per capita incidence (Jelliffe and Stanfield, 1978).

b. Mode of Transmission

Hymenolepis nana eggs can contaminate hands, be trapped on particulate matter, or be aerosolized and accidentally ingested. Because no interme-

Table II
Ectoparasites of Rodents with Zoonotic Potential[a]

Species	Disease in humans	Laboratory host	Agent
Mites			
Obligate skin mites			
Sarcoptes scabiei subspecies	Scabies	Mammals	
Nest inhabiting parasites			
Ornithonyssus bacoti	Dermatitis, murine typhus	Rodents and other vertebrates, including birds	WEE,[b] SLE[c] virus, *Rickettsia mooseri*
Liponyssoides sanguineus	Dermatitis, rickettsial-pox	Rodents, particularly *Mus musculus*	*Ricksettsia akari*
Haemogamasus pontiger	Dermatitis	Rodents, insectivores, straw bedding	
Haemolaelaps casalis	Dermatitis	Birds, mammals, straw, hay	
Eulaelaps stabularis	Dermatitis, tularemia	Small mammals, straw bedding	*Francisella tularensis*
Trixacarus caviae	Dermatitis	Guinea pigs	
Ixodids (ticks)			
Dermacentor variabilis	Irritation, RMSF,[d] tularemia tick paralysis, other diseases	Wild rodents, cottontail rabbits, dogs from endemic areas	*Rickettsia rickettsia, F. tularensis*
Amblyomma americanum	Irritation, RMSF,[d] tularemia	Wild rodents, dogs	
Ixodes scapularis	Irritation, possible tularemia	Dogs, wild rodents	
Ixodes spp.			
Fleas			
Xenopsylla cheopsis	Dermatitis, plague vector, *H. nana, H. diminuta*	Mouse, rat, wild rodents	
Nasopsyllus fasciatus	Dermatitis, plague vector, *H. nana, H. diminuta,* murine typhus	Mouse, rat, wild rodents	
Leptopsylla segnis	*H. diminuta, H. nana,* murine typhus vector	Rat	Harbors salmonella

Source: Modified from Yunker (1964).

[a]Found in laboratory animals that cause allergic dermatitis or from which zoonotic agents have been recovered in nature.

[b]WEE, western equine encephalitis.

[c]SLE, St. Louis equine encephalitis.

[d]RMSF, Rocky Mountain spotted fever.

diate host is required, the eggs readily infect reciprocal hosts (Faust and Russell, 1970).

c. Clinical Features

Well-nourished persons essentially present no symptoms, but the infection can be noted in the proglottids, or ova, seen in the stool. In other persons, symptoms include headaches, dizziness, anorexia, inanition, pruritus of the nose and anus, periodic diarrhea, and abdominal distress. Convulsions have also occurred.

d. Prevention and Control

Strict personal hygiene, appropriate laboratory uniforms, and use of disposable gloves and face masks when handling contaminated bedding and feces are the precautions against this infection.

B. Roundworms

Although *Syphacia obvelata* is ubiquitous in both wild and laboratory mice, no reliable reports of infection in humans exist.

VIII. ARTHROPOD INFESTATIONS

Liponyssoides sanguineus, the house mouse mite, and *Ornithonyssus bacoti,* the tropical rat mite, are the only vectors of human disease. *O. bacoti* is seen in laboratory mice (Fox, 1982); *L. sanguineus* has only been identified on wild mice (see Table II). Bites from these mites — as well as those from another mouse mite, *Haemolaelaps casalis* — cause allergic dermatitis in humans (Fig. 1). Fleas are seldom found in laboratory mice but are common parasites of feral rodents. The Oriental rat flea, *Xenopsylla cheopis,* and another flea, *Nasopsyllus fasciatus,* naturally infest both mice and rats; they are vectors for murine typhus. That *X. cheopis* easily establishes itself in animal facilities can be demonstrated by the bites two students received in animal rooms housing mice (Yunker, 1964).

The house flea, *Leptopsylla segnis,* bites humans and is a vector for plague and typhus, serious diseases in humans. *L. segnis* also serves as an

---

Fig. 1 Maculopapular dermatoses in humans associated with mite and flea bites. (a) Tropical rat mite; (b) flea (courtesy of American College of Laboratory Animal Medicine and Washington State University College of Veterinary Medicine); (c) cheyletiella mite. Reproduced from Fox *et al.* (1984).

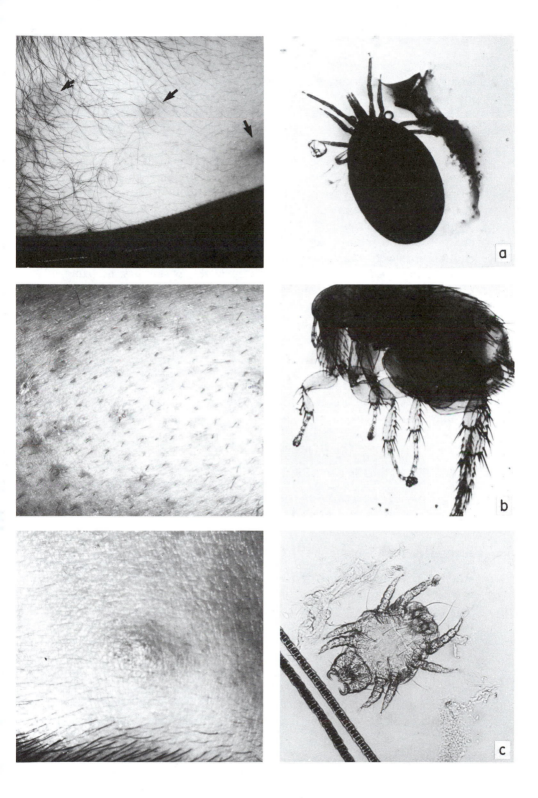

a

b

c

intermediate host for the rodent tapeworms *H. nana* and *H. diminuta,* to which humans are susceptible. This house flea's irritating bite causes allergic dermatitis.

IX. BITES

Over a two-year surveillance period from 1971 to 1972, 196,684 animal bites were listed by 15 reporting areas throughout the United States (Moore *et al.,* 1977). Uncategorized rodent bites accounted for 4% of specified bites. Because of tradition and public emotion, rabies is the primary reason that animal bites are investigated, but rodent bites (especially from wild rats) present other serious public health hazards, especially in impoverished areas where feral rodents abound. In addition to pain, anxiety, and disfigurement, there is the possibility of bacterial infection from such organisms as *Pasteurella* spp., *Clostridium tetani, S. moniliformis,* and *Sp. minus.* Reported incidences and severity of laboratory rodent-associated bites are few, except for published cases of ratbite fever and *Pasteurella* infections (Hubbert and Rosen, 1970).

Depending on the nature of the wound and the health status of the animal inflicting the bite, medical attention may be required. Minor rodent bite wounds should be cleaned thoroughly and topically treated. All laboratory personnel working with animals should maintain current tetanus immunizations (Institute of Laboratory Animal Resources, 1978).

X. ALLERGIC SENSITIVITIES

The following discussion focuses on mice as one example of the many animals that produce allergic sensitivities.

A. Reservoir and Incidence

Allergic skin and respiratory reactions are quite common in laboratory workers handling mice. Hypersensitivity reactions to mouse dander and urine are serious occupational health problems. Numerous people are constantly exposed to laboratory mouse allergens because of the large numbers of mice used in biomedical research. The notion that only rabbit and cat danders produce laboratory animal-related asthma has been disproved; the mouse is now incriminated in producing this allergic response (Rajka, 1961; Newman-Taylor *et al.,* 1977; Lincoln *et al.,* 1974).

Hypersensitivity reactions include nasal congestion, rhinorrhea, sneezing, itching of the eyes, angioedema, and asthma, along with skin

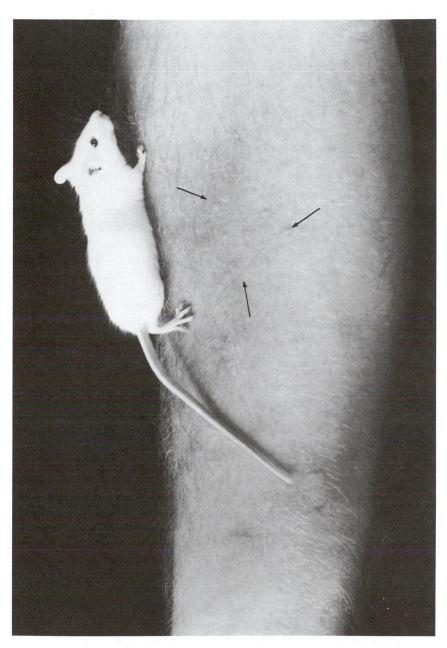

Fig. 2 Small wheals on the midforearm (arrows) and a large wheal adjacent to the tip of the tail of the mouse in the skin of a patient sensitive to mice. Reproduced from Foster *et al.* (1982).

manifestations such as localized urticaria and eczema (atopic dermatitis). Skin wheals and flare reactions appeared in eight mouse-sensitive subjects tested with mouse pelt extracts (Ohman *et al.,* 1975; Figs. 2 and 3). Extract fractions with the electrophoretic mobility of albumin produced maximal skin allergenic activity. Figures 2 and 3 illustrate typical wheal and flare reactions on the skin of a patient hypersensitive to mouse urine. A mouse whose feet were contaminated with urine walked across a patient's arm and produced these lesions.

Intense itching is often manifested where urine or serum has touched the skin (Ohman, 1978). Patients may have a delayed reaction, such as asthma, coming on at night following daytime exposure. Familial predisposition (atopy) to some allergic disorders suggests that inheritance plays a role in the pathogenesis of atopic diseases (Gupta and Good, 1979), although members of the same family may manifest atopy in different ways, some with asthma, others with eczema. The location of the shock organ (i.e., skin, mucous membranes, or respiratory or gastrointestinal tracts) determines clinical manifestations of atopy (Criep, 1976).

Mouse dander (Sorrell and Gottesman, 1957; Lincoln *et al.,* 1974) and mouse urine (Newman-Taylor *et al.,* 1977) appear to be the major antigen sources for personnel working with mice. All of Newman-Taylor's five patients had a history of hay fever or asthma; four of them had handled mice. Symptoms appeared within one year in four patients and after four years in the fifth. Animal exposure rapidly produced rhinitis and conjunctivitis, followed by urticaria when the animal's urine-contaminated feet touched the patients' skin. All five patients developed asthma from a few weeks to two years after being exposed to the animals. Allergen tolerance decreased rapidly. At first, asthmatic episodes occurred several hours after exposure, but eventually attacks came within minutes. When the patients were separated from the animals for a few days, their clinical symptoms disappeared.

Levy (1974) quantitated mouse protein allergic activity and found that albumin, the major component of mouse skin extracts, was highly allergenic in some patients allergic to mice. Additional allergens, such as serum and urine, have been located by Siraganian and Sandberg (1979) and Schumacher (1980). Potent allergens reside within the major urinary complex (MUP) of mouse urine. In three mouse strains, purified MUPs bound to IgE antibodies cross-reacted extensively among themselves and with allergens within dust from a mouse room. This study suggests that laboratory personnel may become sensitized to urinary protein dispersing from mouse cage litter (Schumacher, 1980).

Other laboratory antigens causing allergic reactions include mold and aerosolized food proteins (Patterson, 1964).

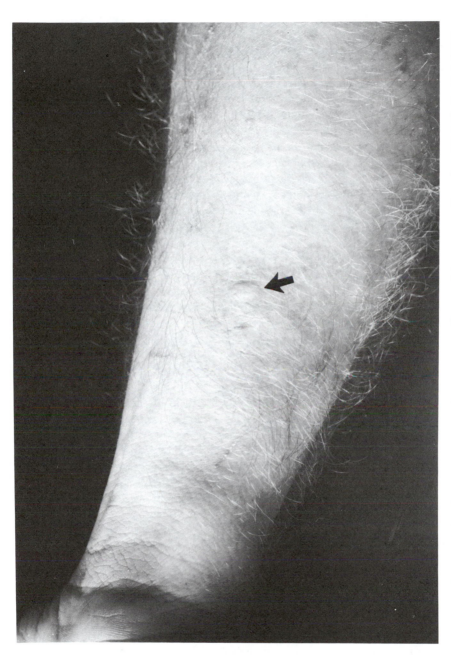

Fig. 3 Large wheal and flare in the skin (arrow) of a patient sensitive to mice. Reproduced from Foster et al. (1982).

B. Pathogenesis

Because allergic sensitivities are the most common significant health hazard in mouse-associated employee activity, the pathogenesis is discussed in some detail.

The pathogenesis of immediate hypersensitivity is initiated by an interaction of mast cells and/or basophils that release preformed chemical mediators such as histamine, serotonins, and heparin. After appropriate sensitization, basophils or mast cells generate other mediators, such as the slow-reacting substance of anaphylaxis (SRS-A; Gupta and Good, 1979). These mediators act as messengers between primary target cells and secondary effector cells or tissues. Effector cells (such as eosinophils, platelets, T lymphocytes, and monocytes) then amplify or modulate the inflammatory host responses, including smooth muscle contraction, vascular dilatation, and increased vascular permeability. Such allergic reactions are often classified as Type I.

Type II reactions occur when an IgG or IgM antibody reacts with an antigen on a target cell, activating complement, which causes cell lysis (Lutsky and Toshner, 1978). Type II reactions are most often seen when drugs act as the antigen and, therefore, are relatively unimportant in people working with laboratory rodents.

Type III allergic reactions are characterized by damage initiated by immune complexes. These complexes activate the complement system, enhancing the inflammatory response. This Arthus reaction produces vasculitis initiated by the deposition of immune complexes of antigen and immunoglobulin (IgG) on the vessel endothelium. Examples include serum sickness, delayed tuberculin hypersensitivity, and hypersensitivity pneumonitis. Laboratory workers who develop asthma several hours after being exposed to mice may have Type III reactions.

Type IV allergic reactions are cell mediated. Antigens are deposited locally and react with sensitized T lymphocytes, which release certain cell-free factors (lymphokines). Type IV reactions include homograft rejection, graft-versus-host reactions, and allergic-contact dermatitis. Type IV reactions may occur when mouse dander, urine, or serum produce erythema and pruritus locally on the skin (Sorrell and Gottesman, 1957; Lincoln *et al.,* 1974).

C. Diagnosis

One must establish a clinical diagnosis and incriminate etiological factors in defining occupational allergic disease resulting from working with mice. Careful detailed histories of patients' complaints and clinical symptoms must be evaluated. Pinning down the appearance of clinical symptoms concomitant to or following environmental exposure narrows the number of allergens to be considered. Nonoccupational exposure to potential allergens must also be taken into account. Family allergy history is also important because atopy predisposes a person to Type I allergic reactions. Physical examinations must be thorough and well documented. Repeat examinations are often performed when the patient is not suffering an acute allergic attack.

Repeated pulmonary function tests and radiological examinations often help, especially when lungs are the target organ. Although rarely indicated and difficult to evaluate, bronchial challenge tests, together with pulmonary function tests, may detect the etiological allergen.

Skin testing with suspected antigens often identifies the hypersensitivity. Patients with Type I sensitivity to animal dander almost always react positively to skin tests performed properly.

Useful laboratory tests include complete blood count; radioallergosorbent test (RAST) to measure immunoglobulins and IgE antibody specific to one allergen; nasal smear for eosinophilia; and serum precipitants to specific allergens. *In vitro* RAST, however, is less sensitive and no more specific than the skin test. Direct eosinophil count is often elevated in the presence of nasal allergy and almost always elevated in patients with asthma.

D. Treatment and Prevention

Pharmacological agents often relieve the allergic response associated with exposure to mice. Useful agents include antihistamines, sympathomimetic agents, corticosteroids, and bronchodilators. Effective pharmacological agents for long-term use include antihistamines for allergic rhinitis, allergic conjunctivitis, and allergic skin reactions. Adrenergic agonists, cromolyn sulfate, and xanthines sometimes help asthmatic patients.

Immunotherapy helped one laboratory worker sensitive to mice (Sorrell and Gottesman, 1957). In this form of therapy, systemic administration of etiological antigens in increasing dosages produces hyposensitivity to animal proteins in patients but may not be recommended in highly sensitive individuals because it can cause uncomfortable local and systemic reactions. There is also serious risk of inducing anaphylaxis in a patient (Gupta and Good, 1979). Treating patients with animal dander extract, however, is probably no riskier than treating them with pollen extracts.

Complete avoidance of the offending antigen is the treatment of choice in preventing allergic reactions to mice. When this is not feasible, other avenues of treatment and control must be considered (Lutsky and Toshner, 1978). Reducing direct animal contact, increasing room ventilation, employing filter caps on animal cages, using exhaust hoods when working with mice, and wearing protective clothing, masks, and respirators all contribute to diminishing allergic response to rodents as well as to other laboratory animal species.

XI. CONCLUSION

Modern laboratory animal management — routine disease surveillance, proper sanitary regimens, acceptable personal hygiene, and personnel health monitoring — limits any zoonotic or health hazard laboratory mice might present. Animal facilities designed to keep out wild rodents and other vermin preclude the introduction of animal and human pathogens into the laboratory environment. Careful design of caging and airflow dynamics within animal rooms minimizes exposure to allergens.

References

Ajello, L., Bostick, L., and Cheng, S. (1968). The relationship of *Trichophyton quinckeanum* to *Trichophyton mentagrophytes*. *Mycologia* **60**, 1185–1189.

Alteras, I. (1965). Human infection from laboratory animals. *Sabouraudia* **3**, 143–145.

Anderson, L. C., Leary, S. L., and Manning, P. J. (1983). Rat-bite fever in animal research laboratory personnel. *Lab. Anim. Sci.* **33**, 292–294.

Arkless, H. A. (1970). Rat-bite fever at Albert Einstein Medical Center. *Penn. Med. J.* **73**, 49.

Armstrong, C. (1963). Lymphocytic choriomeningitis. *In* "Diseases Transmitted from Animals to Man" (T. G. Hull, ed.), pp. 723–730. Springfield, Illinois: Thomas.

Armstrong, C., Wallace, J. J., and Ross, L. (1940). Lymphocytic choriomeningitis: Gray mice, *Mus musculus*. A reservoir for the infection. *Public Health Rep.* **55**, 1222.

Barkin, R. M., Guckian, J. C., and Glosser, J. W. (1974). Infections by *Leptospira ballum*: A laboratory-associated case. *South. Med. J.* **67**, 155–176.

Baum, S. G., Lewis, A. M., Jr., Wallace, P. R., and Huebner, R. J. (1966). Epidemic nonmeningitic lymphocytic-choriomeningitis-virus infection — An outbreak in a population of laboratory personnel. *N. Eng. J. Med.* **17**, 934–936.

Besch-Williford, C., and Wagner, J. E. (1982). Bacterial and mycotic diseases of the integumentary system. *In* "The Mouse in Biomedical Research" (H. L. Foster, J. D. Small, and J. G. Fox, eds.), Vol. II, pp. 55–76. New York: Academic Press.

Biggar, R. J., Woodall, J. P., Walter, P. D., and Haugie, G. E. (1975). Lymphocytic choriomeningitis outbreak associated with pet hamsters. *J. Am. Vet. Med. Assoc.* **232**, 494–500.

Birnbaum, W., Shenberg, E., and Torten, M. (1972). The influence of maternal antibodies on the epidemiology of leptospiral carrier state in mice. *Am. J. Epidemiol.* **96**, 313–317.

Blackmore, D. K., and Francis, R. A. (1970). The apparent transmission of staphylococci of human origin to laboratory animals. *J. Comp. Pathol.* **80**, 645–651.

Boak, R. A., Linscott, W. D., and Bodfish, R. E. (1960). A case of *Leptospirosis ballum* in California. *Calif. Med.* **93,** 163–165.

Booth, B. H. (1952). Mouse ringworm. *Arch. Dermatol. Syphilol.* **66,** 65–69.

Borst, J. G. G., Ruys, A. C., and Wolff, J. W. (1948). Eeen Geval van *Leptospirosis ballum. Ned. Tijdschr. Geneeskd.* **92,** 2920–2922.

Brown, C. M., and Parker, M. T. (1957). Salmonella infection in rodents in Manchester. *Lancet* **273,** 1277–1279.

Brown, R. Z., and Gorman, G. W. (1960). The occurrence of leptospirosis in feral rodents in southwestern Georgia. *Am. J. Public Health* **66,** 682–688.

Brown, T. M., and Nunemaker, J. C. (1942). Rat-bite fever: A review of the American cases with reevaluation of etiology: Report of cases. *Bull. Johns Hopkins Hosp.* **70,** 201–327.

Burgdorfer, W. (1980). The spotted fever-group diseases. *In* "CRC Handbook Series of Zoonoses" (J. J. Steele, ed.), Vol. II, pp. 279–301. Boca Raton, Florida: CRC Press.

Centers for Disease Control (CDC) (1965). "Zoonoses Surveillance: Leptospirosis," Report No. 7, p. 25. Atlanta: U.S. Public Health Service.

Centers for Disease Control (CDC) (1966). "Zoonoses Surveillance: Leptospirosis Annual Summary," p. 3. Atlanta: U.S. Public Health Service.

Centers for Disease Control (CDC) (1976). "Salmonella Surveillance: Annual Summary," Report No. 126. Atlanta: U.S. Department of Health, Education and Welfare, Centers for Disease Control.

Cetin, E. T., Tahsinoglu, M., and Volkan, S. (1965). Epizootic of *Trichophyton mentagrophytes (interdigitale)* in white mice. *Pathol. Microbiol.* **28,** 839–846.

Chmel, L., Buchvald, L., and Valentova, M. (1975). Spread of *Trichophyton mentagrophytes* Var. Gran. infection to man. *Int. J. Dermatol.* **14,** 269–272.

Christie, A. B., Chen, T. H., and Elberg, S. S. (1980). Plague in camels and goats: Their role in human epidemics. *J. Infect. Dis.* **141,** 724–726.

Cole, J. S., Stroll, R. W., and Bulger, R. J. (1969). Rat-bite fever. *Ann. Intern. Med.* **71,** 979.

Collins, M. J., and Parker, J. C. (1972). Murine virus contaminants of leukemia viruses and transplantable tumors. *J. Natl. Cancer Inst. (US)* **49,** 1139–1143.

Cotchin, E., and Roe, F. J. C. (1967). Fungal diseases of rats and mice. *In* "Pathology of Laboratory Rats and Mice," pp. 681–732. Philadelphia: Davis.

Criep, L.-H. (1976). "Allergy and Clinical Immunology." New York: Grune & Stratton.

Davey, D. G. (1962). The use of pathogen free animals. *Proc. R. Soc. Med.* **55,** 256–262.

Davies, R. R., and Shewell, J. (1964). Control of mouse ringworm. *Nature (London)* **202,** 406–407.

Dolan, M. M., Kligman, A. M., Kobylinski, P. G., and Motsavage, M. A. (1958). Ringworm epizootics in laboratory mice and rats; experimental and accidental transmission of infection. *J. Invest. Dermatol.* **30,** 23–25.

Dove, W. E., and Shelmire, B. (1932). Some observations on tropical rat mites and endemic typhus. *J. Parasitol.* **18,** 159.

Ducan, P. R., Thomas, A. E., and Tobin, J. O. (1951). Lymphocytic choriomeningitis. Review of ten cases. *Lancet* **1,** 956–959.

Dvorak, S., and Otechenasek, M. (1964). Geophites zoophilic and anthropophilic dermatophytes: A review. *Mycopathol. Mycol. Appl.* **23,** 23–25.

Faust, E. C., and Russell, P. F. (1970). "Craig and Faust's Clinical Parasitology," 8th ed., pp. 528–529. Philadelphia: Lea & Febiger.

Flynn, R. J. (1973). "Parasites of Laboratory Animals." Ames: Iowa State University Press.

Fox, J. G. (1982). Outbreak of tropical rat mite dermatitis in laboratory personnel. *Arch. Dermatol.* **118,** 676–678.

Fox, J. G., and Beaucage, C. M. (1979). The incidence of Salmonella in random-source cats purchased for research. *J. Infect. Dis.* **139,** 362–365.

Fox, J. G., and Brayton, J. B. (1982). Zoonoses and other human health hazards. *In* "The Mouse in Biomedical Research" (H. L. Foster, J. D. Small, and J. G. Fox, eds.), Vol. 2., pp. 404–411. New York: Academic Press.

Fox, J. G., Newcomer, C. E., and Rozmiarek, H. (1984). Selected zoonoses and other health hazards. *In* "Laboratory Animal Medicine" (J. G. Fox, B. J. Cohen, and F. M. Loew, eds.), p. 639. New York: Academic Press.

Frenkel, J. K. (1973). Toxoplasmosis: Parasite life cycle, pathology and immunology. *In* "The Coccidia" (D. M. Hammond and P. C. Long, eds.), pp. 343–410. Baltimore: University Park Press.

Friedmann, C. T. H., Spiegel, E. L., Aaron, E., and McIntyre, R. (1973). *Leptospirosis ballum* contracted from pet mice. *Calif. Med.* **118,** 51–52.

Galton, M. M., Menges, R. W., Shotts, E. B., Nahmias, A. J., and Heath, C. (1962). "Leptospirosis" (Publ. No. 951). Atlanta: U.S. Department of Health, Education, and Welfare, Public Health Service, Centers for Disease Control.

Geller, E. H. (1979). Health hazards for man. *In* "The Laboratory Rat" (H. J. Baker, J. R. Lindsey, and S. H. Weisbroth, eds.), Vol. 1, pp. 402–207. New York: Academic Press.

Gilbert, G. L., Cassidy, J. F., and Bennett, N. M. (1971). Rat-bite fever. *Med. J. Aust.* **2,** 1131–1134.

Gillespie, R. H., and Timoney, J. G. (1981). "Hagan and Bruner's Infectious Diseases of Domestic Animals," 7th ed., pp. 170–181, 758–772. Ithaca: Cornell University Press.

Greenberg, M., Pellitteri, O. J., and Jellison, W. L. (1947). Rickettsialpox, a newly recognized disease. III. Epidemiology. *Am. J. Public Health* **37,** 860.

Gregg, M. B. (1975). Recent outbreaks of lymphocytic choriomeningitis in the United States of America. *Bull. W.H.O.* **52,** 549–553.

Gupta, S., and Good, R. A., (eds.) (1979). "Cellular, Molecular and Clinical Aspects of Allergic Disorders." New York: Plenum Press.

Habermann, R. T., and Williams, F. P. (1958). Salmonellosis in laboratory animals. *J. Natl. Cancer Inst. (US)* **20,** 933–941.

Heath, C. W., Jr., and Alexander, A. D. (1970), Leptospirosis. *In* "Joseph Brennerman's Practice of Pediatrics" (V. C. Kelley, ed.), Vol. 2, Chapter 26B, pp. 1–5. New York: Harper.

Higa, H. H., and Fujinaka, I. T. (1976). Prevalence of rodent and mongoose leptospirosis on the island of Oahu. *Public Health Rep.* **91,** 171–177.

Hinman, A. R., Fraser, D. W., Douglas, R. D., Bowen, G. S., Kraus, A. L., Winkler, W. G., and Rhodes, W. W. (1975). Outbreak of lymphocytic choriomeningitis virus infections in medical center personnel. *Am. J. Epidemiol.* **101,** 103–110.

Hoag, W. G., and Rogers, J. (1961). Techniques for the isolation of *Salmonella typhimurium* from laboratory mice. *J. Bacteriol.* **82,** 153–154.

Hoag, W. G., Strout, J., and Meier, H. (1964). Isolation of *Salmonella* spp. from laboratory mice and from diet supplements. *J. Bacteriol.* **88,** 534–536.

Holden, F. A., and MacKay, J. C. (1964). Rat-bite fever—An occupational hazard. *Can. Med. Assoc. J.* **91,** 78.

Holmgren, E. G., and Tunevall, G. (1970). Case report: Rat-bite fever. *Scand. J. Infect. Dis.* **2,** 71.

Hotchin, J. E., and Benson, L. M. (1973). Lymphocytic choriomeningitis. *In* "Infectious Diseases of Wild Mammals" (J. W. David, L. N. Karstad, and D. O. Trainer, eds.), pp. 153–165. Ames: Iowa State University Press.

Hubbert, W. T., and Rosen, M. N. (1970). *Pasteurella multocida* infection due to animal bite. *Am. J. Public Health* **60,** 1103–1117.

Hudson, B. W., Quan, S. F., and Goldenberg, M. I. (1964). Serum antibody response in a population of *Microtus californicus* and associated species during and after *Pasteurella pestis* epizootics in the San Francisco Bay area. *Zoonoses Res.* **2,** 15–23.

Hughes, W. T. (1981). *Pneumocystis carinii. In* "Principles and Practice of Infectious Disease" (G. L. Mandell, R. G. Douglas, and J. E. Bennett, eds.), pp. 2137–2142. New York: Wiley.

Institute of Laboratory Animal Resources, National Research Council (1978). "NIH Guide for the Care and Use of Laboratory Animals" (DHEW Publ. No. (NIH) 78-23). Bethesda: U.S. Department of Health, Education and Welfare, National Institutes of Health.

Jelliffe, D. B., and Stanfield, J. P. (1978). "Diseases of Children in the Subtropics and Tropics," pp. 532–433. London: Arnold.

Johnson, K. M. (1982). Viral hemorrhagic fevers. *In* "Textbook of Medicine" (J. B. Wyngaarden and L. H. Smith, Jr., eds.), 16th ed., pp. 1686–1695. Philadelphia: Saunders.

Kaufman, A. F. (1966). Pets and salmonella infection. *J. Am. Vet. Med. Assoc.* **149,** 1655–1661.

Kaufman, A. F., Mann, J. M., Gardiner, T. M., Heaton, F. M., Poland, J. D., Barnes, A. M., and Maupin, G. O. (1981). Public health implications of plague in domestic cats. *J. Am. Vet. Med. Assoc.* **179,** 875–878.

Kawamata, J., Yamanouchi, T., and Lee, H. W. (1980). Outbreaks of "epidemic hemorrhagic fever" in animal laboratories in Japan. *UCLAS Symp. 7th, 1979,* 235–238.

Kean, B. H. (1972). Clinical toxoplasmosis—50 years. *Trans. R. Soc. Trop. Med. Hyg.* **66,** 549–571.

Kessel, J. F. (1923). Experimental infection of rats and mice with the common intestinal amoebae of man. *Univ. Calif. Berkeley, Publ. Zool.* **20,** 409–430.

Krempl-Lamprecht, L., and Bosse, K. (1964). Epidermophyton floccosum (Harz) Langeron und Milochevitsch als Spontaninfektion bei Mäusen. *Kleintier-Prax.* **9,** 203–207.

Lasser, K. H., Lewin, K. J., and Ryning, F. W. (1979). Cryptosporidial enteritis in a patient with congenital hypogammaglobulinemia. *Hum. Pathol.* **10,** 234–240.

Lee, H. W., Lee, P. W., and Johnson, K. M. (1978). Isolation of the etiologic agent of Korean hemorrhagic fever. *J. Infect. Dis.* **137,** 298–308.

Lee, P. W. (1982). New haemorrhagic fever with renal syndrome-related virus in indigenous wild rodents in the United States. *Lancet* **ii,** 1404.

Lehmann-Grube, F. (1971). Lymphocytic choriomeningitis virus. *Virol. Monogr.* **10,** 88–118.

Levine, N. D. (1973). "Protozoan Parasites of Domestic Animals and of Man," 2nd ed. Minneapolis: Burgess.

Levine, N. D. (1980). Some corrections of coccidian (Ampicomplexa:Protozoa) nomenclature. *J. Parasitol.* **66,** 830–834.

Levy, D. A. (1974). Allergic activity of proteins from mice. *Int. Arch. Allergy Appl. Immunol.* **49,** 219–221.

Lincoln, T. A., Bolton, N. E., and Garrett, A. W. (1974). Occupational allergy to animal dander and sera. *J. Occup. Med.* **16,** 465–469.

Lindorfer, R. K., and Syverton, J. T. (1953). The characterization of an unidentified virus found in association with line 1 leukemia. *Proc. Am. Assoc. Cancer Res.* **1,** 33–34.

Loosli, R. (1967). Zoonoses in common laboratory animals. *In* "Husbandry of Laboratory Animals" (M. L. Conalty, ed.), pp. 307–325. New York: Academic Press.

Lutsky, I., and Toshner, D. (1978). A review of allergic respiratory disease in laboratory animal workers. *Lab. Anim. Sci.* **28,** 751–756.

McGill, R. C., Martin, A. M., and Edmunds, P. N. (1966). Rat bite fever due to *Streptobacillus moniliformis. Br. Med. J.* **1,** 1213–1214.

MacKenzie, D. W. R. (1961). *Trichophyton mentagrophytes* in mice: Infections of humans and incidence amongst laboratory animals. *Sabouraudia* **1,** 178–182.

Margard, W. L., Peters, A. C., Dorko, N., Litchfield, J. H., and Davidson, R. S. (1963). Salmonellosis in mice — Diagnostic procedures. *Lab. Anim. Care* **13,** 144–165.

Marples, M. J. (1967). Nondomestic animals in New Zealand and in Rarotonza as a reservoir of the agents of ringworm. *N. Z. Med. J.* **66,** 299–302.

Maurer, F. D. (1964). Lymphocytic choriomeningitis. *Lab. Anim. Care* **14,** 414–419.

Mescon, H., and Grots, I. A. (1974). The skin. *In* "Pathologic Basis of Disease" (S. L. Robbins, ed.), pp. 1374–1419. Philadelphia: Saunders.

Messel, J. L., Perem, D. R., Meligno, C., and Rubin, C. E. (1976). Overwhelming watery diarrhea associated with *Cryptosporidium* in an immunosuppressed patient. *Gastroenterology* **70,** 1156–1160.

Moore, R. M., Jr., Zehmer, B. R., Moultrop, J. I., and Parker, R. L. (1977). Surveillance of animal-bite cases in the United States, 1971–1972. *Arch. Environ. Health* **32,** 267–270.

Morbidity and Mortality Weekly Report (1980). Human Salmonella isolates — United States, 1978, surveillance summary. *Morbidity and Mortality Weekly Report* **28,** 618–619.

Neal, R. A. (1950). An experimental study of *Entamoeba muris* (Grassi 1879); its morphology affinities and host parasite relationship. *Parasitology* **40,** 343–365.

Newcomer, C. E., Anver, M. R., Simmons, J. L., and Nace, G. (1982). Spontaneous and experimental infections of the African clawed frog *(Xenopus laevis)* with *Chlamydia psittaci. Lab. Anim. Sci.* **32,** 6.

Newman-Taylor, A., Longbottom, J. L., and Pepys, J. (1977). Respiratory allergy to urine proteins of rats and mice. *Lancet* **ii,** 847–848.

Nichols, E., Ridge, M. E., and Russel, G. G. (1953). The relationships of the house mouse and the house mite *(Allodermanyssus sanguineus)* to the spread of rickettsialpox. *Ann. Intern. Med.* **39,** 92–101.

Ohman, J. L. (1978). Allergy in man caused by exposure to mammals. *J. Am. Vet. Med. Assoc.* **172,** 1403–1406.

Ohman, J. L., Lowell, F. C., and Bloch, K. J. (1975). Allergens of mammalian origin. *J. Allergy Clin. Immunol.* **55,** 16–24.

Owen, D. (1978). Attempted transmission of *Entamoeba coli* to specified-pathogen-free rodents. *Lab. Anim.* **12,** 79–80.

Parker, J. C., Igel, H. D., Reynolds, R. K., Lewis, A. M., Jr., and Rowe, W. P. (1976). Lymphocytic choriomeningitis virus infection in fetal, newborn, and young adult Syrian hamsters. *Infect. Immun.* **13,** 967–981.

Patterson, R. (1964). The problem of allergy to laboratory animals. *Lab. Anim. Care* **14,** 466–469.

Paegle, R. D., Tweari, R. P., Bernhard, W. N., *et al.* (1976). Microbial flora of the larynx, trachea and large intestine of the rat after long term inhalation of 100 percent oxygen. *Anesthesiology* **44,** 287–290.

Place, E. H., and Sutton, L. E. (1934). Erythema arthriticum epidemicum (Haverhill fever). *Arch. Intern. Med.* **54,** 659–684.

Poiley, S. M. (1970). A survey of indigenous murine viruses in a variety of production and research animal facilities. *Lab. Anim. Care* **20,** 643–650.

Poland, J. D., and Barnes, A. M. (1979). Plague. *In* "CRC Handbook Series in Zoonoses and Mycotic Diseases" (J. H. Steele, ed.), Vol. I, pp. 517–597. Boca Raton, Florida: CRC Press.

Povar, M. L. (1965). Ringworm *(Trichophyton mentagrophytes)* infection in a colony of albino Norway rats. *Lab. Anim. Care* **15,** 264–265.

Raffin, B. J., and Freemark, M. (1979). Streptobacillary rat-bite fever; a pediatric problem. *Pediatrics* **64,** 214–217.

Rajka, G. (1961). Ten cases of occupational hypersensitivity to laboratory animals. *Acta Allergol.* **16,** 168–176.

Reese, N. C., Current, W. L., Ernst, J. V., and Barley, W. S. (1982). Cryptosporidiosis of man and calf: A case report and results of experimental infections in mice and rats. *Am. J. Trop. Med. Hyg.* **31,** 226–229.

Refai, M., and Ali, A. H. (1970). Laboratory acquired infection with *Keratinomyces ajelloi*. *Mykosen* **13,** 317–318.

Richter, C. P. (1945). Incidence of rat bites and rat-bite fever in Baltimore. *J. Am. Med. Assoc.* **128,** 324–326.

Robbins, S. L. (1974). Infectious disease. *In* "Pathologic Basis of Disease" (S. L. Robbins, ed.), pp. 396–400. Philadelphia: Saunders.

Rogosa, M. (1974). *Streptobacillus moniliformis* and *Spirillum minor*. *In* "Manual of Clinical Microbiology" (E. H. Lennette, E. H. Spaulding, and J. P. Truant, eds.), 2nd ed., pp. 326–332. Washington, DC: American Society of Microbiology.

Roughgarden, J. W. (1965). Antimicrobial therapy of rat-bite fever. *Arch. Intern. Med.* **116,** 39–54.

Sanford, J. P. (1982). Plague. *In* "Textbook of Medicine" (J. B. Wyngaarden and L. H. Smith, Jr., eds.), 16th ed., pp. 1521–1523. Philadelphia: Saunders.

Schachter, J., and Dawson, C. R. (1978). "Human Chlamydial Infections." Littleton, Massachusetts: PSG Publishing.

Schumacher, M. J. (1980). Characterization of allergens from urine and pelts of laboratory mice. *Mol. Immunol.* **17,** 1087–1095.

Shults, F. S., Estes, P. C., Franklin, J. A., and Richter, C. N. (1973). Staphylococcal botrymomycosis in a specific-pathogen-free mouse colony. *Lab. Anim. Sci.* **23,** 36–42.

Siraganian, R. P., and Sandberg, A. L. (1979). Characterization of mouse allergens. *J. Allergy Clin. Immunol.* **63**, 435–442.

Skinner, H. H., and Knight, E. H. (1971). Monitoring mouse stocks for lymphocytic choriomeningitis virus — A human pathogen. *Lab. Anim.* **5**, 73–87.

Soave, O. A., and Van Allen, A. (1958). LCM in a mouse breeding colony. *Proc. Anim. Care Panel* **8**, 135–140.

Sorrell, A. H., and Gottesman, J. (1957). Mouse allergy: Case report. *Ann. Allergy* **Nov.– Dec.** 662–663.

Stemmermann, G. N., Hayashi, T., Glober, G. A., Oishi, N., and Frenkel, R. I. (1980). Cryptosporidiosis report of a fatal case complicated by disseminated toxoplasmosis. *Am. J. Med.* **69**, 637–642.

Stoenner, H. G. (1954). Application of the capillary tube test and a newly developed plate test to the serodiagnosis of bovine leptospirosis. *Am. J. Vet. Res.* **15**, 434–439.

Stoenner, H. G. (1957). The laboratory diagnosis of leptospirosis. *Vet. Med. (Kansas City)* **52**, 540–542.

Stoenner, H. G., and Maclean, D. (1958). Leptospirosis (ballum) contracted from Swiss albino mice. *Arch. Intern. Med.* **101**, 706–710.

Stoenner, H. G., Grimes, E. F., Thraikill, F. B., and Davis, E. (1958). Elimination of *Leptospira ballum* from a colony of Swiss albino mice by use of chlortetracycline hydrochloride. *Am. J. Trop. Med. Hyg.* **7**, 423–426.

Stoll, N. E. (1947). This wormy world. *J. Parasitol.* **33**, 41–46.

Stone, W. B., and Manwell, R. D. (1966). Potential helminth infections in humans from pet or laboratory mice and hamsters. *Public Health Rep.* **31**, 647–653.

Storz, J. (1971). "Chlamydia and Chlamydial-Induced Diseases." Springfield, Illinois: Thomas.

Stott, J. A., Hodgson, J. E., and Chaney, J. C. (1975). Incidence of salmonellae in animal feed and the effect of pelleting on content of enterobacteriaceae. *J. Appl. Bacteriol.* **39**, 41–46.

Strangeways, W. I. (1933). Rats as carriers of *Streptobacillus moniliformis. J. Pathol. Bacteriol.* **37**, 45–51.

Sulkin, S. E. (1961). Laboratory acquired infections. *Bacteriol. Rev.* **25**, 203–209.

Sulzer, C. R., Harvey, T. W., and Galton, M. M. (1968). Comparison of diagnostic techniques for the detection of leptospirosis in rats. *Health Lab. Sci.* **5**, 171–173.

Taylor, M. J., and MacDowell, C. E. (1949). Mouse leukemia. XIV. Freeing line I from a contaminating virus. *J. Natl. Cancer Inst. (US)* **17**, 233–245.

Tobin, J. O. (1968). Viruses transmissible from laboratory animals to man. *Lab. Anim.* **3**, 19.

Torten, M. (1979). Leptospirosis. *In* "CRC Handbook Series in Zoonoses" (J. H. Steele, ed.), Vol. I, pp. 363–421. Cleveland: CRC Press.

Turner, L. H. (1970). Leptospirosis III. *Trans. R. Soc. Trop. Med. Hyg.* **64**, 623–646.

Tyzzer, E. E. (1907). A sporozoan found in the peptic glands of the common mouse. *Proc. Soc. Exp. Biol. Med.* **5**, 12–13.

Umenai, T., Lee, P. W., Toyoda, T., Yoshinaga, K., Horiuchi, T., Lee, H. W., Saito, T., Hongo, M., Nobunga, T., and Ishida, N. (1979). Korean hemorrhagic fever in staff in an animal laboratory. *Lancet* **i,** 1314–1315.

Van der Waaij, D., Zimmerman, W. M. T., and Van Bekkum, D. W. (1963). An outbreak of *Pseudomonas aeruginosa* infection in a colony previously free of this infection. *Lab. Anim. Care* **13,** 46–51.

Voge, M., and Heyneman, D. (1957). Development of *Hymenolepis nana* and *Hymenolepis diminuta* (Cestoda: Hymenolepididae) in the intermediate host *Tribolium confusum*. *Univ. Calif., Berkeley, Publ. Zool.* **59,** 549–580.

Wardle, R. A., and McLeod, J. A. (1952). "The Zoology of Tapeworms." Minneapolis: University of Minnesota Press.

Wayson, N. E. (1972). An epizootic among meadow mice in California, caused by the bacillus of mouse septicemia or of swine erysipelas. *Public Health Rep.* **42,** 1489–1493.

Wescott, R. B. (1982). Helminths. *In* "The Mouse in Biomedical Research" (H. L. Foster, J. D. Small, and J. G. Fox, eds.), Vol. II, pp. 373–403. New York: Academic Press.

Williams, L. P., Vaughn, J. B., Scott, A., and Blanton, V. (1969). A ten-month study of *Salmonella* contamination in animal protein meals. *J. Am. Vet. Med. Assoc.* **155,** 167–174.

Wolf, F. W., Bohlander, H., and Ruys, A. C. (1949). Researches on *Leptospirosis ballum* — The detection of urinary carriers in laboratory mice. *Antonie van Leeuwenhoek* **15,** 1–13.

Yager, R. H., Gochenour, W. S., Jr., Alexander, A. D., and Wetmore, P. W. (1953). Natural occurrence of *Leptospira ballum* in rural house mice and in an opossum. *Proc. Soc. Exp. Biol. Med.* **84,** 589–590.

Yunker, C. E. (1964). Infections of laboratory animals potentially dangerous to man: Ectoparasites and other arthropods, with emphasis on mites. *Lab. Anim. Care* **14,** 455–465.

Part IV
Experimental Protocol

7
Experimental Design

Mikelis G. Bickis
Department of Mathematics
University of Saskatchewan
Saskatoon, Saskatchewan

I. Introduction
   A. The Concept of Experimental Design
   B. Chapter Overview
II. Principles of Experimental Design
   A. Observational and Experimental Units
   B. Randomization and Cryptotaxy
   C. Replication
   D. Stratification
   E. Criteria for Evaluating Experimental Designs
III. Guidelines for Designing Experiments
   A. Designs for Screening Studies
   B. Design of Dose-Response Experiments
   C. Studies with *in Utero* Exposure
   D. Experiments with Mixtures of Chemicals
   E. Experiments for Studying Mechanisms
IV. Practical Considerations
   A. Procedures for Randomization
   B. Conclusion

I. INTRODUCTION

The proper design of experiments is of utmost importance in ensuring the scientific integrity of any toxicological testing program. A poorly designed experiment will not yield much useful information even if it is attacked by the most powerful weapons of toxicological, pathological, or statistical expertise. Moreover, the interpretation of such experiments can be problematic or misleading. The interpretation of well-designed experiments, on the other hand, is often straightforward and can make good use of valid and efficient procedures of statistical data analysis. In this chapter, an exhaustive review of the theory and practice of experimental design is not given for there are many good texts available on this subject (Cox, 1958; Anderson and McLean, 1974; Box et al., 1978; Gart *et al.*, 1986). Rather, my purposes are to discuss the fundamental principles of experimental design in the context of *in vivo* toxicity testing and to present guidelines for some of the more usual types of toxicological studies.

The appropriate design for an experiment depends on both the study objective and the nature of the toxicological response of interest. Most toxicological experiments are performed for screening xenobiotics for possible toxicity/carcinogenicity, for estimating dose–response relationships, or for examining mechanisms of toxic/carcinogenic action. It is not always easy to categorize a particular experiment into one of these classes because often researchers hope to get more than one kind of information from the same experiment. Thus, if a particular compound is found toxic in a screening study, the investigator may want to estimate the risks at low doses, which requires knowledge of the dose–response relationship. Similarly, an investigative experiment on the joint action of several chemicals might also be used for screening purposes.

Toxicological experiments are commonly classified as involving acute, subchronic, or chronic exposure. This distinction is not too important from a design point of view because the same considerations apply to all classes. However, long-term experiments do provide additional complications that are of little consequence in experiments of briefer duration. A more important distinction is the nature of the response variable. Thus, investigative experiments on fetotoxicity will, in general, require different design strategies from those involving carcinogenicity.

A. The Concept of Experimental Design

At the planning stage of a toxicological experiment, the investigator has in mind a population of test animals and a set of chemical treatments whose effects are to be studied. Depending on the situation, the "target" population may be as specific as a particular batch of a particular strain of mouse or as general as all mammals. The set of treatments might comprise various doses of a particular compound or a whole family of compounds and mixtures. Before the investigator can proceed, he or she must select specific animals and specific treatments with which to perform the experiment.

The experimental design consists of three things: a specification of the animals and treatments to be included in the experiment; a rule defining the allocation of particular treatments to particular animals; and a description of the variables to be measured.

The preceding description is actually too simplistic unless one interprets the terms *animal, treatment,* and *variable* in the most general sense. The experiment is actually not performed on a particular set of animals but on a particular set of animals in a particular environment. Thus, the first part of the experimental design should specify the animals together with their environment, which includes, among other things, cages, feed, handling, lifespan, necropsy, and pathology. Similarly, treatment refers not only to a specified dose of a particular chemical but also includes such factors as route of administration, frequency of dosing, and adjustments for changes in body weight. Furthermore, the description of the variables should specify what is to be observed and when these observations are to be made. In practice, many of these factors are not explicitly stated as part of the design but are subsumed under the standard operating procedures of the laboratory or research program. However, the experiment cannot be considered well designed if any of these matters are left to be decided by happenstance.

The experimenter is free to fix a number of parameters at the design stage of the study. The most obvious parameter is the total number of animals to be used. It is intuitively clear that a greater number of animals will lead to more informative experimental results. A second parameter is the number of treatment groups and the particular dosing regimen to be applied to each group. The dosing regimen depends on the objectives of the study. The selection of the actual dose levels may be a difficult problem — particularly selection of the highest dose. Once the dosing regimens have been established and the total number of animals has been decided, there remains the question of animal allocation. Traditionally, an equal number of animals have been assigned to each treatment group, although in some situations an unbalanced allocation may be a preferable strategy.

A crucial part of any experimental design is proper randomization. This procedure both protects against biases due to unsuspected confounding factors and provides a basis for statistical inference. To appreciate the nature and importance of experimental randomization, we must first understand the statistical principles of experimental design.

Because biological organisms are inherently variable, we would not expect to observe the same responses from all individuals in an experiment even if the experimental conditions were identical for them. It follows that in the case of an experiment in which the effects of several sets of experimental conditions are compared, there will be some uncertainty about what portion of any observed differences can be ascribed to the experimental treatments, and what portion is due to this inherent variability. Thus, the significance of the results will have to be judged by statistical criteria. Adopting terminology from the physical sciences, we will designate this variability that appears to compromise the unambiguous interpretation of experimental results as *experimental error,* although this phenomenon usually has nothing to do with errors of measurement as such.

B. Chapter Overview

In the following section, we will explain the fundamental principles of experimental design, including randomization, replication, and stratification, and discuss how these considerations contribute to the validity and efficiency of toxicological experiments. Section III presents guidelines for designing some particular types of study. In the first subsection, we look at screening studies and at how to control false negative rates. Design considerations for dose–response studies are presented in the next subsection, including the problem of low dose extrapolation. In the remaining subsections, experiments involving *in utero* exposure, experiments with mixtures of chemicals, and specialized experiments for studying mechanisms of action are discussed. Section IV provides practical advice about the implementation of the procedures discussed in this chapter and offers some concluding comments.

II. PRINCIPLES OF EXPERIMENTAL DESIGN

The purpose of experimental design is to maximize the information provided by the test system, given operational feasibility and restraints on resources. In order for this purpose to be achieved, biases in the experiment that will vitiate the conclusions must be eliminated, experimental error must be reduced, and provisions must be made for the assessment of experimental error. These requirements can be satisfied through proper application of randomization, replication, and stratification.

A. Observational and Experimental Units

Before these techniques can be used, one must have a proper understanding of the fundamental concepts of observational unit and experimental unit. As used in this chapter, the term *experimental unit* refers to the largest portion of the experimental material that is treated as a unit. This simple concept is the source of much confusion in the design of experiments and is fraught with ambiguity. Much of the ambiguity stems from divergent understanding of the word *treated*. A few examples can clarify this definition.

In a feeding study with multiple caging, the cage rather than the individual animal forms the experimental unit because, although it is the animal that consumes the treatment, the treatment is applied by the experimenter to the cage; and more importantly, the experimenter cannot distinguish the treatments given to different animals in the same cage. A more subtle example involves an experiment with a volatile substance in which different treatments are maintained in different cage racks. In this case, the entire cage rack becomes the experimental unit. Although the treatment may be actually applied to individual cages, all cages in the rack are constrained to the same treatment; hence, once more, one cannot distinguish the treatments given to different animals in the same cage rack.

It is possible for an experiment to be performed in which several different hypotheses will be examined. In such cases, different aspects of the experiment may require different definitions of experimental units, as the following more complicated example illustrates. A number of female rats are assigned to either a test or control diet and are then bred. After weaning, four pups of each litter are retained; two are put on the maternal diet and two on the opposite diet. The purpose of the experiment is to determine both *in utero* and postweaning effects of the test compound. Consider now an arbitrary litter of four pups. Regardless of how the maternal diets are assigned, all the pups will have been exposed to the *same in utero* treatment. Comparisons between control and test animals are thus necessarily comparisons between entire litters; therefore, the magnitude of any differences must be gauged against variation among litters treated alike. Thus, for purposes of assessing *in utero* effects, one must consider the complete litter as the experimental unit. However, any animal, regardless of its maternal diet, can be assigned either postweaning diet. Hence, comparisons between test and control postweaning diets do not involve comparison of entire litters. In this case, the individual pup is the experimental unit.

A concept often confused with experimental unit is *observational unit*. This is the unit of experimental material that is actually observed. In most *in vivo* toxicology studies, the observational unit would appear to be the individual animal. However, the unit depends on what is being looked at. For hematology, the unit will be the blood sample, for histopathology, the slide. In the case of multiple caging, the observational unit for food consumption will be the cage.

Recognizing what constitutes the experimental unit is a critical first step in the design of any experiment. This exercise can be facilitated if the animals are considered as a series of "black boxes", each with a number of inputs and outputs. The inputs are any factors that may affect the experimental results. Some may be controlled by the experimenter, such as chemical dose, date of sacrifice, and diet; others may be beyond control, such as feed contaminants, environmental gradients, and epizootics. The outputs are the observations made of the units. Two "black boxes" belong to different experimental units if both their inputs and outputs are independent.

Independence of inputs requires that any variation in the input of one unit does not affect the input of any other unit unless it affects all units uniformly. For example, an error in dosing should affect only a single unit; therefore, in a feeding study, animals housed in a single cage and feeding from the same container must all belong to the same experimental unit. However, variation in the constituents of the feed does not affect the definition of the experimental units provided that all animals are receiving the same feed.

Independence of outputs requires that information about one unit does not provide any information about the other. Suppose, for example, that a pathologist knows that two animals were receiving the same treatment. Information gleaned from the examination of one animal might then be used in the diagnosis of the other. In this situation, the two animals cannot be considered as separate experimental units.

Another way of clarifying the definition of the experimental unit is to consider the relationships among the units in the absence of treatment effects. The experimental units should be *exchangeable* in the sense that each experimental unit should have the same relationship to all other experimental units. If it appears that the putative experimental units form clusters of units, such that units within a cluster resemble each other more than units in different clusters, then each cluster should be considered an experimental unit. Alternatively, the clusters can be used as blocks in the experimental design (the use of blocks is discussed in Section II,D). In practice, neither animal populations nor experimental environments are sufficiently homogeneous to satisfy the exchangeability criterion automatically. However, exchangeability can be achieved by incorporation of randomization into the experimental design.

B. Randomization and Cryptotaxy

Toxicological experiments are not of much use if their scientific validity is in question. In addition to the controls required to ensure scientific integrity (see Chapter 8), the study must have statistical validity. This concept means that statements based on statistical analysis of the results are true. Although there may be extreme cases in which the interpretation of a bioassay will be obvious even to the layperson, the more typical situation involves appreciable variability; therefore, conclusions will generally be of a statistical nature. Thus, the lack of statistical validity can render the entire experiment uninterpretable.

1. Randomization

Statistical validity requires that experimental units to be compared for assessment of treatment effects do not differ in any respect that may introduce bias into the comparison. If factors that may affect such comparisons are recognized, their effect can be minimized by matching animals on this basis. An example of such an approach is the so-called *litter-matched design* in which one animal in a litter is given a control treatment and its littermate is given a test chemical. However, even this procedure does not eliminate all accidental differences. It is quite possible that, of two animals from the same litter on the same treatment, one may develop a tumor while the other one may not. Moreover, there are many possible factors that may influence a particular animal's propensity for exhibiting a toxicological response. The investigator may have knowledge of some of these factors, but cannot always control them. More seriously, there may be influences that the investigator may not even suspect, yet their effect can induce spurious differences among the treatment groups.

The technique of randomization ensures that such influences do not vitiate the validity of the study. With this technique, assignment of treatments to experimental units is done at random, although certain restrictions may be placed on the possible assignments. Biases may still exist in specific comparisons, but the properties of the randomization process ensure that these biases will average out in statistical statements. Furthermore, randomization guarantees the exchangeability of experimental units, which is required for statistical inference.

The definition of exchangeability implies that the experimental units are precisely those entities that are randomized. It is important to recognize that all aspects of the experimental unit must take part in the randomization. In a toxicological experiment, the experimental unit includes not just the animal but also the animal's environment and all observations taken on it. In particular, the position of the animal's cage in the experimental room forms part of the experimental unit, as does the necropsy and the histopathology examination. All these parts of the experiment should be randomized.

A specific study dramatizes this problem. In an experiment to assess the carcinogenicity of allura red, animals were assigned to treatment groups at random. However, housing of the treatment groups was systematic: all animals on the control diet were placed in contiguous cages in one cage rack at one end of the experimental chamber. Animals on the low dose were similarly placed in a block of contiguous cages next to the controls, followed by animals on the middle dose. Finally, animals given the high dose were placed at the far end of the room, mostly on the far side of the last cage rack. Analysis of the results revealed significant differences in mortality between the front and back of the cage racks (Lagakos and Mosteller, 1981), suggesting the possibility of some environmental gradient that affected survival. Because the groups on increasing dose levels also followed this gradient, it was impossible to distinguish the effect of treatment from the effect of position. Such a problem would not have arisen had the cage positions of the animals been assigned at random.

Suppose now that the histopathological examination is also done in the same systematic sequence. As the pathologist is examining the slides, he or she may begin to notice certain unfamiliar anomalies. However, as the pathologist progresses through the samples, one anomaly becomes more and more clearly defined until it is recognizable at a glance. It stands to reason that the animals whose slides are near the end of the sequence would be more likely to have this anomaly detected than would the animals whose slides were near the beginning. If the animals near the end are in the group given the high dose, there is the possibility of an artifactual treatment effect appearing. This artifact can be aggravated if the pathologist, expecting a treatment effect, examines the slides from the treated animals with greater diligence.

2. Cryptotaxy

A safeguard akin to randomization is the coding of treatment information so that no one directly involved in the experiment knows what treatment each individual animal is receiving. This ignorance should extend from the principal investigator, to the animal care personnel, to the pathologist. Randomization ensures that nothing in the experimental environment will differentially affect the treatment groups. Because the personnel involved in the study are part of that environment, ignorance of the treatment groups will ensure that all animals are handled equivalently.

Protocols mandating such ignorance are standard in clinical trials, and called "blind" or "double blind". The noun *cryptotaxy* (adjective *cryptotaxic*) is coined to designate this property in bioassays. Far from being standard, cryptotaxy is still the exception rather than the rule in most toxicological experiments and is, moreover, the subject of considerable controversy (Fears and Schneiderman, 1974; McConnell et al., 1985; Arnold et al., 1988). Most of these discussions center around the advantages and disadvantages of blind or "masked" pathology versus the traditional "open" approach. In some discussions, the idea of blind pathology seems to degenerate into a conspiracy to keep the pathologist in the dark about everything concerning the study and to ask for histopathological diagnoses based on anonymous coded slides. The concept of cryptotaxy, however, does not single out the pathologist as the vulnerable party to biased evaluations. Rather, the principle requires all experimental units to be handled identically throughout the course of the experiment. The surest way of implementing this ideal is to hide any distinguishing information from *all* study personnel. In this way, experimental data can speak for themselves, without the possibility of prejudice.

Although there is no consensus on the relative importance of such rigor, rational consideration of the issues involved leads one to conclude that strict scientific validity does require cryptotaxic experiments. In toxicological experiments, particularly in chronic ones, there are many interactions between study personnel and experimental animals. Furthermore, many indicators of toxicity, such as clinical signs and diagnosis of lesions, are at least partly subjective. Thus, many opportunities exist for the staff to bias the results unconsciously. Such a concern may be very serious in experiments with large mammals, such as primates, in which various interventions, such as treatment for disease, may be mandated. Different criteria for deciding on therapy or sacrifice may be used inadvertently, depending on the animal's treatment group. Moreover, some animals may even sense subtle psychological signals from their handlers, a particular concern of investigators studying behavioral effects.

It follows that pathology, both gross and histological, should also be done blindly. This requirement does not mean that the pathologist is expected to diagnose lesions with no information other than a numbered slide. Obviously, all tissues of an animal, as well as its whole clinical history, should be available for the pathologist to arrive at a diagnosis. However, nowhere in this history should there be any indication of the animal's experimental treatment. Indeed, the pathologist need not even know that the animals come from different treatment groups. All animals should be considered equivalent *a priori* so that diagnosis can be made strictly on the basis of what can be observed, without reference to any prior expectations. For this reason, animals should be presented to the pathologist in a random order.

3. Some Objections

There are, nonetheless, disadvantages to both randomization and cryptotaxy, which are sometimes put forth as arguments against these procedures. Most disadvantages are associated with the increased expenses of meticulous record keeping and staff time requirements. However, this price must be paid for ensuring the scientific validity of the experiment. Moreover, many problems can be solved by careful advance planning.

Among the objections raised against randomization are the increased chance of dosing errors and the possibility of cross-contamination due to spillage of feed or excreta. A procedure for handling the difficulty of dosing errors is outlined in Section IV. The second is a more serious concern. Design modifications of cages or cage racks may be required. Sometimes, particularly if the test chemical is volatile, physical separation of treatment groups may be the only feasible arrangement. In such a case, it is important to recognize that an entire block of contiguous cages in a treatment group constitutes a *single* experimental unit. In addition, the design of the experiment, its analysis, and its interpretation are all materially different from those of an experiment with individually randomized cages.

Randomization sometimes is said to be unnecessary in toxicological bioassays because great efforts are taken to ensure the uniformity of the controlled laboratory environment. However, perfect uniformity is unachievable, and practical uniformity has never been demonstrated. Even if it were shown conclusively that animal rooms have no appreciable gradients in temperature or air quality, there would remain the possibility that cage location can be related to psychological stress, which may promote the development of neoplasia (Riley, 1981). For example, location of the cages relative to light sources has been shown to induce differential pathology (Bellhorn, 1980). Thus, the appeal to carefully controlled conditions as an alternative to randomization may be ill-founded. However, proper randomization provides for scientific validity without requiring environmental homogeneity.

Pathologists often object to cryptotaxy for a number of reasons, one of which is that it appears to cast doubt on their professional integrity. Because this is not a text on the social psychology of scientists, this point will not be pursued. An apparently more valid objection is that, without knowledge of which animals are treated and which are controls, the pathologist will have no idea what abnormalities to expect and among which animals to seek them. This is precisely the point. The pathologist should examine all tissues with equal diligence, even if it may appear to be "wasteful" to spend time looking for abnormalities in control animals.

Moreover, no pathologist should beg the question by looking for precisely those anomalies that appear to distinguish treated animals from controls because this distinction may be fortuitous. Only if anomalies are identified *without reference to treatment groups* can the conclusion of treatment effects be validly maintained.

Randomization and cryptotaxy are particularly important for experiments that will receive public scrutiny, such as those that will be used for making regulatory decisions. These procedures not only ensure scientific validity, but they also make visible the concern for objectivity.

C. Replication

In order for an experimental inference to have scientific import, it must be repeatable. A unique result has only anecdotal interest. Replication is a technique whereby the repeatability of a result is assessed.

Replication is not achieved from multiple observations on the same animal, nor is it necessarily present when several animals are placed in each treatment group. To have replication, it is essential that there be a number of experimental units on the same treatment. Statistical significance of the result is assessed by comparing the differences among treatment groups with the variation found among experimental units in the same group. Such a comparison is defensible only if the exchangeability criterion is satisfied. For this reason, a design in which each treatment appears only in a contiguous group of cages really has no replication, regardless of the number of animals in each group.

The simplest form of replication is achieved when a number of experimental units in each treatment group is provided and the units are assigned to treatments at random. This procedure leads to the so-called *completely randomized design,* which appears to be the most commonly used in toxicological research. This design is simple to set up and analyze. Its statistical analysis is transparent; the raw data provide a valid picture without the need for elaborate statistical adjustments. However, this design is not always easy to implement operationally; therefore, it is often corrupted in actual experiments.

An alternative to the completely randomized design is the *randomized block design.* For this design, experimental units are partitioned into replicates, each of which contains as many units as there are treatment groups. Within each replicate, treatments are assigned to the units at random. Consider an experiment with five treatments in which four cage racks are available. Each side (front or back) of the rack is able to accommodate five rows of up to seven cages. An experiment utilizing 200 animals can be set up as follows: 50 cages per rack can be arranged into

Mikelis G. Bickis

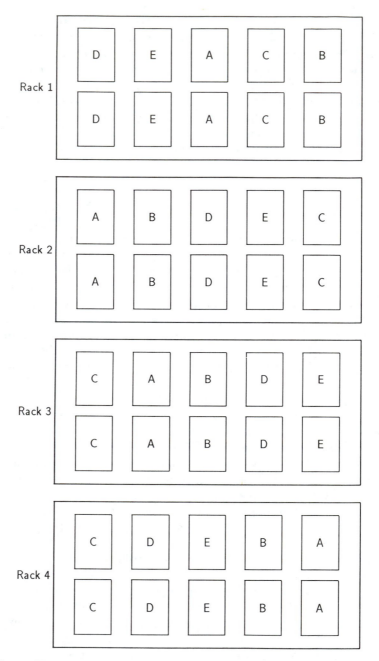

Fig. 1 Top view of a possible cage arrangement of an experiment with five treatments and 200 animals. Note that the four cages under the top one shown receive the same treatment.

five vertical columns, each column consisting of five cages at the front of the rack and five more adjacent cages at the back of the rack (Fig. 1). After the test animals are randomly assigned to the cages, a treatment group can be randomly assigned to a column of cages, under the restriction that each rack gets exactly one column on each treatment. With this design, the column of 10 cages forms the experimental unit, and each cage rack forms a replicate (or *block*). Note that arrangement of similarly treated cages in columns reduces the problem of cross-contamination.

One advantage of the randomized block design is that exchangeability is required only among units in the same replicate. Thus, there is no difficulty in having different racks in different rooms or in starting the experiment at different times. A disadvantage of this design is that there is no direct estimate of variability because one does not have exchangeable units on the same treatment. Note that, in the example, variation among the 10 cages in a column does *not* form a valid estimate of experimental error because these cages are not exchangeable. In a randomized block design, experimental error has to be estimated indirectly as the variation of differences between treatments across replicates. Such an estimate can be justified by the exchangeability of replicates.

A disadvantage of both the completely randomized and the randomized block designs is that there is only one estimate of experimental error available. Therefore, no possibility of verifying the exchangeability assumption exists. A solution to this problem is to run a number of distinct completely randomized experiments. Each experiment can then be considered as a replicate of a randomized block design. To allow ready comparisons of the experiments, they should all follow the same protocol. Aside from this restraint, there need be no attempt to keep the repetitions uniform. In fact, it can be advantageous to make them as diverse as possible. They can be run in different rooms at different times, perhaps even in different laboratories with different strains of animals.

There are at least two advantages to replicating experiments in this manner. First, it allows one to address the question of treatment–replicate interaction. Does the effect of the treatment depend on the replicate? If it does not, then there is some assurance of the repeatability of the results. If, on the other hand, it does, then one is forced to examine the reason for this inconsistency. There may be factors present in some replicates that modify the effect of the treatments. Such factors can, for example, be contaminants in the test compound or the feed, genetic makeup of the animals, or differences in the experimental environment.

The second advantage, which is particularly relevant to carcinogenicity assessments, is derived from the first. There is the increased chance of discovering a susceptible subpopulation or a synergistic set of conditions. Because the toxicological manifestation of the test compound may depend on the presence of other (often unknown) factors, either in the test animals themselves or in their environment, there is generally a higher probability[1] of detecting any effects if a number of repetitions are run under various conditions.

D. Stratification

As already mentioned, the inherent variability of biological organisms leads to the possibility that any observed differences between treated and control individuals can be fortuitous. To reduce the probability of such a spurious difference, it is best to have the test and control animals as similar as possible. Any group of experimental units selected on the basis of similarity is called a *stratum* or *block*. If animals in the same block are given different treatments, then there is less chance of the observed differences being due to the inherent variation, allowing one to be more sure of the significance of the result. Because comparisons are made *within* the block, differences with animals in other blocks are of no concern. The replicates discussed in the previous section can be considered as blocks.

The criteria used for selecting blocks should be motivated by the investigator's knowledge of what can reasonably affect the response of interest. Animals can be blocked by pedigree, reducing genetic variation within a block. Another popular blocking factor is body weight, so that differences in vigor are not confounded with the treatment effects. An obvious blocking factor for chronic studies is cage position. For example, one bank of cages can constitute a block. If the response of interest involves a measurement that has appreciable day-to-day variation, then "day of observation" should be a blocking factor. And, of course, a block can be defined by a combination of blocking factors.

An extreme type of blocking, which defines the individual animal as the block, leads to the so-called *repeated measures design*. Such a design is possible in the case of acute reversible toxicity experiments in which there is no aftereffect and each animal can, in turn, be used as both control and treated subject. (It goes without saying that a random proce-

---

[1] The actual probability of detecting such an effect depends on several parameters, one of which is the size of the experiment. If the experiment has sufficient replication so that the false negative rate is no greater than the false positive rate (see Section III,A) and the error degrees of freedom are not too few (>30), then a "shotgun" approach (at least for responses with an approximately normal distribution) involving a variety of small replicates under different conditions is more likely to determine whether a test compound *may* be toxic than is one large replicate under arbitrarily selected homogeneous conditions. The advantage of the shotgun approach, of course, is dependent on a correct data analysis that accounts for the inherent stratification (see Section II,D).

dure implemented independently for each animal should determine which treatment is applied first.) Provided that the danger of cross-contamination can be avoided, such a design might also be used in skin-painting studies in which one side of the animal is painted with the test substance and the other side with a vehicle control. Similarly, the dose dependence of the pharmacokinetics of a rapidly eliminated test chemical can be studied if the same animal is given various doses over a period of time. In this instance also, the sequence of dose levels should be randomized.

In most toxicological experiments, however, an animal can be used only once, in which case the smallest possible block is a pair of animals chosen to be as similar as possible. Distributing the members of a litter among the different treatments gives a *litter-matched design* in which the blocks are litters of animals.

Stratification is not without its disadvantages. Since blocks are different *a priori,* comparisons between blocks do not provide information about experimental error. It is thus possible that, although a blocked design may have a smaller experimental error, it may not offer much assurance about how small that error is. This paradoxical situation may arise if the number of experimental units is small. Another problem that may occur, particularly in chronic studies, is the possibility of losing part of the block because of premature death or autolysis. This eventuality diminishes the value of data on the other animals in the block.

E. Criteria for Evaluating Experimental Designs

The first requirement of any experiment is that it should be able to provide the information needed. In particular, it should be free from biases, such as those caused by lack of randomization, and it should have a sufficient number and variety of treatment groups to enable identification of the quantities of interest. There will, however, be many designs satisfying these requirements, and one needs some criterion for choosing among them. Such criteria are provided by the measures of sensitivity and efficiency.

The *sensitivity* of an experiment measures how well small differences can be detected. For experiments such as screening studies, in which the ultimate goal is a decision, the sensitivity is often quantified by the *false negative rate.* That is, the experimenter decides what magnitude of effect is of practical concern, and determines the probability of *not* detecting such an effect by the given experiment. For experiments such as dose–response studies in which the goal is the estimation of some parameter, the sensitivity can be measured by the standard error of the estimate, or preferably, by the expected width of a confidence interval.

All things being equal, experiments with more animals will tend to be more sensitive. There will in many cases, however, be a particular design that will be the most sensitive among all designs with that number of animals. This design, which gives the maximum information per animal, is called the *optimal* design. Optimal designs are not generally used, however, for a number of reasons. First, it often happens that the optimal design depends on parameters that cannot be known until the experiment is completed. Second, the experiment may be carried out for a number of purposes, and the design that is optimal for one purpose may not be optimal for another. Finally, the optimal design may be unworkable because of operational constraints.

A useful quantity in comparing designs is *efficiency*. When expressed as a percentage, the efficiency of a design can be thought of as the number of animals that would be as sensitive in an optimal experiment as in an experiment with *this* particular design and 100 animals. Thus, the efficiency of a design gives the relative amount of information provided per animal.

Two desirable properties of designs are *robustness* and *ruggedness*. Experimental designs are generally constructed on the basis of either prior knowledge or a set of reasonable assumptions and are implemented by means of a rigid protocol. A design is robust if it maintains reasonable efficiency even if the basis of its construction departs somewhat from the truth. A design is rugged if it is not compromised by minor deviations from the protocol.

In the planning of an experiment, robustness and efficiency sometimes have to be traded off. The choice of design depends, among other things, on the cost of the experiment and on the accuracy of prior information. Efficiency is an important consideration in expensive experiments but may be a minor concern in situations in which the marginal cost of adding more animals is small. Robust and rugged designs should be used in innovative research, because there is little basis for constructing an optimal design and changes of protocol may well be required.

III. GUIDELINES FOR DESIGNING EXPERIMENTS

A. Designs for Screening Studies

1. False Positive and False Negative Rates

In a screening study, the purpose of the experiment is to arrive at a decision as to whether the test compound does or does not exhibit a toxic effect. Two types of error are possible in the making of such a decision: an innocuous chemical may be declared to be toxic or a toxic chemical may be considered harmless. The probabilities of those two types of error are often called "false positive" and "false negative" rates, respectively. These rates depend on both the experimental design and the decision procedure used. False positive rates are traditionally controlled by testing the data for statistical significance. It is then the function of the experimental design to control the false negative rate.

Since the false negative rate also depends on the inherent variability of the response of interest, information from previous studies is required before an experiment can be properly designed. Such information may be difficult to find, however, because researchers often do not publish standard deviations of their observations. Handbooks such as those of Altman and Dittmer (1972) and Mitruka and Rawnsley (1981) may be helpful in this regard, although their documentation of variability is not always adequate. If information on variability cannot be found, then a pilot study, perhaps involving only control animals, is advised. Although an accurate determination of variability requires hundreds of observations, a small pilot experiment of approximately 30 animals can provide an upper confidence limit on the standard deviation from which a bound on the false negative rate of the primary experiment can be estimated.

Although the false positive rate is generally controlled by testing for statistical significance, its effective size can also be affected indirectly by the design. Toxicologists typically record many different response variables on each experimental unit, whereas the commonly used significance tests bound the false positive rate on the assumption that only a single response is actually analyzed. Repeated reliance on such tests over the large number of response variables measured in a toxicological experiment can inflate the false positive rate of the entire experiment to an unacceptable level. One way of addressing this difficulty is through the use of multivariate statistical methods. These techniques, however, will fail if there are too few experimental units. At the very least, the experiment should have as many experimental units as it has variables, counting both response variables (e.g., survival time) and design variables (e.g., dose). Applying multivariate techniques to such a minimal experiment will, however, give very large false negative rates. A good rule of thumb is that the total number of animals should exceed twice the number of distinct variables being measured.

2. Sample Size Determination with Dichotomous Data

The determination of the number of animals required to control the false negative rate is generally a complex procedure, and a professional statistician should be engaged for this purpose. However, the procedure is fairly straightforward in the simplest case of a completely randomized design in which the response is dichotomous (e.g., appearance of a particular lesion). The procedure is outlined in detail next to illustrate the thought processes required for such an exercise. A brief discussion of the case with continuous data is given in Section III, A, 4. More detail, both conceptual and technical, can be found in Gart *et al.* (1986) and Healy (1987).

A false negative is least likely if the control and treated response rates are as different as possible. Thus, an optimal design will have only two treatment groups: a control group and one at the highest practicable dose. In chronic experiments, this highest dose is the maximum tolerated dose (MTD; Chapter 9) because exceeding this dose can reduce the sensitivity by causing premature death of the treated animals. It is usual to allocate an equal number of animals to control and treated groups, even though such an allocation is not always optimal. The optimal allocation depends on precise knowledge of the expected response rates in both control and treated groups, but the whole motivation for the experiment is precisely the *lack* of this knowledge.

The two-group experiment is not very robust for a chronic study because exceeding the MTD can compromise the whole experiment. One or two intermediate dose levels are thus advisable, even if they reduce efficiency. The actual efficiency may depend on the shape of the dose–response curve, but for a linear relationship the efficiency of a design is proportional to the variance of the dose levels. Thus, a design with three treatment groups (control, MTD/2, and MTD) is approximately 67% efficient, whereas one with four treatment groups (control, MTD/4, MTD/2, MTD) is approximately 55% efficient.

Once the treatment groups have been chosen, the size of the experiment must be determined to guarantee a sufficiently low false negative rate. A thorough approach to this problem can become very complex because one must balance all the consequences of false negatives and false positives against the various costs of the study. Consequently, this very important step of planning an experiment is too often addressed in vague terms, and the final number of animals used is rather arbitrary. The following approach, although somewhat simplistic, should impart some rationality to this exercise.

First, the experimenter must select an "indifference point" in the range of possible responses. This indifference point is an excess response rate at the MTD for which the consequences of the two types of error (false negative and false positive) are equal. In other words, if the true difference between responses at the MTD and the control are at this hypothetical level, then the hazard of the compound is perfectly balanced

Table I

Number of Animals in Each Group Required to Maintain Both False Positive and False Negative Rates below 5%[a]

Excess response at MTD (%)	Response in control group (%)			
	0	1	10	20
5	181	295	979	1546
10	89	121	289	423
15	59	74	147	202
20	44	52	92	121
25	34	40	65	82

[a] Fisher's exact test with equal-sized groups on control and on MTD was used.

against any losses due to alleged toxicity. The choice of an indifference point is not an easy matter. Such a choice involves the considerations of the compound's benefits, the seriousness of the toxic response, and, not the least, what fraction of the MTD corresponds to actual exposure levels. Although a certain subjectivity is unavoidable, a statement of the indifference point allows an honest evaluation of the experiment's conclusions.

Table I lists the number of animals required in each treatment group to give an experiment in which both the false positive and false negative rates are equal to 5%. Note that these numbers depend on the control response rate as well as on the excess rate at the MTD. Since a 5% rate of false positives is generally accepted, using the number of animals required for an excess rate equal to the indifference point will give an experiment in which the probabilities of the two types of error match the seriousness of their consequences. From Table I, one can see that a considerably larger experiment is required to detect toxic responses that have a high spontaneous rate of occurrence. It is not very feasible to detect those effects with an excess response rate of less than 5%.

3. Including Time-to-Event Data

The preceding discussion refers to the sensitivity required for an experiment in which only a dichotomous response is observed. Such a response can be death or morbidity in acute studies, appearance of a specific pathological sign in subchronic studies, or presence of malignant neoplasms at necropsy in chronic studies. In many such situations, the dichotomous nature of the response merely represents a convenient reduction of the actual data that can, in fact, be further quantified. Thus, instead of just noting the presence of a pathological sign, one can record and analyze its severity; instead of just noting death or the appearance of a malignancy, one can record the time at which it took place.

Recording the time of the event is of particular concern in chronic carcinogenicity studies, because neglecting to do so can seriously impair the proper analysis and interpretation of the experiment. Several biases are possible if one looks at only the lifetime tumor incidence as an indicator of carcinogenicity (Gart *et al.*, 1979; Peto *et al.*, 1980; Bickis and Krewski, 1985).

The first problem arises because the test compound can increase the mortality of the animals at the MTD and, thereby, reduce the time at which they are at risk of developing tumors. On the other hand, earlier deaths can lead to earlier detection of internal tumors and, thereby, give the illusion of a shorter latent period. Although these two biases tend to compensate for each other, the extent of this compensation cannot be determined unless both time and cause of death are recorded for each animal. Another possibility is that the test compound does not increase lifetime tumor incidence but merely reduces the latent period. Such a case will go undetected if only incidence data is analyzed.

A further difficulty with carcinogenicity tests is the ambiguity of the response of interest. Except for skin and possibly mammary tumors, the only time established is "time of death with tumor". Of more interest is "time of tumor appearance" or "time of death from tumor", but these data are often unobservable. Estimates of these quantities are possible, however, if periodic sacrifices of a fraction of the experiment are scheduled for necropsy so that the prevalence of tumors among apparently healthy animals can be determined (Berlin *et al.*, 1979; Kalbfleisch *et al.*, 1983; Turnbull and Mitchell, 1984).

In principle, the recording of time-to-event data increases the sensitivity of the experiment because more information is collected. In practice, however, the loss in efficiency due to dichotomization is small, except in situations in which the control response rate is high. Thus, the main reason for collecting this information is to control the possible biases discussed previously. In those situations (e.g., acute studies) in which these biases do not arise, the dichotomous data may be quite adequate (Gart and Tarone, 1987).

4. Sample Size Determination with Continuous Data

In the case of a continuous response variable, the determination of sample size is based on the same principles as in the case of a dichotomous response, except the technical details are different. As an example, consider the case of two equally sized groups, one on control and one on test compound, in which the response variable follows a normal distribution. For definiteness, we suppose that a toxic effect is one that *reduces* the value of this variable. The modification to the case of an increasing effect is straightforward.

The required sample size now depends not on the magnitude of the control response but on its variability. This variability is most conveniently expressed in terms of the *coefficient of variation,* defined as the ratio of the standard deviation to the mean.[2] The essential quantity for determining the sample size is the ratio of percent reduction at the indifference level to the coefficient of variation. This quantity, which is called *eccentricity,* measures how much overlap there is between the control and treated populations and, thus, how easy it is to distinguish them.[3] If the eccentricity is large, then it is unlikely for any control individual to have a lower value than a treated individual. The effect can be clearly seen even with a small experiment. If the eccentricity is small, however, then there may be many control individuals who have levels lower than some treated individuals. It will require a large sample to establish that an apparent depression of the response variable is unlikely to have been due to chance. A large experiment will be required in situations in which a slight but consistent depression of a response variable is of biological significance.

Table II lists the number of animals required in each group to maintain both false positive and false negative rates below 5% as a function of the eccentricity for a completely randomized design with two treatments. Suppose, for example, that we want to design an experiment in 6-month-old male rats to detect a weight loss of 5%. If the coefficient of variation of body weight is known to be 3%, then the eccentricity will be $5/3 = 1.67$. As Table II indicates, between 7 and 11 animals will be required in each group. A parameter such as blood cholesterol, however, may have a coefficient of variation as high as 36%. A 5% reduction will give an eccentricity of only $5/36 = 0.14$. Over 1000 animals per group will be required for adequate sensitivity with a completely randomized design.

---

[2] The coefficient of variation is often expressed as a percentage.

[3] One can equivalently express this distinguishability in terms of the *percent overlap.* Suppose that one wants to determine a threshold level of the response such that individuals with lower levels will be deemed to be in the affected population, whereas those with a higher level will be deemed to be in the unaffected population. In addition, suppose that the threshold is chosen to maximize the separation between the two populations. Then the percent overlap is defined as the percentage of unaffected individuals deemed to be affected plus the percentage of affected individuals deemed to be unaffected.

Table II
Number of Animals in Each Group Required to
Maintain Both False Positive and False Negative
Rates below 5%[a]

Eccentricity	% Overlap	Number of animals
0.10	96	2166
0.20	92	542
0.30	88	242
0.40	84	136
0.50	80	88
0.60	76	61
0.70	73	45
0.80	69	35
0.90	65	28
1.00	62	23
1.50	45	11
2.00	32	7
2.50	21	5
3.00	13	4
4.00	5	3
5.00	1	3
6.00	0.3	2

[a] One-sided t test with equal-sized groups on control and on
test treatment was used.

Such an experiment, can be made more efficient by stratification. If the
animals can be initially grouped into blocks having similar cholesterol
levels, then the variation *within* a block is relevant for determining the
required sample size.

B. Design of Dose-Response Experiments

If the purpose of an experiment is to estimate the dose – response curve or
some aspect of it, then an experiment with only two treatment groups is
generally inadequate. A sufficient number of dose levels are needed to
define the shape of the relationship clearly. If the mathematical form of
the relationship is definitely known to come from a two-parameter family, such as the logistic or multihit (Krewski and Van Ryzin, 1981), one
can in fact estimate the relationship solely from an experiment at two
appropriately selected doses (Krewski *et al.,* 1986a). In practice, however,
one rarely has assurance that a postulated mathematical model is the
correct one; hence, robustness becomes a more important consideration
than optimality.

A parameter that is often of interest in experiments with dichotomous responses is a particular quantile of the dose–response curve. That is, for some number p, one wants to estimate that dose at which a fraction p of the population will respond. A dose in which p is equal to 0.5 is usually referred to as the median effective dose (ED_{50}), or median lethal dose (LD_{50}) if the response is death, which is a common way of quantifying the result of an acute toxicity test. In carcinogenicity trials, one is more likely to be interested in the quantile for a small value of p, say 10^{-6}, which is then called a low-dose extrapolation. However, Sawyer et al. (1984) used an analogous quantity called the TD_{50}, defined as the chronic dose inducing tumors in 50% of the animals living a standard lifespan, to quantify the potency of carcinogens.

1. Estimation of ED_{50} or Other Quantile for Acute Studies

Estimation of the ED_{50} is more efficient if the dose groups bracket this response rate. If there is no prior indication of this value, then the only recourse is to choose a fairly large number of dose levels spread over a wide range. Sometimes it might be advantageous to perform an initial estimation in a pilot experiment using only a few animals in each group. The estimate can then be refined in a second experiment.

Finney (1971) recommends that, if there are only a few animals available (fewer than 30 in total), the doses for estimating the ED_{50} should be chosen to approximate response rates of 10, 50, and 90%. For larger experiments, less extreme doses are more efficient; therefore, with over 100 animals per group, one should aim for the 30, 50, and 70% response points. In experiments in which the approximate dose range is well known and the shape of the dose–response curve is of no particular interest, three dose levels are probably sufficient if the response does not occur spontaneously. If there is an appreciable probability of spontaneous response, however, then a control group must be included as well.

In acute tests, the possibility exists for sequential procedures. That is, instead of simultaneously treating a group of animals, one treats one animal at a time then adjusts the dose for the next animal, depending on the outcome of the trial. Bruce (1985) has discussed application of such a technique. McLeish and Tosh (1983) and Wu (1985) have offered theoretical discussions of the statistical properties of these methods and their efficient implementation.

2. Low-dose Extrapolation for Chronic Studies

For situations in which low dose extrapolation is based on a conventional mathematical model, the question of experimental design has been much studied. Although optimal designs exist, their exact implementation requires knowledge of the dose–response relationship one is trying to estimate. The most useful designs in such situations are robust ones. Krewski *et al.* (1984c) examined the efficiency for a number of designs for 50 actual doses–response curves from published data. For model-based extrapolation, this empirical study suggests that a good practical design involves four treatment groups including a control, an MTD, and two other doses equally spaced between them. The preferred method is to place approximately twice as many animals at the intermediate doses as at the extreme ones. Portier (1981) came to similar conclusions using Monte Carlo methods.

These results should not be considered definitive, however, because recent research casts doubt on the appropriateness of model-based extrapolation. Linear extrapolation procedures, which are not sensitive to the choice of a particular mathematical model of the dose–response relationship, are becoming more generally recommended (Krewski *et al.*, 1984b, 1986b). More research needs to be done to determine designs that are advantageous for linear extrapolation.

As with the case of screening studies, the number of animals required for a sufficiently sensitive study is of interest. It is difficult to provide such a number because it will depend on many parameters. An important consideration is the ratio of the expected dose in the population at risk to the MTD. A general principle is that if the response being studied is totally absent in the experimental animals, then an upper 95% confidence limit on the risk is three times the reciprocal of the number of treated animals. Thus, if we assume that *one* in a million is an acceptable risk, the size of the treated dose group should be at least *three* million times the ratio of environmental dose to experimental dose if linear extrapolation is used. If, in fact, the experimental animals do exhibit responses, then the confidence limit on the low-dose risk will be higher; thus the dose groups ought to be at least twice that size to ensure adequate prediction of virtual safety. For example, if the MTD is 10,000 times the anticipated human exposure, then 300 animals per treatment group may be adequate if neither treated nor control animals show any response. If, on the other hand, the anticipated usage will lead to exposures of 1% of the MTD, then at least 30,000 animals per treatment group will be needed to assure adequate precision — clearly an impractical situation (Clayson and Krewski, 1986).

C. Studies with *in Utero* Exposure

Experiments in which test animals are exposed to a xenobiotic *in utero* are generally done for one of two purposes: to study effects on reproduction, which would include not only effects on reproductive physiology but also mutagenicity and teratogenicity, or to assess toxicity/carcinogenicity due to lifetime exposure, beginning at conception.

1. Reproductive Studies

The design of experiments on reproductive toxicology follows the same general principles as other toxicological studies. The only distinction is that the response of interest involves the reproductive system. It is important, however, to properly identify the experimental unit. Since, in most cases, the test treatment will be applied to females before, during, or after conception, these maternal animals constitute the experimental unit. Thus, in planning a teratology study, the number of fetuses does not matter as much as the number of mothers. It follows that accurate records must be kept of the maternal source of each fetus.

In some *in vivo* assessments of mutagenicity, such as the dominant lethal test, the test compound is administered to males before they are bred to see if it causes mutations during spermatogenesis. In such cases, the males become the experimental unit. Males are often bred with a number of females; this strategy sometimes generates quite a large set of data. If a male is bred with a number of females over a period of weeks following treatment, it may be possible to examine which stage of spermatogenesis is affected. However, the precision of the experiment depends primarily on the number of males used. Use of several females per male should not be considered a form of replication.

2. Two-Generation Studies

Friedman (1970) was the first to suggest the need for chronic studies in which the test compound is administered to the experimental animals perinatally. In such experiments, the parent (F_0) generation is dosed for some time prior to mating, and the females are maintained on the treatment throughout pregnancy and lactation. After weaning, the animals of the second (F_1) generation are themselves treated with the test compound for their lifetime.

Such a testing procedure is reasonable because it mimics the human situation. Food additives and many environmental contaminants are often consumed throughout one's lifetime. It is thus possible for a child to receive a xenobiotic or its metabolites either via the placenta or from its mother's milk. Possibly the fetus or infant may be at greater risk for a number of reasons: the immature organism may be inherently more susceptible to the compound, the dose may be increased because of concentrating effects of the placenta or mammary glands, or another chemical may be present because of placental or fetal metabolism. Furthermore, the toxic effects of perinatal exposure may express themselves differently from those of adult exposure.

There are several examples. Diethylstilbestrol (DES) given to women during pregnancy causes vaginal tumors in their daughters (Forsberg, 1981), although no such effect has been reported in the mothers. In several rodent studies (Tisdel et al., 1974; Arnold et al., 1980; Taylor et al., 1980), the incidence of bladder tumors in rats exposed to saccharin in utero was somewhat greater than that in rats exposed only after weaning. In a more recent study (Schoenig et al., 1985), in utero exposure did not appear to play much of a role in carcinogenesis; however, it was suggested that exposure during lactation might have an effect.

In planning a two-generation study, one must bear in mind its appropriateness and cost. It has been estimated (Grice et al., 1981) that a two-generation study will cost 12–18% more than a conventional chronic one. Added cost will not be well spent if the study is not appropriate. First, one must consider whether the human subpopulation at risk includes pregnant women. Second, one must ask to what extent the placental/fetal/lactation physiology and pharmacodynamics of the test animals resemble those of humans. If they are radically different, then the extrapolation of the two-generation study to humans can be problematic.

a. Dose Selection

The selection of dose levels presents special problems in two-generation studies. Consideration must be given to the doses given premating, during pregnancy, during lactation, and to juvenile and adult offspring. The maximum tolerated dose might not be appropriate for the dams if such a high level adversely affects reproduction. On the other hand, adjusting the dose during the course of the study complicates the estimation and interpretation of a dose–response relationship.

Ideally, females should be in a state of pharmacokinetic equilibrium before mating. Pharmacokinetic studies may be necessary prior to the two-generation study to establish the rate and length of dosing required to achieve this state. Estimation of the effective dose to the fetus can also be achieved in such studies. In addition, prior studies of teratogenicity and reproductive toxicity should be required to ensure that the highest dose given to the females does not affect their fertility or the viability of their offspring.

b. Mating

If the possibility exists that the potential toxicity is due to mutagenic effects occurring during spermatogenesis, then both sexes should be treated prior to mating. If only *in utero* prenatal effects are of interest, however, it is sufficient to dose only the females. In such a situation, repeated use of the same male can reduce the genetic variation in the F_1 generation.

Ideally, pairs of animals to be mated should be selected randomly, which may be difficult to realize in some species in which incompatibilities may arise. Infertility due to mating failure may be acceptable in large experiments but can be disastrous in primate studies in which animals are few and expensive. Some deliberate shuffling of the original pairings may be unavoidable.

Random pairings can be restricted by design. If several animals from several sources are being tested simultaneously, one may want to keep mating within the source. If litter information is available on the F_0 animals, then one may want to either ensure or exclude sibling mating. Restricted randomization can also make multiple use of males to reduce experimental error. In such a design, paternity is used as a blocking factor, enabling more genetic similarity between the animals on different treatments.

As an example, consider an experiment in which the *in utero* effects of several levels and types of polychlorinated biphenyls (PCBs) on monkeys will be examined. There are nine females in each of five treatment groups and nine males available. Each male is to be mated with one female from each dose group. Because several days are required for each mating, impregnation of all females may be spread over a period of time. To avoid the possibility of pregnancies in different dose groups occurring at different times (and thereby introducing an extraneous factor in treatment comparisons), the allocations of males to females should not be done entirely at random. Instead, a mating scheme shown in Table III should be set up. The order in which the nine males can be selected for mating for each dose group is specified in the table. The males can be divided randomly into a group of five and a group of four. Because the matings will alternate between these two groups, a male will not be required to mate with two females too closely in succession.

The actual allocations of females to males can be done dynamically. At any time period, the first unmated female in a dose group to menstruate can be paired with a male assigned to that dose group. However, mating of the next female in that dose group should not be allowed until one female from each of the other dose groups has been mated. If there are only four males in the second group, there will be a dose group without matings in alternate periods. Thus, for example, the second mating in dose group 3 will not take place until the third period, that is, until all the other dose groups have completed their second mating. Because the

Table III

A Mating Scheme for Balancing 9 Males across 5 Treatment Groups and 10 Time Periods

	Males to be mated				
			Dose group		
Period	1	2	3	4	5
1	5	3	8	4	7
2	1	6	(wait)	9	2
3	3	4	5	7	8
4	2	(wait)	6	1	9
5	4	5	7	8	3
6	6	1	9	2	(wait)
7	7	8	4	3	5
8	(wait)	9	2	6	1
9	8	7	3	5	4
10	9	2	1	(wait)	6

mating scheme does not assign a male to a specific female, there is enough flexibility to allow some adjustments for incompatibility. If a mating is unsuccessful, then the female can be retired and another from that dose group brought in. The retired female can be paired with another male at a later time.

Note that the design of this experiment could have been simpler had there been 10 males and 50 females. This example illustrates how an ingenious design can accommodate operational constraints and still satisfy the requirements of validity and efficiency. Setting up such designs and analyzing the results of such experiments require a high level of expertise, however, and a professional statistician should be consulted.

c. Litter Distribution

In two-generation experiments involving rodents or other animals with multiple births, remember that the litter, not the individual F_1 animal, is the experimental unit. In general, for a given number of F_1 animals, the most efficient design is one in which each F_1 animal comes from a different litter. Such an experiment is more expensive because more F_0 animals are needed. However, because F_0 animals are retained for a relatively short period of time, the added cost is not a large percentage of the total cost of the experiment.

When littermates are admitted to the F_1 phase, the loss in sensitivity is a function of the intralitter correlation of the response under study (Krewski et al., 1984a). This intralitter correlation can be due to several phenomena: genetic similarity in susceptibility to the test chemical, similarity in intrauterine or postpartum environments, or interlitter variation in the effective dose reaching the fetus. This last factor can be studied pharmacokinetically. Grice *et al.* (1981) reported experiments in which three chemicals (saccharin, amaranth, and styrene) were administered to pregnant rats; the fetal absorption of these chemicals displayed intralitter correlations of 0.7, 0.3, and 0.9, respectively. Although the intralitter correlation of the toxic *response* may not necessarily be that high, the magnitude of these correlations does point to the need to take litter effects into account.

Grice *et al.* (1981) have recommended taking one animal of each sex per litter. Such a selection will allow valid significance tests of sexes separately without adjustments for litter effects. However, if information from the sexes is combined, then the intralitter correlation should be taken into account.

The actual selection of animals for the F_1 phase should be done at random to avoid possible biases. In addition, litters should be randomly culled to a maximum of eight pups at four or five days of age to equalize the stress on the dam and to prevent the natural selection of more vigorous offspring.

There may be experiments in which the selection of more than one animal per litter is indicated. This would be the case, for example, if the intralitter correlation of the response in question is itself a study objective. If one wanted to distinguish perinatal from postweaning effects, then two animals per litter can be chosen, one to receive the test treatment after weaning, the other to receive a control treatment.

The possibility of selection bias is increased if several pups per litter are chosen. If there is some small treatment effect, either on fertility or on postpartum survival, then the larger litters will tend to have animals that are more resistant to the treatment. If the F_1 generation is selected solely from litters of a given size, then the apparent effect of the treatment can be reduced. Such a possible bias was noted by Lagakos and Mosteller (1981) in their review of the chronic carcinogenicity of allura red, in which only litters with more than three pups of each sex were admitted to the F_1 phase.

D. Experiments with Mixtures of Chemicals

Currently, most screening studies are performed on one specific chemical, and there is a deliberate attempt to keep other xenobiotics out of the environment or feed of the test animals. However, because human populations are exposed to a diverse cocktail of environmental contaminants, food additives, and drugs, it is important to be able to study the joint action of a number of chemicals simultaneously (Selikoff and Hammond, 1977). Such experiments will not only indicate interactions among chemicals but, if well designed, can also reduce the overall cost of a screening program (Simon, 1980).

The phenomenon of a mixture being more potent than anticipated from its constituents is commonly called *synergism*. There is insufficient space in this chapter to discuss in any depth the difficulties in the precise definition and interpretation of this concept. A good summary, although in a different context, can be found in Morse (1978). However, one should always bear in mind that a bioassay can detect only what is called "phenomenological synergism" in which two (or more) compounds *appear* to be enhancing each other's effects. Such an observation does not imply that there is, in fact, a chemical or toxicological interaction between the compounds, nor does the absence of synergism preclude a genuine interaction.

Standard designs for examining the effects of combinations of chemicals are the so-called factorial designs. One chooses a certain number of levels of each chemical, then applies all the combinations of these levels. If one chooses control plus k_1 levels of compound A and control plus k_2 levels of compound B, then one has an experiment with $(k_1 + 1)(k_2 + 1)$ treatments, of which one is control, k_1 are pure compound A, k_2 are pure compound B, and the remainder are mixtures of the two compounds. This procedure can in theory be carried out with any number of compounds, although in practice it can become unwieldy if the number of test compounds is large. For example, with only five compounds, each at control and two dose levels, 243 different treatment groups are required. However, in a factorial experiment, the number of experimental units per group need not be very large. In fact, efficiency is maintained as long as the total number of animals minus the number of treatment groups is not too small. Thus, the experiment with 243 treatment groups and two animals per group has about the same sensitivity as an experiment with three treatment groups and eighty animals per group. Nonetheless, in an exploratory experiment in which the interactions of many compounds are being investigated, it may be unnecessary to examine all possible combinations. Important insight may be gained by a suitably selected subset of combinations. The choice of this subset is a complex and crucial matter and should be made by an experienced statistician.

Standard factorial designs may not be that useful in experiments in which large toxic effects are anticipated, particularly if the response is dichotomous. If most of the animals already show signs of toxicity to a single chemical, then any additional effect due to other chemicals may be difficult to quantify. There will consequently be little information in the combinations of high doses. Moreover, in chronic carcinogenicity studies, the combination of several chemicals, each at the MTD, can easily exceed the MTD for the mixture. A possible approach in such situations can be to reparametrize the treatments in terms of total dose and proportions of various chemicals. If there is prior information on the relative potencies of the several chemicals, then the total dose can be standardized to give equal expected responses regardless of the proportions. Finney (1971) has outlined procedures for implementing such designs for dichotomous responses and Cornell (1981) has done the same for quantitative responses.

There has been a resurgence of interest in toxicological experiments involving mixtures. A series of such experiments is reported by Elashoff et al. (1987) and Fears et al. (1988, 1989). A good review of the many issues involved has been published by the National Research Council (1988) of the United States.

E. Experiments for Studying Mechanisms

If the purpose of an experiment is to investigate some mechanism of toxicity or carcinogenicity, then the design will have to be custom made to suit the particular problem. In all cases, the general principles discussed previously will apply. In addition, it is important to consider in advance whether the experiment will, in fact, answer the question asked. A good mental exercise is to imagine what the expected results will be under alternative hypotheses and whether these alternatives can be distinguished by the treatment groups.

As an example, consider an experiment that is to determine whether compound X is a promoter of carcinogenesis. The hypothesis indicates that, among animals in which carcinogenesis has been initiated, those that are chronically exposed to this substance should have an excess of neoplasms compared to those not so exposed. However, to examine this hypothesis, it is not adequate to treat a group of animals with an initiator, then randomly split the group such that half remain on a control treatment and half receive the putative promoter. In an experiment of this nature, one will not be able to distinguish whether compound X is a promoter or a complete carcinogen itself. To make that distinction, one will also need a group receiving compound X in which carcinogenesis is not initiated.

Whenever an innovative experiment is planned, a professional statistician should be consulted before the design is finalized. Otherwise, the investigator may find that the experiment produces nothing but a mass of costly, uninterpretable data.

IV. PRACTICAL CONSIDERATIONS

A. Procedures for Randomization

The effective use of randomized and cryptotaxic experiments requires that the procedures be carefully implemented to avoid the tedium of handling a complicated arrangement of treatments. A suggested way of implementation is presented in this section. The basic requirements are a computer equipped with a sorting program and a program for selecting random permutations of integers, a printer, and a supply of fanfolded gummed labels.

The first step in implementation is to define the caging sequence. After the cages have been numbered, a random permutation of the numbers 1 to n, where n is the number of cages, is generated. As each animal is removed from the shipping container, it is placed in the cage number corresponding to the next number in the permuted list. This cage number becomes the unique identifier of that animal for the duration of the experiment. All documents used for recording data use that number, and no other designation. Cryptotaxy is thus ensured.

This principle can be suitably modified for special requirements. There is no problem with affixing location information, such as cage rack and row, for convenience of finding the cage. To minimize the chance of transcriptional errors, check digits can be added to the cage numbers (e.g., a digit equal to the iterated sum of the other digits can be inserted between the last two digits; therefore, cage 179 becomes 1789, cage 25 becomes 275, but cage 265 does not exist). If multiple caging is used, the randomized list of cage numbers will have to contain repetitions and the animals within a cage will have to be distinguished, perhaps by letter codes (A, B, C, etc.).

If blocking is required, then cage numbers can be subdivided into blocks. These generally are defined by ranges of cage numbers, although other blocking procedures are possible. The cage numbers are now rearranged according to another random permutation in which a different permutation is chosen for each block. With this random sequence of cage numbers in hand, treatments groups are assigned systematically to the cages. A master list can then be sorted by cage numbers to designate the treatments to be applied to each cage. This master list, however, should not be consulted during the course of the study. Ideally, it should be sealed until all results have been collected.

Actual dosing can be implemented from a computer printout of gummed labels for each treatment group indicating which cage numbers will receive the designated treatment. These labels should be given to a "dosing technician", not otherwise involved in the study, who will prepare the treatments in individual dose containers and label them with the preprinted labels. After the technician has rearranged the containers in the order of the cage numbers, he or she will give them to the dosing personnel. Dosing personnel will apply the doses one cage at a time, verifying in each case that the number on the dose container corresponds to the number on the cage.

The computer can also prepare a supply of blank forms containing the cage numbers in their natural sequence. Any data collected during the course of the study, from food consumption to pathology, can be recorded on such forms. A more sophisticated and expensive approach is to have an on-line data capture system in which all data is directly entered into the computer. Because mistakes in computer data entry leave no traces, such a system has to be carefully designed to prevent unauthorized modification of data. One approach is to keep a perpetual log of all transactions. To maintain cryptotaxy, it should also be impossible to recover treatment information from such a system until the study is terminated.

B. Conclusion

In this chapter, the principles involved in designing useful toxicological experiments, using the methods of randomization, replication, and stratification have been considered. These methods ensure that the experiment is *valid,* in the sense of telling nothing but the truth, and *efficient,* in the sense of telling the whole truth.

In designing an experiment, one must keep in mind its purpose. Guidelines can be given for designing experiments for screening chemicals, for estimating dose–response relationships, and for investigating mechanisms of action. However, in a field as complex as toxicology, it is not possible to give simple rules that will exactly specify the design of every desired experiment. Consideration must be given to what is operationally feasible, as well as to what is sound subjective scientific judgment on such questions as the magnitude of the MTD, the use of *in utero* exposure, and the evaluation of mixtures.

Toxicological experiments are costly and time-consuming and usually involve many persons, both professional and technical. The value of an entire experiment hinges on the soundness of the experimental design. It is essential for all study personnel to be made aware of the necessity of randomization, cryptotaxy, and meticulous data recording. Without this awareness, one may view some procedures outlined in this chapter as nothing but a bureaucratic nuisance, and the temptation to shortcut the system becomes great. Thus, the entire validity of a study may be compromised.

All aspects of an experimental design should be explicitly incorporated into the final protocol and reviewed by a statistician who can anticipate the data analysis procedures and any problems they may cause. Nothing should be left to chance, except of course, the actual randomization.

References

Altman, P. L., and Dittmer, D. S. (1972). "Biology Data Book." Bethesda: Federation of American Societies for Experimental Biology.

Anderson, V. L., and McLean, R. A. (1974). "Design of Experiments: A Realistic Approach." New York: Marcel Dekker.

Arnold, D. L., Moodie, C. A., Grice, H. C., Charbonneau, S. M., Stavric, B., Collins, B. T., McGuire, P. F., Zawidzka, Z. Z., and Munro, I. C. (1980). Long-term toxicity of ortho-toluenesulfonamide and sodium saccharin in the rat. *Toxicol. Appl. Pharmacol.* **52,** 113–152.

Arnold, D. L., Farber, E., and Krewski, D. (1988). Carcinogenicity testing: Histopathology and the blind method. *Comments Toxicol.* **2,** 67–80.

Berlin, B., Brodsky, J., and Clifford, P. (1979). Testing disease dependence in survival experiments with serial sacrifice. *J. Amer. Stat. Assoc.* **74,** 5–14.

Bickis, M., and Krewski, D. (1985). Statistical design and analysis of the long-term carcinogenicity bioassay. *In* "Toxicological Risk Assessment, I" (D. B. Clayson, D. Krewski, and I. Munro, eds.), pp. 125–147. Boca Raton, Florida: CRC Press.

Bellhorn, R. W. (1980). Lighting in the animal environment. *Lab. Anim. Sci.* **30,** 440–450.

Box, G. E. P., Hunter, W. G., and Hunter, J. S. (1978). "Statistics for Experimenters. An Introduction to Design, Data Analysis, and Model Building." New York: Wiley.

Bruce, R. D. (1985). An up-and-down procedure for acute toxicity testing. *Fund. Appl. Toxicol.* **5,** 151–157.

Clayson, D. B., and Krewski, D. (1986). The concept of negativity in experimental carcinogenesis. *Mutat. Res.* **167,** 233–240.

Cornell, J. A. (1981). "Experiments with Mixtures: Designs, Models, and the Analysis of Mixture Data." New York: Wiley.

Cox, D. R. (1958). "Planning of Experiments." New York: Wiley.

Elashoff, R. M., Fears, T. R., and Schneiderman, M. A. (1987). The statistical analysis of a carcinogen mixture experiment I: The liver carcinogens. *J. Nat. Cancer Inst.* (US) **79,** 509–526.

Fears, T. R., and Schneiderman, M. A. (1974). Pathologic evaluation and the blind technique. *Science* **183,** 1144–1145.

Fears, T. R., Elashoff, R. M., and Schneiderman, M. A. (1988). The statistical analysis of a carcinogen mixture experiment II: Carcinogens with different target organs, N-Methyl-N'-nitro-N-nitrosoguanidine, N-butyl-n-(4-hydroxybutyl)nitrosamine, dipentylnitrosamine and nitrilotriacetic acid. *Toxicol. Ind. Health* **4,** 221–255.

Fears, T. R., Elashoff, R. M., and Schneiderman, M. A. (1989). The statistical analysis of a carcinogen mixture experiment III: Carcinogens with different target systems, Aflatoxin

B1, N-butyl-n-(4-hydroxybutyl)nitrosamine, lead acetate, and thiouracil. *Toxicol. Ind. Health* **5**, 1–24.

Finney, D. J. (1971). "Probit Analysis." Cambridge: Cambridge University Press.

Forsberg, J. G. (1981). Permanent changes induced by DES at critical stages in female development: 10 years experience from human and model systems. *Biol. Res. Pregnancy* **2**, 168–175.

Friedman, L. (1970). Symposium on the evaluation of the safety of food additives and chemical residues. II. The role of the laboratory animal study of intermediate duration for evaluation of safety. *Toxicol. Appl. Pharmacol.* **16**, 498–506.

Gart, J. J., Chu, K. C., and Tarone, R. E. (1979). Statistical issues in interpretation of chronic bioassay tests for carcinogenicity. *J. Natl. Cancer Inst. (US)* **62**, 957–974.

Gart, J. J., Krewski, D., Lee, P. N., Tarone, R. E., and Wahrendorf, J. (1986). "Statistical Methods in Cancer Research, III. The design and analysis of long-term animal experiments." *IARC Sci. Publ.* **79**.

Gart, J. J., and Tarone, R. E. (1987). On the efficiency of age-adjusted tests in animal carcinogenicity experiments. *Biometrics* **43**, 235–244.

Grice, H. C., Munro, I. C., Krewski, D. R., and Blumenthal, H. (1981). *In utero* exposure in chronic toxicity carcinogenicity studies. *Food Cosmet. Toxicol.* **19**, 373–379.

Healy, G. F. (1987). Power calculations in toxicology. *Alternat. Lab. Anim.* **15**, 132–139.

Kalbfleisch, J. D., Krewski, D. R., and Van Ryzin, J. (1983). Dose–response models for time-to-response toxicity data. *Can. J. Stat.* **11**, 25–49.

Krewski, D., and Van Ryzin, J. (1981). Dose response models for quantal response toxicity data. *In* "Statistics and Related Topics" (M. Csorgo, D. A. Dawson, J. N. K. Rao, and A. K. Md. E. Saleh, eds.), pp. 210–231. New York: North-Holland.

Krewski, D., Brennan, J., and Bickis, M. (1984a). The power of the Fisher permutation test in 2 × k tables. *Commun. Statist. Simula. Computa.* **13**, 433–448.

Krewski, D., Brown, C., and Murdoch, D. (1984b). Determining "safe" levels of exposure: Safety factors or mathematical models. *Fund. Appl. Toxicol.* **4**, S383–S394.

Krewski, D., Kovar, J., and Bickis, M. (1984c). Optimal experimental designs for low dose extrapolation. II. The case of non-zero background. *In* "Topics in Applied Statistics" (Y. P. Chaubey and T. D. Dwivedi, eds.), pp. 167–191. Montreal: Concordia University Press.

Krewski, D., Bickis, M., Kovar, J., and Arnold, D. L. (1986a). Optimal experimental designs for low dose extrapolation. I. The case of zero background. *Utilitas Mathematica* **29**, 245–262.

Krewski, D., Murdoch, D., and Dewanji, A. (1986b). Statistical modelling and extrapolation of carcinogenesis data. *In* "Modern Statistical Methods in Chronic Disease Epidemiology" (S. H. Moolgavkar and R. L. Prentice, eds.), pp. 259–282. New York: Wiley-Interscience.

Lagakos, S., and Mosteller, F. (1981). A case study of statistics in the regulatory process. *J. Nat. Cancer Inst. (US)* **66**, 197–212.

McConnell, E. E., Van Ryzin, R. J., Ward, J. M., and Glocklin, V. C. (1985). 'Blinded' slide reading vs. individual slide evaluation, assignment of cause of death, relevance of animal dose to human dose. *In* "Proceedings of the Symposium on Long-Term Animal Carcinogenicity Studies: A Statistical Perspective," pp. 9–25. Washington, DC: American Statistical Association.

McLeish, D., and Tosh, D. (1983). The estimation of extreme quantile in logit bioassay. *Biometrika* **70,** 625–632.

Mitruka, B. M., and Rawnsley, H. M. (1981). "Clinical Biochemical and Hematological Reference Values in Normal Experimental Animals and Normal Humans". New York: Masson.

Morse, P. M. (1978). Some comments on the assessment of joint action in herbicide mixtures. *Weed Science* **26,** 58–71.

National Research Council (1988). "Complex Mixtures." Washington, DC: National Academy of Sciences.

Peto, R., Pike, M. C., Day, N. E., Gray, R. G., Lee, P. N., Parish, S., Peto, J., Richards, S., and Wahrendorf, J. (1980). Guidelines for simple, sensitive significance tests for carcinogenic effects in long-term animal experiments. *IARC Monogr. Suppl.* **2,** 311–426.

Portier, C. J. (1981). Optimal bioassay design under the Armitage–Doll multi-stage model (Institute of Statistics Mimeo Series). Chapel Hill: Department of Biostatistics, University of North Carolina.

Riley, V. (1981). Psychoneuroendocrine influences on immunocompetence and neoplasia. *Science* **212,** 1100–1109.

Schoenig, G. P., Goldenthal, E. I., Geil, R. G., Frith, C. H., Richter, W. R., and Carlborg, F. W. (1985). Evaluation of the dose response and *in utero* exposure to saccharin in the rat. *Food Chem. Toxicol.* **23,** 475–490.

Sawyer, C., Peto, R., Bernstein, L., and Pike, M. (1984). Calculation of carcinogenic potency from long-term animal carcinogenesis experiments. *Biometrics* **40,** 27–40.

Selikoff, I. J., and Hammond, E. C. (1977). Multiple risk factors in environmental cancer. *In* "Environmental Cancer" (H. F. Kraybill and M. A. Mehlman, eds.), pp. 467–483. New York: Hemisphere.

Simon, W. (1980). Avoiding megamouse experiments. *J. Toxicol. Environ. Health* **6,** 907–910.

Taylor, J. M., Weinberger, M. A., and Friedman, L. (1980). Chronic toxicity and carcinogenicity to the urinary bladder of sodium saccharin in the *in utero*-exposed rat. *Toxicol. Appl. Pharmacol.* **54,** 57–95.

Tisdel, M. O., Nees, P. O., Harris, D. L., and Derse, P. H. (1974). Long term feeding of saccharin in rats. *In* "Symposium: Sweeteners" (G. E. Inglett, ed.), pp. 145–158. Westport, Connecticut: Avi.

Turnbull, B. W., and Mitchell, T. J. (1984). Nonparametric estimation of the distribution of time to onset for specific diseases in survival/sacrifice experiments. *Biometrics* **40,** 41–50.

Wu, C. F. J. (1985). Efficient sequential designs with binary data. *J. Am. Stat. Assoc.* **80,** 974–984.

8

Selection and Quality Control Aspects of Test Animals

Douglas L. Arnold
Toxicology Research Division
Bureau of Chemical Safety
Food Directorate
Health Protection Branch
Health and Welfare Canada
Ottawa, Ontario

Harold C. Grice
CANTOX, Inc.
Nepean, Ontario

I. INTRODUCTION

Hygienic procedures to minimize the inadvertent introduction of pathogens into animal facilities and the spread of zoonotic diseases are described in Chapter 5. Procedures to monitor animals upon their arrival and during the conduct of the study regarding health status and latent disease are discussed in this chapter. Latent diseases may only become evident because of the stress imposed by the testing procedures (i.e., exposure to the test substance, environmental variables, and various study manipulations), but they may necessitate termination of a study. Acquisition of a healthy laboratory animal from a reputable vendor is a requisite for all toxicological studies. Because the cost of animals in a toxicological testing program usually represents less than 5% of the total cost of the study (Box, 1974), inappropriate frugality is not cost-effective.

149

The utility of an animal monitoring program is negated if animal facilities are not properly maintained and appropriate husbandry procedures are not followed. Animal care personnel have a primary role in this regard (see Chapters 3 and 17). Consequently, it is necessary for these personnel to be familiar with the study objectives and aware of their respective responsibilities (Arnold *et al.*, 1978).

A basic disease surveillance program should be carried out by all laboratories conducting subchronic or chronic studies, although the comprehensive program detailed in this chapter is probably not undertaken routinely by most laboratories. The objectives of such a program are:

1. to ascertain the vendor's ability to supply animals of acceptable quality,
2. to facilitate early detection of latent diseases,
3. to minimize the occurrence of communicable diseases.

II. THE ANIMAL

Although nonhuman primates are increasingly being used in certain types of toxicological study, for reasons of economics, familiarity, and availability of historical data, rodents still constitute the primary test species. Many international agencies have suggested the use of other species, but little progress has been made to date identifying suitable alternative species (Arnold and Grice, 1978). Consequently, most comments contained herein are more germane to rodents. A suggested reading list for other species can be found at the end of this chapter.

The choice of potential animal vendors must be evaluated with criteria designed to meet the experimental objectives. These criteria should be determined in consultation with a specialist in laboratory animal medicine or with the veterinarian for the in-house animal colony. Consideration should be given to the animal data, the vendor's animal facilities, and the animals in transit.

A. Animal Data

A supplier should be able to provide data on the genetic background of each animal strain, which includes confirmation of the strain's integrity (Festing, 1974) as well as information concerning the strain's age, weight range, lifespan, behavioral peculiarities (such as docility or intractability), and availability. Depending on the duration and type of toxicological study, other desirable data may include a growth chart for use in detecting abnormal growth patterns, history of subtle subclinical abnormalities, historical data concerning the incidence of spontaneous tumors, disease problems such as enteritis, nephrosis, cardiomyopathy, and hydronephrosis, biochemical peculiarities, such as elevated serum lactic dehydrogenase (LDH) levels that may suggest the presence of latent diseases (Notkins, 1965; Riley, 1975, 1981), and number, type, and frequency of visible genetic mutations. These data are often affected by age and sex and should be employed accordingly.

Sources of historical information other than that provided by the supplier include published reports and information from other laboratories with experience involving the strain in question. However, data from other laboratories may be dissimilar (Clayson, 1962; *Toxicology Forum on Saccharin,* 1977; Sher, 1982).

B. Vendor's Animal Facilities

A visit to a potential vendor's animal facilities to evaluate the quality control program, husbandry techniques, health monitoring procedures, type of staff employed, and general appearance of the facilities may be desirable. Specific items of concern include environmental control, watering system, dietary factors, housing, and bedding.

To provide some degree of continuity and to minimize stress on the animals when they are first received from the vendor, environmental conditions (temperature, humidity, light cycle, and number of air changes per hour) and such husbandry procedures as the vendor's feeding schedules should be known by the purchaser. However, during the in-house quarantine period, several environmental factors may of necessity require gradual alteration to coincide with the experimental requirements.

The type of water surveillance in use at the vendor's facilities to monitor bacterial content (e.g., *Pseudomonas aeruginosa* and coliforms), possible chemical (e.g., halogenated hydrocarbons) or pesticide contamination, and concentration of calcium carbonate ($CaCO_3$; hardness) should be ascertained.

The supplier should provide information concerning the type of diet used (i.e., chow, open or closed formula, certified, cubes or ground), any changes in the source or type of diet, the feeding method (i.e., restricted intake or *ad lib.*), and whether the diet is monitored for bacteria or contaminants (e.g., heavy metals, mycotoxins, estrogenic activity, or pesticides). The vendor should also advise the purchaser of any rodenticides or insecticides used within the breeding facility because animals may inadvertently ingest or inhale these agents as a result of feed or bedding contamination or aerosolization.

Information concerning the type of housing (single or group) and bedding used by the supplier will be more relevant to some research programs than to others because bedding may be treated with or naturally contain enzyme inducers. Wood chip bedding should be analyzed for pentachlorophenol (PCP), a wood preservative used by the furniture industry.

C. Animals in Transit

Shipping procedures must be directed toward protecting the research animals from exposure to unwanted pathogens (e.g., sendai virus and *Mycoplasma* spp.) and minimizing shipment stress. Vendors will provide shipping containers of varied construction to withstand the rigors of travel. In addition, polyester fiber filters may be used to minimize the exposure of research animals to pathogenic organisms. Steps must be taken to reduce dehydration of research animals during transit (Weisbroth *et al.*, 1977).

Institutions and animal suppliers should have vans specifically equipped to transport laboratory animals in a fully controlled environment. Such vehicles should be easy to decontaminate and disinfect. The responsibility of the driver should not be limited solely to transporting animals. Ideally, the driver should be trained in all aspects of animal care and handling, via either an internal instructional program or one under the auspices of the Canadian Association for Laboratory Animal Science or the American Association for Laboratory Animal Science.

Ordering animals from more distant suppliers requires that the animals be shipped via public carrier, usually by airplane. A supplier should provide the flight number and times of departure and arrival to speed the collection of the animals at their destination because most airports do not have facilities to accommodate laboratory animals properly. Due to the occasional departure of public carriers from their schedules, the purchaser can request that public carrier personnel telephone upon the animals' arrival.

When laboratory animals are shipped via public carrier, their husbandry during transit is beyond the control of the supplier and the investigator, which is an area of continuing concern. Historically, there have been many instances in which animals were left without proper protection during inclement weather or containers were crushed and the animals asphyxiated; however, many countries have passed legislation to preclude such occurrences.

Once the available suppliers have been evaluated and one or two are selected who have the strain and quality of animal desired, it is necessary to order a few animals of different ages from a supplier and subject them to an intensive health screening program similar to that subsequently described. This aids in determining the effectiveness and reliability of the supplier's quality control program.

III. RECEIPT AND QUARANTINE

Ideally, to minimize the concerns of animal care, each animal facility should have a receiving and quarantine area for the exclusive use of incoming animals. Such a facility should be physically separated from the other animal housing facilities. The receiving area should have sufficient floor space to accommodate each animal shipment, as well as bench space, storage facilities, and equipment necessary for an adequate assessment of each animal's health. The design of the receiving area should include good ventilation and facilitate efficient and frequent cleaning and sanitizing operations. Use of sanitizing agents that jeopardize the integrity of the animal for research purposes is contraindicated.

The animal receiving area should be used primarily as a place to initially screen animals and reject those that are undesirable. The examining team might consist of the driver who received the animals at the vendor or airport, an animal technician, and a veterinarian or veterinary technician. A more detailed examination is conducted during the quarantine period.

Standard procedures used in the receiving area include counting, weighing, and examining the animals for overt signs of disease as well as for ectoparasites. Shipping containers should be examined for defects or damage and their contents scrutinized for signs indicative of diarrhea. Each animal should be examined for any other signs of disease. If the animals are clinically asymptomatic, they are transferred to a quarantine room.

The receiving area can then be thoroughly cleaned or sanitized. Disposable materials should be bagged, removed from the area, and stored or incinerated as dictated by in-house procedures and municipal requirements.

For most laboratory animals, the required quarantine period is 2–4 weeks; however, for feral animals and monkeys, up to 8 weeks may be required (Canadian Council on Animal Care, 1984). Once experience has demonstrated that a particular vendor provides quality animals, the animals may be moved directly to their test rooms following the initial observation. The quarantining of newly received animals is undertaken to provide a period in which the veterinarian can more extensively evaluate the animals' health and identify disease processes and etiological agents while minimizing their possible introduction into the colony. The veterinarian may use clinical laboratory tests and the pathologist's findings to assist in this endeavor. Selected use of prophylactic or therapeutic regimens should be undertaken only during the quarantine period, because such treatments are generally not compatible with many experimental protocols using rodents.

When a quarantine period is not used, several days must be set aside in order for the animals to adjust to their new environment while recovering from the stress of shipment (Weihe, 1965; Grant *et al.*, 1971; Sontag *et al.*, 1976).

Regardless of whether a quarantine period is or is not used, the following procedures should be implemented to reduce the inadvertent introduction and/or spread of communicable diseases within the facility.

1. House only one species in each room.

2. House similar species from different suppliers, or similar species from the same supplier shipped at different times, in different rooms. Ideally, separate rooms should also be used whenever a supplier ships animals from more than one of the supplier's animal production rooms, even though such animals may be contained in one shipment (Loew, 1980).

3. Thoroughly sanitize each room whenever a group of animals is removed.

4. Establish and adhere to procedures concerning the flow of personnel, supplies, and equipment. Ideally, all personnel attending the animals should either service only one group of animals or use protective clothing in an attempt to assure the integrity of each group (room) of animals (Loew, 1980).

5. Have 100% exhausted air with individual temperature and humidity controls monitored daily in each room (Fox, 1977).

6. Use monitoring devices on washing equipment to ensure that water temperature is appropriate (i.e., $>83°C/180°F$) for sanitation of test cages, cage racks, water bottles, and sipper tubes.

7. Ensure that used water bottles are never refilled; they should be washed and sanitized prior to reuse. Automatic watering systems must be checked daily to confirm their proper functioning. Water samples must be tested periodically for microbiological organisms and chemical contaminants.

8. Sponge walls weekly and wet-mop floors daily, preferably with a disinfectant, although some disinfectants may be contraindicated in certain situations. Walls and floors should also be monitored for the presence of microbiological organisms to determine efficiency of disinfec-

tants. Floor drains and waste containers require special attention because they act as microbiological reservoirs.

9. Have locker room facilities available to personnel to permit removal and storage of personal clothing, including shoes. Only suitable garments provided by the research facility should be worn in the animal rooms. Footwear should consist of safety shoes with steel toes and skid-resistant soles and heels. The prescribed footwear and outer garments should not be taken or worn outside the locker room and animal quarters, except when the garments are sent for laundering or during emergency situations that require evacuation of the animal facilities. In the latter situation, specific procedures must be established for reentry. Although a commercial laundry is acceptable for many experimental situations, in-house laundering of clothing contaminated with potentially toxic or carcinogenic agents is essential. Alternatively, disposable coveralls, gloves, head cover, mask or respirator, and shoe covers may be more appropriate.

10. Animals housed in shoe box cages should be transferred at least once a week to clean sanitized cages. The pullpapers under suspended wiremesh cages should be changed at least once a day and the cages sanitized every other week. Test chemicals that cause diuresis or diarrhea will necessitate alterations in these schedules.

11. Preventative maintenance on the ventilation system and other mechanical equipment should be scheduled and performed at prescribed intervals. Additionally, air filters and humidifiers should be changed or monitored at frequent intervals. Such "intrusions" into the test animal's environment should be recorded in appropriate log books.

12. In recent years, various types of laminar flow systems have been introduced in an attempt to provide "clean rooms", particularly for chronic studies. Air enters the room from the ceiling and is directed downward in a vertical, laminar flow fashion. The air is collected at the floor level and recycled through high efficiency particulate air (HEPA) filters prior to being reintroduced at the ceiling. Such systems are particularly useful for reducing the incidence of pulmonary lesions (Duprat *et al.*, 1983).

Unless caused by latent viruses, an outbreak of disease among animals within 3 days of their arrival is generally attributable to an endemic disease present in the supplier's colony. With such a short incubation time, it is unlikely that the animals were exposed to the disease in transit. However, a disease condition that may not have been clinically apparent in the vendor's colony can be activated by such in-transit stresses as cold, heat, or dehydration.

The initial step in implementing a quarantine program is the establishment of precise standard operating procedures (SOPs) to be followed upon receipt of the animals. Technicians executing the program should have a thorough understanding of all procedures to be followed, including who is to be contacted for problems beyond their responsibility.

The preexperimental acceptance testing to be conducted during the quarantine period can vary, depending on study objectives. However, the toxicologist, the veterinarian, and the laboratory animal care specialist together should define the acceptance testing program. One of the initial steps is to determine the number of additional animals to be ordered for the disease evaluation program, usually 10% in excess of study requirements. In addition to having the SOPs available prior to the arrival of the animals, it is necessary to have data recording sheets or microprocessor software available to record required data, ascertain that specimen acquisition was accomplished, etc.

Obviously, if some animals in the shipment appear to be ill upon arrival, they should be removed immediately and prepared for the examination described subsequently. If the animals appear healthy when received, they should be taken to the quarantine room. The animals used for the disease surveillance program should then be randomly selected from all the animals available and divided into two groups. Half the animals selected should be used in connection with the initial disease surveillance program conducted during the quarantine period, whereas the remaining half should be distributed equally among all treatment groups for subsequent disease surveillance. Although these animals are housed within the same room and racks as the test animals are, they should be designated as animals to be used only for purposes of disease surveillance. At preselected intervals (possibly quarterly or semiannually as appropriate), some proportion of these animals should be killed and examined in the same manner as those killed upon receipt.

Initial items to determine are an animal's body weight followed by an examination for ectoparasites, which, for rodents, include those listed in Table I. For nonhuman primates, such information as date and place of origin, details about previous tuberculosis testing, and previous medications administered to the animal is of interest. This is followed by clinical examinations, the frequency of which might be once a week throughout the quarantine period for feral animals and should include a review of some or all of the following items.

1. Eyes: Observe for discharge, inflammation, edema, presence of eyelashes; do photosensitivity and opthalmic evaluation.
2. Nares: Observe for discharge and inflammation.
3. Mouth: Observe for unusual salivation, color of mucous membrane,

Table I
Possible Ectoparasites in Rodents

Organism	Mouse	Rat
Mites		
Bdellonyssus bacoti	x	x
Myobia musculi	x	
Myocoptes musculinus	x	
Myocoptes romboutsi	x	
Notoedres muris		x
Psorergates simplex	x	
Radfordia affinis	x	
Lice		
Polyplax serrata	x	
Polyplax spinulosa		x

appearance of gingiva and tongue, and status of teeth. For nonhuman primates, the lesions of herpes B virus usually develop on the tongue, but the mucous membranes of the inner lips, gums, and conjuctiva can also be involved (Canadian Council on Animal Care, 1984).

4. Skin and hair coat: Observe for drying or flaking skin, erythema or pustular lesions, thinning or loss of hair, and hyperpigmentation.

5. Body/muscles: Observe general muscular development and tone, prominence of body protrusions, flexibility of joints, and hydration state.

6. Lymph glands: Palpate inguinal, axillary, popliteal, and submandibular nodes for enlargement or abnormalities.

7. Abdomen: Palpate for tenderness, organ enlargement or abnormalities, and excess fluid.

8. Heart and lungs: Evaluate heart and respiratory rate by stethoscopic ausculation.

9. Digits: Observe for arthritis, callous formation, and abnormalities of the nails and nail beds.

10. Body temperature.

11. Blood samples: Perform hematological evaluation including hemoglobin, hematocrit, RBC, WBC, differential counts, platelet counts, and coagulation screening test. In addition, nonhuman primate blood should be screened for parasites (see Chapter 18). Biochemistry profile is not often obtained during the initial health assessment; however, such clinical chemistry data may provide useful background information. Storage of excess sera in a sera bank may be useful as a future reference. For additional information, see Chapter 19.

12. Endoparasites: For nonhuman primates, which are obviously too

costly to kill for purposes of a disease surveillance program, collect and examine fecal and urine samples. However, rodents should be killed and examined for the endoparasites listed in Table II.

13. Pathogenic bacteria: Examine throat and fecal swabs for organisms in nonhuman primates; obtain samples for bacteriological evaluation from specific organs in rodents. Samples should include tracheal or nasopharyngeal washings for specific identification of *Mycoplasma* sp. and intestinal washings for identification of potential pathogens (Table III).

14. *Mycoplasma* organisms: Examine for *Mycoplasma pulmonis* (in lungs, trachea, uterus, middle ear) by culture and fluorescent antibody

Table II
Possible Endoparasites in Test Animals

Organism	Location[a]	Mouse	Rat	Monkey
Ancylostoma spp.	GI			x
Aspiculuris tetraptera	C, CA	x	x	
Balantidium spp.	GI			x
Capillaria hepatica	L	x	x	
Cysticercus fasciolaris	L (larval stage)	x	x	
Eimeria spp.	Epithelial cells of CA, C, I	x	x	
Entamoeba muris	C, CA, D, I, J	x	x	x
Eperythrozoon coccoides	Blood	x		
Esophagostomum spp.	GI			x
Giardia muris	CA, D, J	x	x	x
Haemobartonella muris	RBC	x	x	
Hepatozoon muris	L	x	x	
Heterakis spumosa	C, CA	x	x	
Hexamita muris	CA, D, I, J	x	x	
Hymenolepis diminuta	D, J	x	x	
Hymenolepis microstoma	D, L (bile ducts)	x		
Hymenolepis nana	D, I, J	x	x	
Klossiella muris	K	x		
Necator spp.	GI			x
Strongyloides	GI			x
Syphacia muris	C, CA	x	x	
Syphacia obvelata	C, CA	x	x	
Toxoplasma gondii	b	x	x	
Trichosomoides crassicauda	B, K, U		x	
Trypanosoma duttoni	Blood	x		
Trypanosoma lewis	Blood		x	

[a] B, bladder; CA, cecum; C, colon; D, duodenum; GI, gastrointestinal tract (stool); I, ileum; J, jejunum; K, kidney; L, liver; U, ureter; RBC, red blood cell.

[b] Cysts in reticuloendothelial and central nervous systems; trophozoites in epithelial cells and gut.

Table III
Possible Bacterial Pathogens in Test Animals

Organism	Location	Mouse	Rat	Monkey Throat swab	Monkey Rectal swab
Aeromonas spp.					x
Bacillus piliformis	Histological demonstration in liver sections	x	x		
Bordetella bronchiseptica	Lungs, bronchi, middle ear	x	x	x	
Campylobacter spp.					x
Citrobacter freundii	Colon	x			
Corynebacterium kutscheri	Nasopharynx, lungs, kidney, liver, lymph nodes	x	x		
Diplococcus pneumoniae				x	
Hemolytic E. coli					x
Hemophilus influenza				x	
Klebsiella pneumoniae	Lungs, other organs	x	x	x	
Mycobacterium tuberculosis				x	
Pasteurella multocida	Lungs, conjunctiva, bladder, skin, brain	x	x	x	
Pseudomonas pneumotropica	Lungs, nasopharynx, conjunctiva, uterus	x	x	x	
Pseudomonas aeruginosa	Majority of tissues, middle ear	x	x		
Salmonella (all types, especially *S. typhimurium* and *enteriditis*)	Lungs, liver, spleen, other organs	x	x		x
Shigella spp.					x
Staphylococcus aureus (coagulase +)	Cornea, lungs, conjunctiva	x	x	x	
Streptococcus group A, type 50 or type D	Lungs, liver digestive tract, cervical lymph nodes	x	x		
Streptococcus pneumonia	Lungs, nasopharynx, middle ear	x	x		
Streptobacillus moniliformis	Nasopharynx, middle ear, conjunctiva, articulations	x	x		

(FA) techniques, for *Mycoplasma arthritidis* by culture, and for other *Mycoplasma* spp.

15. Pathogenic fungi profile: Examine for *Microsporum* spp. and *Trichophyton* spp. on the skin and hair of both the mouse and rat.

16. Viral profile: Perform serological testing by complement fixation (CF), hemagglutination inhibition (HI) technique, enzyme-linked immunosorbent assay (ELISA), or indirect immunofluorescence (IFA) for the viral agents listed in Table IV. For rhesus monkeys, tuberculin testing or retesting should be undertaken; be concerned about such viruses as SV40, SV5, foaming virus, and herpesvirus simiae as well.

17. Histopathological review: Examine all major rodent organs (skin, eye, brain, trachea, lungs, heart, liver, kidney, spleen, intestine, reproductive tract, skeletal muscles, bone marrow, pancreas, adrenals, urinary bladder, central nervous system) and all grossly abnormal areas of dermal, supportive, or skeletal tissues.

18. Special techniques: Some inapparent infections may be activated by certain types of experimental manipulation, such as the use of surgical techniques or immunosuppressive agents. *Pseudomonas* infection in mice and rats may be activated by irradiation or immunosuppressive chemicals. *Hemobartonella muris* and *Eperythrozoon coccoides* are usually inapparent infections of limited pathogenicity that may be more apparent

Table IV
Possible Viral Organisms in Rodents

Organism	Mouse	Rat
Ectromelia (ECTRO)	x	
Encephalomyelitis (GDVII)	x	x
Kilham rat virus (KRV)		x
Lymphocytic choriomeningitis (LCM)	x	x
Minute virus of mice (MVM)	x	x
Mouse adenovirus (MAD)	x	
Mouse hepatitis (MHV)	x	
Papova virus (K virus)		
Pneumonia virus of mice (PVM)	x	x
Polyoma (Poly)	x	
Rat corona virus and sialodacryoadenitis virus (SDA)		x
Reovirus type 3 (REO-3)	x	x
Sendai (Send)	x	x
Toolan H-1 (H-1)		x
Epizootic diarrhea (EDIM)	x	
Cytomegalovirus (MCMV)	x	
Hantaal	x	x

following splenectomy, concurrent viral infection (e.g., MHV), or daily examination of Giemsa stained blood smears. Inapparent murine leukemia, cytomegalovirus, *Pneumocystis carinii,* and *Bacillus piliformis* may be activated by irradiation, prolonged administration of corticosteroids, and immunosuppressive agents (e.g., azathioprine).

19. Disease transmission studies: A disease process may have advanced to the point at which macrophage invasion is so extensive that the organism responsible for the condition cannot be identified histopathologically or by typical clinical laboratory techniques. In such a situation, one can identify the agent by inoculating an aliquot of a homogenate of the diseased tissue into a member of the same species that is free of the suspected organism. Subsequently, the inoculated animal needs to be killed for a definitive diagnosis.

20. Other considerations: The only animals that might not be examined in such detail are those to be used for an acute study with a short observation period. Ideally, however, it is preferable to incorporate a health monitoring program in all experimental protocols (see Chapter 17).

Equally important aspects of any disease surveillance – health monitoring program include such measures as:

1. ascertaining that various perishable supplies and reagents have not deteriorated or become contaminated and reordering all supplies in a timely and efficient manner on correct forms.

2. maintaining a schedule for cleaning the physical plant (e.g., animal rooms and receiving areas) and laboratory equipment (e.g., scales and pH meters).

3. maintaining a log of all chemical and clinical laboratory work undertaken, with details about who performed each test, as well as the test results, including blanks, standards, and controls, and ascertaining concurrently that all required work sheets are properly filled out and specimens properly labeled and stored.

4. undertaking a quality control program in which qualified individuals ascertain that all procedures have been performed and recorded according to the study protocol and SOPs.

IV. CONCLUDING COMMENTS

A disease surveillance program should be implemented prior to and during all toxicological tests. However, because of the resource (money and personnel) implications for toxicological tests of longer duration, such a program becomes mandatory. The objectives of such a program are obvious: early detection of latent diseases before they confound experimental results; minimization of the introduction of unwanted parasites and pathogens into the animal quarters; providing quality control data for each supplier of laboratory animals.

References

Arnold, D. L., Fox, J. G., Thibert, P., and Grice, H. (1978). Toxicology studies. I. Support personnel. *Food Cosmet. Toxicol.* **16**, 479–484.

Arnold, D. L., and Grice, H. (1978). The use of the Syrian hamster in toxicological studies, with emphasis on carcinogenesis bioassay. *Prog. Exp. Tumor Res.* **24**, 222–234.

Box, P. G. (1974). Standards for Procuring High Quality Animals for Research. *2nd Charles River Int. Symp. Lab. Anim. Milano, Italy.*

Canadian Council on Animal Care (1984). "*Guide to the Care and Use of Experimental Animals,*" Vol. II. Ottawa: Canadian Council on Animal Care.

Clayson, D. B. (1962). "Chemical Carcinogenesis," p. 55. London: Churchill.

Duprat, P., Jensen, R., Owen, R., Fabry, A., and Conquet, P. (1983). The effect of environment and environmental monitoring on toxicology studies. *In* "The Importance of Laboratory Animal Genetics, Health and the Environment in Biomedical Research" (E. C. Melby Jr. and M. W. Balls, eds.), pp. 183–191. New York: Academic Press.

Festing, M. F. (1974). Genetic reliability of commercially-bred laboratory mice. *Lab. Anim.* **8**, 265–270.

Fox, J. G. (1977). Clinical assessment of laboratory rodents on long term bioassay studies. *J. Environ. Pathol. Toxicol.* **1**, 199–226.

Grant, L., Hopkinson, P., Jennings, G., and Jenner, F. A. (1971). Period of adjustment of rats used for experimental studies. *Nature, London* **232**, 135.

Loew, F. M. (1980). Considerations in receiving and quarantining laboratory rodents. *Lab. Anim. Sci.* **30**, 323–329.

Notkins, A. L. (1965). Lactic dehydrogenase virus. *Bact. Rev.* **29**, 143–160.

Riley, V. (1975). Mouse mammary tumors: Alteration of incidence as apparent function of stress. *Science* **189**, 465–467.

Riley, V. (1981). Psychoneuroendocrine influences on immunocompetence and neoplasia. *Science* **212**, 1100–1109.

Sher, S. P. (1982). Tumors in control hamsters, rats and mice: Literature tabulation. *CRC Crit. Rev. Toxicol.* **10**, 49–79.

Sontag, J. M., Page, N. P., and Saffiotti, U. (1976). "Guidelines for Carcinogen Bioassay in Small Rodents" (DHEW Publ. No. (NIH) 76-801.) Washington, DC: Department of Health, Education and Welfare.

Toxicology Forum on Saccharin (1977). Omaha: University of Nebraska Medical Center.

Weihe, W. H. (1965). Temperature and humidity chromatograms for rats and mice. *Lab. Anim. Care* **15**, 18–28.

Weisbroth, S. H., Paganelli, P. G., and Salvia, M. (1977). Evaluation of a disposable water system during shipment of laboratory rats and mice. *Lab. Anim. Sci.* **27**, 186–194.

Additional Reading

Baker, H. J., Lindsay, J. R., and Weisbroth, S. H. (1979). "The Laboratory Rat." New York: Academic Press.

Benirschke, K., Garner, F. M., and Jones, T. C. (1978). "Pathology of Laboratory Animals," Volumes I & II. New York: Springer-Verlag.

Bhatt, P. N., Jacoby, R. O., Morse, H. C., New, A. E. (1986). "Viral and Mycoplasmal Infections of Laboratory Rodents - Effects on Biomedical Research." Orlando, Florida: Academic Press.

Bourne, G. N. (1975). "The Rhesus Monkey." New York: Academic Press.

Fiennes, R. N. (1972). "Pathology of Simian Primates." Basel: S. Karger.

Foster, H. L., Small, J. D., and Fox, J. G. (1981). "The Mouse in Biomedical Research." New York: Academic Press.

Fox, J. G. (1987). "Laboratory Animal Medicine." London: Academic Press.

Greene, C. E. (ed.) (1984). "Clinical Microbiological and Infectious Diseases of the Dog and Cat." Philadelphia: Saunders.

Hamm, T. E., Jr. (ed.) (1986). "Complications of Veral and Mycoplasmal Infections in Rodents to Toxicology Research and Testing." New York: Hemisphere.

Harkness, J. E., and Wagner, J. E. (1983). "The Biology and Medicine of Rabbits and Rodents." Philadelphia: Lea & Febiger.

Hine, J. M., and O'Donoghue, P. M. (1979). "Handbook of Diseases of Laboratory Animals." London: Heinemaisn.

Kalter, S. S. (1984). "Viral and Immunological Diseases in Non-Human Primates." New York: Alan R. Liss.

Melby, E. C., Jr., and Back, M. W. (1983). "Importance of Laboratory Animal Genetics, Health, and the Environment in Biomedical Research." London: Academic Press.

Needham, J. R. (1979). "Handbook of Microbiological Investigations for Laboratory Animal Health." New York: Academic Press.

Povey, R. C. (1985). "Infections and Diseases of Cats: A Clinical Handbook." Guelph, Ontario: Centaur Press.

Tuffery, A. A. (1987). "Laboratory Animals: An Introduction for New Experimenters." New York: Wiley.

Wallach, J. D., and Boeuer, W. J. (1983). "Diseases of Exotic Animals." Philadelphia: Saunders.

Part V
Conducting a Study

9
Oral Ingestion Studies

Douglas L. Arnold
Toxicology Research Division
Bureau of Chemical Safety
Food Directorate
Health Protection Branch
Health and Welfare Canada
Ottawa, Ontario

I. INTRODUCTION

From a historical perspective, there have traditionally been three major types of oral ingestion studies; acute, subchronic, and chronic. These studies are primarily differentiated by the length of time that the test substance is administered in the feed or drinking water, or via gavage. In the acute study, the test substance is either administered to the test animals as a single bolus dose or as a series of small doses during a 24-hour period. The animals are then observed during the next 14 days for toxic affects.

Subchronic rodent studies usually consist of several experiments. The initial studies require only a few days or weeks and are often termed subacute studies. The subsequent experiments require 90 to 120 days. A slight variation in this general format consists of feeding the test substance for X days followed by a recovery period of Y days during which only the control diet is fed. The objective of these studies is to ascertain the toxicological consequences of continuous dosing.

The chronic study encompasses a major portion of the test species lifespan, usually 18 months for mice and hamsters and 24 months for rats. The objective of the chronic study is to determine the long-term effects of continuous dosing.

A major concern with any test substance is whether it has tumorigenic potential. Consequently, a fourth type of oral ingestion study is the cancer bioassay, which is somewhat of a misnomer because the comparison is usually between the control (untreated) and treated groups versus a comparison between a test substance and a positive standard. A true cancer bioassay, wherein one group receives a positive "standard" carcinogen for comparison purposes, is seldom conducted due to economic and safety considerations. However, regulatory agencies allow those who submit toxicological data to combine the chronic study with the modern day version of the cancer bioassay. Such a study is usually entitled a chronic/carcinogenicity study. Developmental toxicity, reproductive, and metabolic studies are other types of oral ingestion studies that are discussed in subsequent chapters.

Acute, subchronic, and chronic/carcinogenicity studies are performed sequentially. Data gained from the acute experiment regarding toxicological affects (i.e., dose and effect information, target tissues and organs) are used in the design of the protocol for subchronic studies, whose data, along with that from other toxicological studies, are used to establish the protocol for the chronic/carcinogenicity study.

II. PRETEST CONSIDERATIONS FOR ORAL INGESTION STUDIES

A. Available Data

Prior to the administration of any test substance to an experimental animal, it is necessary to review all its toxicological, chemical, and physical properties. For a new test substance, the data may be limited to a quantification of impurities and its physical and reactive properties. A search of the scientific literature for data concerning chemicals of a similar structure may provide some indication of potential toxicological effects. A note of caution however: the reduction of a specific double bond with a chemical like aflatoxin reduces its tumorigenic potential by 150 times (Wogan and Shank, 1971).

B. Purity and Stability Data

Prior to the start of any toxicological testing program, the purity and stability of a test substance must be ascertained. It is necessary to determine the stability of a test substance and its impurities under various storage conditions as well as within the dosing media. Although such an undertaking is relatively straightforward for a food additive containing a few minor impurities, this task can be quite complex when pesticide formulations, cosmetics, or other consumer products of diverse composition are tested. Impurities have on occasion been suspected or found to contribute to toxicological findings (Moore and Courtney, 1971; Weil et al., 1973; Toth et al., 1977; Arnold et al., 1983); consequently, a different synthesis procedure or a reformulation of a product can dramatically affect toxicological findings. Conversely, the procedure used to synthesize or formulate a product for toxicological testing may be different from the one used during the pilot plant portion of the developmental process or from the synthesis–formulation procedures used for the commercial preparation, which may introduce, reduce, or delete other impurities.

C. Species Selection

Ideally, the species used for testing should metabolize and excrete the test substance in a similar manner to humans (Weil, 1972; International Agency for Research on Cancer, 1980). However, metabolic data from humans are seldom available until the toxicological testing or safety evaluation program is nearing completion.

The mouse, rat, and dog are the usual species selected for oral ingestion studies, but the rodent is the predominant species for the following reasons.

1. Economics: low purchase and housing costs allow for the use of a relatively large sample size, thereby enhancing statistical sensitivity.
2. Historical data: a considerable amount of biochemical and pathological information is available regarding rodents that served as control animals in previous tests. Spontaneous tumor incidence data are particularly important when data are evaluated from studies in which a change in the apparent incidence rate and/or time of appearance of

the spontaneous tumors was the major toxicological affect (Tarone *et al.*, 1981; Task Force of Past Presidents, 1982; Clayson, 1987). Studies in which the incidence rate of spontaneous tumors is "high" are almost impossible to evaluate and are often considered flawed because of the "background noise".

3. Husbandry: rodents are amenable to frequent handling (Arnold *et al.*, 1977) and dosing by gavage. Their inability to vomit is a useful characteristic.

One disadvantage of using some rodent species is that they are coprophagous animals. Such a practice results in the test animal receiving more than the intended amount of test substance and/or its metabolites, which may alter intestinal flora or result in the induction of various enzymes. Such happenings complicate the assessment of any dose-effect relationship and extrapolation of the findings to humans.

The monkey is increasingly being used in toxicological feeding studies. Supporting rationale for its use often includes its phylogenetic proximity to humans. However, there is little metabolic evidence to suggest that the monkey is a more relevant surrogate for humans than rodents are because the monkey is a herbivore. Some have concluded that monkeys are unsuitable surrogates for evaluating the toxicity of many agents (Gehring *et al.*, 1973). Regardless of the species chosen, whenever there is a marked interspecies or sexual difference with respect to toxicological responses to a test substance, studies should be undertaken to determine the "cause" of the difference prior to the initiation of any chronic studies.

D. Test Species' Age

In general, the use of rapidly growing or young adult animals when the study is initiated is appropriate. The potential use or exposure of the test substance to animals of a specific age group may be dictated; that is, specific drugs or consumer products may be used only for infants or adults.

Determining an animal's precise age is often difficult. Most researchers working with rodents attempt to circumvent this problem by using test animals within a specific weight range.

E. Mode of Test Substance Administration

Administration of test substances in the acute and some shorter-term oral ingestion studies is usually via gavage, but administration in feed or drinking water or via capsule is occasionally done. Gavaging requires a reasonable amount of skill when young animals are used. The advantage of gavage administration is knowing the precise amount of test substance administered. Gavage administration is often the only alternative for test substances having a very high vapor pressure; it reduces the contamination of the laboratory environment (Fox and Helfrich-Smith, 1980; Keene and Sansone, 1984; Sansone and Fox, 1977; Sansone *et al.*, 1977) and is useful for nonpalatable substances. However, prolonged gavaging of test animals may lead to secondary stress-related responses. The experience of the U.S. National Cancer Institute/National Toxicology Program (NTP) has also shown that the vehicle and/or the volume of vehicle used during chronic gavage studies may have appreciable effects on study results and their interpretation (Nutrition Foundation, 1983; National Toxicology Program, Board of Scientific Counselors, 1984).

When the gavaging technique is used for acute tests, the feed is withheld for a period of time prior to dosing, allowing the animal's stomach to empty. Typically, feed is withheld from the rabbit and rat for 12–16 hr, the mouse and hamster for 4–6 hr, and the dog for 20–24 hr. (National Academy of Sciences, 1977). Feed withdrawal is an attempt to reduce the interanimal variation because a full digestive tract will alter absorption and, eventually, the pharmacokinetic characteristics of a test substance following its bolus administration (see Chapter 13). However, in some situations, fasting also increases the toxicity (i.e., lower LD_{50} value) of orally administered drugs (Kast and Nishikawa, 1981).

Administration of the test substance in known amounts to a larger animal can be accomplished by use of a gelatin capsule, and monkeys can be trained to self-administer their own doses. Maintaining the integrity of the gelatin capsule requires the preparation of a nonaqueous dosing solution based on the solubility properties of the test substance and the use of a flavoring agent to mask the taste of the test substance.

For the preparation of aqueous dosing solutions, the chemicals' solubility in water may be enhanced by a slight rise in temperature or alteration in the pH. Carboxymethylcellulose, acacia, or tragacanth may also be beneficial for preparing a suspension, but emulsions with vegetable oils or lecithin may not be completely satisfactory if homogenous mixtures cannot be maintained until the dosing process is completed. Lipid-soluble compounds are best administered in vegetable oil or polyethylene glycol, however, their volumes should be minimized due to laxative and possible biological effects (Nutrition Foundation, 1983; National Toxicity Program, Board of Scientific Counselors, 1984). Solvents such as alcohol, glycerine, and glycols (Davidow and Hagan, 1955) as well as various thickening and suspending medias (National Academy of Sciences, 1975; Zbinden, 1979) may exert their own pharmacological and biochemical activities and should be avoided. More recently, microencapsulation is favored for some experimental situations (Melnick et al., 1987).

The volume of a dosing solution should not exceed 10 ml/kg of body weight per day for a rodent and preferably should be in the 5 ml/kg of body weight or less range. With larger volumes, the stomach's capacity _nay be exceeded and some of the dosing solution will either end up in the intestine or be aspirated into the lungs due to the back pressure during the gavaging process.

When the diet is used as the dosing media, it usually consists of a commercial "mash" or ground commercial cubes so that a more uniform composition is obtained. The alternative of coating the outside of the cubes with the test substance is a less desirable method. Because of the mash's powdery nature, it is often necessary to add corn oil as a dust suppressant at a level up to 4%. The mash may be repelleted, but this may alter heat-labile nutrients and/or the test substance (i.e., heat degradation, evaporation, interaction with various nutrients, etc.). For test materials whose physical properties are such that they are not easily dispersed in the feed, it may be necessary to first dissolve the test substance in an organic solvent or oil in order to achieve homogeneous mixing. In such situations, the diet will require sufficient mixing to ensure homogeneity and allow for vaporization of the organic solvent. Care must be taken to ensure that the solvent and test substance do not covolatize and that the control diet is prepared in a similar fashion.

Although it is not a common practice to administer test substances in drinking water, the administration of beverages and beverage components may dictate the use of drinking water as a vehicle. Occassionally, practical necessity dictates the use of drinking water also. Regardless of the administration mode, homogeneity of mixing and test substance stability should be ascertained by analysis at appropriate intervals.

In most oral ingestion studies, the feed and water are supplied *ad libitum*. However, to ascertain the amount of test substance ingested, there is a need to quantitate the amount of vehicle (feed or water) consumed. This task is not facilitated by rodents that tend to spill their feed, by monkeys that often throw their feed out of their cage, or by many watering bottles currently available. In addition, as a consequence of *ad libitum* feeding, most test animals tend to become obese as they get older. Some regulatory agencies have begun to question whether *ad libitum* feeding during rodent studies is appropriate for toxicological tests, especially long-term ones (Department of Health and Social Security, 1982). This question arose from nutritional studies that clearly demonstrated that a reduction in caloric intake results in lower body weight with less body fat, lower incidence of spontaneous tumors, and increased longevity

(Ross, 1961; Ross et al., 1970; Ross and Bras, 1971; Nolen, 1972). However, caloric restriction may also lead to a reduction in the incidence of some induced tumors (Tannenbaum and Silverstone, 1957).

F. Pharmacokinetics

The bolus dose inherent with gavaging raises concerns about the administered volume, differential uptake of the test substance from aqueous as opposed to nonaqueous solutions, and any associated pharmacokinetic and metabolic alterations. There are quantitative data to indicate that continued use of the gavaging technique alters toxicological manifestations of chemicals when compared to dietary administration (Arnold et al., 1979; Weil et al., 1973); which may be due in part to induction of metabolic enzymes, (Nutrition Foundation, 1983; National Toxicology Program, Board of Scientific Counselors, 1984).

Absorption of test substances from oils is thought to proceed in a manner similar to other lipophilic substances wherein the lipophilic substance is first solubilized by the bile salts. Absorption is presumed to be passive and dependent on a concentration gradient established at the enterocyte membrane (Nutrition Foundation, 1983). Unlike aqueous solutions that are absorbed into the portal systems and immediately pass through the liver ("first pass effect" at which time they may be detoxified or enzymatically altered), lipophilic solutions are transported via the mucosal lymphatic system and enter the systemic circulation via the superior cava. Therefore, a significant portion of a test substance administered in oil may not pass through the liver during its initial or first pass circulation within the animal via the portal system, thereby exposing target organs to concentrations of the test substance different from those that would occur if it were administered in an aqueous solution. Withey et al. (1983) also found a significant decrease in the rate and extent of uptake of low molecular weight alphatic chlorinated hydrocarbons administered in an oil solution as opposed to an aqueous solution. For additional information, see Chapter 13.

G. Dose Selection

The selection of appropriate doses for any toxicity study is a demanding proposition, especially as study duration increases (International Life Sciences Institute, 1984). Care must be taken to ensure that the high dose level does not exceed the homeostatic capabilities of the test animal to metabolize, transport, and excrete the test substance. When the capacity to perform these functions is exceeded, artifactual responses can occur. Ideally, the doses in most toxicological studies are usually uniform multiples or are logarithmically spaced. As a general rule, the top dose level should induce a toxicological effect and the lowest dose should be a reasonable multiple above the anticipated human exposure. The magnitude of the multiple will vary depending on whether a drug, food additive, or environmental contaminant is being tested. Although the highest dose employed should result in toxic effects, it makes little sense to feed relatively innocuous substances at excessively high dosages simply to induce toxic effects. Generally, the highest dose level should not exceed 5% of the diet. For the test substance that has no nutritive value, there is concern about nutrient dilution; for substances that have nutritive value, there is concern about imbalancing the diet. If it is necessary to administer large amounts of a test substance in the diet, a semipurified diet should be considered because its composition can be modified to a greater extent without adversely affecting nutritional quality than a chow diet can. When the concentration of the test substance in the diet is so high, making the diet nutritionally imbalanced, the resulting state of malnutrition can cause a variety of blood and organ changes undistinguishable from those observed with some drugs (Zbinden, 1963).

For dietary studies, the test substance can be included as a constant percentage (w/w) of the diet or at a concentration that provides a consistent mg of test substance intake per kg of body weight. The latter requires weighing the animals and adjusting the concentration of the test substance in the diet on a weekly basis for the first 3 or 4 months of the study then at least biweekly thereafter. The major difference between the two procedures is that when animals are fed at a constant dietary percentage, their intake of the test substance is much higher per kg of body weight during the animals' most rapid growth phase. A similar situation also occurs in developmental studies in which the lactating rat will ingest considerable more feed during the initial week of lactation than during the final week. However, adjusting dietary concentrations in the lactating situation presents a concern regarding data interpretation and extrapolation because lactating humans also increase their food consumption.

H. Frequency of Dosing

As with the route of dosing, the frequency of dosing should be similar to that of humans. For drugs, the anticipated dosing schedule may be known and a dosing frequency for the test animals devised, but seldom are animals dosed more than once a day. Food additives or contaminants may be ingested throughout the day (noncaloric sweeteners contained in beverages and snacks), in bolus dosages periodically during meals (solvents and other materials that may migrate from food packaging materials), or in feed in which additives can be only guessed at (pesticides on produce due to the availability of fresh produce in North American markets throughout the year from many sources). However, for studies in which the test substance is added to the diet, there is general concurrence that it be administered continuously for the duration of the study. It should be noted that rodents normally ingest their feed by "continuous nibbling," whereas humans usually ingest their food as discrete meals. For materials administered by capsule or gavage, some have indicated that an acceptable practice is not to administer them on the weekends for economic reasons (Zbinden, 1963). Simplistically, such a scheme results in a 28.6% decrease in exposure as well as a 48-hour recovery period each week. Some have attempted to modify the situation by determining the quantity of test substance that would be consumed during a seven-day period and divide it into five equal doses. This purely mathematical procedure cannot be recommended as acceptable methodolgy (Benitz, 1970). The greater quantity of test substance administered with each of the five dosages, as opposed to the seven, may have significant pharmacological implications for a myriad of test substances (see Chapter 13).

I. Housing

Many animals used for toxicological testing live in a colony type of situation in their natural habitat. Consequently, some toxicologists suggest that individually housed animals are more "stressed" than those housed in groups, and such stress may result in artifactual toxicological effects (Balazs et al., 1962; Hatch et al., 1963; Steplewski et al., 1987; Wiberg et al., 1966). Although this may be true for nonhuman primates that have been captured in the wild, standard laboratory rodents have been housed in a laboratory environment for an extensive number of generations and the practice of handling laboratory rodents frequently appears to have overcome some of these problems (Arnold et al., 1977). In addition to the statistical considerations, in which the cage is used as the experimental unit (see Chapter 7), individual housing has several advantages, as indicated in Chapter 17. In addition, the animals' macro- and microenvironmental considerations should not be overlooked (Fox, 1977; Weihe, 1971; Lane-Petter, 1963).

J. Quality Control

One aspect of most toxicological studies that may not receive sufficient attention is the quality of the animal received from the vendor (see Chapter 8; Fox et al., 1979).

III. THE RANGE FINDING TEST

Test substances can be arbitrarily divided into two types: (1) the "new" test substance for which toxicological data is essentially nonexistent and (2) the test substances for which some toxicological data exists but additional data are required. The following discussion primarily involves the testing of new chemicals. Each test substance should be recognized as a unique entity, and the toxicological testing program developed for it should be customized. Rigid adherence to standardized protocols for toxicological testing is discouraged. However, the design of any toxicological test is often a compromise between an all-encompassing experiment and those components that can be practically achieved in view of time and resource constraints (Zbinden, 1963).

Previously, with a new test substance, a range finding study was conducted prior to initiation of an acute study, which has become somewhat synonymous with the determination of the median lethal dose (Davidow and Hagan, 1955; "PMA takes position," 1983) or the LD_{50} (i.e., that dose of a test substance resulting in lethality to 50% of the test population). The LD_{50} concept was originally proposed by Trevan in 1927. The test was developed as a biological method for standardization of drug potency. The drugs tested included digitalis extracts, insulin, cocaine, and diptheria toxin. In the intervening years for reasons that are not apparent, there seemed to be a need to determine an LD_{50} for a multitude of chemicals. Due to the biological variability within any test population, determination of an LD_{50} value is associated with some degree of uncertainty (Müller and Kley, 1982). Therefore, the LD_{50} value is always listed in the toxicological literature as a numerical value with a calculated confidence limit. However, many seem to have forgotten that the quantitation of LD_{50} results are only attempts to provide relative rankings for substances that elicit a spectrum of biological responses that include lethality. Trevan (1927) realized that LD_{50} values are not absolute or constant in the same manner as a chemical's physical properties are. In addition to the sample size effecting the LD_{50} confidence limits, there are numerous reports about differences attributable to strain (genetics; Brown, 1964), to environmental variables, and to protocol practices (Craver et al., 1950; Allmark, 1951; Griffith, 1964; Balazs, 1970; Hunter et al., 1979).

A range finding study provides general information on a test substance's acute clinical manifestations and relative lethality so that an appropriate dose range can be selected for the acute study. Currently, the emphasis is to diminish the use of the acute test for the "accurate" determination of an LD_{50} or ED_{50} value in lieu of more thorough evaluation of toxicological manifestations (Sperling, 1976; Griffin, 1981; Rowan, 1981; Zbinden and Flury-Roversi, 1981; Baß et al., 1982; Müller and Kley, 1982; Schütz and Fuchs, 1982; Weil, 1983; Gad et al., 1984; Uvarov, 1984; Rowan and Goldberg, 1985; Zbinden, 1986). However, for some chemicals in commerce, there is still a requirement to determine an LD_{50} value for safety labeling purposes (Rowan, 1981; Zbinden, 1986).

Most toxicologists agree that any test substance that is not lethal when administered acutely at a concentration of 5 g/kg of body weight is essentially not toxic (Hodge and Sterner, 1949; Gleason et al., 1957). Consequently, the initial dose in a dose ranging study might be 2 g/kg of body weight; however, greater caution should be exercised for test substances that are caustic, acidic, or suspected irritants. For the most efficient use of test animals, one should dose only two to three animals of each sex at this level then observe the animals for toxicological manifestations. If a lethal dose has been administered, the animals will usually die within 24–72 hours. With nonlethal doses, the animals should be observed for at least 14 days after dosing and possibly for 21 days for evidence of delayed toxic effects. If consecutive dosage levels are then chosen based on the previous results, the time to complete the range finding study is excessively prolonged; therefore, the use of two to three animals of each sex per dose up to four widely spaced dosages is a reasonable compromise.

The test substance is administered via gavage to randomly selected animals from the available test population whose feed, but not water, has been removed for a period of time, as previously mentioned. The dose or dosing solution is prepared according to the anticipated procedures for the acute study. The animals' weights are determined so that animals of different weights are dosed at the desired concentration (X g of test substance/kg of body weight). Following dosing, an animal is returned to its cage with ad libitum access to feed and water. A monitoring program is immediately initiated at 15- to 30-minute intervals after dosing. The interval between observations should increase during the postdosing period. By the end of the two-week observation period, a minimum of two to three observations per day may suffice. The observation period may be extended if signs of delayed toxicity become evident. Each observation period should include handling the animal while examining it for various clinical signs of toxicity and behavioral change(s). Additionally, body weight and feed consumption are determined at least weekly, and all observed clinical signs followed to ascertain whether they are reversible. Time of onset and/or reversibility must be accurately recorded.

All animals should be necropsied. For animals dying within the first 24 hours after gavaging, particular attention should be given to the esophagus for signs of perforation and to the lungs for signs of blood and/or dosing solution. Occasionally, blood will appear in the nostrils of an animal whose esophagus has been perforated. Extra animals should be available to replace any animals that may be accidentally killed. Histological examination of the tissues, particularly in the high dose group, may help to identify the major target organs.

IV. THE ACUTE TEST

The number of animals to be used for an acute test will be a function of the mathematical procedure chosen to calculate the LD_{50} value (Deichmann and LeBlanc, 1943; Armitage and Allen, 1950; Horn, 1956; Schütz and Fuchs, 1982; Bruce, 1987; van Noordwijk and van Noordwijk, 1988) and/or the accuracy desired (Trevan, 1927). Most procedures require a minimum of four or five dose levels with three to five animals per dose, whereas older methods prescribe up to ten animals per dose. The larger test groups will improve the accuracy of the LD_{50} value and will be more typical of the test population at large.

Dose levels are chosen to cover the 10% to 90% mortality range because some mathematical tests do not allow for the inclusion of zero or 100% mortality results. Doses are often spaced at log intervals for most LD_{50} calculation procedures.

The objectives of the acute study are to:

1. determine the relative acute toxicity (LD_{50} value) of the test substance for comparison with other chemicals and/or for labeling purposes;
2. determine the clinical manifestations elicited by the test substance;
3. determine which organ or organ systems are affected;
4. determine the relative minimal lethal dose;
5. determine the slope of the dose-response curve (when the toxic effect, in this case lethality, is plotted against dose);
6. determine the danger of accidental ingestion of a large quantity of drug or test substance (compare "PMA takes position," 1983; British Toxicology Society, 1984);
7. provide assistance in the determination of a dose range for the repeat dose studies to follow (National Technical Information Service, 1980).

The acute study itself is conducted in a similar manner to the range finding study.

1. The feed is withdrawn, but access to water is allowed.
2. The animals are weighed just prior to dosing.
3. The dosing formulation is prepared.

4. The animals are dosed and returned to their cages with *ad libitum* access to feed and water.
5. The animals are observed frequently for the first few hours then three or four times a day during the remainder of the observation period, which should last at least 14 days. Behavioral tests may be undertaken (Gad, 1982). The time of onset, severity, and duration of all toxic signs and manifestations are recorded. Typical items for observation include animal motor activity, respiration character and rate, salivation, anorexia, vomiting in nonrodent species, changes in excrement, changes in the condition of coat, changes in posture, pupillary reaction, discharge from lacrimal glands, discharge from urinary and intestinal tracts, and changes in pulse and heart rates in larger animals (see Chapter 17).
6. All animals are necropsied and the survivors of the highest dose should be histologically examined as should all that succumb after 72 hours on test.

V. REPEATED DOSING STUDIES

A. The 14- to 28-Day Study

The 14- to 28-day study is the initial in a series of studies wherein a test substance is administered repeatedly and usually daily. It provides the first substantive indication of how rapidly an animal is able to metabolize and excrete the test substance. Consequently, the purposes of this study are to:

1. determine if there is cumulative toxicity;
2. determine what organ system(s) is/are affected;
3. determine if there are toxicological manifestations in addition to those seen during the acute study;
4. determine the dosages (i.e., toxic and with no apparent effect) for the 90-day study.

A minimum of three dose groups plus a control group is required, but four or five dosage levels should probably provide more than a proportional increase in toxicological information. Each sex is treated as a separate experiment, and the dosages are often different between the sexes. The top dose should result in some toxicological affects, whereas there should be no apparent toxicological effect from the lowest dose.

During the conduct of the study, data concerning feed and water consumption and body weight gain should be collected. In addition, the typical observations performed during the acute study should also be undertaken. Upon termination, the animal's weight should be determined and one of several options should be chosen in an attempt to characterize the toxicological effects.

1. Obtain blood samples from each animal for hematological and clinical chemistry evaluation; necropsy all animals and determine the weight of the major organs. Initially, to enhance efficiency, one might conduct only histopathological evaluations on the high dose and control animals. If treatment-related histopathological effects are observed in the animals on the highest dose, then the animals of the next to the highest dose and so forth are examined until no treatment effects are found.
2. Euthanize half the test animals and perform the tasks indicated in the previous option. Feed the remaining animals control diet for a period of time to ascertain whether the various toxicological effects are reversible, which is termed a reversibility study. At the end of this observation period, the animals should be evaluated as stated in the first option.
3. As a variation of option two, sacrifice some animals, usually five per group, and determine the concentration of the test substance and/or its metabolite(s) in selected organs. Give the remaining animals the control diet for a period of time. This option is more analytical in nature than the second. Upon completion of this observation period, the analytical procedures as well as those procedures indicated in the first option are repeated.

When a dose-response curve is plotted, the data are often such that the highest dose may occassionally result in a less or a more severe toxicological effect than is predicted by the lower doses. Such observations may be due in part to such competing factors as a lack of nutrition due to dietary dilution or unpalatability of the test substance in the diet; secondary toxicological effects may be due to the higher dose (i.e., metabolic overload) or to physiological or pharmacological stresses.

B. The 90-Day Study

In a 90-day study, the dosage levels are often lower than those in a 14- to 28-day study. For chemicals like saccharin, which are metabolically inert and readily excreted, there will be only minimal differences between the dose levels and the cumulative toxicity effects observed in the 28- and 90-day studies. However, for substances that bioaccumulate (i.e., their concentration in body tissues increases with time on test), like heavy metals and halogenated hydrocarbons, there will be significant increases in the toxicological effects at similar dose levels with increasing study duration. Pharmacokinetic studies are useful in this regard, but their duration are often of insufficient length to indicate the full extent of bioaccumulation.

As dose levels decrease in these longer studies, toxicological effects may become more subtle. Consequently, with the advent of micromethods for evaluating hematological and clinical biochemistry parameters (see Chapters 18 and 19), it is not uncommon for periodic blood and/or urine samples to be obtained. However, even with the availability of micromethods, the stress inherent in animal capture and the attainment of specimens at periodic intervals should dictate the use of a satellite group for sampling to preclude synergistic effects between stress and toxicological effects. One advantage of monitoring the same animal continuously is that a consistent outlier can be more easily dealt with during data evaluation. Conversely, pathological and/or other differences between the satellite and nonsatellite groups may complicate data evaluation.

A major objective of this study, like the 28-day study, is the determination of an apparent no-effect dose and the establishment of dosages for the next study in the sequence. As with all toxicological studies, the highest dose level should induce a frank toxicological effect when administered at a reasonable dosage (i.e., ≤5% of the diet).

The three possible options listed for the 28-day study should also be considered when the 90-day study is complete. Parameters monitored during subchronic studies often include most of the following: immunological and neurological behavioral testing; organ function testing or other physiological monitoring; biochemical testing in addition to serum chemistry; hematological evaluation; urinary analysis; ophthalmologic evaluation; as well as food and water intake, body weight determination; and clinical observations. Postmortem aspects include gross observations, bone marrow and spleen assessments, organ weights, and light and/or electron microscopy.

VI. THE CHRONIC TOXICITY AND CANCER BIOASSAY STUDIES

There are essentially two types of long-term feeding studies, as previously described in the introduction. A third type is the two-generation protocol wherein the female parent is fed the test substance for approximately three to four months prior to breeding on a one-to-one basis with a male parent receiving the same treatment. Test substance administration is continued throughout breeding, gestation, and nursing. Consequently, the infant is exposed to the test substance and the dam's metabolites *in utero* and via the breast milk until weaning (Grice *et al.,* 1981). Such a testing protocol may be pragmatically appropriate because humans are exposed to many xenobiotics from conception until death.

One of the most difficult decisions in the design of a chronic toxicity/ carcinogenicity study is the selection of appropriate dosages, particularly the highest dose level (International Life Sciences Institute, 1984). Two concerns in this regard are survivability and decreased weight gain.

Survivability The doses for the chronic toxicity/cancer bioassay should be so chosen that there is no statistical significant differences between the survivability among test groups, other than for a carcinogenic or tumorigenic response. If survivability is significantly lower in the treated groups than in the controls for reasons other than carcinogenicity, there is a possibility that the test animals may not survive the latent period, especially if the test substance is a weak carcinogen.

Decreased weight gain Ideally, one is attempting to administer the test compound at the highest dose possible without exceeding the generally accepted guidelines concerning decreased weight gain; that is, growth rate in the test group should not be suppressed more than 10% of the control group's during the duration of the study (International Agency for Research on Cancer, 1980). As previously noted, a decreased weight gain resulting from a caloric restriction due to a lack of palatability or dilution of the diet by the test substance may result in a decreased incidence of spontaneous and possible treatment-induced tumors.

More recently, various agencies have been recommending that such additional parameters as pathological alterations and clinical laboratory measurements also should be considered in the dose-selection process of the highest maximum tolerated dose (MTD; National Toxicity Program, Board of Scientific Counselors, 1984; U.S. Interagency Staff Group on Carcinogens, 1986). One problem in this regard is the lack of an accepted definition for MTD (Haseman, 1985).

Three treated groups and a control group are the minimal number of groups required for an acceptable chronic toxicity study; however, the use of mathematical models to quantify risk have a greater sensitivity when more groups are included on the response portion of the dose-response curve.

Prior to the finalization of any chronic study protocol, it is highly desirable that the following information be available.

1. The test animals' ability to absorb, excrete, and metabolize the test substance following single and multidosing regimes (i.e., pharmacokinetic study results).

2. The tissues or organ systems in which the test substance or its metabolites accumulate and/or result in histopathological damage, to include excessive cellular proliferation.
3. Whether the metabolic/excretion "patterns" change as the amount of test substance administered increases; that is, is the animal able to metabolize the test substance in the manner seen at lower dosages, or are new metabolites found, or is a higher percentage of the administered dose excreted unchanged? When either of these changes occur, the administered dose has resulted in a "metabolic overload", and the metabolic break point has been exceeded. Usually, the metabolic break point should not be exceeded. If humans are found to metabolize the test substance in a manner analogous to exposing the test species to dosages that exceed the test species' metabolic break point, then it is appropriate to include such a dosage group in the study. However, this author is unaware of any chemical that illustrates this point.
4. The results from the shorter-term feeding studies, the reproductive and teratogenic studies, as well as the results from any satellite studies conducted for the purpose of mechanism elucidation.

Many guidelines for a chronic study outline that studies in which mice and rats are used should last for a minimum of 18 and 24 months, respectively, and that the survival rate at this time must be at least 50%, with unscheduled losses (due to autolysis, "lost animals", etc.) being less than 10% (International Agency for Research on Cancer, 1980) to encourage good husbandry techniques. Recently, a controversy has arisen in the scientific literature regarding the duration of a chronic toxicity study for drugs. Apparently, in an attempt to reduce the confounding of study results arising from spontaneous tissue lesions due to aging and/or environmental factors, some regulated institutions are seeking to have the duration of the chronic studies reduced to 12 months or less whereas others maintain that nonneoplastic, pathological lesions have been found to have a latent period of more than one year (Frederick, 1986; Lumley and Walker, 1985, 1986). Although 6- to 12-month studies are of sufficient duration to detect most toxic effects, they are not of sufficient duration to encompass the latent period for most tumorigenic/carcinogenic test substances.

Parameters to be monitored during a chronic study will depend on the objectives of the study. If invasive techniques, like blood sampling, are required or stressful situations, such as the use of metabolic cages, are necessary, the inclusion of satellite groups specifically for this purpose should be part of the experimental design. The minimal number of parameters that should be followed during a chronic study include:

1. Body weight: preferably weekly, but weekly for the first 13 to 15 weeks

on test then biweekly for the next 30 to 40 weeks and monthly thereafter is generally viewed as a minimal monitoring requirement.
2. Feed or water consumption: individual consumption is the most useful
   for health monitoring and study evaluation considerations. They
   should be determined at similar intervals as body weight.
3. Clinical examinations: maintenance of a clinical file for each animal is
   needed to follow the course of any disease or toxic state and is required
   by the pathologist during the gross and microscopic evaluation (see
   Chapter 17).
4. Pathological examination: gross necropsy and microscopic evaluation
   are needed (see Chapter 20).

The last component of any toxicological test is summarization of data,
with evaluation and extrapolation of the findings to humans. As pointed
out in Chapter 25, various considerations inherent in the design of an
experiment will have a direct bearing on the interpretation of experimental results.

VII. CONCLUDING COMMENTS

In the framework of toxicological testing, oral ingestion studies encompass a series of tests whose primary differentiation involves duration.
The final study is the chronic/carcinogenicity study that involves a major
portion of the test species' lifespan and, from a regulatory point of view,
may be the feeding study with the greatest implications for human
exposure and health.

The magnitude of any toxicological study is limited by resources. More
recently, ethical concerns about animal usage have resulted in a con-
certed effort to obtain more quality information from each test animal
and to monitor ever more subtle parameters as opposed to such quantal
responses as mortality. Concurrently, study personnel are now better
qualified to undertake these tasks, and their efforts have been aided by
various technological advances described throughout this text.

In the future, we will probably see this evolutionary process continue
in the direction of monitoring ever increasing subtle toxicological
changes at dosage levels more closely approximating human exposure
concentrations. Technological advances will probably permit multiana-
lyte determinations from a single small specimen. Such technology will
require less operator involvement, hopefully less stress on the experimental animal due to the smaller specimen required, and dramatic increases
in the amount, quality, and validity of toxicological data. However, the
ability of electronic gadgetry to quantify and analyze an ever increasing
array of items with greater accuracy may have some limitations regarding
extrapolation of such results to the ultimate test species — humans.

References

Allmark, M. G. (1951). A collaborative study on the acute toxicity testing of several drugs. *J. Am. Pharm. Assoc.* **40**, 27–31.

Armitage, P., and Allen, I. (1950). Methods of estimating the LD_{50} in quantal response data. *J. Hyg. Camb.* **48**, 298–322.

Arnold, D. L., Charbonneau, S. M., Zawidzka, Z. Z., and Grice, H. C. (1977). Monitoring animal health during chronic toxicity studies. *J. Environ. Pathol. Toxicol.* **1**, 227–239.

Arnold, D. L., Krewski, D., and Munro, I. C. (1983). Saccharin: A toxicological and historical perspective. *Toxicology* **27**, 179–256.

Arnold, D. L., Moodie, C. A., McGuire, P. F., Collins, B. T., Charbonneau, S. M., and Munro, I. C. (1979). The effect of orthotoluenesulphonamide and sodium saccharin on the urinary tract of neonatal rats. *Toxicol. Appl. Pharmacol.* **51**, 455–463.

Baβ, R., Günzel, P., Henschler, D., König, J., Lorke, D., Neubert, D., Schütz, E., Schuppan, D., and Zbinden, G. (1982). LD_{50} versus acute toxicity: Critical assessment of the methodology currently in use. *Arch. Toxicol.* **51**, 183–186.

Balazs, T. (1970). Measurement of acute toxicity. *In* "Methods in Toxicology." (G. E. Paget, ed.), pp. 49–81. Oxford: Blackwell Scientific Publications.

Balazs, T., Murphy, J. B., and Grice, H. C. (1962). The influence of environmental changes on the cardiotoxicity of isoprenaline in rats. *J. Pharm. Pharmacol.* **14**, 750–755.

Benitz, K. -F. (1970). Measurement of chronic toxicity. *In* "Methods in Toxicology" (P. E. Paget, ed.), pp. 82–131. Oxford: Blackwell Scientific Publications.

British Toxicology Society (1984). British Toxicology Society Working Party on Toxicity — A new approach to the classification of substances and preparations on the basis of their acute toxicity. *Hum. Toxicol.* **3**, 85–92.

Brown, A. M. (1964). Strain and sex differences in response to drugs. *In* "Evaluation of Drug Activities: Pharmacometrics" (D. R. Lawrence and A. L. Bacharach, eds.), pp. 111–123. New York: Academic Press.

Bruce, R. D. (1987). A confirmatory study of the up-and-down method for acute oral toxicity testing. *Fund. Appl. Toxicol.* **8**, 97–100.

Clayson, D. B. (1987). The need for biological risk assessment in reaching decisions about carcinogens. *Mutat. Res.* **185**, 243–269.

Craver, B. N., Barrett, W. E., and Earl, A. E. (1950). Some requisites to making LD_{50}s from different laboratories comparable. *Arch. Ind. Hyg. Occup. Med.* **2**, 280–283.

Davidow, B., and Hagan, E. C. (1955). Acute toxicity. *Food, Drug Cosmet. Law J.* **10**, 685–694.

Deichmann, W. B., and LeBlanc, T. J. (1943). Determination of the approximate lethal dose with about six animals. *J. Ind. Hyg. Toxicol.* **25**, 415–417.

Department of Health and Social Security (1982). "Guidelines for the Testing of Chemicals for Toxicity," Report on Health and Social Subjects, 27. London: Her Majesty's Stationery Office.

Fox, J. G. (1977). Clinical assessment of laboratory rodents on long term bioassay studies. *J. Environ. Pathol. Toxicol.* **1**, 199–226.

Fox, J. G., and Helfrich-Smith, M. E. (1980). Chemical contamination of animal feeding systems: Evaluation of two caging systems and standard cagewashing equipment. *Lab. Anim. Sci.* **30**, 967–973.

Fox, J. G., Thibert, P., Arnold, D. L., Krewski, D. R., and Grice, H. C. (1979). Toxicology studies. II. The laboratory animal. *Food Cosmet. Toxicol.* **17**, 661–675.

Frederick, G. L. (1986). The necessary minimal duration of final long-term toxicologic tests of drugs. *Fund. Appl. Toxicol.* **6**, 385–394.

Gad, S. C. 1982. A neuromuscular screen for use in industrial toxicology. *J. Toxicol. Environ. Health* **9**, 691–704.

Gad, S. C., Smith, A. C., Gramp, A. L., Gavigan, F. A., and Derelanko, M. J. (1984). Innovative designs and practices for acute systemic toxicity study. *Drug Chem. Toxicol.* **7**, 423–434.

Gehring, P. J., Rowe, V. K., and McCollister, S. B. (1973). Toxicology: Cost/time. *Food Cosmet. Toxicol.* **11**, 1097–1110.

Gleason, M. N., Gosselin, R. E., and Hodge, H. C. (1957). "Clinical Toxicology of Commercial Products." Baltimore: Williams and Wilkins.

Grice, H. C., Munro, I. C., Krewski, D. R., and Blumenthal, H. (1981). *In utero* exposure in chronic toxicity/carcinogenicity studies. *Food Cosmet. Toxicol.* **19**, 373–379.

Griffin, J. P. (1981). Referring to the paper by Zbinden and Flury-Roversi. *Arch. Toxicol.* **49**, 99–103.

Griffith, J. F. (1964). Interlaboratory variations in the determination of acute oral LD_{50}. *Toxicol. Appl. Pharmacol.* **6**, 726–730.

Haseman, J. K. (1985). Issues in carcinogenicity testing: Dose selection. *Fund. Appl. Toxicol.* **5**, 66–78.

Hatch, A., Balazs, T., Wiberg, G. S., and Grice, H. C. (1963). Long-term isolation stress in rats. *Science* **142**, 507.

Hodge, H. C., and Sterner, J. H. (1949). Tabulation of toxicity classes. *Am. Ind. Hyg. Assoc. J.* **10**, 93–96.

Horn, H. J. (1956). Simplified LD_{50} (or ED_{50}) calculations. *Biometrics* **12**, 311–321.

Hunter, W. J., Lingls, W., and Recht, P. (1979). Intercomparison study on the determination of single administration toxicity in rats. *J. Assoc. Off. Anal. Chem.* **62**, 864–873.

International Agency for Research on Cancer (1980). Long-term and short-term screening assays for carcinogens: A critical appraisal. *IARC Monogr. Suppl.* **2**, 21–83.

International Life Sciences Institute (1984). "Current Issues in Toxicology Sponsored by the ILSI. The Selection of Doses in Chronic Toxicity/Carcinogenicity Studies." and "Age Associated (Geriatric) Pathology: Its Impact on Long-Term Toxicity Testing." Basel: S. Karger.

Kast, A., and Nishikawa, J. (1981). The effect of fasting on oral acute toxicity of drugs in rats and mice. *Lab. Anim.* **15**, 359–364.

Keene, J. H., and Sansome, E. B. (1984). Airborne transfer of contaminants in ventilated spaces. *Lab. Anim. Sci.* **34**, 453–457.

Lane-Petter, W. (1963). The physical environment of rats and mice. *In* "Animals for Research: Principles of Breeding and Management." (W. Lane-Petter, ed.), pp. 1–20. New York: Academic Press.

Lumley, C. E., and Walker, S. R. (1985). The value of chronic animal toxicology studies of pharmaceutical compounds: A retrospective analysis. *Fund. Appl. Toxicol.* **5**, 1007–1024.

Lumley, C. E., and Walker, S. R. (1986) A critical appraisal of the duration of chronic animal toxicity studies. *Regul. Toxicol. Pharmacol.* **6**, 66–72.

Melnick, R. L., Jameson, C. W., Goehl, T. J., and Kuhn, G. O. (1987). Application of microencapsulation for toxicology studies. I. Principles and stabilization of trichloroethylene in gelatin-sorbitol microcapsules. *Fund. Appl. Toxicol.* **8**, 425–431.

Moore, J. A., and Courtney, K. D. (1971). Teratology studies with the trichlorophenoxy acid herbicides 2,4,5-T and Silvex. *Teratology* **4**, 236.

Müller, H., and Kley, H.-P. (1982). Retrospective study on the reliability of an "Approximate LD_{50}" determined with a small number of animals. *Arch. Toxicol.* **51**, 189–196.

National Academy of Sciences (1975). "Principles for Evaluating Chemicals in the Environment," pp. 141–142. Washington, DC: National Academy of Sciences.

National Academy of Sciences (1977). "Principles and Procedures for Evaluating the Toxicity of Household Substances" (Publication 1138), pp. 10–17. Washington, DC: National Academy of Sciences.

National Technical Information Service (1980). "Proceedings of the Workshop on Subchronic Toxicity Testing," p. 20. Denver, Colorado: National Technical Information Service.

National Toxicology Program (1984). "Report of the NTP Ad Hoc Panel on Chemical Carcinogenesis Testing and Evaluation." Washington, DC: Board of Scientific Counselors, U.S. Department of Health and Human Services, Public Health Service.

Nolen, G. A. (1972). Effect of various restricted regimens on the growth, health and longevity of albino rats. *J. Nutr.* **102**, 1477–1494.

Nutrition Foundation (1983). "Report of the Ad Hoc Working Group on Oil/Gavage in Toxicology Meeting," (Arlington, Va.) Washington, DC: Nutrition Foundation.

Pharmaceutical Manufacturer's Association (1983). PMA (Pharmaceutical Manufacturers Association) take position on LD_{50} test. *ILAR News* **26**, 30–32.

Ross, M. H. (1961). Length of life and nutrition in the rat. *J. Nutr.* **75**, 197–210.

Ross, M. H., and Bras, G. (1971). Lasting influence of early caloric restriction on prevalence of neoplasms in the rat. *J. Natl. Cancer Inst. (US)* **47**, 1095–1113.

Ross, M. H., Bras, G., and Ragbeer, M. S. (1970). Influence of protein and caloric intake upon spontaneous tumor incidence of the anterior pituitary gland of the rat. *J. Nutr.* **100**, 177–189.

Rowan, A. N. (1981). The LD_{50} test: A critique and suggestions for alternatives. *Pharm. Technol.* **5**, 65–66, 80–86, 89–90, 92–94.

Rowan, A. N., and Goldberg, A. M. (1985). Perspectives on alternatives to current animal testing techniques in preclinical toxicology. *Annu. Rev. Pharmacol. Toxicol.* **25**, 225–247.

Sansone, E. B., and Fox, J. G. (1977). Potential chemical contamination in animal feeding studies: Evaluation of wire and solid bottom caging systems and gelled feed. *Lab. Anim. Sci.* **27**, 457–465.

Sansone, E. B., Losikoff, A. M., and Pendleton, R. A. (1977). Potential hazard from feeding test chemicals in carcinogen bioassay research. *Toxicol. Appl. Pharmacol.* **39**, 435–450.

Schütz, E., and Fuchs, H. (1982). A new approach to minimizing the number of animals used in acute toxicity testing and optimizing the information of test results. *Arch. Toxicol.* **51**, 197–220.

Sperling, F. (1976). Nonlethal parameters as indices of acute toxicity. Inadequacy of the acute LD_{50}. *In* "Advances in Modern Toxicology: New Concepts in Safety Evaluation" (M. A. Mehlman, R. E. Shapiro, and H. Blumenthal, eds.), Vol. I, pp. 177–191. Washington, DC: Hemisphere.

Steplewski, Z., Goldman, P. R., and Vogel, W. H. (1987). Effect of housing stress on the formation and development of tumors in rats. *Cancer Lett.* **34**, 257–261.

Tannenbaum, A., and Silverstone, H. (1957). Nutrition and the genesis of tumours. *In* "Cancer" (R. W. Raven, ed.), Vol. I, pp. 306–334. London: Butterworth.

Tarone, R. T., Chu, K. C., and Ward, J. M. (1981). Variability in the rates of some common naturally occurring tumors in Fischer 344 rats and (C57B1/6N × C3H/HeN)F₁(B6C3F₁) mice. *J. Natl. Cancer Inst. (US)* **66**, 1175–1181.

Task Force of Past Presidents (1982). Animal data in hazard evaluation: Paths and pitfalls. *Fund. Appl. Toxicol.* **2**, 101–107.

Toth, B., Wallcase, L., Patil, K. Schmeltz, I., and Hoffman, D. (1977). Induction of tumors in mice with the herbicide succinic and 2,2-dimethylhydrazide. *Cancer Res.* **37**, 3497–3500.

Trevan, J. W. (1927). The error of determination of toxicity. *Proc. R. Soc. London Ser. B* **101**, 483–514.

U.S. Interagency Staff Group on Carcinogens (1986). Chemical carcinogens: A review of the science and its associated principles. *Environ. Health Perspect.* **67**, 201–282.

Uvarov, D. O. (1984). Research with animals. Requirement, responsibility, welfare. *Lab. Anim.* **19**, 51–75.

van Noordwijk, A. J., and Noordwijk, J. (1988). An accurate method for estimating an approximate lethal dose with few animals, tested with a Monte Carlo procedure. *Arch. Toxicol.* **61**, 333–343.

Weihe, W. H. (1971). The significance of the physical environment for the health and state of Adaptation of laboratory animals. *In* "Defining the Laboratory Animal," pp. 353–378. Washington, DC: National Academy of Sciences.

Weil, C. S. (1972). Guidelines for experiments to predict the degree of safety of a maternal for man. *Toxicol. Appl. Pharmacol.* **21**, 194–199.

Weil, C. S. (1983). Economical LD₅₀ and slope determinations. *Drug Chem. Toxicol.* **6**, 595–603.

Weil, C. S., Woodside, M. D., Bernard, J. B., Condra, N. I., King, J. M., and Carpenter, C. P. (1973). Comparative effect of carbaryl on rat reproduction and guinea pig teratology when fed either in the diet or by stomach intubation. *Toxicol. Appl. Pharmacol.* **26**, 621–638.

Wiberg, G. S., Airth, J. M., and Grice, H. C. (1966). Methodology in long-term toxicity tests: A comparison of individual versus community housing. *Food Cosmet. Toxicol.* **4**, 47–55.

Withey, J. R., Collins, B. T., and Collins, P. G. (1983). Effect of vehicle on the pharmacokinetics and uptake of four halogenated hydrocarbons from the gastrointestinal tract of the rat. *J. Appl. Toxicol.* **3**, 249–253.

Wogan, G. N., and Shank, R. C. (1971). Toxicity and Carcinogenicity of aflatoxins. *In* "Advances in Environmental Science and Technology" (J. N. Pitts and R. L. Metcalf, eds.), pp. 321–350. New York: Wiley.

Zbinden, G. (1963). Experimental and clinical aspects of drug toxicity. *In* "Advances in Pharmacology" (S. Garattini and P. A. Shore, eds.), pp. 1–112. New York: Academic Press.

Zbinden, G. (1979). Application of basic concepts to research in toxicology. *Pharmacol. Rev.* **30**, 605–616.

Zbinden, G. (1986). Acute toxicity testing, public responsibility and scientific challenges. *Cell Biol. Toxicol.* **2**, 325–335.

Zbinden, G., and Flury-Roversi (1981). Significance of the LD₅₀ test for the toxicological evaluation of chemical substances. *Arch. Toxicol.* **47**, 77–99.

10
Inhalation Studies

William M. Snellings
Union Carbide Corporation
Danbury, Connecticut

Darol E. Dodd
Bushy Run Research Center
Export, Pennsylvania

Handbook of
In Vivo Toxicity Testing

189

I. INTRODUCTION

As stated in previous chapters, techniques in toxicity testing, particularly in inhalation testing, are evolving rapidly. One must understand that for inhalation systems there is no universal design. The art is relatively new, and normally one laboratory builds on what another has developed.

Tight control of certain environmental parameters in the inhalation chamber, such as temperature, humidity, airflow, and pressure, is difficult to maintain by conventional air-conditioning and ventilation systems. The maintenance of a constant chamber concentration of a test compound and the continuous analytical monitoring of the test atmosphere are operations that require dependable and precise instrumentation. Inhalation laboratories today use equipment, such as pumps, flow metering devices, analytical instruments, inhalation chambers, and filtration systems, made by several different manufacturers. In this chapter, we do not discuss the multitude of inhalation system designs nor the many different equipment manufacturers but present a few system designs that have been proved to work.

Focus is on facility planning, including environmental control and chamber and ventilation system designs. In addition, procedures used to generate, analyze, and then remove the test compound before exhausting the chamber air safely into the atmosphere are reviewed. Finally, safety equipment and procedures are discussed as an integral part of the complete inhalation operation.

II. ROOM DESIGN

Chamber rooms in which only acute exposure studies are conducted may be designed differently from rooms for longer-term inhalation studies. Because lethal concentrations of test compounds are often generated in acute studies, additional safety precautions may be necessary. For example, both the chamber and the generation system may be placed in an exhaust hood for acute studies.

Rooms containing the inhalation chambers, animals, and analytical instrumentation should be close to each other. Animals are not routinely housed in the chambers during nonexposure times for three reasons:

1. If the ventilation system fails, temperature, humidity, and oxygen content will fall outside acceptable ranges much faster in a small chamber than they will in a large room.
2. If the test compound adheres to the walls of the inhalation chamber and animal cages, then animals are exposed to a relatively high concentration of the test compound, usually for 6 hours during the expo-

sure period, and to a low concentration for 18 hours. The question then becomes to what concentration(s) are the animals really exposed?

3. If the inhalation chamber becomes dirty, cleaning the chamber may involve high pressure spraying and increased humidity levels that can affect the stable environment of the animals.

The inhalation exposure room can contain all the exposure chambers plus the control chamber, or each separate inhalation room can contain one chamber. Naturally, the multiple chamber room is cheaper to build and operate and, with respect to room environmental conditions, all animal groups can be treated the same. However, room air may have to be analyzed to demonstrate that the room has not become contaminated by "off-gassing" from the exposed animals. Off-gassing refers to contaminated air that can enter the room either from the animals' bodies or from their exhalation. If this appears to be a significant problem, the room exhaust rate may have to be increased or the animals may have to be permanently maintained in the chambers.

For studies lasting 3 months or longer, housing the animals in the same room as the chambers may be more practical than moving the animals to a separate room because there is less chance of contaminating the connecting corridors with test compounds. The possibility of spreading communicable diseases also is minimized. However, this consideration needs to be weighed against the increased difficulties of conducting routine maintenance and cleaning of the chambers and equipment in the same room that houses the animals.

A very practical safety addition for each chamber room is to have an exhaust hood containing a sink. These areas can be used for preparation of the test compound and for cleaning any contaminated equipment, like the vapor or aerosol generator. If these operations are conducted in the chamber room, the chances for cross-contamination of the test compound to other parts of the laboratory facility are minimized. Moreover, these hoods can be equipped with low and high speed fans; therefore, if an accidental spill or leak of the test compound occurs in the room, the high speed fan can be used as an emergency room exhaust. At all other times, the fan is operated in the low speed mode and functions as a part of the room exhaust system. For safety reasons, the hood fan should have the low-high speed switch located outside the chamber room.

The following items have proved to be beneficial and cost-effective:

1. Catwalks around a bank of tall chambers so that ladders are not necessary for inspection of aerosol or vapor generation equipment.
2. Chemical drain lines located in the floor of the rooms attached to each

chamber so that chambers can be washed and effluent disposed of safely.

3. Animal food containers that can be mounted on a wall rack because all food should be removed from animal cages prior to exposure.

4. Two doors for each chamber room so that there is more than one exit in case of an emergency, such as a fire or an accidental spill. (Doors should be located so as to help control the flow of people within the chamber room. For example, people involved with the operation of aerosol or vapor generation equipment can use one door; people connected with animal care operations can use the other door.)

5. Five chambers in each bank of chambers so that considerable flexibility can be incorporated in the study design.

Current Organization for Economic Co-operation and Development (OECD;1981) guidelines for subchronic and chronic inhalation studies state that there should be at least three test groups and a control group. The extra chamber (fifth one) can be very beneficial when the results of previous studies are inconclusive, therefore, making it difficult to select three proper target exposure concentrations for the longer-term study. The addition of an extra test group can facilitate the determination of the minimal effect or no-observable-effect level with only a little additional effort. Furthermore, the fifth chamber is necessary if either a vehicle, solvent, or another negative control group is required for a study. Moreover, because one of the major rate-limiting steps in starting new inhalation studies is the development of an aerosol or vapor generation system, preparation for the next study can be started in the extra chamber while the current study is still in progress. A separate chamber exhaust for the fifth chamber is required in this design because of the potential hazards associated with mixing different test compounds in a common chamber exhaust system.

As discussed in the next section, the shape of the chambers to be used will appreciably affect the room design. For instance, a subfloor several feet below ground level may have to be incorporated to contain certain types of chambers. Lastly, the room should be big enough to allow sufficient air space between chambers so that the heat from one chamber does not affect the temperature in an adjacent chamber.

III. CHAMBER DESIGN

Excellent discussions on chamber design have previously been published, in particular Fraser et al. (1959), Drew and Laskin (1973), Drew (1978), Leong (1981), and MacFarland (1983). An early consideration in chamber design is the determination of whether a nose- or head-only exposure system (Fig. 1) is more appropriate than a whole-animal or whole-body exposure system for specific testing needs. For example, for sensory irritation evaluation, head-only chambers have been specifically designed so that respiratory rate can be monitored (Alarie, 1966).

Recent designs and uses of different nose-only systems have been reported by Green *et al.* (1984), Leach *et al.* (1984), Phalen *et al.* (1984), and Klimisch *et al.* (1987). The advantages of nose-only over whole-body exposure systems are:

1. Less of the test compound is needed because chamber volume is smaller and, consequently, filtration of the chamber exhaust can be more easily accomplished.
2. There is no additional exposure of the animals to the test compound due either to absorption through the skin or to ingestion via grooming when the compound adheres to the fur or skin.
3. There is less chance of worker exposure to the test compound upon removal of the animals from the exposure chamber.

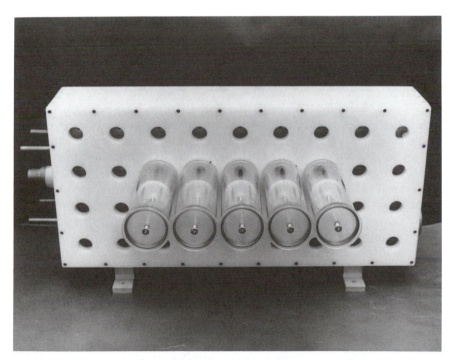

Fig. 1 Nose-only chamber (IN-TOX Products, Albuquerque, New Mexico) with animal restraint tubes. Maximum number of animals that can be exposed is 72.

4. Biological samples (e.g., blood) can be easily obtained during a pharmacokinetic or metabolic study.
5. Inhalation dosimetry and respiratory functions, such as respiratory rate and tidal volume, can be assessed during exposure (Landry *et al.*, 1983).
6. The time required for chamber equilibration to be 99% of the desired concentration is considerably less than for the larger whole-body exposure chambers. This can be an advantage if the total exposure time is an hour or less.

The disadvantages of nose-only exposures include the following:

1. Does not mimic an industrial exposure situation in which additional exposure occurs due to skin contact
2. Causes stress to the animals because of the restraints used to confine them during exposure
3. Increases labor requirements during chamber loading and unloading of animals and for equipment cleanup
4. Results in inability to assess ocular irritancy because the test compound does not come in direct contact with the eyes

Several questions have been raised concerning exposure concentration in the nose-only and whole-body types of exposures. What is the true exposure concentration for animals that "bury" their nose under another animal when multiply housed in a whole-body aerosol study? A study by Ulrich and Marold (1979) indicated that there was no difference in the blood levels of a chemical between singly and multiply housed rats in whole-body aerosol studies. What is the true exposure concentration for an animal that moves in the restraint tube of a nose-only exposure, thereby altering the concentration in the breathing zone of the animal? LaBauve *et al.* (1983) have reported that simple modifications to the exposure system can reduce or eliminate this problem. Does the respiratory rate or tidal volume change with added stress and/or heat created from restraint procedures used in the nose-only exposure system? A study by Mauderly (1986) indicated that elevated minute volume can occur in the first 45 minutes of nose-only exposures. This effect can be minimized by conditioning the animals to repeated tube confinement before the actual treatment period (Mauderly, 1986). For certain nose-only exposure systems, will the animals at one end of the chamber be exposed to a lower concentration of the test compound or a different test compound (i.e., rebreathing effects) than the animals at the other end of the chamber? Cannon *et al.* (1983) have designed a chamber for which this is reported not to be a problem. These questions and others are currently being investigated.

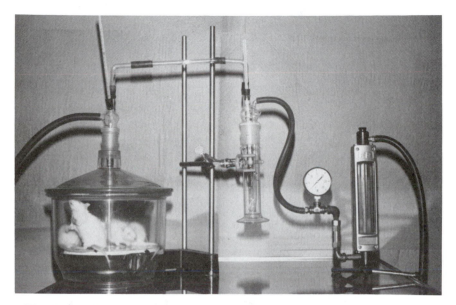

Fig. 2 Simple exposure system for acute testing under dynamic exposure condition. Rats are exposed in a 9-liter desiccator to a substantially saturated vapor.

Whole-animal exposure chambers can be made successfully in different shapes and out of different materials (Fraser *et al.,* 1959; Drew and Laskin, 1973; MacFarland, 1983). In the design of the chamber shape, one objective is to obtain the greatest volume of exposure chamber for the smallest external surface area, which ideally is a sphere. The principle behind this design is to get the greatest number of animals in a chamber with the least amount of wall surface. The amount of wall area and the material from which the walls are made are important because of the potential loss of test compound from the atmosphere due to adsorption. However, spherically designed chambers are not practical when the large amount of floor space required and the difficulty incurred in manufacturing curved stainless steel and glass are considered.

Chambers for acute inhalation studies have included modifications to glass containers such as aquariums (Barrow and Steinhagen, 1982), bell jars, and desiccators (Fig. 2). These chambers have been used for inhalation testing under dynamic (constant airflow) or static (stationary air) exposure conditions. Special chamber features for static exposures have included an air-lock or sliding drawer mechanism for the quick introduction of the animals into substantially saturated vapors and an internal fan to facilitate vaporization and chamber distribution (Fig. 3).

One of the first modern whole-animal exposure chambers was made at the University of Rochester and is frequently referred to as the "Roches-

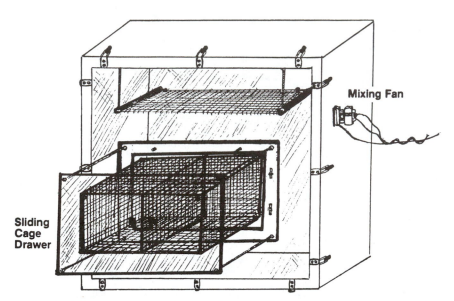

Fig. 3 Simple exposure system for acute testing under static exposure conditions. Test compound is placed in tray adjacent to a fan at top of chamber. A sliding drawer mechanism on the front wall of the 120-liter chamber allows for the quick introduction of rats or mice into a substantially saturated concentration of the test compound vapor.

ter Chamber". This chamber, a hexagonal prism fitted with hexagonal pyramids at the top and bottom, was designed to be aerodynamically similar to a wind tunnel (Leach *et al.,* 1959). Currently, a more routinely used modification of that design is a four-sided hedron with pyramid-shaped top and bottom (Fig. 4). Hinners *et al.* (1968) have described this design in detail.

A popular configuration for the air and test compound inlet section of the top pyramid is a short cylinder with a tangential feed tube. Other designs have been discussed by Beethe (1978). Moss *et al.* (1982) have demonstrated that, when the test material is thoroughly mixed with air in the chamber inlet, a more uniform distribution of the test material occurs within the chamber. For good mixing conditions or turbulent airflows, the Reynolds Number should be greater than 3,000 [$R = vdw/\mu$ where v = velocity of fluid (ft/sec); d = diameter of pipe (ft); w = density of fluid (lb/cu ft); μ = absolute viscosity of fluid (lb/sec · ft)]. For example, for a 3-in diameter inlet duct, the critical velocity to prevent laminar flow is 120 ft/min (Alden and Kane, 1970). Sometimes a deflection tube, venturi, or screen at the chamber inlet is needed to produce the necessary turbulence for complete mixing (Carpenter and Beethe, 1980).

Hinners *et al.* (1968) have reported that the slope of the pyramidal

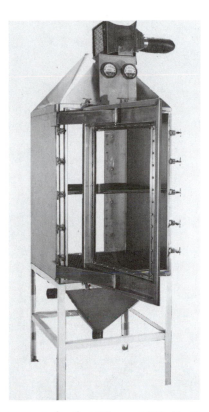

Fig. 4 Whole-body exposure chamber (Young and Bertke Co., Cincinnati, Ohio) with pyramidal top and bottom (1.5 m³). Chamber can be used for both vapor and aerosol studies. Door design insures a leak-proof seal.

chamber top is more important than the slope at the bottom for obtaining good chamber distribution of the test compound. They have recommended that the slope of the top funnel be no less than 50 degrees from the horizontal. However, the slope often is dictated by height limitations placed on the chamber because of room dimensions. Consequently, the chamber inlet may require deflectors or diffusers to create a more uniform distribution of the test compound within the breathing zone of the animals. It is also desirable to have some method of cleaning the inside of the chamber easily. Fabricating a sloping bottom so that the cleaning solution can be conveniently collected and drained accomplishes this.

The degree of difficulty in loading animals into or out of the chamber must be considered in the chamber design. A hydraulic lift or ramp may be necessary to get cages or cage carriers into a Hinners-type chamber.

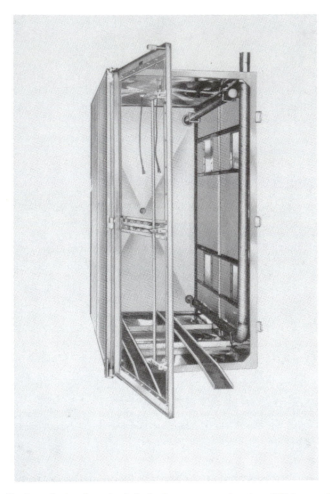

Fig. 5 Rectangularly shaped whole-body exposure chamber (Wahman, Timonium, Maryland). Fold-up ramp is shown that allows for easy walk-in entry of animal cage carriers. Chamber (4.3 m³) can be used for gas and vapor studies.

This problem may be alleviated if the room is designed with a sunken floor to hold the pyramidal bottom of the chamber and, therefore, allow floor-level entry into the chamber.

A very simply designed rectangular chamber for gas and vapor studies (Fig. 5) has three advantages:

1. It is the best design for housing the greatest number of animals in the least volume. As a result, less test compound is required, and chamber room size requirements are not as large.

2. The construction is simple, which keeps the purchase price low.
3. Because of the walk-in entry, special room design or ramps are not needed.

The major disadvantage in this chamber design is that it is not suitable for aerosol studies because of the difficulty in cleaning the chamber and the manifold system that introduces the test compound into the chamber.

The inlet manifold at the top of the chamber is a 2 ¾-in duct with thirty-two $\frac{11}{32}$-in evenly spaced holes. This duct extends horizontally the length of one chamber wall. The diameter of the duct as well as the number of holes can be changed as long as one half of the cross-sectional area of the duct is approximately equal to the sum of the area of all the holes. This allows for an even airflow from each hole. Along the bottom of the chamber is a similarly designed duct for chamber exhaust. In this type of chamber design, insertion of metal trays between levels of animal cages to collect excrement is actually beneficial to the uniform chamber distribution of the test compound. These collection trays are a definite advantage because they prevent contamination (e.g., metabolites) of animals at lower levels.

Collection trays can also be used in horizontal flow inhalation chambers (Ferin and Leach, 1980); however, uneven chamber concentration distribution has been reported for certain test materials in this type of chamber (Hemenway and MacAskill, 1982). Moss *et al.* (1982) have reported on a multitiered 2 m³ vertical flow inhalation chamber in which collection pans and other air deflectors are used in a way that allows the energy from the moving air to provide the necessary mixing, resulting in improved chamber distribution characteristics (Yeh *et al.*, 1986).

For safety purposes, special "live-in" glove boxes can be used. These are attached to inhalation chambers (Fig. 6) so that a door between the glove box and chamber can be opened following each exposure of the animals to the test compound, and the animals can be transferred from chamber to glove box. By using the gloves attached to the portholes, the worker does not come in direct contact with the animals. This procedure is especially helpful in whole-body exposures to dust because, following the exposure, the animals' fur and cages are often loaded with the test compound. Opening chamber doors results not only in personnel becoming exposed to the test compound but also in contamination of the room. Furthermore, if the animals are then transferred to an animal room, the corridor to this room will also become contaminated. Often, this contamination problem is not fully appreciated unless the chemical can be easily detected (e.g., by fluorescence using a UV source). This chamber and glove box arrangement can also be used for vapor studies in which the

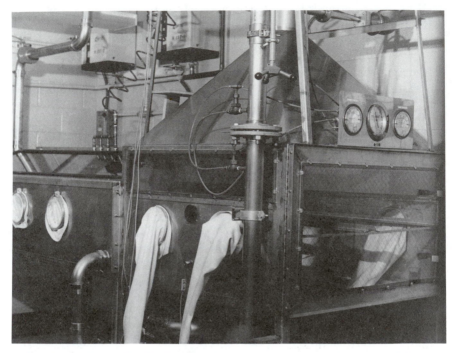

Fig. 6 Inhalation chamber (1 m³) with glove ports and a glove box attached. Animals can be removed from the chamber to a housing area without the worker coming in direct contact with them.

compound is expected to be highly toxic at low concentrations, thus eliminating the need for special protection equipment during the removal of the animals from the chambers. Moreover, with highly toxic compounds, a safer procedure may be to place a smaller inhalation chamber and the generation equipment within this chamber; in this way, all handling of the test compound can be done through the glove ports.

Size requirements of the inhalation chambers depend on the objectives of the testing facility. If the spectrum of studies includes the use of multiple species, it is desirable to have large chambers to expose all species at the same time in order to reduce cost and ensure the same exposure conditions for each species. However, care should be taken not to design too large a chamber. Usually, with larger chamber sizes, generation of high aerosol or vapor concentrations becomes more costly and sometimes impossible unless multiple aerosol or vapor generators are used. Additionally, all heating, cooling, humidification, and filtration equipment will require sufficient capacity to condition larger volumes of air. Chambers that are approximately 4 to 5 m³, as those just described, are well designed for subchronic and chronic studies (240 rats) as well as for developmental toxicity studies (30 rats and 24 rabbits). For 9- and 90-day studies (10 to 20 rats and/or mice per sex), 1 to 2 m³ chambers have proved to be sufficient.

A "rule of thumb" employed is that the total animal volume should not exceed 5% of the chamber volume (McFarland, 1976). One can make a rough estimate of the animal volume by assuming that the weight in grams of the animals corresponds to the volume in milliliters. However, it appears that an animal volume of not more than 1% to 2% of the total chamber volume is more desirable than the 5% mentioned previously. Even when the outside walls of an inhalation chamber are cooled to decrease the heat load within the chamber resulting from the animals' body heat (Bernstein and Drew, 1980), a 5% animal volume may necessitate a considerable increase in chamber airflow to maintain temperature and humidity at an acceptable and uniform level within the chamber.[1]

Another item that should be considered in chamber design is the type of materials used for chamber construction. For testing most compounds, chambers should be made of stainless steel and glass. A recommended grade of stainless steel is type 304 or 316 (type 302 is prone to weld decay). Type 316 has molybdenum added, which slightly improves its resistance to chlorides and sulphur acids. Stainless steel greater than 18 gauge may be too thin and, therefore, may flex when the chamber airflow is turned on. It is recommended that the door as well as one chamber wall or wall insert be made of glass so that animals can easily be observed. For safety purposes, glass with embedded wire mesh should be used.

Lighting is an important consideration, although chambers do not need an internal light source because the recommended glass inserts allow adequate light if inhalation rooms are well lighted. Also, a light source in the chamber is not usually effective in illuminating all levels of the chamber equally and can be a safety concern if not correctly sealed or shielded.

To ensure against leaks, chambers must have good seals around windows and doors as well as adequate door latches. Daily monitoring of chamber pressure with a simple manometer may provide an adequate check for leaks. Alteration in chamber pressure may be the first sign of a damaged seal or of an improperly latched door. Depending on a change in chamber airflow may not be a reliable indicator even for a substantial

[1] Chambers should not be designed with a common wall nor should they be placed immediately adjacent to each other. Sufficient airflow around the chamber must be allowed, thereby decreasing the heat load of the chamber.

chamber leak because airflow is usually measured in the exhaust duct; consequently, the exhaust air volume will remain the same but the air inlet volume will be split between the inlet duct and the leak. All gaskets and seals should be made of materials that will not react with the chemicals to be tested. Although there are no universally accepted materials, silicone-based sealants and butylene rubber gaskets are popular. Windows can have a stainless steel strip covering the gasket material around the window edge. This reduces the surface area of the gasket material which is in direct contact with the test compound. Special care should be taken with the gasket around the door because it is more difficult to maintain.

Certain features should be present in every chamber. One of these is analytical sampling ports. It is recommended that one large port (2 to 3 in. in diameter) be installed in which several sample lines can be placed for testing compound distribution within the chamber.

Another recommended feature is a drain for removal of waste water collected during chamber cleanup. To prevent backflow of gases from the waste storage tank into the inhalation chamber (which operates under negative pressure relative to the tank), a shutoff valve on the drain is necessary. Water traps should not be used because the test compound may react with the water in the trap. A careful check should be made before the start of each exposure session to ensure that this drain valve is closed; if it is not, it is possible that the airflow in the chamber may be at a normal setting, yet some chamber intake air may be coming from nondesirable sources. It is recommended that a feed disposal unit be installed in this waste-water line to grind up feces or animal feed, particularly if the animals live in the chamber. Because the feed disposal unit can produce an aerosol of the waste water, removal of the animals from the chamber or capping of the line is recommended whenever the disposal unit is in operation. Another suggestion is to place wire mesh over the drain in the bottom of the chamber to block the exit of any animal that may escape from its cage during exposure.

If the animals are to live in the chambers, a drinking-water supply line should be included. For exposure periods of six hours or less, no drinking water system within the chamber is necessary to maintain the health status of the animals. Chambers may also need a separate water supply line for internal cleaning. Chamber cleaning systems usually are not effective unless hot water can be used at a high pressure. Caution must be taken if workers spray the chamber walls with the chamber door open because the spray can aerosolize any test compound adsorbed onto the walls, causing personnel to be exposed. To prevent exposure to personnel, a rotating garden sprinkler system, installed at the top of the chamber, can provide an inexpensive chamber cleaning system for water-soluble compounds.

All chambers should be connected to a neutral ground. This may be of benefit in some dust studies in order to dissipate static charge buildup, which can cause the test compound to become attracted to the chamber walls. Furthermore, with potentially explosive test compounds, it is necessary to ground all parts of the vapor generator and chamber inlet because, at certain concentrations, the test compound may be ignitable by static electricity. If exposure concentrations must be close to the explosive level of the test compound, special precautions must be taken (Pullinger *et al.*, 1979). Even animal carriers must be grounded because the rubber wheels on these carriers may prevent the dissipation of static charge buildup.

Finally, animal exposure cages can be one of the most costly items of the inhalation laboratory. Therefore, it is practical to have the chamber and chamber doors large enough so that existing exposure cages and cage carriers can easily be transferred into and out of the chamber.

IV. CHAMBER CONCENTRATION DISTRIBUTION ANALYSIS

The chamber concentration of a test compound at different locations in a chamber is usually determined to check the distribution characteristics of the chamber. Because of significant differences in design of nose-only and head-only chambers, each with potentially different distribution characteristics, this discussion is limited to whole-body exposure chambers.

After the installation of new chambers, a concentration distribution analysis should be performed with a full load of animals in one of the chambers. This analysis for gases or vapors (toluene can be used) may include a 15-point check of the test chemical concentration if animals are located on three or more levels within the chamber. This entails a 5-point (4 corners of the plane and the center) analysis at three different horizontal levels (top, middle, and bottom), all placed within the breathing zone of the animals. Prior to actual animal testing, a 9-point distribution (four corners of two horizontal planes located at the top and bottom of the chamber and one sample point at the center of the chamber, which is the normal location of the sampling probe) is more than sufficient for confirming distribution analysis. If all animals are located on one level, a 5-point distribution is appropriate.

Although differences in distribution characteristics among different gases or vapors are usually negligible, for major studies like a subchronic or chronic experiment, data should be obtained with the actual compound being tested. For confirmation of the distribution characteristics, one test chamber may be checked before the start of a study. This chamber should have a full load of animal cages but contain no animals. During the study, this chamber may be checked with a full load of animals.

For an accurate analysis during distribution testing, multiple samples at each sampling position should be taken. A mean concentration ($\pm$ standard deviation) is calculated for each position. Then a mean ($\pm$ standard deviation) of these means is calculated along with the coefficient of variation. For most gases or vapors, an acceptable coefficient of variation among the different sampling points should be less than 5%. For aerosols, this depends greatly on the particular compound. Naturally, this type of distribution testing is started after the theoretical time is reached for the chamber concentration to reach equilibrium. What cannot be assessed by this type of distribution analysis is whether certain areas take a longer time to become equilibrated. However, this problem can be resolved by determining the time it takes each point to reach the target concentration. Two possible explanations for poor chamber distribution are incomplete mixing of the test material in air or chamber leaks. For a discussion on correct chamber design and critical velocities for effective mixing, refer to Section III on chamber design. If a low concentration value for a particular area is obtained in the distribution analysis, the adjacent walls, windows, and doors must be checked for possible leaks.

Leaks in large chambers can be found by the following method. Someone must be closed inside the chamber with the chamber inlet air shut off. Then the chamber exhaust is carefully increased until a slight negative pressure (approximately ½ in. water) is obtained. The person inside the chamber can then check for leaks by applying liquid soap (e.g., Snoop® liquid, NUPRO Co., Willoughby, Ohio) to suspected areas and watching for bubbles to form. For smaller chambers, leaks can be detected with the Halogen Leak Detector (model 5000, TIF Instruments, Inc., Miami, Florida) if the inlet and exhaust ducts are closed off and a slight positive chamber pressure is created by the introduction of Freon® gas. This type of detector is battery operated, portable, inexpensive, and quite sensitive. Elimination of leaks is important because, if the leak is significant, there may be less than a normal amount of air diluting the test compound before it enters the breathing zone of the animals. Therefore, some animals may be exposed to concentrations of the test compound that are higher than the target concentration.

V. VENTILATION SYSTEM

Animal and analytical working areas should have once-through ventilation rather than recirculating room air. Requirements for a chamber ventilation system include the ability to set and maintain constant chamber airflow over a range of low flow rates ($\sim$ 5 air changes per hour) to high flow rates ($\sim$ 40 air changes per hour). Air change is defined as chamber airflow per hour divided by chamber volume. This terminology is misleading. Because of air mixing, a numerical value of 1 does not mean that one complete exchange of new air has taken place in the chamber. Refer to MacFarland (1976) for a more detailed discussion.

Designs of chamber ventilation systems are usually modifications of one of two different systems, one called a *pull* and the other a *push-pull* ventilation system. With these systems, air in the chamber can be displaced by "pulling" (i.e., by creating negative pressure on the exhaust side of the chamber) or by "pushing" (i.e., by displacing positive pressure on the inlet side of the chamber).

In a pull system, only one chamber exhaust fan is necessary for ventilation in a bank of chambers. The main advantage of this type of system is that it is fairly simple to design and construct because the air "pulled" through the chamber comes from the same room in which the chambers are located, thereby eliminating the need for two separate heating/cooling systems, one for the room and one for the chambers. The disadvantages of a pull ventilation system are several. Alteration of airflow in one chamber will change the airflow in other chambers. Naturally, this problem can be eliminated with the use of a separate exhaust fan on each chamber but at additional cost and with increased maintenance. As the chamber airflow rates increase or as the resistance in the inlet duct increases (e.g., by the addition of an inlet duct filter), the negative pressure in the chamber also increases, resulting in potential stress on the animals.

However, with the push-pull ventilation system, these kinds of problems are not as severe. Chamber airflows can be maintained within each chamber by keeping a constant pressure (relative to the room) in both the inlet and exhaust ducts. Constant pressure is accomplished by static pressure sensors that control airflow valves in these ducts. Therefore, if the airflow of any chamber is modified, then the inlet and exhaust duct sensors will respond independently by signaling the airflow valves to open or close, thereby maintaining the same static pressure as before the modification. Consequently, neither airflow nor chamber pressure is significantly altered in the remaining chambers.

The term *push-pull system* can be somewhat misleading because, in some systems, pressures in both the chamber inlet and exhaust duct, relative to the room, are negative; however, air passes through the chamber because the exhaust duct is at a greater negative pressure than the inlet duct. Therefore, in the push-pull and pull systems, the test compound can safely be introduced into the chamber inlet duct and contained in the chamber because both are under negative pressure relative to the room.

VI. ENVIRONMENTAL CONTROL

Perhaps two of the most difficult tasks in any inhalation facility are controlling the environmental and ventilation systems. Engineering needs are not just an adaptation of conventional heating, ventilation, and air-conditioning (HVAC). For the relatively small rooms or chambers used in an inhalation facility, a low volume HVAC system is more appropriate than a high volume system because it is cheaper to build and operate; however, the ability to stabilize temperature and humidity fluctuations under certain conditions may be difficult. The following points describe some problems in the area of environmental control.

A. Temperature

Acceptable chamber temperature ranges have been established in different guidelines: OECD (1981) has recommended $22°C \pm 2°$; FIFRA (1982), $22°C \pm 2°$; TSCA (1987), $24°C \pm 2°$. These temperature ranges are not difficult to maintain unless the number of animals is close to 5% of the chamber volume or the test compound requires substantial heating because it evaporates at a high temperature.

To calculate the basal (inactive) metabolic rate of an animal, the equation $M = 6.6W^{0.75}$ can be used, where M = Btu/hr/animal and is a function of weight (W) and W = lb/animal (Strock and Koral, 1965). For the average total heat loss from the animals to the environment over a 24-hour period of a normal animal activity, Gorton *et al.* (1976) have recommended that the basal rate be multiplied by 2.5. From calculations of the animals' basal metabolic rate coupled with the normal allowances for heat gains and losses due to lights and ventilation, it would appear that the heat load in the chamber would be so great that very high ventilation rates and/or very low incoming air temperature would be necessary to maintain the animals within a normal temperature range. This overestimate can be due to the fact that the stainless steel walls of a Hinners' inhalation chamber have been shown to be effective at removing as much as 90% of the animal heat, whereas the airstream only removes 10% (Bernstein and Drew, 1980). Consequently, lowering the room temperature in which the inhalation chambers are situated may result in acceptable chamber temperatures without having to increase chamber airflow or decrease incoming air temperature.

Maintenance of a stable chamber temperature can be accomplished by a modulating process of cooling then reheating the chamber supply air. For example, in the summer, the outside air can be cooled below a set temperature point and then heated to the desired temperature. Conventional air-conditioning using only cyclic cooling can result in considerable chamber temperature variations.

B. Relative Humidity

Probably the most difficult task of an HVAC system is to maintain the relative humidity within acceptable ranges at all times of the year. The acceptable relative humidity ranges of the chamber environment have also been established in different guidelines: OECD (1981) has recommended 30% to 70%; FIFRA (1982) and TSCA (1987), 40% to 60%. Maintenance of stable relative humidity can be a problem when the weather changes appreciably in a relatively short period of time, for example, from a cool night (with air of low water vapor content) to a hot morning (when the humidity is high because of dew evaporation).

A problem that can occur in removing large amounts of water vapor by cooling the air is that the condensate can freeze on the cooling coil. One approach to solving this problem is to combine in series two dehumidification systems, one operating by cooling and condensing the water vapor and the other by absorbing the water vapor onto a desiccant. For the latter, the desiccant may be contained in a rotary mechanism that continuously rotates through a heating element that reactivates the desiccant (Cargocaire Engineering Corporation, Amesbury, Massachusetts).

As with chamber temperature, relative humidity can be maintained if the water content of the incoming air is lowered below the dew point and then steam is added back to the air to bring it to an acceptable level. The combination of the two-step dehumidification system and the modulating procedures for temperature and relative humidity are very effective in maintaining a stable environment.

Two modifications that have proved beneficial in maintaining a more constant level of humidity within the chambers consist of the placement of the humidity sensor for feedback control in the exhaust air duct (downstream of the filter in an aerosol chamber system) rather than in the inlet air duct and the insertion of a flow arrester (e.g., a small orifice plate) in the steam line. The use of a wick, which absorbs the bolus of steam from the humidifier to allow for slow evaporation, is not recommended because of the potential for bacterial growth on the wick. These modifications will slow down the response of the system.

One may also consider using electric vaporizers for humidification rather than a boiler system. Because of the possible contamination of the chamber air due to chemicals used to treat water in the boiler (e.g., corrosion inhibitors), electric vaporizers may be preferred.

C. Monitoring Temperature and Relative Humidity

Testing guidelines vary on the frequency of monitoring and recording temperature and relative humidity. For example, TSCA (1987) guidelines have recommended continuous monitoring and recording every 30 minutes, whereas FIFRA (1982) guidelines have recommended recording at least once every 60 minutes. Usually, there is no problem regarding instrumentation for chamber temperature measurement; however, relative humidity determination can be difficult because sensors used for water vapor detection are often affected by the test compound in the chamber. One of the cheapest and most accurate methods of determining relative humidity is with dry and wet bulb thermocouples, but this system requires time-consuming calculations and extra maintenance (e.g., one thermocouple must remain wet). On the other hand, some detectors (i.e., organic and inorganic crystals that sense moisture) require no special preparation and provide a direct readout in percent relative humidity, but they can be damaged by the vapors of certain test chemicals.

To measure relative humidity using wet-dry bulb thermocouples, the wet bulb must have the air moving across the probe. The air velocity necessary for an accurate measurement is not attainable in the chamber but is in the chamber exhaust duct (Fig. 7). Consequently, one must determine the moisture content of the air in the exhaust duct (intercept of wet bulb and dry bulb temperature on a psychrometric chart) then transform it to the relative humidity in the chamber using the dry bulb temperature value for the chamber (from intercept, move horizontally on a psychrometric chart to chamber temperature and read relative humidity). It should be noted that large quantities of water may be required to keep the wick wet if the relative humidity of the exhaust duct air is below 50% or if chamber airflow rates are high.

D. Filtration of Chamber Inlet Air

A common air-filtration system for the inlet air contains a prefilter or "roughing" filter, followed by an activated carbon filter that is followed

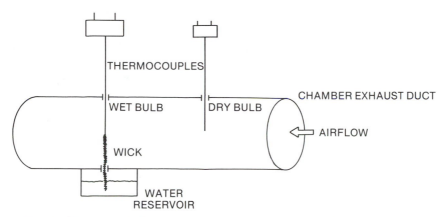

Fig. 7 Thermocouple (K-type) placement in chamber exhaust duct for relative humidity determination. The reservoir should contain distilled water.

by a standard high efficiency particulate (HEPA) filter. A standard HEPA filter is designed to remove particles greater than 0.3μ. The purpose of the prefilter is to trap large particles, so that the HEPA filter does not become clogged so frequently. The HEPA filter is placed after the carbon filter in order to trap any carbon dust particles. Refer to Section VIII on chamber exhaust for additional information on filtration.

E. Noise Control

Installation of noise-reduction equipment, for example, a baffle system like a muffler, may be necessary. A muffler can be inserted into the exhaust duct between the exhaust fans and the chambers. As a guide, maximum sound levels of 62 to 65 DB (A scale) within the chamber are acceptable. However, because stressful, high frequency noise can be perceived by certain animal species and not by humans, it is necessary to make sure that animals in the chamber show normal behavior and body weight gains. This is, perhaps, as important as keeping sound levels within the above-stated ranges.

F. Monitoring and Alarm System

For inhalation chamber temperature and humidity, wet and dry bulb probes can be attached to a data logger that can scan each probe continuously. If there is a deviation in temperature beyond a preset range, the data logger will print these values along with the time of day. Otherwise, the data logger will print the wet and dry bulb temperatures on an hourly basis.

The testing guidelines (e.g., OECD, 1981) have stated that continuous monitoring of chamber temperature and humidity is necessary. Incorporation of a reliable scanning system with notification of deviations from defined limits, as just described, is a practical approach to this requirement.

Certain environmental controls not only have alarm capabilities but also have fail-safe mechanisms incorporated into their operation. For example, if the temperature of the air from the heating duct of the room drops below a low temperature limit, an alarm will sound. If no action is taken within a short period of time, the airflow to the room will automatically shut off. This prevents extreme stresses to the animals from incoming cold air and freezing of the steam coils. Rooms large enough to have space for chambers and animal housing usually can maintain an oxygen level that will be unaffected by a temporary shutdown of airflow. An upper limit temperature alarm functions similarly. If the temperature exceeds a certain upper limit, as in a fire situation, the room airflow system will automatically shut down.

G. Important Considerations for Environmental Control Systems

Backup equipment or the ability to divert conditioned air from one set of chambers not being used to another are important considerations in the design of environmental systems. Some examples of this for a push-pull ventilation system are depicted in Fig. 8. In this figure, two banks of chambers are shown, each having its own air inlet, air-conditioning system, and air exhaust system. The numbers encircled in the figure refer to the following numbered sections on equipment redundancy or alternative procedures.

1. Instead of a backup air-conditioning unit for each bank of chambers (total of four units), only three air-conditioning units are set in series such that any two can be operated at one time. Rotation of the units will allow for normal and preventive maintenance.
2. If any part of the ventilation system fails (i.e., heating, air-conditioning, or filtration) and there is no backup equipment, either bank of chambers can be used if the two ventilation systems are interconnected.
3. Exhaust fans have an electrical interrupt switch such that when one fan fails, due to electrical power or belt failure, the other fan will switch on immediately. At the same time, a pneumatic valve closes the duct to the nonfunctional fan to prevent back draft through this fan.

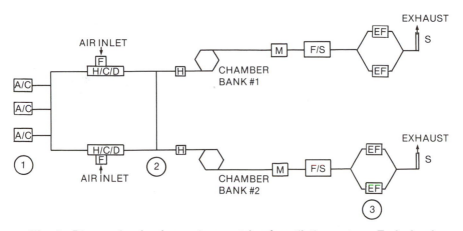

Fig. 8 Diagram for chamber environmental and ventilation systems. Each chamber bank contains five chambers connected to a common inlet and exhaust duct for that chamber bank. A/C, air-conditioning units; F, filtration; H, humidification; M, muffler; F/S, filtration/scrubber; EF, exhaust fan; S, stack.

Naturally, cost of redundant equipment versus cost incurred because of downtime of the chambers or disruption of an ongoing experiment has to be evaluated. Short interruptions in a subchronic or chronic study may have little bearing on the results of the test, but interruption in a developmental toxicology or short-term study may result in having to repeat the study.

Another important consideration in environmental control is what types of valve and damper controls are the most appropriate in an HVAC system. Electrical control systems may be more costly and more difficult to operate primarily because a separate motor is required to operate each valve or damper; whereas only air pressure is necessary to control functional components in a pneumatic control system.

VII. CHAMBER AIR AND AIRFLOW

Methods have been described on how to condition the air entering the chamber (refer to Section VI on environmental control). Briefly, the air is first filtered to remove contaminants and then adjusted for temperature and moisture content. Introduction of a test compound to the air entering the chamber may alter the air temperature or relative humidity. For example, the glass evaporator described later in this chapter (refer to Section IX on vapor and gas generation) is designed so that all air coming into the chamber passes through it. Therefore, heat applied to the evaporator will warm the incoming air. To compensate for this additional source of heat, the air entering the evaporator may have to be adjusted in order for the resulting air at the breathing zone of the animals to be within the desirable temperature and relative humidity ranges. There are certain cases, however, particularly during this generation of aerosols, in which the relative humidity range recommended by the guidelines may not be practicable.

To select a suitable chamber airflow, several factors must be considered. Turbulent mixing of the test material in air should occur for good chamber distribution of the test material (refer to Section III on chamber design for a discussion on critical velocity for turbulent airflows). The oxygen concentration should not fall below 19%. Heat and humidity generated by the animals should not increase substantially. Contaminants, such as ammonia, produced from the bacterial action on animal excreta, should be kept to a minimum concentration. Barrow and Dodd (1979) measured chamber ammonia concentrations as a function of chamber airflow and animal volume. Increasing the chamber airflow resulted in lowering the chamber ammonia concentrations for a given animal volume.

The amount of test compound available or the expense and labor of cleaning the test compound from the atmosphere may be the limiting factors for selection of a suitable chamber airflow. Perhaps the most important consideration for chamber airflow selection is the amount of time required for the chamber concentration to reach equilibrium (final concentration), which is dependent on chamber airflow. A general equation for chamber concentration buildup (or decay) was derived by Silver (1946). The exponential form of the equation describing the rise in concentration is $C = (W/F)[1 - \exp(Ft/V)]$, where C is the concentration in the chamber after time (t); W is the weight of the test compound introduced per minute; F is the total airflow through the chamber; and V is the chamber volume.

By rearranging this equation, one can calculate the time necessary to reach a percentage (P) of the chamber equilibrium concentration: $P = 100[1 - \exp(-Ft/V)]$. When a percentage value is selected, the equation collapses to the simple form $t_p = K(V/F)$, where t_p equals the time required to attain a percentage of the equilibrium concentration and K becomes a constant determined by the percentage value. For example, the time required to reach 99% of the equilibrium concentration is termed t_{99}, and the constant (K) from the equation $t_p = K(V/F)$ equals 4.605. Likewise, the time to reach 85% of the chamber equilibrium concentration (t_{85}) can be calculated by using the value of 1.897 for K. MacFarland (1976) has recommended that the selection of chamber airflow meets the condition that the duration of exposure be at least 13 times t_{99}. Thus, for a chamber volume of 1,000 liters and an exposure time of six hours, a chamber airflow of at least 166 liters/minute would be recommended. Most inhalation toxicologists realize the advantages in selecting a chamber airflow that gives a low t_{99} value. In general, for whole-body exposure chambers, an airflow of 10 to 15 air changes (chamber volume) per hour is appropriate; but for nose-only exposure chambers, a minimum flow of twice the minute volume times the number of animals exposed is suggested.

Current OECD (1981) guidelines have stipulated a continuous monitoring of chamber airflow or at least a frequent recording of airflow. There are several ways to measure chamber airflow, but an orifice meter placed on the intake or exhaust duct of the chamber is a simple and popular procedure. An orifice meter should be positioned at least five pipe (duct) diameters upstream from a bend in the pipe and at least ten pipe diameters downstream from a bend. The orifice meter measures rate of flow as opposed to total flow. When an orifice plate (or restriction) is placed in an airstream duct, a differential pressure is created. The pressure on the upstream side of the orifice plate is greater than the pressure on the downstream side. Throat taps are strategically placed on each side of the orifice plate for measurement of pressure. One tap needs to be positioned a half pipe (duct) diameter downstream from the orifice meter and the other tap placed one pipe diameter upstream from the orifice meter (Partridge, 1952). A differential pressure gauge (Magnehelic® gauge, Dwyer Instruments, Inc., Michigan City, Indiana) may be connected to the taps. If factors such as orifice diameter, pressure differential, static pressure, and orifice flow constants are determined, then the velocity of air passing through the orifice plate can be calculated. Although a theoretical calculation of chamber airflow may be derived from an orifice meter, this device is usually used as a relative measure of airflow and does not provide accurate flow data.

Reliable standards for more accurate assessments of chamber airflow are dry gas meters or airflow transducers, such as the type made by Autotronic Controls Corporation, El Paso, Texas. The transducer has a rotating shaft in which the number of revolutions is dependent on airflow. Once positioned in the intake or exhaust duct of a chamber, the transducer is capable of giving continuous measurement of airflow. A disadvantage of placing any airflow monitor in an exhaust duct is its susceptibility to corrosion by the test compound. To save expense, one transducer can be used to calibrate several (or all) chambers in a facility. However, each chamber needs an orifice meter. A calibration curve plotting pressure drop across the chamber orifice plate as opposed to airflow

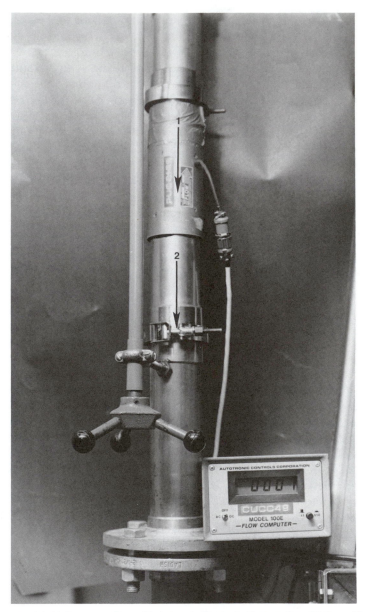

Fig. 9 (1) Airflow transducer (Autotronic Controls Corporation, El Paso, Texas). (2) Tri-Clover® clamps (Ladish Co., Kenosha, Wisconsin) allow for easy insertion of the transducer into the duct for calibrating chamber airflow.

data from the transducer can be produced for each chamber. For convenience, the transducer may be adapted so that it can be easily installed in a chamber duct. Figure 9 shows a transducer positioned in the chamber exhaust duct with Tri-Clover® clamps (Ladish Co., Kenosha, Wisconsin). Calibration checks can be made prior to, during, or following study exposures. Chamber airflow can be precisely regulated if gate valves are placed in the chamber duct system. A valve that requires at least five revolutions before it is fully opened or closed allows precise control of chamber airflows. For easy operation and safety, the handles of the gate valves can be extended so that all valve changes can be made at ground level.

Another popular instrument for measuring chamber airflow is a mass flowmeter. Mass flowmeters work on the principle of measuring the heat transferred by the gas, in this case, air. Three factors determine the transfer of heat: the number of molecules (mass flow) passing the heat source, the amount of heat added to the air, and the heat capacity of air (approximately 0.288 calories/liter/°C). Because the thermal sensor of the mass flowmeter detects the number of air molecules flowing across its surface, direct measurements are made irrespective of temperature and pressure conditions. However, when mass flow is converted to volumetric flow, a correction for air temperature and pressure is necessary. Manufacturers (e.g., Kurz Instruments, Inc., Monterey, California) of mass flowmeters will provide a calibration curve that takes into account the cross-sectional area of the pipe where the flowmeter is to be installed as well as the heat capacity of air. Portable mass flowmeters must be properly positioned and aligned in an air duct to give precise readings. The sensors of mass flowmeters are subject to damage by test chemical atmospheres and are expensive to replace; therefore, a system in which the flowmeters can be easily installed and removed, such as the Tri-Clover® clamp system described earlier, is recommended.

Chamber airflow measurements may also be assessed with a pitot tube connected differentially to a manometer. However, a pitot tube positioned in an exhaust duct can be clogged by animal dander. Also, to obtain accurate (± 2%) readings requires correct location and precise alignment of the pitot tube in the air duct. Another way of obtaining a continuous recording of chamber airflow is to insert a pressure transducer between taps of an orifice meter. The electronic signal produced by the pressure transducer is then traced on a recorder. Calibration curves of electronic signal response versus airflow can then be generated.

When measuring chamber airflow, one must take into consideration any extra air that may be introduced into the chamber by generation of the test compound, by sampling of the test compound, or by chamber leaks. Airflow data are commonly measured from the exhaust side of the chamber to take into consideration all possible additions or subtractions of airflow. MacFarland (1981) has given a hypothetical example in which a sampling pump increased the total chamber airflow and subsequently led to a lower chamber concentration of the test compound. Significant deviation in chamber airflow during an exposure can jeopardize the validity of a study if not detected quickly. Perhaps the simplest indicator for an emergency situation is a differential pressure sensor that reacts by sounding an alarm to changes in pressure within the chamber inlet duct.

VIII. CHAMBER EXHAUST

A popular method of cleaning the contaminated air from a chamber or a bank of chambers that have a common exhaust duct is to filter the exhaust. A common filtration system contains a prefilter or "roughing" filter, followed by a standard HEPA filter or an activated carbon filter. The purpose of the prefilter is to trap large particles, such as animal dander and hair, so that the HEPA filter does not become clogged so frequently. Although an activated carbon filter is highly effective in adsorbing and retaining many gases and vapors, it is not able to remove all of them. Activated charcoal has a low capacity for retaining ammonia or formaldehyde. The charcoal may, however, be chemically impregnated to increase its retaining capacity for a particular gas or vapor. For example, the impregnation of activated carbon with triethylene diamine enhances the trapping of methyl iodide. Information on the types, specifications, and typical properties of commercially made impregnated carbons is readily available in brochures and technical bulletins printed by the manufacturers (e.g., Barnebey Cheney, Columbus, Ohio).

A filtration system often requires a considerable amount of maintenance, but there are several features that can be added to a system to make it more convenient and manageable. For example, a bag-in, bag-out HEPA filter provides protection for the individuals responsible for changing the filter and transporting it to a suitable disposal area. A differential pressure gauge can be placed across each HEPA filter to monitor replacement frequency of the filter. As the HEPA filter becomes clogged, the pressure drop across the filter increases. This may cause a problem in maintaining constant chamber airflow. Therefore, frequent readings of the differential pressure gauges are recommended to keep chamber operators aware of pressure fluctuations in the exhaust duct.

To check the efficiency of a charcoal filter, analytical sampling of the air downstream of the filter is necessary. The sampling should be done periodically because the theoretical calculation of quantity of charcoal needed to reduce the concentration to a particular level is not always accurate. The difference between the theoretical and actual value for filter "break through" may be due to several factors, such as the gradual sloughing of the adsorbed test compound, particularly if the chamber airflow is left on during the 18 hours (assuming 6-hour exposure) when the test compound is not being generated. In this case, the amount of charcoal needed may be less than the theoretical calculated amount.

Consideration must be given to the quantity of carbon required for safe filtration, the time required before changing the medium, and the degree of uncertainty about whether the filtration medium will work. For rough estimating purposes, for every pound of pure test material to be trapped, four to six pounds of charcoal are needed. If the airflow through the filter is not of sufficient contact time (e.g., two seconds or longer), more charcoal may be necessary.

Instead of used charcoal filters being replaced with new filters, a refillable charcoal filter can be purchased and the charcoal bed replaced when needed. The housing of this filter should be of durable material, such as stainless steel. Also, used carbon can be reactivated by high temperature oxidation or stripped by steam; however, the costs for these methods can be high and should be weighed against the costs for off-site disposal as a toxic waste.

A filtration system will not be adequate for some vapors and gases because activated charcoal lacks the ability to adsorb and retain some test compounds, and unrealistically large charcoal beds are required to remove these compounds. In addition to filtration, air washing or scrubbing is another process that eliminates undesirable vapors and gases. Good design practice is to recirculate the scrubbing medium at approximately 10 to 15 gal/min/sq ft of scrubber cross section if the scrubber column is 18 in or less. Effective filtration by air washing or scrubbing is not just limited to water-soluble gases and vapors. Selectivity for enhanced chemical retention can be made by altering the pH of the water; however, the scrubber (e.g., Heil Process Equipment Division, Avon, Ohio) will have to be designed with suitable plumbing and interior surface, such as epoxy, to prevent corrosion from caustic agents. An example of how water treatment enhances retention is that of an 8% sodium hydroxide solution in a spray-type washer. The solution effectively extracts most airborne sulfur dioxide, whereas the solubility of sulfur dioxide in untreated water is less than 10% at 25°C. If a wide variety of vapors and gases are to be generated in an inhalation facility, a filtration system and an air scrubber can be placed in series (Fig. 10). The drawbacks to having an air scrubber alone are inefficiency in chemical scrubbing, cost, maintenance, and problems associated with disposal of waste

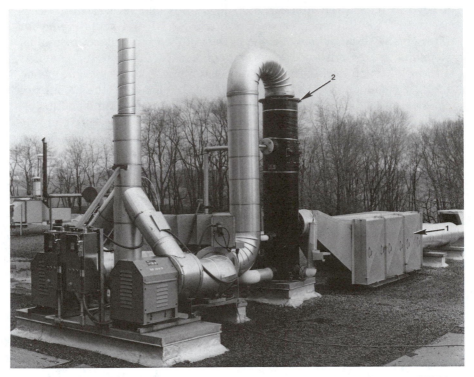

Fig. 10 Test compound is removed from chamber exhaust by (1) filtration (HEPA and activated carbon) and/or (2) scrubbing.

water. Proper safety equipment must be installed for the storage and disposal of the waste water.

Total elimination or destruction of chamber exhaust, if possible, can be very costly. Because of the high chamber concentrations required for some toxicity studies or because of extremely low odor threshold concentrations of some test compounds, different exhaust treatment systems may be necessary. In these cases, other alternatives of chamber exhaust treatment should be considered. However, even with a combination of two or three procedures, decreasing exhaust concentrations by three orders of magnitude may be the best that is attainable. Incineration of the chamber air can be as much as 99.9% efficient in destruction of organics but can be the most costly means of treatment. In addition, the oxidative products may still have to be removed before allowing the exhaust air to enter the atmosphere. The different types of incinerator equipment available include flame, fume, and catalytic incinerators.

Modification to existing boilers or incinerators can be a more economical approach to treat the chamber exhaust but will probably not be as effective as the other types of incinerators listed.

Methods of treatment that are nondestructive but do assist in decreasing the ground concentration levels of the test material include increasing the stack height and routing the exhaust to a stack that has heated air to aid in thermal dispersion. In addition, many chamber exhaust systems are designed to pull much more air than what comes from a bank of chambers having a common exhaust duct. The extra air or "makeup" air keeps the pressures within the exhaust duct constant and dilutes the test compound coming from the chambers. An effective way of diluting the chamber exhaust is to add the diluting air after the chamber exhaust air has been treated by filtration or scrubbing. Therefore, a smaller volume of air is treated, which allows for slower airflows and, consequently, more effective treatment.

Exhaust stack height and wind speed contribute to the dilution of the exhaust. A cautionary comment: in the design of an exhaust system, place the system an adequate distance (and downstream of prevailing winds) from any air intake duct. For dispersion estimates from an exhaust stack, refer to Turner (1974). From these equations, a concentration of the test compound can be determined at a given distance for a given wind speed and stack emission rate.

IX. VAPOR AND GAS GENERATION

For generation of vapors, a multitude of methods exist (Miller *et al.*, 1980; Potts and Steiner, 1980; Decker *et al.*, 1982). The important features of a well-designed vapor generator are a large surface area for liquid evaporation, a variable controlled heating element, and an ability to create turbulent mixing within the generator and conduct the generated vapors into the chamber with air or appropriate diluent gas (usually nitrogen). One generator that has proved successful for a variety of both low and high boiling liquids is a heated spiral-grooved glass tube (Fig. 11) that has the test compound flowing countercurrent to the chamber airflow (Carpenter *et al.*, 1975). The heating element is a curled nichrome wire that is wrapped around the spiral grooves and extends the length of the tube. Connected to the nichrome wire is a variable transformer. The temperature in the evaporator is maintained at the lowest level sufficient to vaporize the liquid. All air entering the chamber travels through the tube. To protect personnel working around the heated glass tube from burns, a glass jacket covers the tube. For safe operation, the test material

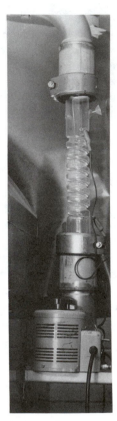

Fig. 11 Heated spiral-grooved, glass tube vapor generator used to vaporize low and high boiling liquids. Glass jacket cover has been removed.

must not be heated close to its autoignition point, and consideration of safe operation during equipment failure (e.g., loss of heat or breakage of evaporator column) should be made before testing is initiated. Two important modifications have been made on the original design by Carpenter *et al.* (1975). First, a glass tube (approximately 5 mm in diameter) runs about one third the distance along the inside of the spiral-grooved evaporator and is open near the top of the evaporator where it is attached. A thermocouple can be placed inside the 5-mm glass tube, and the temperature within the evaporator can be monitored. Also, clamps have been installed on both ends of the chamber air intake duct where the evaporator is to be placed. In order to produce a good seal, flanges have been added to both ends of the glass evaporator. This feature allows easy removal of the evaporator for cleaning purposes or for insertion of another type of liquid evaporator.

One type of liquid evaporator, which has a large surface area for vaporization, utilizes a hot countercurrent airstream to vaporize the liquid instead of applying heat directly to the liquid–surface interface (Fig. 12). The large surface area is achieved by a long, rotating stainless steel tube tilted 10 to 20 degrees from a horizontal position so that the metered liquid test compound flows down the tube by gravity. The primary use of this type of liquid evaporator has been for the vaporization of test compounds that decompose or polymerize if heated directly.

There are situations in which the vapor of concern must be generated from a parent test compound of different physical and/or chemical composition. For example, in thermal decomposition inhalation studies, vapors are evolved from heating solid test compounds. We have used a tubular furnace generator that can be heated to very high temperatures (e.g., 600°C) for the production of monomer vapors from liquid dimer test compounds. The furnace (Lindberg® Furnace, General Signal, Watertown, Wisconsin) has an oven length of 12 in. with an oven diameter of 1 in. A 1-in. (diameter) by 18-in. (length) quartz tube is placed in the hollow cylinder of the furnace. Within the tube are several smaller quartz tubes of 2 mm (diameter) by 12 in. (length) to increase the surface area and allow "cracking" of the dimer to the monomer. The liquid test compound is metered into one end of the tube, and nitrogen gas is passed through it to carry the vapor to the chamber air intake duct for further dilution of the vapor-nitrogen mixture with air. If the test material is a

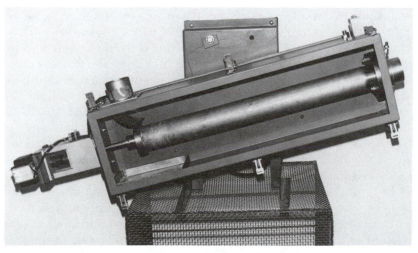

Fig. 12 Vapor generator used to vaporize mixtures and test compounds that decompose if heated directly. The test compound flows down the inside of the rotating tube until it is vaporized by warm air passing through the tube.

solid (e.g., menthol, napthalene, paradichlorobenzene, or paraformalde-hyde), a stainless steel container (McMaster Carr Supply Co., New Brunswick, New Jersey) placed in an industrial oven is often used to vaporize the test compound. Air or nitrogen gas lines are connected to the stainless steel container to carry the vapor to the chamber air intake duct.

The procedure for generating a vapor by first aerosolizing the liquid test material and then heating the aerosol conducting tube to evaporate the droplets (or allowing the droplets to evaporate at ambient tempera-tures) has been used. However, caution must be taken because the com-plete elimination of the test material aerosol may be difficult to achieve. Furthermore, methods used to check the presence of an aerosol in the exposure atmosphere may not be reliable, particularly when a volatile aerosol is sampled. This concern is important because differences in toxic effects for some solvents have been noted (personal observation) when animals were exposed to a vapor atmosphere generated by a heated glass evaporator as opposed to being exposed to a vapor-aerosol mixture gener-ated by aerosolizing methods.

The delivery of liquid test compound to an evaporator must be done by a highly reliable pump. The pump should be spark proof, resistant to chemical attack, and capable of delivering solutions of widely varying viscosities as well as not contaminate the test compound. Two depend-able pumps are the piston type (Fluid Metering, Inc., Oyster Bay, New York) and the syringe type (Sage Instruments, Orion Research, Cam-bridge, Massachusetts) generally used for high flow (ml/min) and low flow (μl/min) deliveries, respectively. Both types of pumps can be pur-chased with continuous variable flow control, which allows the amount of test compound delivered into the evaporator to be accurately and pre-cisely metered. The delivery lines leading into or away from the pumps should be made of inert material. Usually Teflon® or stainless steel lines and fittings are employed. Prior to operation, the input and output sides of the pumps can be pressure tested with SNOOP® liquid (NUPRO Co., Willoughby, Ohio) to check for leaks.

The piston pump requires a reservoir of the liquid test compound to be placed a few inches above the pump head. The test compound must then be siphoned into the pump head. Because siphoning the test compound may be hazardous, a ball valve can be placed on the end of the delivery line away from the reservoir. With a syringe temporarily attached adja-cent to the ball valve, the delivery line can be filled and the ball valve closed. After the delivery line is attached to the inflow side of the pump head, the ball valve can be opened. Piston pumps that operate in forward and reverse gears are recommended because, at the end of the vapor generation, the liquid test compound can be pumped back into the reservoir with less likelihood of chemical spills. Also, weight or volume of the test compound delivered during exposure can be easily measured in this manner (for calculating nominal chamber concentration).

A syringe pump requires little maintenance, and pump operation is simple. Reliable performance can be ensured by removing all air bubbles from the syringe and the delivery line and by selecting a syringe size so that the plunger is not withdrawn from the barrel more than about 70% of its length. This is to avoid the possibility of buckling between the barrel and the plunger, which might cause a sudden surge in test compound delivery and, consequently, promote overexposure of the animals in the chamber.

Both the piston-type and the syringe-type pumps need to be calibrated with the liquid test compound prior to generating test chamber atmospheres. Small differences among calibration curves of various test compounds do exist for any pump, presumably due to differences in the test compounds' specific gravity and viscosity. Also, friction between a glass barrel and a plunger changes with use. The stroke volume of a piston pump may also change due to wear on the plunger and/or the cylinder. Calibration curves commonly consist of pump settings or determination of liquid flow rates. By measuring the volume delivered by the pump with a stopwatch, one can determine the liquid flow rate. For greater accuracy, the weight of the test compound delivered over a defined time period can be determined. Accurate flow rates can be assessed if several minutes or possibly hours are allowed to pass before the recording of volume collected and if duplicate or triplicate recordings are made. After data points are established, linear regression statistics may be applied and a slope and Y intercept calculated. Once the calibration curve is constructed, a desired flow rate can be set on the flow control dial of the pump.

Maintenance of pumps is usually minimal; however, cleaning is recommended on a daily basis during use. The appropriate cleaning solvent depends on compatibility with the test compound, but warm water or acetone is often used. The seals of the piston pumps should be checked frequently because volatile organic liquids tend to dry the seals, which causes stiffening and cracking.

Several liquid test compounds are highly volatile, reactive, and flammable, and, therefore, require a unique method to generate vapors prior to introduction into the inhalation chambers. One procedure is to keep the test compound in a stainless steel cylinder equipped with a pressure relief valve (which should be safely vented), a pressure gauge, and metering valves (Fig. 13). A filling tube extends from the bottom of the cylinder to the union with the ball valves. The cylinder is then joined to a

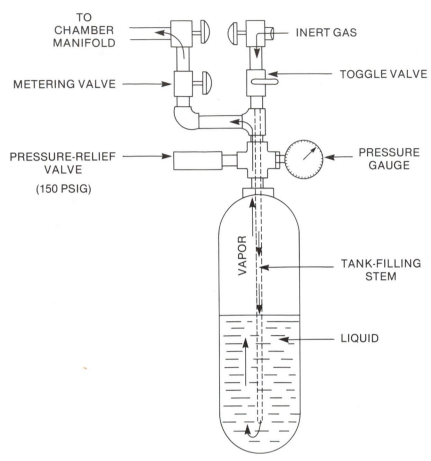

Fig. 13 Vapor generator used for highly volatile, reactive, or flammable test compounds.

stainless steel manifold line that leads to flowmeters attached to the air intake ducts of individual chambers. Due to the latent heat of vaporization, the manifold line may have to be thermally controlled, and, if so, proper grounding is required. A nitrogen (or suitable carrier gas) supply is attached to the filling tube. A "one-way" flow valve may be placed between the nitrogen supply and the cylinder to prevent overpressurization of the test compound cylinder. When the chamber flowmeters are opened, the nitrogen pushes the vapors of the cylinder head space into the manifold line, and the resultant nitrogen–test compound vapor mixture is delivered into the chamber air intake duct. This procedure was used to deliver vapor-air mixtures of methyl isocyanate, a highly volatile, reactive, and flammable chemical (Dodd *et al.*, 1986). The cylinder has to be temperature regulated in order to control the vapor pressure of the test compound.

The goal of this setup is to maintain a constant vapor concentration in the manifold line. However, there are several assumptions that have to be made before a vapor concentration of test compound in the manifold line can be calculated. The degree of saturation between the test compound and the carrier gas may be less than 100% and will vary for any given temperature, thus lowering the cylinder head space vapor concentration. If accuracy is a prerequisite, then an analytical determination of the test compound in the manifold line will give the inhalation toxicologist a concentration value from which to calculate appropriate chamber airflow and test compound flow rates to obtain a desired chamber concentration.

Dilution of pure gases is the simplest procedure for generating test atmospheres in a dynamic exposure system. Schematically, a gas cylinder of known concentration of a test compound is connected to a flowmeter, which is attached to the chamber intake duct. If the flow rate of the test compound is assumed to be far less than that of the chamber air, the following equation can be used: $ppm_1 \cdot$ flow rate$_1 = ppm_2 \cdot$ flow rate$_2$, where ppm_1 and flow rate$_1$ are the cylinder concentration and flow rate for the test compound, respectively, and ppm_2 and flow rate$_2$ are the target chamber concentration of the test compound and chamber airflow rate, respectively. The units for flow rate must be the same for both sides of the equation.

Use of high quality, chemical-resistant rotameters (Fischer and Porter Co., Warminster, Pennsylvania) for the delivery of test gases is recommended. To decrease the potential for accidental breakage of the glass tube in the rotameter, a protective shield (e.g., a plastic tube) may be placed around the flowmeter. Although calibration curves are usually supplied by the manufacturers, rotameters are routinely calibrated with air at standard atmospheric conditions (70°F, 760 mmHg) by measuring volume displacement with time. Air volume is usually measured by single or continuous displacement methods. For single displacement procedures, a soap bubble meter or simple spirometer is frequently used. Dry gas meters (Singer-American Meter Division, Philadelphia, Pennsylvania, or Rockwell International, Pittsburgh, Pennsylvania) or wet test meters (GCA Precision Scientific Co., Chicago, Illinois) are examples of instruments used for measurement of continuous displacement of air volume. Following calibration with air, minor corrections for specific test compound flow may then be made. For example, to correct for test gas density, the calculation $F(0.0012/\rho)^{1/2}$ can be used, where F is the airflow in ml/min and ρ is the density of the test compound in g/ml. This equation is most appropriate if the viscosity of the test compound is close to that of air. If atmospheric conditions other than 70°F and 760 mmHg exist, then the calculation $F[(P/14.7) \cdot (530/T)]^{1/2}$ may be employed, where P is the absolute pressure in lb/sq in and T is the temperature in °R (°R = °F + 460) of the test gas. Again, this equation is most appropriate if the conditions of test compound flow are not too radically different from standard atmospheric conditions. Experimentally, test gas flow through a rotameter may be measured with a primary standard flow device, such as a soap bubble meter. Also, when using soap bubble meters, be sure to vent the test compound to an exhaust hood properly, and avoid using flow rates of less than 1 to 2 ml/min because the accuracy declines due to gas permeation through the soap film (Nelson, 1972).

If test gas densities are radically different from that of air (e.g., arsine, Freon, or dichlorosilane) and accuracy of flow is critical, then mass flowmeters are recommended for delivery. The principle of operation of a mass flowmeter was previously discussed in Section VII on chamber air and airflow. Manufacturers supplying the test gas (e.g., Linde Union Carbide, Somerset, New Jersey) frequently sell the most appropriate mass flowmeter with calibration curves. Mass flowmeters are best controlled with a mass flow controller. A throttling solenoid valve and a potentiometer are added to the mass flowmeter in order to control it automatically. The user simply dials in the desired flow setting. However, a change in the test gas supply pressure (most controllers are calibrated at a given pressure) or a change in the back pressure will alter the balance between the potentiometer and the solenoid valve, resulting in inaccurate flows. Mass flow controllers can be used for blending two or more gases to produce a test exposure mixture.

Leaks around the test gas cylinder, regulator, rotameter, flow lines, and fittings can be checked by several means. One is to apply SNOOP® liquid (NUPRO Co., Willoughby, Ohio) around all unions when the delivery system is under pressure. Bubbles from leaks will form within a few seconds even at low pressures (15 psig). Another check for slow leaks is to close the delivery system under about 10 psig of pressure and record the pressure with a pressure gauge attached to the delivery system. The sealed delivery system should be allowed to stand overnight and the pressure on the pressure gauge recorded the following morning. If a leak exists, the pressure in the delivery system in the morning will be less than that of the preset value.

Because the delivery of gaseous test compounds is under positive pressure conditions, one important safety feature in the generation methodology is to place a solenoid valve between the regulator of the test compound cylinder and the flowmeter. When a sudden alteration in chamber pressure occurs, the solenoid valve should automatically close, thereby stopping the test compound flow. This precautionary measure may prevent worker exposure to the test compound and protect the animals in the inhalation chamber from overexposure when chamber airflow is inadvertently lost.

Not all vapor inhalation exposures are dynamic where the airflow and introduction of the test material into the chamber are continuous. A static exposure system is of great practical value in terms of vapor generation because a limited amount of test material is required and procedures for conducting the exposures are simple. For example, the test material may be introduced into a chamber with a glass syringe. This procedure was used to produce high vapor concentrations of methyl isocyanate for animal exposure (Dodd et al., 1987). However, there are several drawbacks to a static exposure system (e.g., loss of maintaining suitable environmental conditions, decay of test material concentration), and differences in acute toxicity between static and dynamic exposures occur for some test materials (Dodd et al., 1988).

X. AEROSOL GENERATION

The primary objective for the toxicological assessment of aerosols is the introduction of inhalable particles into the exposure chamber. Inhalable particles for humans have been defined by the Health Effects Research Laboratory of the EPA as particles ≤ 15 μm aerodynamic equivalent diameter (Miller et al., 1979). Of particular importance are particles $\leq$ 2.5 μm in diameter, because these particles are believed to enter the gas exchange region of the respiratory tract (i.e., the alveoli). This section is limited to a description of only a few aerosol generation systems. For a much broader introduction to aerosol generation, refer to the textbooks edited by Liu (1976), Willeke (1980), and Hinds (1982).

One of the most popular devices for generating dust particles is the Wright Dust Feeder (Wright, 1950). Similar in principle is the Timbrell Dust Generator (Timbrell et al., 1968). The major limitations for use of the Wright Dust Feeder (WDF) are the physical and/or chemical characteristics of the test compound; specifically, hygroscopic materials, fine fibers, and particles of large diameters (> 20 μm) will clog the feeder. In addition, the suitability of the WDF depends on the packing quality of the test compound. The test compound is compressed into a sample cup at pressures up to several thousand pounds per square inch. For some test compounds, these high pressures will alter the size or shape of the particles and may make them nonrespirable. Two means to control chamber concentration with the WDF are to adjust the airflow through the feeder and to alter the test compound delivery rate by changing the gear ratio of the feeder. Newer WDF models have variable speed motors to control particle output more precisely. To prevent excessive clogging of the WDF, a few minor modifications may be helpful. These modifications can best be followed with a parts manual from one of the manufacturers of the WDF (e.g., BGI Inc., Waltham, Massachusetts). Removal of the jet (part DF.206) and of the impactor plate on the air outlet nozzle (part SA.504) and slight reaming of the air outlet nozzle and the nozzle that is part of the leadscrew spigot assembly (part SA.176) will decrease clogging of the WDF. These modifications may slightly alter the particle size distribution within the inhalation chamber.

When a solid particle test compound does not pack well, a brush dust feeder may be used for generating dust atmospheres (Milliman et al., 1981). This device appears to work well with fly ash. Its only serious limitation may be a loss of output with the use of highly cohesive test compounds. In addition, a wide variety of dusts and fibrous aerosols may be generated with a fluidized bed aerosol generator (Willeke et al., 1974; Marple et al., 1978; Agarwal and Nelson, 1981; Carpenter and Verkes, 1980). Three commercially available fluidized bed generators are ones manufactured by GCA Environmental Instruments (GCA Corporation, Bedford, Massachusetts), IN-TOX Products (Albuquerque, New Mexico), and TSI, Inc. (St. Paul, Minnesota). A well-designed fluidized bed aerosol generator may deagglomerate the test compound to provide a more constant output of particle size. For example, fluidized bed aerosol generators are particularly well suited for generating asbestos aerosols (Willeke et al., 1974). There are many designs for the mechanisms of particle feeding these generators (Marple et al., 1978; Sussman et al., 1985). A drawback of fluidized bed generators is that electrical charges may be imparted to the particles. One approach to neutralize the charges (Liu and Pui, 1974) is to pass the particles through an ion field (e.g., krypton-85). Sealed nickel tubes containing the krypton gas (similar to Amersham Capsule X162, Amersham Inc., Arlington Heights, Illinois) can then be inserted into a stainless steel holder similar in design to that described by Teague et al., 1978. The krypton-85 neutralizer, once assembled, should be placed between the aerosol generator and the chamber air inlet. Because of the radioactive gas, a license must be obtained from the U.S. Nuclear Regulatory Commission.

If aerosols are to be formed from a liquid test compound or from suspensions of an insoluble or colloidal agent, then nebulizers are commonly used for droplet generation. Selecting the proper nebulizer depends on the desired exposure concentration and particle size, the duration of exposure, and the physical and chemical properties of the test compound. The Laskin nebulizer (Drew *et al.,* 1978) is available with one to four aspirator tubes. The article by Drew *et al.* (1978) describes a single aspirator tube nebulizer, but the results may be extrapolated to a multiple aspirator tube design. The purpose of multiple tubes is to increase aerosol production. The stainless steel construction of the Laskin nebulizer makes it suitable for generating organic or reactive aerosols at high concentrations. To increase the duration of aerosol generation at a given operating pressure (without refilling the reservoir), the aspirator tube can be lengthened to approximately 3 in. from the original 1-in. design, and the angle of the tip of the aspirator tube changed from 45 to 15°.

A liquid aerosol generator that has been useful for a wide range of test compounds and also provides high aerosol output is the stainless steel air atomizer made by Spraying Systems Co. (Wheaton, Illinois). For some chamber designs, these atomizers (i.e., setup no. 1A; 1650 fluid cap, and 64 air cap) can be directly mounted at the top of the chamber. However, a chamber distribution analysis (Section IV) will have to be performed to demonstrate uniformity of aerosol distribution. To produce a more consistent size of aerosol in the chamber, the air atomizer can be mounted in a glass chromatographic tank to remove by impaction the larger formed droplets. The smaller and more uniform size droplets can then be carried to the air inlet venturi for introduction of the test compound into the chamber. With the atomization tank, the impacted test compound can also be collected and continuously recirculated if desired.

The Solo-Sphere® nebulizer (McGraw Respiratory Therapy, Inc., Irvine, California) utilizes the Babington principle (Litt and Swift, 1972) and, like the Laskin nebulizer, has a high output. However, it may not be suitable for organic materials due to its plastic construction. Also, it should not be used with suspensions of particles because the nebulizer may become clogged. Since Solo-Sphere® nebulizers are mass produced, each has slightly different operating characteristics and, therefore, calibration data must be obtained for each nebulizer used in a study. If only a limited amount of test compound is available, nebulizers of smaller output, such as a Dautrebande (Dautrebande, 1962) or a Lovelace (IN-TOX Products, Albuquerque, New Mexico) may be used. A typical output for the Lovelace nebulizer is 50 μl/min at an airflow rate of 1.2 liter/min.

The operating characteristics of compressed air nebulizers have been studied by several investigators; one study is that of Mercer *et al.* (1968). The most important operating parameters are pressure and flow rate, aerosol output, and particle size distribution. To measure the flow rate (usually in liters/min) at several pressures, a pressure gauge is placed on the compressed filtered air line attached to the inlet of the nebulizer, and airflow is measured downstream from the nebulizer. For aerosol output measurement, the nebulizer and its contents are weighed before and after generation. By determining the volume of solution consumed by the nebulizer with time, one can calculate the nebulizer flow rate. For determination of particle size distribution, see Section XI on aerosol characterization.

The aerosol concentration in the exposure chamber may be regulated by varying the airflow through the nebulizer, the amount of diluting air added to the system (i.e., chamber airflow), and the concentration of the test compound in the nebulizer. These variations may change the mass output and/or the particle size distribution of the nebulizer. Also, the continuous recirculation of a diluted test compound may evaporate the diluent causing an increase in the concentration of the test compound in the reservoir over time. Two possible solutions to this problem are to generate aerosols from a very large reservoir of diluted test compound to "buffer" any concentration changes that may occur due to evaporation or allow only a one-time pass (continuous feed) of the diluted test compound through the nebulizer. Miller *et al.* (1981) have described additional equipment and procedures used to conduct EPA acute inhalation tests.

A final consideration of aerosol generation procedures is to introduce the aerosol, once it has been formed, into the inhalation chamber properly. To ensure particulate mixing (refer to Section III on chamber design for a discussion of critical velocity for turbulent mixing), it is recommended to position a venturi mixer immediately upstream of the chamber. The most critical sizes of the venturi mixer are the cone angles. It is important that all edges be smooth to prevent impaction of the test compound. The aerosol is introduced into the throat of the mixer, which can be constructed of Plexiglas® or Lucite®.

XI. AEROSOL CHARACTERIZATION

This section is limited to a description of only a few methods and procedures of aerosol characterization. A broader discussion of this area can be found in textbooks edited by Mercer (1973), Liu (1976), Lundgren *et al.* (1979), or Hinds (1982) and in a review article by Lippmann (1970). As is discussed in Section XII on chamber concentration analysis, the concentration of nonvolatile aerosols in the chamber is usually measured by gravimetric means. However, there are many types of mixtures and formulations that require other analytical methods to determine the chamber concentration because the information gained by gravimetric means applies to the weight of all components combined in a test compound mixture or formulation, not to an individual active component. For example, pesticide formulations frequently have vehicles of low volatility, and the vehicle will impact on the filter with the test compound of concern. Nominal concentrations, calculated from nebulizer output, must not be relied on to characterize exposure conditions (Miller *et al.,* 1981).

To characterize the aerosol in an exposure chamber requires representative sampling and correct transportation of the aerosol to the measuring instrument. Fissan and Schwientek (1987) have summarized some of the more important effects to consider when aerosols are being sampled and transported. To reduce particle losses and changes during transport, Fissan and Schwientek (1987) have said to make the sampling tubes as short as possible; to arrange the tubes vertically and without bends; to use grounded metallic tubes; and to avoid temperature gradients, changes in the thermodynamic state of the aerosol, and coagulation.

Particle size distribution can be assessed by several techniques, including sedimentation, impaction, microscopy, and velocimetry. If a testing inhalation facility plans to conduct several aerosol studies per year, then the purchase of a particle size analyzer providing rapid, yet accurate data will prove to be of economic value. An example of one such instrument is the TSI APS Model 3300 or 3310 Aerodynamic Particle Sizer (TSI Inc., St. Paul, Minnesota) that measures the aerodynamic size of particles in the 0.5 to 15 μm range. This instrument provides real-time measurements of the size distribution of an aerosol by using laser beam optics (Agarwal *et al.,* 1981). The instrument is linked to a computer with a printer and gives size distribution results within seconds. Because the instrument is a single particle counter, one limitation is overloading the analyzer when the production of high concentrations is desired. Therefore, for high concentration exposures, such as 5 mg/L required for acute "limit" tests (TSCA, 1987), this analyzer is of no value. However, TSI, Inc. has designed a sampling diluter (TSI Model 3302) that is reported to reduce aerosol concentrations by 20:1 or 100:1 without altering the size characteristics of the aerosol (Remiarz and Johnson, 1984). The performance of this diluter remains under scientific evaluation.

Most inhalation toxicologists are familiar with the multistage cascade impactor, which is an inertial aerosol sampler invented by May (1945). Cascade impactors such as the seven-stage Mercer (Mercer *et al.,* 1970), the eight-stage Andersen Mark I (Andersen 2000, Inc., Atlanta, Georgia), the ten-stage Sierra Series 210 (Sierra Instruments, Inc., Carmel Valley, California), or the Lovelace Multi-Jet (Newton *et al.,* 1977) are popular devices and provide a detailed measurement of the particle size distribution. When a cascade impactor is being used, the sampling time is a critical parameter in particle sizing. This is because sampling for too short a time will produce little change in the weight of the substrates, whereas sampling for too long a time will overload the stages and change the operating characteristics of the instrument (Mercer et al., 1970). Generally, the minimum loading for a ten-stage Sierra Series 210 cascade impactor should be 0.2 to 0.5 mg per stage, and the maximum should not exceed 1 to 2 mg for dry particles. Higher loadings may be possible with some liquid aerosols because of greater entrainment of the particles on the filter stages.

Various collection substrates are available from manufacturers, for example, fiberglass filters, cellulose filters, and stainless steel discs. The Mercer impactor (also called the Lovelace impactor, available from IN-TOX Products, Albuquerque, New Mexico) can be used at low sampling flow rates, which may be advantageous when a small chamber with a low chamber airflow is sampled for aerosol concentrations. However, the Mercer impactor is a single-jet design, whereas a multijet design may be more suitable for sampling solid particles. The Andersen four-stage minicascade impactor has been tested for characterization of aerosols in exposure chambers at low sampling flow rates, and results were satisfactory (Martonen et al., 1982).

A thorough calibration must be performed for each cascade impactor to determine sizing parameters and wall losses. Wall losses are primarily attributed to particle settling, which decreases with smaller particle size. For example, particles smaller than about 1 to 2 μm in diameter will, in general, produce negligible wall losses. Particles of uniform size (monodisperse aerosols) may be used to calibrate aerosol analyzers and generators. Berglund and Liu (1973) have described a vibrating orifice monodisperse aerosol generator capable of generating aerosol standards from a variety of solid and liquid materials. The generator is available from commercial sources (TSI Model 3050, TSI, Inc., St. Paul, Minnesota). Polystyrene microspheres (Duke Scientific, Palo Alto, California) are commercially available; however, adequate dilution of the microspheres is necessary for proper characterization (Raabe, 1968).

There are several errors inherent in the methods of interpreting cascade impactor data (Mercer, 1965). One generally accepted method, although laborious, is to plot on log-probability paper the effective cutoff diameter (ECD) as the ordinate and the cumulative percentage less than (or greater than) size range by weight as the abscissa for each stage of the impactor. Effective cutoff diameters are supplied by the manufacturer of the impactor. A particle density of 1.0 g/cc is assumed so that particle size can be reported as equivalent aerodynamic diameters. A line is then fitted to the plotted values. The ECD corresponding to 50 cumulative % (ECD_{50}) is read from the graph. This is the mass median aerodynamic diameter (MMAD). The ECD corresponding to 84.1 cumulative % ($ECD_{84.1}$) is also determined from the curve, and the geometric standard deviation (σg) is calculated from the ratio of $ECD_{84.1}/ECD_{50}$. These two values, MMAD and σg, are useful to characterize particle size distribution for toxicology studies. Generally, the particle size distribution is always presented in graphic form because determination of the percentage of a sample above or below a concerned particle size can be rapidly done upon visual inspection.

To assist in determining the aerodynamic size of an aerosol with a cascade impactor, chemical analysis may be employed. Sodium fluorescein is an orange-red powder, freely soluble in water, with a detection limit as low as 0.02 ppm under ultraviolet light (493.5 nm). Fluorescein can be used to estimate particle size distribution of a liquid test compound if a small amount of it is mixed into the test compound. The assumption must be made that fluorescein mixes homogeneously and does not greatly change the properties of the test compound being generated as a liquid aerosol. After an aerosolized test compound–fluorescein mixture is sampled with a cascade impactor, each stage of the impactor is thoroughly and volumetrically rinsed and the concentration of fluorescein determined. The particle size distribution can then be calculated. Fluorescein can also be used to check for wall losses of an impactor. If parts of the impactor other than collection plates are rinsed, collection efficiency can be estimated. Finally, nebulizer characteristics can be assessed with sodium fluorescein solutions. In particular, evaporative losses of the solvent can be estimated by monitoring the increase in concentration of the nebulizer contents with time.

XII. CHAMBER CONCENTRATION ANALYSIS

Analysis of chamber atmospheres is a critical function in an inhalation study. Two popular methods for the analysis of gas or vapor concentrations are infrared spectrometry and gas chromatography. For aerosol concentrations, a gravimetric determination is commonly performed. In fact, there are numerous analytical methods available for inhalation studies. However, the purpose of this discussion is not to describe analytical methods *per se* but to describe specific systems and procedures that will aid the inhalation toxicologist in the monitoring and analysis of chamber atmospheres. For example, the advantages of automatic chamber sampling far outweigh those of manual (syringe or impinger) chamber sampling. An automatic sampling system is one in which the samples of several different chamber atmospheres are pulled through sample lines at low flow rates (e.g., 100 to 300 ml/min), the sample stream is selected automatically, and the selected sample is injected into the analytical instrument. Automatic chamber sampling decreases humanpower needs, increases sampling precision, and allows a greater number of samples to be analyzed during an exposure. To avoid reaction between the test compound and the sample lines of an automatic sampling system, Teflon® lines are recommended. However, some vapors and gases will adsorb to sample lines or penetrate sample lines, subsequently, lower than expected chamber analytical values will result.

A simple test to determine whether a vapor or gas will adsorb to the sample line is to place a gas standard of known concentration of the test compound on the end of the sampling line inside the chamber, then initiate the automatic sampling procedure. If the analytical results are much lower than expected, adsorption losses should be suspected.

Vapors generated from test compounds that have high boiling points tend to adsorb to chamber sampling lines. One approach to solving the adsorption problem is to heat the entire sample line from the chamber to the analytical instrument. Keeping the sample loop, sample valves, and other parts of the analytical introduction system heated is also recommended. Another approach is to purge the sample line continuously with the chamber atmosphere. The continuous purging may help saturate the adsorption sites on the sample lines so that the vapor or gas stream entering the analytical instrument is in equilibrium with the chamber concentration.

An analytical system may be calibrated in many ways. However, the analytical chemists' adage "standards like samples" should be closely followed during calibration of inhalation analytical instrumentation. That is, if the exposure chamber atmosphere sample is a gas or vapor, the calibration standards should be a gas or vapor. It is preferable to avoid using liquid standards if at all possible, because liquid standards are injected directly into the analytical instrument and do not "calibrate" or check the operation of the sample introduction system. The sample introduction system may include several meters of sample lines and numerous valves, filters, and connectors, all of which may interact with the sample or simply malfunction. A gas or vapor standard will serve to check the operation of the entire analytical system.

In general, dynamic gas standards are preferable to static standards because dynamic generation techniques allow fresh standards to be prepared continuously. In this procedure, a fresh supply of standard gas is constantly purging all contact surfaces and reducing or eliminating adsorption losses.

A useful dynamic method of preparing gas standards utilizes diffusion and permeation devices. With this technique, small amounts of vapor are constantly and reproducibly added to a flowing airstream by diffusion of the vapor through a capillary or permeation polymer device. The temperature of these diffusion and permeation devices must be controlled to $\pm$ 0.1°C to maintain 1% accuracy. Temperature, airflow rate, type and thickness of polymer, length of device, diameter of diffusion path, and number of devices may all be varied to prepare different vapor concentrations. The diffusion rate is determined gravimetrically. Disadvantages include the inability to generate high concentrations of many test compounds and the difficulty in generating standards if the test compound is a mixture. Because the technique depends on vapor pressure phenomena, only a single relatively pure compound may be placed in any one device, although several devices may be used simultaneously and each device may contain a different compound.

Other convenient and useful gas standard generation methods include pure or diluted gas concentration cylinders, "head space" standards based on vapor pressure versus temperature data (pure compounds), and bag-mix standards. Bag-mix gas standard preparation requires the introduction of small, but accurately known volumes of a gas or volatile liquid into an inert container containing a known volume of air. A nonrigid container such as a Tedlar® bag (SKC Inc., Eighty Four, Pennsylvania) is useful for standard preparation when large amounts of standard gases are needed, as with automatic sampling systems. Limitations of this method depend on the chemical and physical properties of the particular test compound in question. Vapor pressure and reactivity must be considered prior to standard preparation. If the compound does not volatilize readily at room temperature or if it is highly reactive or adsorptive, inaccurate concentrations may be obtained with preparation procedures like these. Even with these limitations, static bag mixes have wide utility. Gas standard calibration confirms accurate calibration not only of the gas chromatographic or infrared detector but also of the sample introduction system.

Many infrared gas analyzers have closed-loop calibration systems into which liquid samples of undiluted test compounds are injected into a defined chamber volume and vaporized. This is essentially a static preparation method similar to the bag-mix method previously discussed. Some systems constantly circulate the air, which may help vaporize the liquid. In addition, heated systems are available. Adsorption effects are still possible as with any static generation system. Also, the entire analytical introduction system is not necessarily calibrated with this closed-loop calibration technique. However, there is no reason why gas standards prepared dynamically cannot be used for the infrared calibration.

For dust or nonvolatile liquid aerosol studies, gravimetric analysis is usually a simple and straightforward method to determine chamber concentrations. If gravimetric analysis is inappropriate, the test compound will have to be trapped with impingers in a solvent solution and then analyzed by a spectrophotometric, gas chromatographic, or liquid chromatographic procedure. To trap the test compound efficiently, a second or third impinger in series may have to be added. The removal of a chamber air sample for analysis requires calibration of the sampling device (e.g., flowmeters or critical orifice meters) to obtain an accurate assessment of sample volume. Appropriate methods for transporting aerosol are discussed in Section XI on aerosol characterization.

Some test agents are formulations consisting of both nonvolatile and volatile components. Because of the complexity of many formulations, gravimetric analysis may be the most appropriate method for determining chamber aerosol concentration during animal exposure. Yet, the volatile components of the formulation may be partially or entirely lost due to evaporation either during generation of the aerosol atmosphere or during the collection of atmosphere samples (or both). To correct for this loss and provide an estimate of the formulation concentration in the chamber during exposure, a correction factor must be determined. One approach is to prepare a standard curve of wet (freshly spiked) filter weights as opposed to dry (desiccated and/or oven-dried) filter weights of the test material formulation. The dry filter weights provide an estimate of nonvolatile components of the formulation. The correction factor(s) obtained from the standard curve can be used to calculate the estimated formulation concentration in the chamber. The correction factor is applied to the gravimetric sample filter weight obtained during animal exposure. The gravimetric filters are then dried under procedures similar to those used for preparing the dry filter weights for the standard curve. Caution should be exercised when the appropriate drying time (the time at which there is a negligible change in subsequent filter weighings) is determined, because different components of the formulation have different volatilities and the objective is to measure a defined nonvolatile fraction of the formulation. Furthermore, this procedure provides an estimate and should be used only if other analytical methods for measuring the exposure concentration are not available. The formulation concentration calculated by this method should always be less than the nominal chamber concentration due to uncontrollable losses of the aerosol (described next).

Because measurements of aerosol concentration (e.g., gravimetric) are commonly time-integrated (i.e., samples are taken over a period of time at a fixed sampling flowrate), the stability of aerosol concentration and/

or the detection of aerosol generation problems during an exposure are not easily monitored. Cheng *et al.* (1988) evaluated a real-time aerosol detector (RAM-S, GCA Corporation, Bedford, Massachusetts) to complement standard filtration methods for monitoring the aerosol concentration during an animal exposure. The authors concluded that the results obtained by the RAM-S monitor were reproducible and correlated with mass concentration. However, real-time monitors are not intended to replace gravimetric or chemical analyses because they do not give absolute measurements of aerosol concentration.

Nominal chamber concentrations are easy to calculate and provide useful information for the inhalation toxicologist. A nominal concentration is a time-weighted averaged concentration, which can be calculated by measuring the total amount of test compound delivered during an exposure and dividing this quantity by the total airflow that passed through the chamber. However, nominal concentrations derived from aerosol exposures cannot be relied on to provide accurate exposure concentrations (Miller *et al.*, 1981) due to losses of the aerosol on chamber walls, animal fur, animal cages, etc. Also, the volatility of vehicles in test compound formulations is another cause of aerosol losses.

An analytical-to-nominal concentration ratio is commonly calculated. For gases and vapors, if the nominal concentration is not greatly affected by adsorption losses, an analytical-to-nominal concentration ratio of 0.90 to 1.10 is expected. Analytical-to-nominal concentration ratios below 0.90 usually indicate chamber or sample line adsorption losses and should prompt an additional check of the analytical calibration and the chamber airflow. Analytical-to-nominal concentration ratios above 1.00 are theoretically impossible, but errors associated with both analytical and nominal concentration determinations make a value of 1.10 experimentally possible. Faulty chamber design (e.g., leaks) causes poor chamber distribution of the test compound and also leads to unusually high or low ratio values. A situation in which a high analytical-to-nominal concentration ratio (e.g., 1.3) is obtained but cannot be attributed to calculation errors or chamber design may be due to the physical or chemical properties of the test compound. For example, a gaseous test compound that adsorbs to the sample lines or instrumental sampling loop will have a longer than expected decay time, and normal "washouts" will not remove the agent from the sampling loop. The analytical concentration will consistently climb throughout the exposure period, and the mean analytical value will be much higher than the nominal concentration. Gas standard calibration and heated sampling valves may help to resolve these problems.

A final consideration that is of immeasurable value in saving costs and increasing efficiency is to computerize the analytical systems. Suppose 6 to 12 analyses are obtained for each of four chambers during a six-hour exposure period. For a 90-day study, the number of analyses adds up quickly, and statistical treatment of the data must also be performed. Transmission of analytical data from a microprocessor to a computer provides efficient and accurate treatment of data. The computer software can statistically treat the data and, furthermore, the data can be safely stored (although a hard-copy analysis report for each exposure day's results is recommended). Another feature is to have the computer system capable of initiating an alarm to alert inhalation personnel to "out-of-range" atmospheric conditions in a chamber. A suitable selection of out-of-range concentrations is a deviation greater than ± 10% of the desired (target) chamber concentration.

XIII. ALARMS AND ADDITIONAL SAFETY PROCEDURES

Technology is available for real-time analysis to indicate when a deviation from an acceptable range occurs in the chamber for the test compound concentration, temperature, relative humidity, airflow, and pressure. Moreover, technology is available to correct these parameters automatically if a change beyond an acceptable range occurs.

Reid *et al.* (1981) have discussed several safety procedures followed in an inhalation laboratory, including different alarm systems to indicate interruption in chamber airflow or pressure. As discussed in detail previously, alarms for deviation in chamber airflow (Section VII on chamber air and airflow) or concentration (Section XII on chamber concentration analysis) or alarms for abnormal temperature and humidity (Section VI on environmental control) can result in considerable cost savings. Unfortunately, this is sometimes realized only when a study has to be repeated because of abnormal conditions that went unnoticed because an alarm system was not available.

Additional safety features are sometimes necessary in an inhalation laboratory to avert a potential fire or explosion or to prevent human exposure to the test compound. During evaporation of some test compounds, an improper amount of diluting air may cause a fire or explosion, or the test compound may remain on the animals' fur when personnel remove them from the chamber.

To lessen the chances of an explosion or fire caused by an improper dilution of the test compound in air (as well as preventing an overexposure to the animals), a solenoid switch can be inserted to automatically stop the generation of the test compound when there is an interruption in chamber airflow (previously discussed in Section IX on vapor and gas generation). To lessen the chances of worker exposure upon removal of the animals from the chamber, the worker can put on protective gear. More laboratories are routinely requiring inhalation personnel to wear cartridge-type respirators for unloading the animals from their chambers. This may be a good safety procedure only if the test chemical has good warning properties, if the time for the test chemical to break through the cartridge has been determined for a heavy breathing pattern, and if strict rules about proper fitting, changing, and storage of cartridges are followed. Unfortunately, there is very little or no information on cartridge breakthrough times for many compounds being tested and only limited information on odor thresholds, that is, warning properties (Amoore and Hautala, 1983; Ruth, 1986). Routine use of the mask, even with frequent cartridge changes, may present a false sense of security. Therefore, it is advisable to use as many engineering features as possible to maintain a safe working environment rather than routinely depending on the cartridge-type mask respirators. As discussed in Section III on chamber design, a specially designed chamber with glove ports and attached live-in glove box can provide isolation of the test compound, thereby alleviating the necessity of wearing a respirator and preventing contamination of the immediate work area.

Another measure of safety is to enclose the test compound reservoir and generation equipment (including flowmeters that contain the test compound under positive pressure) in a transparent ventilated box kept at a slightly negative pressure in relationship to the room. However, again, a false sense of security may prevail because the flow through the box would have to be extremely high to contain vapors when the door to the box is open. Instead of opening the door, technicians can adjust all generation equipment through portholes in the walls of the ventilated boxes. The holes are covered by a rubber flap when they are not in use (Fig. 14).

XIV. MISCELLANEOUS MATERIALS AND PROCEDURES

A. Materials

It has been said that good inhalation technicians are good plumbers. Certain types of equipment and materials make the "plumbing job" considerably easier. For example, Poly-Flow® fittings (Imperial-Eastman, Chicago, Illinois) can be used for connecting tubing. Key advantages of these fittings are that they are inexpensive, less likely to slip off plastic tubing, reusable and can be tightened without tools. Another plumbing aid used for sealing areas around glass to metal connections is Apiezon Q® sealing compound (J.G. Biddle Company, Plymouth Meeting,

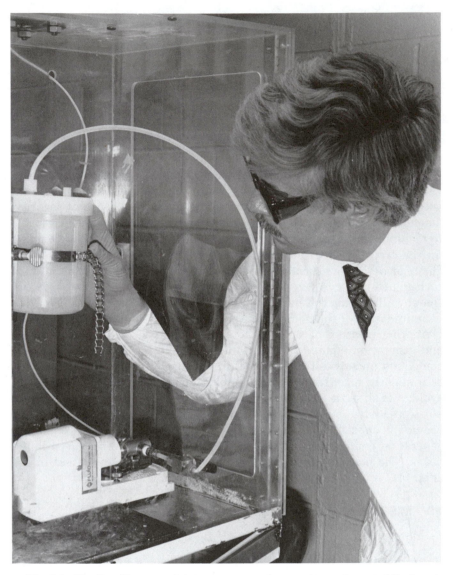

Fig. 14 Ventilated box containing test compound generation equipment. Adjustments to equipment are made through porthole.

Pennsylvania). This compound adheres to metal or glass but can easily be removed without solvents. Common duct tape is also useful as a sealant.

Other equipment or materials that have proved to be useful are as follows:

1. A spray-on material called StripCoat® film (3M, St. Paul, Minnesota) can be used to protect the metal or glass in the chamber from reacting with the test chemical. After the exposures are completed, the film can be peeled off. The key to successful removal of this film is to spray the coating material with a good quality paint sprayer.
2. A handheld laser (Aerotech Helium-Neon Laser, Model LSR-2R, Aerotech, Inc., Pittsburgh, Pennsylvania) can be used to see whether the vapor generator is producing an aerosol (Tyndall beam, Davies, 1975). Naturally, more sophisticated ways are used for actual measurements.
3. Nonpermanent clamp connectors, like Tri-Clover® clamps (Ladish Co., Kenosha, Wisconsin), are relatively leak proof in connecting pipes, whether made of glass or metal, in line with the ventilation system. Despite the high cost of these clamps, they have some significant advantages. These include easy removal of pipes and chambers for decontamination or cleaning purposes and quick insertion of different vapor or aerosol generators and calibration equipment.

B. Procedures

For both rats and mice, normal growth patterns have been demonstrated for animals exposed to control air following removal of both food and water for six hours. There is an adjustment period to this regimen and to the new environment of the inhalation chamber; consequently, mock exposures are recommended prior to administration of the test compound. Water should be drained from the automatic watering system of the animal carriers because a drop of water at the end of a nipple can absorb the test compound. Therefore, in keeping with the practice of low contamination by other routes of administration during a vapor inhalation study (with the exception of skin contact), remove food and water during the time of the exposure period.

Acknowledgments

The authors are particularly grateful to Drs. Dennis R. Klonne and Bernard J. Greenspan for the expertise shared by them on the subjects of aerosol generation and characterization and to Dr. Irvin M. Pritts for his development of the analytical procedures discussed in this chapter. Our appreciation is also extended to Ms. Florence C. Wilt and Ms. Linda L. Farren for their help in preparation of this chapter.

References

Agarwal, J. K., and Nelson, P. A. (1981). A large flow rate fluidized bed aerosol generator. *In* "Proceedings of the Inhalation Toxicology and Technology Symposium" (B. K. J. Leong, ed.), pp. 169–176. Ann Arbor: Ann Arbor Science Publishers.

Agarwal, J. K., Remiarz, R. J., and Nelson, P. A. (1981). An instrument for real time aerodynamic particle size analysis using laser velocimetry. *In* "Proceedings of the Inhalation Toxicology and Technology Symposium" (B. K. J. Leong, ed.), pp. 177–190. Ann Arbor: Ann Arbor Science Publishers.

Alarie, Y. (1966). Irritating properties of airborne materials to the upper respiratory tract. *Arch. Environ. Health* **13,** 433–449.

Alden, J. L., and Kane, J. M. (1970). "Design of Industrial Exhaust Systems," pp. 9–15. New York: Industrial Press.

Amoore, J. E., and Hautala, E. (1983). Odor as an aid to chemical safety: odor thresholds compared with threshold limit values and volatilities for 214 industrial chemicals in air and water dilution. *J. Appl. Toxicol.* **3,** 272–290.

Barrow, C. S., and Dodd, D. E. (1979). Ammonia production in inhalation chambers and its relevance to chlorine inhalation studies. *Toxicol. Appl. Pharmacol.* **49,** 89–95.

Barrow, C. S., and Steinhagen, W. H. (1982). Design, construction and operation of a simple inhalation exposure system. *Fund. Appl. Toxicol.* **2,** 33–37.

Beethe, R. L. (1978). The effects of inlet section configuration and airflow rate on inhalation exposure chamber performances. *In* "Inhalation Toxicology Research Institute Annual Report" (R. F. Henderson, J. H. Diel, and B. S. Martinez, eds.), LF-60, pp. 271–274. Albuquerque: Lovelace Biomedical and Environmental Research Institute.

Berglund, R. N., and Liu, B. Y. H. (1973). Generation of monodisperse aerosol standards. *Env. Sci. Technol.* **7,** 147–153.

Bernstein, D. M., and Drew, R. T. (1980). The major parameters affecting temperature inside inhalation chambers. *Am. Ind. Hyg. Assoc. J.* **41,** 420–426.

Cannon, W. C., Blanton, E. F., and McDonald, K. E. (1983). The flow-past chamber: An improved nose-only exposure system for rodents. *Am. Ind. Hyg. Assoc. J.* **44,** 923–928.

Carpenter, C. P., Kinkead, E. R., Geary, D. L., Sullivan, L. J., and King, J. M. (1975). Petroleum hydrocarbon toxicity studies. I. Methodology. *Toxicol. Appl. Pharmacol.* **32,** 246–262.

Carpenter, R. L., and Beethe, R. L. (1980). Airflow and aerosol distribution in animal exposure facilities. *In* "Generation of Aerosols and Facilities for Exposure Experiments" (K. W. Willeke, ed.), pp. 459–474. Ann Arbor: Ann Arbor Science Publishers.

Carpenter, R. L., and Yerkes, K. (1980). Relationship between fluid bed aerosol generator operation and the aerosol produced. *Am. Ind. Hyg. Assoc. J.* **41,** 888–894.

Cheng, Y. S., Barr, E. B., Benson, J. M., Damon, E. G., Medinsky, M. A., Hobbs, C. H., and Goehl, T. J. (1988). Evaluation of a real-time aerosol monitor (RAM-S) for inhalation studies. *Fund. Appl. Toxicol.* **10,** 321–328.

Dautrebande, L. (1962). "Microaerosols." New York: Academic Press.

Davies, C. N. (1975). European aerosol studies. *In* "Fine Particles, Aerosol Generation, Measurement, Sampling, and Analysis" (B. Y. H. Liu, ed.), p. 5. New York: Academic Press.

Decker, J. R., Moss, O. R., and Kay, B. L. (1982). Controlled-delivery vapor generator for animal exposures. *Am. Ind. Hyg. Assoc. J.* **43,** 400–402.

Dodd, D. E., Fowler, E. H., Snellings, W. M., Pritts, I. M., and Baron, R. L. (1986). Acute inhalation studies with methyl isocyanate vapor. I. Methodology and LC50 determinations in guinea pigs, rats, and mice. *Fund. Appl. Toxicol.* **6,** 747–755.

Dodd, D. E., Frank, F. R., Fowler, E. H., Troup, C. M., and Milton, R. M. (1987). Biological effects of short-term, high-concentration exposure to methyl isocyanate. I. Study objectives and inhalation exposure design. *Environ. Health Perspect.* **72,** 13–19.

Dodd, D. E., Klonne, D. R., Pritts, I. M., Ballantyne, B., and Tyler, T. (1988). Differences in acute toxicity resulting from static and dynamic inhalation exposures to test materials with trace amounts of impurities. *Am. Ind. Hyg. Conf. Abstr.* 99–100.

Drew, R. T. (1978). "Proceedings Workshop on Inhalation Chamber Technology." Upton, New York: Brookhaven National Laboratory.

Drew, R. T., and Laskin, S. (1973). Environmental inhalation chambers. *In* "Methods of Animals Experimentation" (W. I. Gay, ed.), pp. 1–41. New York: Academic Press.

Drew, R. T., Bernstein, D. M., and Laskin, S. (1978). The Laskin aerosol generator. *J. Toxicol. Environ. Health* **4,** 661–670.

Ferin, J., and Leach, L. J. (1980). Horizontal airflow inhalation exposure chamber. *In* "Generation of Aerosols and Facilities for Exposure Experiments" (K. Willeke, ed.), pp. 517–523. Ann Arbor: Ann Arbor Science Publishers.

FIFRA Guidelines (1982). "Pesticide Assessment Guidelines, Subdivision F, Hazard Evaluation: Human and Domestic Animals." Washington, DC: Office of Pesticide Programs, U.S. Environmental Protection Agency.

Fissan, H., and Schwientek, G. (1987). Sampling and transport of aerosols. *TSI J. Particle Instr.* **2,** 3–10.

Fraser, D. A., Bales, R. E., Lippmann, M., and Stokinger, H. E. (1959). "Exposure Chambers for Research in Animal Inhalation" (Public Health Monograph 57). Washington, DC: U.S. Government Printing Office.

Gorton, R. L., Woods, J. E., and Besch, E. L. (1976). System load characteristics and estimation of annual heat loads for laboratory animal facilities. *ASHRAE Trans.* **82,** 107–112.

Green, J. D., Helke, W. F., Scott, J. B., Yau, E. T., Traina, V. M., and Diener, R. M. (1984). Effect of equilibration zones on stability, uniformity, and homogeneity profiles of vapors and aerosols in the ADG nose-only inhalation exposure system. *Fund. Appl. Toxicol.* **4,** 768–777.

Hemenway, D. R., and MacAskill, S. M. (1982). Design, development, and test results of a horizontal flow inhalation toxicology facility. *Am. Ind. Hyg. Assoc. J.* **43,** 1982.

Hinds, W. C. (1982). "Aerosol Technology." New York: Wiley.

Hinners, R. G., Burkart, J. K., and Punte, C. L. (1968). Animal inhalation exposure chambers. *Arch. Environ. Health* **16,** 194–206.

Klimisch, H.-J., Hasenohrl, K., and Hildebrand, B. (1987). Design and experience with head/nose-exposure techniques in a 2-year inhalation study with rats. *In* "The Design and Interpretation of Inhalation Studies," p. 24. Basel: International Life Sciences Institute.

LaBauve, R. J., Stuart, B. O., and Freudenthal, R. I. (1983). The effects of inhalation exposure technique on the LC50 of test compounds. *Toxicologist* **3,** 118.

Landry, T. D., Ramsey, J. C., and McKenna, M. J. (1983). Pulmonary physiology and inhalation dosimetry in rats: development of a method and two examples. *Toxicol. Appl. Pharmacol.* **71,** 72–83.

Leach, C. L., Oberg, S. G., Sharma, R. P., and Drown, D. B. (1984). A nose-only inhalation exposure system for generation, treatment and characterization of formaldehyde vapor. *Am. Ind. Hyg. Assoc. J.* **45,** 269–273.

Leach, L. J., Spiegl, C. J., Wilson, R. H., Sylvester, G. E., and Lauterbach, K. E. (1959). A multiple chamber exposure unit designed for chronic inhalation studies. *Ind. Hyg. Assoc. J.* **20,** 13–22.

Leong, B. K. J. (1981). "Inhalation Toxicology and Technology." Ann Arbor: Ann Arbor Science Publishers.

Lippmann, M. (1970). "Respirable" dust sampling. *Am. Ind. Hyg. Assoc. J.* **31,** 138–159.

Litt, M., and Swift, D. E. (1972). The Babington nebulizer: A new principle for generation of therapeutic aerosols. *Am. Rev. Resp. Dis.* **105,** 308–310.

Liu, B. Y. H. (1976). "Fine Particles: Aerosol Generation, Measurement, Sampling, and Analysis." New York: Academic Press.

Liu, B. Y. H., and Pui, D. Y. H. (1974). Electrical neutralization of aerosols. *J. Aerosol Sci.* **5,** 465–472.

Lundgren, D. A., Harris, F. S., Jr., Marlow, W. H., Lippmann, M., Clark, W. E., and Durham, M. D. (1979). "Aerosol Measurement." Gainesville: University Presses of Florida.

MacFarland, H. N. (1976). Respiratory toxicology. *In* "Essays in Toxicology" (W. J. Hayes, Jr., ed.), Vol. 7, pp. 121–154. New York: Academic Press.

MacFarland, H. N. (1981). A problem and a non-problem in chamber inhalation studies. *In* "Proceedings of the Inhalation Toxicology and Technology Symposium" (B. K. J. Leong, ed.), pp. 11–18. Ann Arbor: Ann Arbor Science Publishers.

MacFarland, H. N. (1983). Designs and operational characteristics of inhalation exposure equipment—A review. *Fund. Appl. Toxicol.* **3,** 603–613.

Marple, V. A., Liu, B. Y. H., and Rubow, K. L. (1978). A dust generator for laboratory use. *Am. Ind. Hyg. Assoc. J.* **39,** 26–32.

Martonen, T., Clark, M., Nelson, D., Willard, D., and Rossignol, E. (1982). Evaluation of a mini-cascade impactor for sampling exposure chamber atmospheres. *Fund. Appl. Toxicol.* **2,** 149–152.

Mauderly, J. L. (1986). Respiration of F 344 rats in nose-only inhalation exposure tubes. *J. Appl. Toxicol.* **6,** 25–30.

May, K. R. (1945). The cascade impactor: An instrument for sampling coarse aerosols. *J. Sci. Instr.* **22,** 187.

Mercer, T. T. (1965). The interpretation of cascade impactor data. *Am. Ind. Hyg. Assoc. J.* **26(3),** 236–241.

Mercer, T. T. (1973). "Aerosol Technology in Hazard Evaluation." New York: Academic Press.

Mercer, T. T., Tillery, M. J., and Chow, H. Y. (1968). Operating characteristics of some compressed air nebulizers. *Am. Ind. Hyg. Assoc. J.* **29,** 66–78.

Mercer, T. T., Tillery, M. I., and Newton, G. J. (1970). A multi-stage, low flow rate cascade impactor. *J. Aerosol Sci.* **1,** 9–15.

Miller, F. J., Gardner, D. E., Graham, J. A., Lee, R. E., Jr., Wilson, W. E., and Bachmann, J. D. (1979). Size considerations for establishing a standard for inhalable particles. *J. Air Pollut. Control Assoc.* **29,** 610–615.

Miller, J. L., Stuart, B. O., DeFord, H. S., and Moss, O. R. (1981). Liquid aerosol generation for inhalation toxicology studies. *In* "Proceedings of the Inhalation Toxicology and Technology Symposium" (B. K. J. Leong, ed.), pp. 121–138. Ann Arbor: Ann Arbor Science Publishers.

Miller, R. R., Letts, R. L., Potts, W. J., and McKenna, M. J. (1980). Improved methodology for generating controlled test atmospheres. *Am. Ind. Hyg. Assoc. J.* **41,** 844–846.

Milliman, E. M., Chang, D. P. Y., and Moss, O. R. (1981). A dual flexible-brush dust-feed mechanism. *Am. Ind. Hyg. Assoc. J.* **42,** 747–751.

Moss, O. R., Decker, J. R., and Cannon, W. C. (1982). Aerosol mixing in an animal exposure chamber having three levels of caging with excreta pans. *Am. Ind. Hyg. Assoc. J.* **43,** 244–249.

Nelson, G. O. (1972). "Controlled Test Atmospheres Principles and Techniques." Ann Arbor: Ann Arbor Science Publishers.

Newton, G. J., Raabe, O. G., and Mokler, B. V. (1977). Cascade impactor design and performance. *J. Aerosol Sci.* **8,** 339–347.

Organization for Economic Co-operation and Development (1981). "Guidelines for Testing of Chemicals," Section 4 - Health Effects. Paris: Organization for Economic Co-operation and Development.

Partridge, F. M. (1952). Fundamentals of orifice measurement. *J. South. Calif. Meter Assoc.* **25,** 207–209.

Phalen, R. F., Mannix, R. C., and Drew, R. T. (1984). Inhalation exposure methodology. *Environ. Health Perspect.* **56,** 23–34.

Potts, W. J., and Steiner, E. C. (1980). An apparatus for generation of vapors from liquids of low volatility for use in inhalation toxicity studies. *Am. Ind. Hyg. Assoc. J.* **41,** 141–145.

Pullinger, D. H., Crouch, C. N., and Dare, P. R. M. (1979). Inhalation toxicity studies with 1,3-butadiene-1. Atmosphere generation and control. *Am. Ind. Hyg. Assoc. J.* **40,** 789–795.

Raabe, O. G. (1968). The dilution of monodisperse suspensions for aerosolization. *Am. Ind. Hyg. Assoc. J.* **29,** 439–443.

Reid, W. B., Klok, J. R., and Leong, B. K. J. (1981). Hazard containment in an inhalation toxicology laboratory. *In* "Proceedings of the Inhalation Toxicology and Technology Symposium" (B. K. J. Leong, ed.), pp. 1–10. Ann Arbor: Ann Arbor Science Publishers.

Remiarz, R. J., and Johnson, E. M. (1984). A new diluter for high concentration measurements with the aerodynamic particle sizer. *TSI Quarterly* **10,** 7–12.

Ruth, J. H. (1986). Odor thresholds and irritation levels of several chemical substances: A review. *Am. Ind. Hyg. Assoc. J.* **47,** 142–151.

Silver, S. D. (1946). Constant flow gassing chambers: Principles influencing design and operation. *J. Lab. Clin. Med.* **31,** 1153–1161.

Strock, C. and Koral, R. L. (1965). "Handbook of Air-Conditioning, Heating and Ventilating." New York: Industrial Press.

Sussman, R. G., Gearhart, J. M., and Lippmann, M. (1985). A variable feed rate mechanism for fluidized bed asbestos generators. *Am. Ind. Hyg. Assoc. J.* **46,** 24–27.

Teague, S. V., Yeh, H. C., and Newton, G. J. (1978). Fabrication and use of krypton-85 aerosol discharge devices. *Health Physics* **35,** 392–395.

Timbrell, V., Hyett, A. W., and Skidmore, J. W. (1968). A simple dispenser for generating dust clouds from standard reference samples of asbestos. *Ann. Occup. Hyg.* **11,** 273–281.

Turner, D. B. (1974). "Workbook on Atmospheric Dispersion Estimates," Office of Air Programs, Pub # AP-26 (NTIS # PB-191-482). Washington, DC: U.S. Environmental Protection Agency.

Ulrich, C. E., and Marold, B. W. (1979). Pulmonary deposition of aerosols in individual and group caged rats. *Am. Ind. Hyg. Assoc. J.* **40,** 633–636.

TSCA Test Guidelines (1987). "New and Revised Health Effects Test Guidelines," Office of Pesticides and Toxic Substances, Report No. 560/6-84-001, Washington, DC: U.S. Environmental Protection Agency.

Willeke, K. (1980). "Generation of Aerosols and Facilities for Exposure Experiments." Ann Arbor: Ann Arbor Science Publishers.

Willeke, K., Lo, C. S. K., and Whitby, K. J. (1974). Dispersion characteristics of a fluidized bed. *J. Aerosol Sci.* **5,** 449–455.

Wright, B. M. (1950). A new dust feed mechanism. *J. Sci. Instr.* **27,** 12–15.

Yeh, H. C., Newton, G. J., Barr, E. B., Carpenter, R. L., and Hobbs, C. H. (1986). Studies of the temporal and spatial distribution of aerosols in multi-tiered inhalation exposure chambers. *Am. Ind. Hyg. Assoc. J.* **47,** 540–545.

11
Dermal Toxicity Testing: Exposure and Absorption

Leonard Ritter
Environmental Health Directorate
Health Protection Branch
Health and Welfare Canada
Ottawa, Ontario

Claire A. Franklin
Environmental Health Directorate
Health Protection Branch
Health and Welfare Canada
Ottawa, Ontario

I. Introduction

II. Acute Dermal Toxicity Testing
   A. Objective
   B. Procedure
   C. Observations

III. Subchronic Dermal Toxicity Testing
   A. Objective
   B. Procedures
   C. Observations
   D. Dermal Irritation Tests
   E. Dermal Sensitization

IV. Percutaneous Penetration
   A. Methods
   B. Principles of the Test Procedures

V. Phototoxicity and Photosensitization

I. INTRODUCTION

Animal models for assessing dermal effects can be divided into two broad categories. The first category includes those studies to measure the percutaneous penetration of toxic chemicals and those to assess the systemic toxicity that may occur following dermal exposure for varying periods of time. The second broad category includes studies in which the skin itself is the direct target organ. The skin either comes in direct contact with the chemical or serves as a target organ for a systemic agent.

In this chapter, several aspects of dermal toxicity are discussed. Topics covered include the need for dermal studies, the fate of absorbed materials, appropriate dosage, selection of test species, and duration of exposure. In addition, the regulatory implications of these test procedures are discussed as well.

Various protocols have been developed to permit studies in both broad categories noted. Protocols discussed in this chapter include tests for assessing systemic effects in animals following their exposure to the chemical at varying lengths of time. In addition, various techniques, both *in vitro* and *in vivo*, used to determine percutaneous penetration are examined. Protocols for assessing target effects on the skin, such as irritation, sensitization, and contact dermatitis, are also presented.

II. ACUTE DERMAL TOXICITY TESTING

A. Objective

Acute dermal toxicity testing assesses the potential hazards associated with a single dermal exposure to a chemical. In Canada and the United States, such testing requirements extend to the safety evaluation of pesticides. The most common endpoint evaluated is the median lethal dose (LD_{50}), or the lethal dose to 50% of the test population, the value of which is determined by procedures based on statistical methods using dose levels which result in mortality rates between 10–90% (Litchfield and Wilcoxon, 1949). Such data are required in both Canada and the United States to support the registration of each new active pesticide ingredient and each new formulation thereof.

B. Procedure

A variety of species including the rat, rabbit, and guinea pig are considered acceptable for testing by many regulatory authorities. Although other species may be considered acceptable, justification for such a selection is invariably required. In all cases, equal numbers of young adult animals of both sexes should be utilized. Untreated control groups are generally considered necessary when the toxicity of the nonactive ingredients is unknown. When the use of vehicles are necessary, aqueous vehicles are preferred. Oils or other suitable vehicles may also be utilized. In all cases, the toxicity of the solvent should be known prior to initiation of the study. When solids are tested, the material should be pulverized and suitably moistened to allow good contact with the skin. Dosages selected should produce a dose-response curve, a range of toxic effects, and mortality. Ideally, the data should permit calculation of an LD_{50} value by a suitable statistical method (Litchfield and Wilcoxon, 1949).

The test material should be applied uniformly to an area approximately equivalent to 10% of the total body surface. Preparation of the test site includes clipping of fur from the dorsal area of the animal's trunk shortly before testing. In addition, in both Canada and the United States, pesticide data requirements may include a test group in which the animal's skin has been abraded in such a way as to penetrate the stratum corneum but not the dermis. Generally, the test chemical is left in contact with the skin for a period of 24 hours and secured in place by a suitable dressing. Wrapped over the dressing is a material, such as rubber or plastic, that retards evaporation of the chemical during the contact period, prevents its loss due to rubbing, and prevents its oral ingestion while the animal is grooming. Following the 24-hour contact period, both the U.S. Environmental Protection Agency (EPA; 1978, 1982) and the Organization for Economic Co-operation and Development (OECD; 1986a, 1986b) guidelines recommend that the test material be removed with a suitable solvent. Removal of the test material following a 24-hour contact period is important to ensure that contact is acute and to minimize the duration and intensity of stress that test animals might experience.

C. Observations

As in any scientific investigation, careful physical observations are of paramount importance. Gross observations should include examination of the skin, fur, eyes, mucous membranes, autonomic and central nervous systems, and behavior. Particular attention should be paid to tremors, salivation, and diarrhea. Observations should be made at least once daily by qualified personnel. Moribund animals should be sacrificed and time of death for all animals should be recorded as accurately as possible. The observation period should be no less than 14 days following treatment and, when possible, should extend until all signs of toxicity have subsided. Detailed histopathology need not be conducted routinely but should include examination of tissues showing evidence of gross pathology during necropsy, particularly in animals that survive more than 24 hours following treatment. Animals that die during the initial 24-hour

Table I
Acute Dermal Toxicity Testing

	Canada	U.S. EPA	OECD
Animals			
Species	Rabbit, rat, guinea pig; others acceptable upon justification	Same as Canada	Same as Canada
Age	Young adult	Same as Canada	Same as Canada
Sex	Male and female	Male and female except females should not be pregnant	Male or female but all the same, preferably the more sensitive; females should be nulliparous and nonpregnant
Test Procedure			
Animals/group	5/sex	5/sex	5/sex
Dose levels	Same as U.S. EPA	At least 3 dose levels appropriately spaced to produce a range of toxic effects and mortality; data calculation of statistically meaningful LD_{50}[a]	Same as U.S. EPA[a]
Controls	Same as U.S. EPA	Only required if toxicity of solvent or carrier unknown; in such cases toxicity is determined first	Not required
Test substance	Same as U.S. EPA	Liquids applied undiluted; solids pulverized and suitably moistened with water or other vehicle	Same as U.S. EPA
Test duration	Same as U.S. EPA	Test material in contact with skin for at least 24 hours; secured in place with a suitable dressing (gauze) and covered with a nonirritating material to retard evaporation; removed with water or appropriate solvent	Same as U.S. EPA

(continues)

Table I *(continued)*

	Canada	U.S. EPA	OECD
Observations			
Observation period	At least 14 days; not terminated until all signs of toxicity have subsided	Same as Canada	Same as Canada
Gross examination	Same as U.S. EPA	Test animals observed at least once daily and all evidence of toxicity recorded; moribund animals sacrificed; body weights recorded at initiation and termination of study	Same as U.S. EPA
Histopathology	Need not be routinely performed on all animals	Same as Canada	Should be considered for all tissues with evident gross pathology in animals surviving more than 24 hours

[a] Both U.S. EPA (1982) and OECD (1986a,b) guidelines provide for limited testing. Specific details can be obtained from the appropriate guideline.

period of an acute study are not likely to show treatment-related pathology. However, valuable pathological information is often derived from animals surviving several days or weeks. Data of this type can be very useful in the implementation of therapy in human poisonings.

Table I summarizes data requirements for acute dermal toxicity testing in Canada and the United States and by OECD.

III. SUBCHRONIC DERMAL TOXICITY TESTING

A. Objective

Subchronic dermal toxicity testing is often carried out to determine the highest dose to which test animals can be exposed for at least 21 days, but not greater than 90 days, without sustaining relevant toxic effects biologically. Generally speaking, data from a subchronic 21-day dermal toxicity study are required when use of the product is likely to result in repeated human dermal exposure. Hazards of this type may be of relevance to persons occupationally exposed to pesticides, or more directly, to cosmetics. Studies of at least 21 daily exposures are considered minimal in such cases. In the United States, only technical grade material need be tested, whereas testing with the formulated product is required if any component of the formulation is likely to increase dermal absorption of the test material or potentiate toxic effects. In Canada, it is desirable to include both a 90-day study carried out with technical grade material and a 21-day study carried out with the formulated product. OECD guidelines (1986a,b) do not specify the exact nature of the material to be tested. Data derived from subchronic dermal studies should establish the toxicity of the product to which consumers may be exposed, hence the final formulation should be tested. Similarly, it needs to be established whether vehicles or formulants confer any direct toxicity or whether formulation components enhance uptake of an active ingredient proved to be toxic; therefore, active ingredients should be tested alone as well. Comparison of formulation and active ingredient test results then allows a more meaningful assessment of overall toxicity of the total product. Unacceptably high toxicity of the overall product, which may be attributable to the carrier, can often be addressed by altering the carrier while maintaining the integrity of the active ingredient and total product.

B. Procedures

A variety of species including the rat and rabbit are acceptable test species in Canada and the United States. OECD guidelines include the guinea pig as well. At least 10 young adults of each sex should be utilized for testing at each dose. A control group (vehicle or untreated) should be included. As with acute studies, doses should be selected to produce a range of toxic responses. Although Canadian guidelines do not specify the number of doses to be utilized, U.S. EPA (1978) and OECD guidelines (1986a,b) require at least three doses. In addition, doses should be selected in such a way to permit estimation of a clear, no-observable-effect level (NOEL) as well as valid statistical analysis. The test material should be applied as a thin film to an exposed area that represents no less than 10% of the total body surface of the test animal. Preparation of the test site should include clipping of fur from the area just prior to initiation of the test then weekly thereafter. Continued maintenance of the test site should be adjusted to accommodate rate of hair growth and any physical abrasion that may develop as a result of fur clipping or application of the test material. In addition, U.S. EPA requires that half the test group have the test site abraded (penetration of the stratum corneum) once a week throughout the study. Experimental conditions for subchronic exposure should attempt to duplicate anticipated human exposure to the chemical under actual conditions. Because human exposure to chemicals under typical conditions is often restricted to working hours, test animals should, therefore, be exposed to a single application of the test material daily for five days a week for no less than three consecutive weeks. The site should be occluded for at least six hours per day with a porous gauze fabric overwrap of nonirritating material, such as plastic, to retard evaporation and prevent oral ingestion.

C. Observations

Careful physical observations are of paramount importance. Daily gross observations should include respiration status, behavioral patterns, and central nervous system effects. Morbidity and mortality rates should also be assessed daily. As repeated dermal application may produce dermal irritancy, dermal irritation should be scored according to a suitable method such as that reported by Draize (1965) and Draize et al. (1944). Food consumption should be evaluated at least once weekly, and body weight should be recorded at initiation of the experiment and once weekly thereafter. Clinical investigations should include routine hematology (see Chapter 18) and biochemistry (see Chapter 19) screens at the beginning and end of the test on a sufficiently large group of animals to provide meaningful results. In addition, specific tests related to the specific type of chemical under investigation may also be advisable. If organophosphates are being tested, cholinesterase may be measured. Particular care should be exercised to ensure that moribund animals are sacrificed. Studies in which more than 10% of the test animals in any one group are autolyzed may be sufficiently compromised to a point that they are no longer useful for the purpose for which they were designed. All test animals should be subjected to routine gross necropsy. Histopathology should be performed on all animals in the high dose and control groups and should include all gross lesions as well as tissue from the brain, pituitary gland, salivary gland, heart, thymus, thyroid, lungs, esophagus, stomach, small and large intestine, adrenals, pancreas, liver, kidneys, testes, urinary bladder, ovaries, spleen, lymph nodes, and any other obviously affected organ. Histopathological requirements for intermediate dosage groups may vary between regulatory agencies, and consultation should be sought prior to initiation of a study.

Table II summarizes data requirements for subacute dermal toxicity testing in Canada and the United States and by OECD.

Table II
Subchronic Dermal Toxicity Testing

	Canada	U.S. EPA	OECD
Animals			
Species	Preferably rabbit; others may be acceptable upon justification	Same as Canada	Rat, rabbit, or guinea pig
Age	Young adult	Same as Canada	Same as Canada
Sex	Both sexes	Nonpregnant female; both sexes	Nonpregnant, nulliparous female; both sexes
Procedures			
Animals/group	Not specified	10/sex/group	Same as U.S. EPA
Dose levels	Not specified	At least 3 dose levels; dose levels selected should be effective but nonirritating[a]	At least 3 dose levels[a]
Controls	Vehicle or untreated control	Same as Canada	Same as Canada
Test substance	Not specified	Liquids should be applied undiluted and solids should be pulverized and suitably moistened	Same as U.S. EPA
Duration	Same as U.S. EPA	5 day/week, at least 6 hr/day, 21, 28, or 90 days; test material should be applied as thin film to exposed area not less than 10% of total body surface; test site occluded with nonirritating material for daily exposure period	Same as U.S. EPA
Observations			
Observation period	Same as U.S. EPA	Animals observed at least once daily by qualified personnel; body weights recorded initially and weekly thereafter	Same as U.S. EPA
Gross pathology	Same as U.S. EPA	All test animals subjected to gross necropsy; moribund animals sacrificed	Same as U.S. EPA

(continues)

Table II (*continued*)

	Canada	U.S. EPA	OECD
Laboratory investigation	Same as U.S. EPA	Full hematology screen at beginning and end of study; biochemistry determinations to include calcium, potassium, serum transaminase, direct and total bilirubin, glucose alkaline phosphatase, urea nitrogen, total protein; others may be required as necessary	Same as U.S. EPA
Histopathology	Same as U.S. EPA	Done on all animals in high dose and control groups; done on affected tissues and organs; additional histopathology may be required on intermediate dose groups if effects are noted in high dose groups	Same as U.S. EPA

[a] Additionally U.S. EPA may require that half the test group have the test site abraded once per week throughout the study.

D. Dermal Irritation Tests

Dermal irritation is the production of a reversible inflammatory response at the site of application following an animal's single, repeated, or prolonged contact with the test material. There is no involvement of the immune system as there is in sensitization. Dermal corrosion is the production of irreversible damage to the skin at the site of application. Substances with a pH of less than 2.0 or greater than 11.5 need not be tested because they are presumed to be highly irritating. Product labels should so indicate this.

The Draize (Draize *et al.,* 1944) or modified Draize test is the standard test required by many regulatory agencies. Information obtained from this test is used for labeling products. Originally, the exposure period was 24 hours but that has since been reduced to 4 hours, following which the application site is washed with water or an appropriate solvent.

1. Modified Draize Test

a. Animals

Both the albino rabbit and guinea pig are the preferred species for this test. At least three rabbits should be used and, depending on the results, more may be necessary. Depilation should be done 24 hours prior to the test by shaving or clipping the dorsal area of the trunk.

b. Test Material

A dose of 0.5 ml of liquid or 0.5 g of solid moistened with enough water or appropriate solvent to ensure good dermal contact is applied. Each animal serves as its own control.

c. Application

The test material is applied to an area of approximately 1 cm^2. It is covered with a gauze patch, and nonirritating tape is used to hold it in place. A semiocclusive dressing should be used to hold the patch in place for the 5-hour duration of the study. Animals should be prevented from ingesting or inhaling the test material. At the end of the exposure period, excess material left on the skin when the patch is removed should be carefully washed off. Some agencies require that abraded skin be used also. This can be done on the contralateral side to the unabraded test area.

d. Clinical Observation

Animals should be examined for signs of erythema and edema in 0.5 to 1 hour after patch removal, then in 24, 48, and 72 hours. The observation period may need to be extended to enable full evaluation of reversibility or irreversibility but normally does not exceed 14 days. Evaluation of the skin reaction should be done according to the scale in Table III.

e. Interpretation

There are many factors that can affect the outcome of the test: occlusion, abrasion, duration of exposure, subjective gradation, application site, the patch itself, and species selection. The rabbit is generally more sensitive than humans to irritants; therefore, care must be taken when test results are extrapolated to humans (McCreesh and Steinberg, 1977). In fact, substances that have been prescreened in animals can be tested in humans. This is indeed done for many chemicals that are intended for dermal use (i.e., cosmetics).

Numerous modifications of the Draize Test and other methods are summarized in a U.S. EPA (1982) report.

Table III
Evaluation of Skin Reactions

Symptom	Irritation reaction[a]
Erythema and eschar formation	
Very slight erythema (barely perceptible)	1
Well-defined erythema	2
Moderate to severe erythema	3
Severe erythema (beet redness) to slight eschar formation (injuries in depth)	4
Total possible erythema score	4
Edema formation	
Very slight edema (barely perceptible)	1
Slight edema (edges of site well defined by definite raising)	2
Moderate edema (site raised 1 mm)	3
Severe edema (site raised more than 1 mm and extending beyond area of exposure)	4
Total possible edema score	4
Total possible score for primary irritation	8

[a] Primary irritation index: 0–2, mild reaction; 3–5, moderate reaction; 6–8, severe reaction.

E. Dermal Sensitization

Dermal sensitization (allergic contact dermatitis) is a delayed immuno-logically mediated response to an antigenic substance. Animals are exposed to the test substance then, after a minimum induction period of one week, are given a challenge exposure to determine whether a hyper-sensitive state has been induced. Sensitization is determined from a comparison of the response to the challenge exposure with that of the initial induction exposure. Erythema and edema observed in animals are similar to those produced by dermal irritants. In humans, itching, vesi-culation, purpura, and necrosis may also be observed. The OECD guide-lines (1986a,b) list seven established guinea pig methods and another less documented (footpad test). All these methods are useful and reliable for predicting human response. These tests can be categorized by route of administration: epicutaneous route (open epicutaneous test and closed patch test), intradermal route (Draize test and Freund complete adjuvant test), or a combination of the two routes (maximization, optimization, split-adjuvant, and footpad tests). Chemicals may act as allergy-inducing agents as well. This process of sensitization occurs when a low molecular weight chemical (hapten) conjugates with normal body protein in the epidermis. The hapten-protein conjugate is then carried to a regional lymph node by lymphatic drainage of the skin, leading to formation of

Table IV
Dermal Sensitization Studies on Guinea Pigs[a]

Test	Draize	Freund's complete adjuvant (FCA)	Mauer optimization	Buehler	Open epicutaneous test	Maximization	Split-adjuvant
Route	Intradermal[b]	Intradermal	Intradermal	Epicutaneous[c]	Epicutaneous	Intradermal and epicutaneous	Intradermal and epicutaneous
No. in test group	20	8–10	10–10	10–20	6–8	20–25	10–20
No. of test groups	1	1	1	1	up to 6	1	1
No. in control group	20	8–10	10–10	10–20	6–8	20–25	10–20
Induction exposure							
Route	Id	Id	Id	Dermal	Dermal	Id and dermal	Id and dermal
No. of exposures	10	5	9	3	20 or 21	1 id, 1 dermal	4
Exposure period	—	—	24 hr	6 hr each	Continuous	—, 48 hr	48 hr each
Patch type	—	—	—	Closed	Open	Closed	Closed
Test group(s)	TS[d]	TS in FCA	TS in FCA	TS	TS	TS, TS + FCA, FCA	TS
Control group	—	FCA only	—	—	Vehicle[e] only	FCA, FCA + V, V	—
Site	Left flank	Right flank	Back	Left flank	Right flank	Shoulder	Shoulder
Frequency	Every 2nd day	Every 2nd day	Every other day	Every 7 days	Daily	0(id), 7 day (dermal)	0, 2, 4, 7 days
Duration	0–18 days	0–8 days	0–21 days	0–14 days	0–20 days	0–7 days	0–7 days
Concentration	2–10 times first concentration	Same throughout	0.1 ml 0.1%	Same throughout	Same per group; different between groups	—	Same throughout

Challenge exposure							
Route	Id	Dermal	Id	Dermal	Dermal	Dermal	Dermal
No. of exposures	1	2	2	1	2	1	1
Day(s)	35	22 & 35	14 & 28	28	21 & 35	21	20
Exposure period	—	—	24 hr	6 hr	—	24 hr	24 hr
Patch type	—	Open	—	Closed	Open	Closed	Closed
Test group(s)	TS	TS	TS	TS	TS	TS	TS
Control group	TS	TS	TS	TS	TS	TS	TS
Site	Right flank	Left flank	Back, new site	Right flank	Left flank	Left flank, TS, right flank vehicle	Shoulder
Concentration	Same as first	4 different	0.1 ml 0.1%	Same as induction	4 different	Same as 2nd induction	Half induction
Evaluation (hr after challenge)	24, 48	24, 48, 72	24 hr	24, 48	24, 48, and/or 72	24, 48	24, 48

[a] Reproduced by permission from Organization for Economic Co-operation and Development (1981).
[b] Id.
[c] Ec.
[d] Test substance.
[e] V.

sensitized lymphocytes in the lymph node. Secondary exposure to the hapten of skin on any skin site that contains sensitized lymphocytes will lead to an allergic response and characteristic alterations of contact dermatitis (leukocyte chemotaxis, vasodilation, and increased vasopermeation).

Unfortunately, no single test seems to be a reliable predictor for all compounds and reproducibility is frequently poor, particularly for weak allergens. The maximization test is more sensitive and, hence, more likely to show a substance to be a sensitizer than the other tests. The epicutaneous tests, however, give better correlations of relative potency *vis a vis* human skin contact. It is virtually impossible to estimate "safe" exposures to contact allergens from guinea pigs alone. Definitive results can be achieved only in a human population.

The principle features of the seven guinea pig studies as summarized in the OECD (1981) guidelines are shown in Table IV. The classical Landsteiner–Draize test is simple and reliable but not sensitive enough to detect weak allergens. Therefore test methods have been modified through the use of various adjuvant techniques to make the guinea pig more susceptible to sensitization. Two tests are presented here in detail: the Draize intradermal test because it is so frequently used and the maximization test because it is sensitive and correlates well with human data.

1. Draize Test

a. Animals

Twenty standard outbred Hartley strain guinea pigs, 300–500 g, are used in each test group and control group. The hair should be removed from the application site by careful shaving.

b. Test Material

A 0.1% solution (suspension or emulsion for solids) in physiological saline, paraffin oil, or propylene glycol is injected intradermally.

c. Induction

A series of 10 intradermal doses (0.05 ml for the first and 0.1 ml for others) are given on alternate days at various sites on the left flank or alternatively, three times a week. Skin reactions should be read 24 hours after each injection. The control group is not injected.

d. Challenge

The challenge is performed on day 35 with a single intradermal injection of 0.05 ml of the test solution in the right flank at approximately the same level as the first induction injection. The readings are taken at 24 and 48 hours. The reaction to the challenge dose is compared to both the inducing dose and the control.

e. Interpretation

The sites are evaluated 24 hours after each injection for diameter, height, and color. A substantially higher than average reaction at the challenge site indicates that the test material is a sensitizer. The purpose of this test is to screen out severe sensitizing materials for human tests.

f. Limitations of Method

The Draize test is not sensitive enough to detect weak sensitizers and cannot be used to test finished bacteriostatic products because of their irritating components. The route of exposure (intradermal) is dissimilar to that of human exposure, and the concentration used does not relate to those to which humans are potentially exposed.

2. Maximization Test

In the maximization test, which was developed by Magnusson and Kligman (1969, 1970) and Magnusson (1975), several potentiating factors have been combined to enhance the likelihood of inducing sensitization in test animals. Both intradermal and epicutaneous exposure are used as well as Freund's complete adjuvant and an irritant if necessary. It is considered to be the most sensitive of all the guinea pig sensitization tests.

a. Animals

Twenty to 25 standard outbred Hartley strain guinea pigs are used in each of the test and control groups.

b. Test Material

The highest nonirritating concentration (1-5% allergen) is used in saline in Freund's complete adjuvant (FCA), and FCA alone. Insoluble substances are made up in paraffin oil, peanut oil, or propylene glycol. Solids are pulverized and incorporated in petrolatum at 25% by weight or at the highest level that will produce mild to moderate irritation.

c. Induction

Intradermal Injections   An aggressive primary stimulation of the immune system is achieved through the use of six intradermal injections. An electric clipper is used on a 4 by 6 cm area over the guinea pigs shoulders. Three duplicate injections are made in a row on each side: (1)

0.1 ml adjuvant alone; (2) 0.1 ml test material in saline; and (3) 0.1 ml test material in FCA. Control animals are tested with FCA, FCA and vehicle, and vehicle. The injection sites should be just within the boundary of the 2 by 4 cm patch.

Topical Application   Seven days later, the test area is reshaved and the test material in petrolatum is applied topically with filter paper to the same sites and wrapped with an occlusive bandage cover for 48 hours. A pretreatment (24 hours prior to testing) of sodium lauryl sulfate is used when the test material is nonirritating.

d. Challenge

Fourteen days after this initial induction period (day 21), the animals are challenged with topical patches occluded for 24 hours on their clipped and shaved flank. The highest nonirritating concentration of the test material, one fifth of that concentration, and the vehicle alone are applied with a 10-cm diameter circular patch over the previously treated site and occluded for 24 hours.

e. Result

The test area is shaved 3 hours prior to being read. Readings are taken with a 4-point scale (see Table III) at 24 and 48 hours after removal of the patch. The frequency of sensitization, not the intensity, is important. The rating of allergenicity is based on the number of animals sensitized. In further reports (Magnusson and Kligman 1977), results were expressed in two ways: (1) by the proportion of animals sensitized and (2) by the intensity of the reaction. This mean response was calculated by summing the numerical reading for all three challenge concentrations and dividing this by the total number of readings, including the negative ones.

f. Value of the Test

Although there are a number of drawbacks to this test (the intradermal injection bypasses the normal skin barrier function, the exposure is dissimilar to that seen in humans), it is the most sensitive test available and generally has a low rate of false negatives. The maximization test has been shown to correlate well with the same test conducted in humans (Magnusson, 1975). Because the human test also bypasses the normal barrier function of the skin, the utility of this test as a screen remains unclear (Table V).

Table V
Maximization Test Grading in the Guinea Pig[a]

Sensitization rate (%)	Grade	Classification
0–8	I	Weak
9–28	II	Mild
29–64	III	Moderate
65–80	IV	Strong
81–100	V	Extreme

[a] From Magnusson and Kligman (1969).

IV. PERCUTANEOUS PENETRATION

Human skin is primarily an excretory organ consisting of four layers: the horny layer or stratum corneum, the epidermis, the dermis, and the subcutis. The outermost layers, the stratum corneum and the epidermis, prevent water loss and retard absorption of chemicals into the body. In general terms, lipid-soluble (lipophilic) substances permeate skin better than water and electrolytes (hydrophilic). The dermis plays an important role in thermoregulation because of its extensive vasculature and sweat glands.

The process of absorption takes place in three steps: penetration of the chemical into a particular layer, permeation (penetration) of the chemical through one layer into another, and resorption or movement of the chemical into capillary or lymph vessels. Bioavailability is the amount and time course of chemical in the bloodstream following resorption. All these factors play a role in the ultimate toxicity of the chemical. A useful summary of the parameters affecting percutaneous penetration is given in Wester and Maibach (1983).

A. Methods

There are numerous ways to measure percutaneous absorption *in vivo*. They can be categorized into procedures used to measure the disappearance of the test material from the surface of the skin, the amount of material in the various layers of the skin or in the whole body, and the amount of material or metabolites in blood (with either radio-labeled or nonlabeled compounds). Other procedures are used to measure the response of sweat glands and capillaries or the production of an inflammatory reaction once the chemical has penetrated to the deeper layers of the skin. These various procedures are well summarized in Schaefer *et al.* (1982).

One of the more widely used and accepted methods, which has the advantages of being quantitative and allowing for reuse of the test animal, was developed by Feldman and Maibach (1969, 1970) and has been used extensively for the testing of drugs and, to a lesser extent, for the testing of environmental chemicals. This procedure can also be conducted with unlabeled compounds if sensitive analytical procedures are available, which definitely increases its suitability for studies conducted in humans.

B. Principles of the Test Procedures

Quantitative estimates of the percutaneous absorption of the test material following dermal application of radio-labeled material can be determined. The test is conducted in two parts. An intramuscular (IM) injection of the test material is given in the first part, urine and feces samples are collected until no radioactivity is detectable. After this washout period, an equivalent dose is applied dermally in the second part of the test. Again urine and feces samples are collected until there is no detectable radioactivity. The total excretion value obtained following IM injection is used to correct for incomplete excretion following dermal application. Similar investigations in which *in vitro* percutaneous absorption models are used are also gaining popularity.

1. Animal Selection

a. Species and Strain

There are wide variations in the structure and pilosity of skin in different species. No study has been able to predict an apparent consistency in the skin of any animal species with the skin of humans (Tregear 1966). Bartek *et al.* (1971, 1972) used six radio-labeled compounds and found that skin permeability was greater in laboratory animals than in humans, with human skin being the least permeable and rabbit skin the most. For caffeine these studies showed inconsistencies in this sequence, with human skin being more permeable than pig skin. Wester and Maibach (1975, 1976a, 1976b) demonstrated that for testosterone, hydrocortisone, and benzoic acid, the skin of rhesus monkeys was similar to that of humans. It is important to be aware of these differences when one chooses the test species. In fact, one should validate the animal model if the data are to be extrapolated to the human situation. Because rhesus monkey skin appears to be the most appropriate model, we use the *Rhesus* species to describe percutaneous testing. However, the procedure can easily be modified for other species.

b. Number and Sex

A number of test monkeys sufficiently large to be statistically acceptable should be used. This seems to vary from four to eight animals per dose group. There does not appear to be a significant difference between the sexes, and because of difficulty in obtaining rhesus monkeys, both sexes are frequently used in each group.

c. Control Animals

Each animal serves as its own control through the use of pre-exposure sampling.

2. Dose Level

Because the monkeys will be reused, every effort should be made to keep the amount of the radio-labeled material as well as the actual amount of the chemical as low as feasible. In order to compare the amount of penetration of various chemicals, the total amount of radioactivity applied should be constant. Radioactivity is usually in the range of 1 to 10 μCi, with the concentration of chemical being approximately 4 μg/cm^2. To achieve these parameters, the area of application will vary depending on the specific activity of the chemical. It does not appear to be critical that the rate of 4 μg/cm^2 be adhered to; in some cases, it is easier to keep the area constant and allow fluctuations in the amount per cm^2. These conditions may be altered if the effects of area or concentration are being studied. The choice of solvent is also important because it can markedly affect skin absorption. The volume of application is usually 100 μl if the solvent dries quickly and less for others. Run off from the application site should be avoided. Generally, acetone or water is used for dermal application, depending on the solubility of the test material, and propylene glycol is used for intramuscular injection.

3. Application

Monkeys are isolated in their holding cage with the collapsing mechanism and sedated with a minimum dose of ketamine. They can then be removed from their cage and carefully placed in a holding chair for the 24-hour period immediately after dosing. Monkeys can be trained to use the chair and do not need to be anesthetized.

Intramuscular injection of the radio-labeled chemical can be given once a monkey is in the chair. Topical application should be made before the monkey is placed in the chair. The fur on the application site can be removed with clippers or with a depilatory cream 24 hours prior to application. In monkeys there appears to be no differences between shaved and unshaved skin in percutaneous penetration of the chemical (Wester and Maibach, 1975), provided that the stratum corneum is not abraded. The choice is thus one of convenience. Care should be taken to ensure that there are no nicks or cuts in the skin at the time of application. A rectangle demarcating the required topical area for application should be drawn on the skin and the application made in even motion all over the delineated area with a microliter syringe. Gentle blowing during this application speeds evaporation and prevents run off. A self-adhesive foam frame should be placed on the outside edge of the delineated area and loosely covered with a nonocclusive gauge patch. The edge of the patch should be secured with adhesive tape. The site may or may not be washed with soap and water at the end of 24 hours in accordance with the individual protocol.

The monkeys should be given feed and liquids while they are chaired to ensure adequate urine flow. At the end of the 24-hour period, the monkeys are placed in a metabolism cage for the remainder of the experiment.

4. Application Site

It has been shown that percutaneous penetration can vary widely with the site of application in humans (Feldman and Maibach, 1967; Maibach *et al.* 1971) and in animals (Wester *et al.,* 1971; Noonan and Wester, 1980). When parathion was used in humans, it was shown that the least amount of penetration occurred through the forearm skin (9%); penetration through the skin on the forehead was 36%; complete penetration occurred through scrotal skin.

When asinphos-methyl was used in both humans and monkeys, a similar relationship was shown with the forehead skin being more permeable than the forearm skin (Franklin, 1985). The abdomen has also been used. The choice of site should be made with these differences kept in mind as well as the impact that the value will have on estimation of the risk.

5. Urine and Feces Collection

Total urinary output should be collected at 4-, 8-, 12-, and 24-hour intervals for the remainder of the experiment. If the samples are prepared for counting immediately, they can be kept at 5°C, otherwise they should be frozen. Feces are collected at 24-hour intervals. The collection period should continue until there is no detectable radioactivity above background. Collecting pans should be carefully rinsed with water before each sample is collected and the washings calculated and added to the urinary counts. The chair, urine collection lines, and trays should be washed every 24 hr, and the washings calculated separately. Solid urine deposits are removed with sulfuric acid.

6. Counting of Urine

Sample volumes are recorded and 4 ml of urine or wash are dispensed into scintillation vials and stored at -20°C until analysis. At that time, 10 ml of scintillation cocktail (Beckman Readisolv MP) are added. The samples are stored in the dark for 24 hours to minimize chemiluminescence. Counting efficiency should be corrected by the external standard ratio (ESR) method.

V. PHOTOTOXICITY AND PHOTOSENSITIZATION

There are several types of dermal toxicity tests outside the scope of this chapter. These include phototoxicity and photoallergic sensitization, urticaria, acne genicity, and changes in skin pigmentation. Although these tests may be important to the evaluation of some topical drugs and cosmetics, animal models are highly specialized and not routinely utilized. Animal models for the study of photosensitivity are perhaps the most commonly used and are described briefly in this section.

The Hartley strain albino guinea pig is most commonly used for photosensitivity studies. Nuchal hair is removed, an appropriate concentration of the test material applied, and the treated area irradiated. The nuchal region is selected due to its lower threshold for erythema than the thoracic and lumbar areas (Morrison *et al.,* 1981). In some cases, a 20% solution of sodium lauryl sulfate has been used as a substitute for ultraviolet B irradiation (Horio, 1976). Ultraviolet (UV) irradiation is most conveniently delivered by fluorescent tubes with a spectral emission in the 320 to 400 nm range. Three to five repetitions of the induction sequence are performed within a one-to-two-week period. Before attempts are made to elicit photosensitivity, a period of two to three weeks is allowed for development of a photoimmune reaction.

The elicitation procedure involves several steps very similar to those of the induction process. Hair is first removed from an appropriate site, the nuchal region being avoided (to minimize false positive reactions). The test material is then applied in duplicate sites. One site is irradiated while the other site, intended to serve as a control, is covered with some suitable opaque material. The test site is then exposed to ultraviolet A radiation and scored 24 hours later. Scoring is graded on the basis of erythema, with no reaction being scored as 0 and maximal erythema as 4.

In general, there appears to be a good correlation between the induction of phototoxic and photoimmunological reactions in both humans and guinea pigs. In this case, the guinea pig model is useful as a rapid screening procedure before such studies are initiated in humans.

Acknowledgments

The authors are grateful to Ms. Cindy Barnes for her assistance in the preparation of the manuscript.

References

Bartek, M. J., LaBudde, J. A., and Maibach, H. I. (1971). Skin permeability in vivo: Rat, rabbit, pig and man. *Clin. Res.* **19,** 358.

Bartek, M. J., LaBudde, J. A. and Maibach, H. I. (1972). Skin permeability in vivo: Comparison in rat, rabbit, pig and man. *J. Invest. Dermatol.* **58,** 114–123.

Canada Department of Agriculture (1984). Registration Guidelines for Registering Pesticides and Other Control Products Under the Pest Control Products Act in Canada. Ottawa: Canada Department of Agriculture.

Draize, J. H., Woodward, G. and Calvery, H. O. (1944). Methods for the study of irritation and toxicity of substances applied topically to the skin and mucous membranes. *J. Pharmacol. Exp. Ther.* **82,** 377–390.

Draize, J. H. (1955). VIII. Dermal toxicity. *Food Drug Cosmet. Law J.* **10,** 722.

Draize, J. H. (1965). "Appraisal of the Safety of Chemicals in Foods, Drugs and Cosmetics — Dermal Toxicity," pp. 46–59. Topeka, Kansas: Association of Food and Drug Officials of the United States.

Feldman, F. J., and Maibach, H. I. (1967). Regional variation in percutaneous penetration of ^{14}C cortisol in man. *J. Invest. Dermatol.* **48,** 181–183.

Feldman, R. J., and Maibach, H. I. (1969). Percutaneous penetration of steroids in man. *J. Invest. Dermatol.* **52,** 89–94.

Feldman, R. J., and Maibach, H. I. (1970). Absorption of some organic compounds through the skin in man. *J. Invest. Dermatol.* **54,** 339.

Franklin, C. A. (1985). "Assessment of Occupational Exposure to Pesticides and Its ACS Role in Risk Assessment Procedures in Canada" (ACS Symposium Series, 29). Washington, DC: American Chemical Society.

Horio, T. (1976). The induction of photocontact sensitivity in guinea pigs without UVB radiation. *J. Invest. Dermatol.* **67,** 591–593.

Litchfield, J. T., and Wilcoxon, A. (1949). A simplified method of evaluating dose-effect experiments. *J. Pharmacol. Exp. Ther.* **96,** 99–115.

McCreesh, A. J., and Steinberg, M. (1977). Skin irritation testing in animals. *In* "Advances in Modern Toxicology: Dermatotoxicology and Pharmacology" (F. N. Marzulli and H. I., Maibach, eds.), Vol. 4, pp. 193–210. New York: Wiley.

Magnusson, B., and Kligman, A. M. (1969). The identification of contact allergens by animal assay. The guinea pigs maximization test. *J. Invest. Dermatol.* **52,** 268–275.

Magnusson, B., and Kligman, A. M. (1970). Identification of contact allergens. *In* "Allergic Contact Dermatitis in the Guinea Pig," pp. 102–124. Springfield, Illinois: Thomas.

Magnusson, B. (1975). The relevance of results obtained with the guinea pig maximization test. *In* "Animal Models in Dermatology" (H. Maibach, ed.), pp. 76–83. Edinburgh: Churchill Livingstone.

Magnusson, B., and Kligman, A. M. (1977). Factors affecting contact sensitization. *Ad. Mod. Toxicol.* **4,** 289–304.

Maibach, H. J., Felman, R. J., Milby, T. H., and Serat, W. F. (1971). Regional variation in percutaneous penetration in man. *Arch. Environ. Health* **23,** 208–211.

Morrison, W. L., Parrish, J. A., Anderson, R. R., and Harris, T. J. (1981). Variations in the erythemal response of guinea pig skin. *Photochem. Photobiol.* **33,** 283.

Noonan, P. K., and Wester, R. C. (1980). Percutaneous absorption of nitroglycerin. *J. Pharm. Sci.* **69,** 365–366.

Organization for Economic Cooperation and Development (1986a). "Guidelines for Testing of Chemicals." Paris: Organization for Economic Cooperation and Development.

Organization for Economic Cooperation and Development (1986b). "Guidelines for Testing of New Chemicals." Paris: Organization for Economic Cooperation and Development.

Schaefer, H., Zesch, A., and Stuttgen, G. (1982). "Skin Permeability." New York: Springer-Verlag.

Tregear, R. T. (1966). "Physical Functions of the Skin." New York: Academic Press.

U.S. Department of Commerce, National Technical Information Service (1982). "Pesticide Assessment Guidelines, Subdivision F, Hazard Evaluation: House and Domestic Animals" (Report PB 83-153916) Washington, DC: U.S. Department of Commerce.

U.S. Environmental Protection Agency (1978). "Proposed Guidelines For Pesticide Registration: Hazard Evaluation. Human and domestic Animals" (Publ. No. 43) p. 3766. Washington, DC: U.S. Environmental Protection Agency.

U.S. Environmental Protection Agency (1982). "Dermatotoxicity," (Rep. 560/11-82-002). Washington, DC: U.S. Environmental Protection Agency.

Wester, R. C., and Maibach, H. I. (1975). Percutaneous absorption in the rhesus monkey compared to man. *Toxicol. Appl. Pharmacol.* **32,** 394–398.

Wester, R. C., and Maibach, H. I. (1976a). Skin penetration — concentration dependence in the rhesus monkey and man. *Clin. Res.* **24,** 268A.

Wester, R. C., and Maibach, H. I. (1976b). Relationship of topical dose and percutaneous absorption in rhesus monkey and man. *J. Invest. Dermatol.* **67,** 518–520.

Wester, R. C., and Maibach, H. I. (1983). Cutaneous pharmacokinetics: Ten steps to percutaneous absorption. *Drug Met. Rev.* **XIV(2).**

Wester, R. C., *et. al.* (1971).

12
Developmental Toxicity Studies[1]

Carole A. Kimmel
Reproductive and Developmental Toxicology Branch/OHEA
U.S. Environmental Protection Agency
Washington, D.C.

Catherine J. Price
Chemistry and Life Sciences
Center for Life Sciences and Toxicology
Research Triangle Institute
Research Triangle Park, North Carolina

I. Introduction

II. Basic Study Design: Developmental Toxicity (Segment II) Study
  A. Basic Protocol
  B. Chemistry and Dosing
  C. Animal Husbandry
  D. Maternal Evaluations
  E. Fetal Evaluations

III. Data Summarization, Analysis, and Interpretation
  A. Data Summarization
  B. Statistical Analysis
  C. Interpretation of Data

IV. Use of Historical Control Data

V. Postnatal Evaluation Studies

VI. Short-Term Screening Systems

I. INTRODUCTION

Developmental toxicity studies (also referred to as teratology or segment II studies) are conducted routinely in the toxicological assessment of foods, drugs, and chemicals. The first guidelines for these studies were promulgated by the U.S. Food and Drug Administration (FDA) in 1966

[1] The views in this chapter are those of the authors and do not necessarily represent the views or policies of the U.S. Environmental Protection Agency.

Handbook of
In Vivo Toxicity Testing

and included three test protocols (segments I, II, and III) for the testing of all new drugs for reproductive and developmental effects. The segment I or the fertility and reproduction study is designed for assessment of a chemical's effects on male and female fertility, general reproductive function, and development of the offspring. This protocol is usually conducted in rats. Males are treated for 60 days and females for 14 days prior to mating as well as during the mating period. Following mating, females are treated until midpregnancy when some are sacrificed to determine pregnancy status and viability of fetuses, or until the end of the lactation period when pups are examined for growth and abnormalities. In the segment II study, which is the main focus of this chapter, test animals are assessed for potential adverse effects from chemical exposure during major organogenesis on embryo/fetal development, including the production of structural alterations (teratogenic effects) [U.S. FDA, 1966; U.S. Environmental Protection Agency (EPA), 1982, 1985]. In the segment III or peri- and postnatal studies, pregnant animals (usually rats) are treated from day 15 of gestation throughout lactation; parturition, litter size and weight, and growth and viability of pups to weaning are observed.

Another protocol used to assess the reproductive and developmental toxicity of new foods, food additives, and pesticides (U.S. FDA, 1970; U.S. EPA, 1982, 1985) is the multigeneration study in which animal exposure to the test product begins several weeks prior to mating and continues throughout the derivation of two or three generations. More than one litter may be derived per generation, one of which may be selected for examination of fetuses prior to term similar to that done in the segment II protocol. Palmer (1981) and Marks (1985) reviewed the historical development of these tests and compared in detail the protocols required by various countries for routine reproductive and developmental toxicity testing. Because guidelines among agencies and among countries may differ or evolve over time, laboratories conducting such studies must design study protocols and plan for the archival storage of study records and biological samples in order to meet the existing requirements of the agency to which the data is to be submitted.

The segment II study protocol was originally implemented in the aftermath of the thalidomide crisis, and emphasis was placed on the detection of malformations in the fetus. Currently, however, concern is raised by any adverse developmental outcome, and the term *developmental toxicity* is used to include any of the four major manifestations of abnormal development: death, malformation, growth alteration, and functional deficit. Although the experimental details are now more precisely defined, the basic protocols are essentially the same as those originally outlined by the U.S. FDA (1966). In addition, the importance of adverse maternal effects and the relationship of adverse maternal and fetal effects are now recognized (Fabro *et al.,* 1982; Kimmel *et al.,* 1987).

In addition to the routine testing procedures used, recent efforts have been made to develop procedures for evaluating postnatal function (e.g., behavior and a variety of organ systems); short-term testing to reduce the number of animals used and the cost of testing; and studies on the mechanism of a test chemical's action, including the effects that occur at the time of agent insult as well as the chain of events (pathogenesis) that results in an adverse outcome. In this chapter, we briefly outline postnatal functional evaluation and short-term tests related to screening but we primarily discuss the conduct of conventional developmental toxicity studies and issues related to technical support requirements, analysis, and interpretation of data that are unique to this field. In particular, the importance and use of historical control data are presented for three laboratory species (CD rat, CD-1 mouse, and New Zealand white rabbit) that have been investigated extensively at the Research Triangle Institute funded by the National Toxicology Program (NTP) and the National Center for Toxicological Research (NCTR). Individual study reports prepared in compliance with the U.S. FDA (1978) good laboratory practice (GLP) regulations provide detailed descriptions of the study design for developmental toxicity evaluations of environmental agents used and implemented in the context of this NTP/NCTR research and testing effort (e.g., see Price *et al.,* 1984a, 1984b). Recommendations for testing, as stated in this chapter, are based on the experience of the authors in this testing program; in some cases, recommendations represent particular techniques that have been adopted in an effort to achieve uniformity.

II. BASIC STUDY DESIGN: DEVELOPMENTAL TOXICITY (SEGMENT II) STUDY

A. Basic Protocol

The standard protocol for the segment II study (U.S. FDA, 1966; U.S. EPA, 1982, 1985) involves timed-mating of healthy laboratory animals, dosing throughout the period of major organogenesis (days 6–15 for rats and mice; 6–18 or 19 for rabbits), and sacrifice just prior to delivery to avoid maternal cannibalization of abnormal pups. Maternal animals are observed throughout gestation. After pregnant females are sacrificed, the uterus is removed, the contents are examined, and the live fetuses are collected and thoroughly examined. Testing is often conducted in at least two species (usually rat or mouse and rabbit). At least three dose levels are recommended along with a concurrent vehicle-treated control group. The recommended number of animals per group is usually 20 rodents, whose pregnancies are confirmed, and 12–15 rabbits. However, to obtain equivalent statistical power, the number of rabbits should be at least the same as the number of rodents. Replication of treatment groups within the study design (e.g., two replicates of 10–15 mated subjects per treatment group) increases the power of the study and strengthens the confidence of data interpretation. All studies conducted for the National Toxicology Program include a replicate study design in which the breeding dates for consecutive replicates are separated by at least two weeks. Animals from the same supplier obtained in the same or different shipments may be used in each replicate.

B. Chemistry and Dosing

1. Chemistry Support Requirements, Safety, and Handling

The procedures summarized in this section are those used in the National Toxicology Program and are described in detail in publications by Jameson and Walters (1984) and Walters and Jameson (1984). The chemical agent to be used in all toxicity studies of that agent should be obtained in large enough supply from a single lot. Chemical analyses should include determinations of purity and stability under appropriate storage conditions. Once the vehicle has been chosen, chemical–vehicle mixing procedures and storage conditions must be established along with procedures for analyzing concentration, homogeneity, and stability of chemical–vehicle formulations. If corn oil is used as a vehicle, peroxide levels should be determined; any batch having a value greater than or equal to 10 meq/kg should be rejected as being rancid. Dosing formulations should be coded so that personnel who administer the agent are unaware of the concentration of the agent in each formulation. There may be practical difficulties with coding suspensions and colored solutions that can be visibly rank-ordered unless opaque vials are used. Predosing and postdosing analyses should be done to verify the concentration of the dosing formulation. If a dosing formulation is found to be outside a range of $\pm$ 10% of the theoretical concentration upon predosing analysis, it should be rejected and replaced with a new formulation. If a bulk chemical is maintained for use over several months, reanalysis of the bulk chemical should be conducted at appropriate intervals to check purity and stability against a reference sample that has been stored at optimum conditions (e.g., $-20\,^{\circ}$C or lower).

Appropriate safety and handling procedures should be instituted during all aspects of the study. Potentially hazardous chemicals should be handled only in laboratory areas especially designed to provide adequate safety. Safety precautions for chemical agents may include, but not be limited to, adequate clothing, masks, goggles or safety glasses, gloves, portable monitoring devices, hoods with adequate air flow for volatile or radioactive materials, established emergency procedures, and adequate ventilation systems in the animal rooms, especially in the cage changing and washing areas. Environmental monitoring of all work areas is important to assure adequate personnel protection. In the laboratory, adequate ventilation should be available to protect personnel from possible inhalation of toxic substances such as formaldehyde used in the tissue fixing solutions.

2. Dosing Procedures

The route of exposure selected for developmental toxicity studies may be based on the route of exposure most likely in humans. In the case of oral exposure, it may be preferable to intubate rather than to administer in diet or drinking water because the dose given can be more precisely controlled. In addition, a higher dose can be delivered via intubation than via the diet or drinking water when palatability or solubility problems occur. Parenteral routes of exposure may include dermal, subcutaneous, intramuscular, intravenous, and intraperitoneal routes. The latter route should be avoided, if possible, because intraperitoneal administration results in bathing of the pregnant uterus as well as in absorption by the abdominal visceral circulation. In rabbits, intraperitoneal injection frequently results in spontaneous abortion. Dermal and inhalation exposure both present unique sets of technical problems that are not discussed in this chapter but are common to other types of toxicity testing [see Phalen (1984) and U.S. EPA (1985) for discussions of inhalation studies; Drill and Lazar (1983) and Kimmel and Francis (1990) for discussions of cutaneous toxicity testing].

For oral intubation or parenteral injection, the volume of dosing solution administered per unit of body weight should be standardized across dose groups and based on daily body weights. Dose volumes of 5 ml/kg (rats), 10 ml/kg (mice), or 1 ml/kg (rabbits) are generally acceptable for oral intubation, although larger volumes may be required for compounds with low solubility. When feed or drinking water is the vehicle, the study should include frequent measurement of the amount of food or water consumed, and spillage should be controlled as much as possible. In some studies, food and/or water consumption may be reduced due to poor palatability of the test compound given in the diet or due to adverse effects on consummatory behavior. In these cases, it may be desirable to include one or more pair-fed control groups in order to determine the relative contribution of consummatory deficits to adverse developmental outcome (see, e.g., Schwetz et al., 1977; Abel et al., 1981). However, the pair-fed animals should be delayed by at least one day in order to match daily intake based on gestational age.

The timing of exposure is a critical consideration in developmental toxicity studies, more so than in any other area of toxicology. This is true because most critical developmental events occur during a very narrow time period in gestation, especially in smaller laboratory species. Thus, the day on which animals are mated and the stage of gestation at dosing must be recorded. Similarly, it is recommended that dosing of all groups be restricted to a particular time of day, with no more than two hours elapsing between dosing of the first and last animals if possible. Although standard evaluation procedures require dosing throughout the period of major organogenesis, it may be necessary to expose the mother prior to implantation or mating to build up a greater body burden if the agent is poorly absorbed or requires a long time to reach a steady state level. On the other hand, if an effect is produced by exposure throughout organogenesis or if an agent is known to induce liver metabolizing enzymes, it may be desirable in subsequent studies to expose animals over shorter segments of organogenesis in an attempt to determine critical periods of exposure and specific types of effects produced.

The preferred vehicle for intubation or injection in developmental toxicity studies is distilled water or 0.9% saline. If the agent is insoluble in water, then the possibility of solubilizing or suspending it homogeneously in a vehicle such as corn oil or carboxymethyl cellulose should be considered. More exotic vehicles should not be used unless historical control data are available or can be collected. Even those vehicles considered biologically inert may have subtle and unexpected consequences.

Positive control agents in developmental toxicity evaluations have often been used for training purposes. They allow researchers to become familiar with different species and their reproductive characteristics and with various malformations that may be encountered, because the types and frequencies of malformations in untreated or vehicle-treated animals is quite limited (Aliverti et al., 1980). However, using a positive control along with the evaluation of every unknown agent is wasteful of time and resources, especially in a laboratory in which studies are conducted on a routine basis. A positive control may be a useful reference if it is a structural analog or if it is expected to have adverse effects similar to those caused by the agent being studied.

C. Animal Husbandry

1. Housing and Environmental Conditions

The care of any live laboratory animal should be administered according to the principles described in the National Institute of Health (1985) *Guide for the Care and Use of Laboratory Animals* and should conform to U.S. Department of Agriculture (1970, 1987) regulations. Incoming animals should be quarantined for an appropriate period (usually 10–14 days) so that their general health status can be assessed. In order to ensure animal quality further, some rodent vendors can provide "viral antibody free" animals from colonies screened for pathogens before shipment. Alternatively, serum can be collected from sentinel animals or from animals at scheduled necropsy and screened for antibodies during quarantine and/or termination of the study (Hamm, 1986). Animals whose pregnancies have been timed can be purchased from suppliers, but the pregnancy rate is not usually as high as when animals are bred in house. Animal holding rooms should be vermin proof; no pesticides, rodenticides, anthelmintics, etc., should be used.

Housing facilities should be equipped with devices for monitoring, recording, and controlling temperature and relative humidity, ideally with individual controls for each animal holding room. Lighting should be controlled by automatic adjustable devices, usually set for a 12:12 hour light-dark cycle. Air exchange should be frequent enough to avoid odor buildup (e.g., 10–12 times per hour). Bedding should be changed 2–3 times per week, and cages changed at least weekly. Food and water should be supplied *ad libitum*. A certified commercial diet appropriate during active reproduction in the test species is recommended unless a laboratory conducts its own dietary analyses. In the latter case, limits should be placed on the range of dietary constituents and contaminants allowed. Distilled or deionized and/or millipore filtered water is preferable for drinking water. If tap water is used, frequent analyses should document the levels of salts and chemicals as well as microbiological contaminants.

2. Animal Requirements

Maternal animals should be young, healthy, virgin females (8–12 weeks of age for mice and rats; 5–6 months of age for rabbits). The acceptable weight range should not be too broad (200–300 g for rats; 20–35 g for mice; 2.5–5 kg for rabbits) because body weight is used as an indicator of toxicity and reproductive performance varies with age and body weight.

Males should be sexually mature; experienced breeders should be used if possible. Following mating, a stratified randomization procedure should be used to assign females to treatment groups based on body weight at mating or at start of treatment. In order to minimize the genetic influence of individual male breeders, the number of females mated with a particular male within each treatment group should be limited, and breeding records should be maintained.

3. Mating Procedures

a. Rats

Several procedures may be used for timed-mating of rats. Vaginal cycles may be followed from cytological evaluations of vaginal smears (Hafez, 1970). The estrous cycle may be staged only on the day of breeding. Alternatively, animals may be placed with males at random with no regard to the stage of the estrous cycle. The latter procedure requires a larger breeding colony because only 20–25% of the females can be expected to mate on a given night (4–5-day estrous cycle). The vaginal lavage can be checked for sperm the morning after breeding. However, if males and females are paired 1:1 and placed in hanging cages with fresh paper underneath, copulation plugs (which in rats do not remain in the vagina) may be detected the next morning under those cages in which insemination has occurred. The pregnancy rate for females in proestrus or estrus (i.e., number of confirmed pregnancies to number of plugs or sperm-positive smears) is usually high in rats, approximately 90%.

b. Mice

Males and females may be cohabited (1–2 females/male) overnight or for shorter periods of time, and copulation plugs, which remain in the vagina in mice, may be detected the next morning (Hafez, 1970). To increase the rate of successful matings, females may be "primed" according to Whitten's (1956) method. In this procedure, a single male mouse is placed in a wire mesh cage inside the home cage of 10 females. Forty-eight hours later, females are placed 1:1 or 2:1 with breeder males overnight, and the vagina is checked for copulation plugs the next morning. The pregnancy rate in primed mice mating 1:1 is approximately 87%.

c. Rabbits

Rabbits may be pair-mated if a doe and buck are placed together and copulation is observed. Another procedure requiring fewer males involves artificial insemination (Hafez, 1970). To induce ovulation, females receive an intravenous injection of pituitary luteinizing hormone (1 mg/kg) or chorionic gonadotropin (100 USP units per animal) no more than two hours prior to insemination. Semen is collected from males that have been trained to use an artificial vagina (Bredderman *et al.*, 1964) in conjunction with a teaser female. Prior to insemination, a sample of the ejaculate from each male is diluted with saline and examined for sperm motility and density. Sperm are counted under a microscope with a hemacytometer or particle counter. A sperm count of at least 28.8×10^7 sperm/ml is recommended for insemination. Females are then inseminated with 0.25 ml of undiluted ejaculate. On the average, two to three females can be inseminated with a single semen collection. The pregnancy rate in New Zealand white rabbits that are artificially inseminated is approximately 90%.

D. Maternal Evaluations

Maternal signs of toxicity are important indicators of chemical effects and should be examined carefully in developmental toxicity studies in order to assess the relative sensitivity of maternal and fetal endpoints. All evaluations should be conducted without knowledge of the test group being examined.

Body weights on given gestation days, particularly during treatment and at term, should be recorded. Body weight gain (e.g., during treatment or throughout gestation) may be a more sensitive indicator of adverse effects because the pregnant animal is increasing in weight throughout gestation and incremental weight changes are more easily detected. Corrected weight gain (i.e., maternal weight gain throughout gestation corrected for gravid uterine weight) indicates the status of the maternal animal alone at sacrifice and is not confounded by any effect of the chemical on litter size and/or litter weight. Maternal weight gain may also be corrected for total litter weight if the gravid uterus is not weighed.

Clinical signs are important qualitative indicators of toxicity. When a chemical is administered in the feed or drinking water, observation for clinical signs once daily at the time of weighing is usually adequate. For routes of administration such as subcutaneous injection or gavage, the study director may designate additional times after dosing for observation when clinical signs are expected to be most pronounced. These observation times are based on the known or expected time course for bioavailability and/or biological response. In some cases, clinical signs may provide a better indicator of maternal toxicity than body weights. Clinical signs may include, but are not limited to, changes in skin, fur, eyes and mucous membranes as well as in respiratory, circulatory, autonomic and central nervous systems, spontaneous motor activity, and other behavioral patterns.

Food and water consumption should be measured daily in those studies in which dietary or drinking water administration of the chemical is used, or when appetite or excretory effects (such as increased gut motility or diuresis) are suspected. Calculation of the amount of chemical consumed on a body weight basis allows a more accurate estimate of dosage.

A gross pathological examination should be made at sacrifice, and organ weights and histopathology may be included when there is suspected target organ toxicity. More extensive pathological assessments are generally included in the acute, subacute, subchronic, and chronic toxicity evaluations.

Maternal animals are typically sacrificed one to two days prior to term to allow thorough evaluation of the uterine contents and to avoid cannibalization of abnormal young. Thus, sacrifices are typically scheduled for gestational day 20 for rats, day 17 for mice, or day 30 for rabbits when "day 0" is considered the day of sperm or plug detection, observed mating, or insemination, as applicable. The uterus is removed at sacrifice, weighed intact, then opened along the antimesometrial border. Implantation sites, resorptions, dead and live fetuses are counted. Live fetuses are removed for further examination and numbered individually so that observations (e.g., weight, external, visceral, and skeletal observations) may be compared for each fetus.

E. Fetal Evaluations

Each live fetus is weighed individually and examined externally for structural alterations. The sex of each may be determined by external examination in some species but should be confirmed during the visceral examination. Two methods are routinely used for visceral examination of fetuses, the freehand razor-blade sectioning technique (Wilson, 1965) or the fresh visceral dissection technique (Staples, 1974; Stuckhardt and Poppe, 1984). The former procedure requires Bouin's fixation prior to sectioning, which precludes skeletal staining of the same fetuses. Therefore, only a portion of each litter is examined, usually one third to one half. With the freehand technique, every other or every third fetus should be selected for visceral or skeletal examination so that fetuses from different uterine positions are represented. The practice of selecting fetuses for visceral examination that have external malformations should be avoided because this may bias the results toward visceral defects, especially if an agent produces a dose-related increase in external anomalies. Prior to the use of the fresh visceral dissection technique, fetuses should be decapitated or anesthetized by placing them on a moist paper towel over a tray of ice, which reduces core body temperature below 25°C (Lumb and Jones, 1973; Blair, 1979). Because the fresh visceral dissection method does not preclude skeletal staining, all fetuses may be examined for external, visceral, and skeletal malformations. A portion or all of the fetuses may be decapitated and the head fixed in Bouin's solution and examined by freehand razor-blade sectioning (Wilson, 1965). Those fetuses to be examined for skeletal defects should be stained with alizarin red S and may be counterstained with alcian blue for examination of both bone ossification and cartilage development (Peltzer and Schardein, 1966; Crary, 1962; Kimmel and Trammell, 1981; Marr et al., 1988).

When unknown agents are tested, a variety of unanticipated structural anomalies may be produced, some of which may be novel even to a highly experienced investigator. In such cases, it is especially important for documentation of anomalies to be as complete as possible (including drawings and/or photographs). Preservation of specimens for archival purposes is also desirable in such cases.

Because there is no generally accepted standard terminology for fetal observations in developmental toxicity studies, each laboratory must develop its own glossary of terms and definitions. Guides to use include lists of observations from historical control data (Palmer, 1971; Banerjee and Durloo, 1973; Perraud, 1976; Stadler et al., 1983; Morita et al., 1987; Charles River Laboratories, 1988), from reference books (Warkany, 1971; Taylor, 1986), from embryology textbooks or atlases (Walker and Wirtschafter, 1957; Wirtschafter, 1960), and from medical dictionaries. Each laboratory must also determine the normal range of variability for the species and strains used and what changes should be considered outside the normal range. This can be especially difficult for any organ or system that continues to develop at the time of observation; for example, renal and skeletal development continues into the early postnatal period (Fritz and Hess, 1970; Woo and Hoar, 1972; Aliverti et al., 1979). Thus, the status of these systems should be recorded for all control and treated groups so that alterations in the developmental status among treated groups can be detected.

Classification of observations as major and minor malformations or variations is a common practice (e.g., Palmer, 1971). However, this classification procedure should be considered only as a convenient tool for examining the effect of a toxic agent.

III. DATA SUMMARIZATION, ANALYSIS, AND INTERPRETATION

A. Data Summarization

The summarization of data for all endpoints, both maternal and fetal should be based on the dam or litter because the dam is the individual treated. Maternal body weights and weight gain during treatment and gestation, as discussed, should be presented along with clinical signs observed, measurements of food and water consumption (total amount of food and water consumed as well as the amount relative to body weight), amount of chemical administered or consumed based on body weight, and any specific organ weights or observational data obtained at necropsy. Maternal pregnancy status at term for each dose group should include the mean number of implantation sites per dam and the mean number and percent (based on implantation number) of resorptions, late fetal deaths, and nonlive implants (resorption plus late fetal deaths) per dam. If treatment was begun prior to implantation, the number of corpora lutea per dam should also be presented. One can calculate the percentage of preimplantation loss by subtracting the number of implantations from the number of corpora lutea, dividing by the number of corpora lutea, and multiplying by 100 for each dam.

The fetal endpoints should include the average number of live fetuses for dams with live litters, the average litter sex ratio (expressed as % males, % females, or ratio of males to females per litter), mean fetal body weight per litter (mean of litter means), and number and percent (based on number of live fetuses) of malformed fetuses per litter (mean of individual litter values). In addition, data for the latter two endpoints can be calculated for each sex individually. The number and percent malformed per litter can be calculated based on the type of examination (i.e., external, visceral, or skeletal) and can be evaluated further by selected individual defects if examination of the raw incidence data indicates an increase in a particular type of defect. If defects are categorized as major or minor malformations or variations, the number and percent per litter (mean of individual litter values) can also be calculated for each category. The combination of resorptions, dead, and malformed fetuses (number and percent based on number of implantations, mean of individual litter values) gives an indication of the incidence of total adversely affected implants. Another way of expressing the data is to calculate the number and percent of litters having one or more resorptions, malformed fetuses, affected implants, etc.

B. Statistical Analysis

Several approaches have been used in the statistical analysis of data from developmental toxicity studies (Weil, 1970; Gaylor, 1978; Haseman and Kupper, 1979; Gad and Weil, 1986). The approach used in our studies conducted for the National Toxicology Program is described in this section. For data collected in each study, a parametric evaluation of the dose effect, replicate effect, and dose × replicate interaction is conducted on selected measures with appropriate analysis of variance (ANOVA) designs. Analyses of the data are carried out with appropriate general linear models (GLM) in the Statistical Analysis System[2] (SAS Institute, 1985a, 1985b). Prior to GLM analysis, an arcsine-square root transformation is performed on all litter-derived percentage data (Snedecor and Cochran, 1967). If differential litter size is thought to be a confounding factor, a weighted analysis of transformed proportions may be used (Haseman and Kupper, 1979). Generally, a dose × replicate design is used and a linear trend test for dose effects is conducted. If no significant dose effects are observed for maternal body weight measurements, then a three-way ANOVA design (dose × replicate × day) with day as a repeated measure is conducted. Data for male and/or female fetal weights and malformations are analyzed with a three-way ANOVA design (dose × replicate × sex) with sex as a repeated measure within litters. Each sex is also evaluated separately in a dose × replicate design.

When significant main effects of dose occur, Williams' multiple comparison test is used (Williams, 1971; 1972). Duncan's multiple range test (Siegel, 1956) or Dunnett's test (SAS Institute, 1985a, 1985b) is used for comparison of exposed groups and controls. A one-tailed test is employed for all pair-wise comparisons except for maternal and fetal body weight parameters and for the percent males per litter, for which a two-tailed test is utilized. The data for any measure that shows a significant dose × replicate interaction is further analyzed for dose effects within each replicate; an analysis of variance procedure and pair-wise comparisons are used where appropriate in this instance. Results yielding nonsignificant dose × replicate interactions are considered as evidence that pooling data across replicates is justified. Nominal scale data (e.g., number and percentage of litters with one or more resorptions, dead and/or malformed fetuses, etc.) are analyzed by the Chi square test for independence for differences among treatment groups. A test for linear trend on proportions is used in conjunction with each Chi square test. When Chi square test results indicate significant dose effects, a one-tailed Fisher exact probability test is used for pair-wise comparisons between each treated group and the vehicle control group. For further details on the statistical approaches used, see Price et al. (1984a, 1984b).

C. Interpretation of Data

When interpreting data from developmental toxicity studies, investigators must consider not only the individual endpoints but also the integration of all maternal and developmental effects and the relationship of

---

[2] SAS Institute, Inc., Box 8000, Cary, NC 27511.

the lowest maternal effective dose to the lowest developmental effective dose. An effect on any of the three major endpoints of developmental toxicity that are assessed in these studies (i.e., death, malformation, growth alteration) is considered to be an adverse developmental effect. Effects on the developing conceptus occurring below doses that are toxic to the maternal animal are of greatest concern. Because the understanding of the relationship between maternal toxicity and developmental effects is limited, one cannot conclude that developmental effects in the presence of mild to moderate maternal effects are secondary to maternal toxicity; rather, one must be concerned about developmental effects that occur in the range of low to moderate maternal toxicity (i.e., doses that produce a slight weight loss up to those causing no more than 10% maternal mortality). Further information on the interpretation of developmental toxicity data and on the risk assessment process may be found in the U.S. EPA's *Guidelines for the Health Assessment of Suspect Developmental Toxicants* (U. S. EPA, 1986a,1989) and *Standard Evaluation Procedure for Teratology Studies* (Chitlik *et al.,* 1985).

IV. USE OF HISTORICAL CONTROL DATA

Interpretation of data from developmental toxicity studies requires a knowledge of the background data for control animals of the species and strain used. Comparison of data from study controls with historical control data may be beneficial; therefore, it is important to have a comprehensive historical control data base available. As indicated earlier, determining the background or spontaneous incidence rate of particular endpoints for each laboratory is important. Comparison of historical data bases between laboratories is useful for determining the variability of such data and may indicate those endpoints most affected by laboratory environments. However, the absence of standardized terminology for fetal defects among laboratories sometimes hampers interlaboratory comparison of incidence data.

Historical data in three species (mouse, rat, rabbit) were accumulated over a four-year period (1980–1983) on NCTR/NTP contracts. Standard criteria were used so that data were comparable from study to study. These data include both the maternal and fetal endpoints that have been discussed and are, therefore, more complete than any in the currently published literature. Tables I and II present the data for vehicle-treated controls (distilled water or corn oil) for CD rats [(COBS) CD® (SD) BR outbred albino rats, Charles River Laboratories, Inc., Kingston, New York]. Tables III and IV present the same data for CD-1 mice [(COBS) CD-1® (ICR) BR outbred albino mice from the same source as for rats].

The data for rats and mice treated with either vehicle are combined because embryo/fetal endpoints from groups treated concurrently with either corn oil or distilled water were similar (George *et al.*, 1988; Price *et al.*, 1988). These findings are in contrast to an earlier retrospective comparison of vehicles from the historical control data suggesting that corn oil administration during organogenesis might be associated with an increased incidence of fetal malformations (rats and mice) and reduced fetal weight (rats; Kimmel *et al.*, 1985b). The data for New Zealand white (NZW) rabbits (Dutchland Laboratory Animals, Inc., Denver, Pennsylvania) are shown in Tables V and VI and are presented for the two vehicles combined.

The cautious use of historical control data even within the same laboratory is urged. In particular, comparison of study control data with the 95% confidence limits of historical data is probably more appropriate than comparison with the mean or, at the other extreme, with the full range of variability for a particular endpoint. If study control data fall within the 95% confidence limits of the historical control data, it may be assumed that the study animals are representative of other animals of that species. Dose-related changes in treated animals versus study controls can be assumed then to be due to treatment. Although standardized procedures may be used in the collection of data accumulated in the historical control data base, subtle changes may occur with time due to genetic alterations in the strain or stock of the species used, changes in environmental conditions both in the breeding colony of the supplier and in the laboratory, and changes in personnel conducting studies and collecting data. Therefore, it is important to examine changes in data over time within the historical data base and to compare study control data with recent as well as cumulative historical data. This can be done in several ways: for example, by plotting incidence data or weights for individual studies or by comparing average values year by year or for smaller increments of time. Any change in laboratory procedure that might affect control data should be noted and the data accumulated separately from previous data. Haseman *et al.* (1984) have recommended criteria for the use of historical control data for carcinogenicity studies that are appropriate for developmental toxicity studies as well.

V. POSTNATAL EVALUATION STUDIES

A number of investigations of the postnatal effects of developmental exposure to agents have been conducted and have indicated the potential for altered function (Rodier, 1978; Adams and Buelke-Sam, 1981; Vorhees and Butcher, 1982; Kavlock and Grabowski, 1983). Great Britain

Table I
Historical Data Summary of Measures for CD Rats Treated with Vehicle on Gestational Days 6 through 15[a,b]

	N	Mean	SEM	Range (min.)	Range (max.)	95% confidence interval (lower)	95% confidence interval (upper)
Maternal body weight (gd 0)[c]	313	236.5	1.1	200.3	294.0	234.3	238.8
Maternal body weight (gd 6)	313	261.6	1.2	210.8	324.8	259.4	263.9
Maternal body weight (gd 11)	313	278.6	1.2	222.2	351.1	276.3	281.0
Maternal body weight (gd 15)	313	298.5	1.3	233.1	366.0	296.0	301.0
Maternal body weight (at sacrifice)	313	356.0	1.6	257.5	444.9	352.8	359.2
Maternal weight gain (gestation)	313	119.5	1.2	42.7	184.7	117.2	121.8
Maternal weight gain (treatment)	313	36.9	0.6	−37.5	64.0	35.6	38.1
Maternal weight gain (corrected)[d]	312	48.1	0.9	−1.0	99.0	46.3	49.9
Gravid uterine weight	312	71.5	0.9	0.6	99.7	69.6	73.3
Liver weight	311	14.94	0.10	9.97	20.49	14.74	15.14
Relative liver weight (% body weight)	311	4.20	0.02	3.33	5.50	4.15	4.24
Corpora lutea per dam	120	15.87	0.24	9.00	25.00	15.39	16.34
Implantation sites per dam	313	13.21	0.16	1.00	20.00	12.90	13.53
Preimplantation loss per dam (%)	120	11.01	1.27	0.00	92.00	8.51	13.52
Resorptions per litter	313	0.59	0.08	0.00	15.00	0.44	0.74
Resorptions per litter (%)	313	5.07	0.73	0.00	100.00	3.62	6.51
Late fetal deaths per litter	313	0.02	0.01	0.00	3.00	−0.01	0.04
Late fetal deaths per litter (%)	313	0.11	0.08	0.00	23.08	−0.04	0.27
Nonlive implants per litter	313	0.61	0.08	0.00	15.00	0.45	0.76

Nonlive implants per litter (%)	313	5.18	0.74	0.00	100.00	3.72	6.65
Affected implants per litter	313	1.03	0.10	0.00	16.00	0.84	1.22
Affected implants per litter (%)	313	8.31	0.83	0.00	100.00	6.67	9.94
Live fetuses per litter[e]	310	12.73	0.16	1.00	18.00	12.42	13.04
Male fetuses per litter[e] (%)	310	48.69	0.89	0.00	100.00	46.94	50.45
Average fetal body weight per litter[e]	310	3.56	0.02	2.77	4.75	3.52	3.60
Average female fetal body weight per litter[e]	308	3.48	0.02	2.57	4.71	3.44	3.52
Average male fetal body weight per litter[e]	309	3.64	0.02	2.90	4.85	3.60	3.68
Malformed fetuses per litter[e]	310	0.43	0.05	0.00	7.00	0.32	0.54
Malformed fetuses per litter[e] (%)	310	3.35	0.44	0.00	54.55	2.49	4.21
Malformed female fetuses per litter[e]	308	0.21	0.03	0.00	4.00	0.14	0.27
Malformed female fetuses per litter[e] (%)	308	3.22	0.56	0.00	75.00	2.12	4.32
Malformed male fetuses per litter[e]	309	0.23	0.03	0.00	4.00	0.16	0.29
Malformed male fetuses per litter[e] (%)	309	3.44	0.50	0.00	50.00	2.46	4.43

[a] Vehicle is distilled water or corn oil, po.

[b] Pregnancy rate, 90%; ratio of number of confirmed-pregnant dams at sacrifice to the total number of mated females × 100. The mating procedure involved pairing 1 female in proestrus or estrus with 1 male overnight and checking for sperm in the vaginal lavage the next morning (day 0 of gestation).

Total number of confirmed-pregnant dams, 313.

Litters with live fetuses, 310; total number of live fetuses, 3946.

Litters with one or more resorptions, 109 (35%).

Litters with one or more late fetal deaths, 3 (1%); late fetal deaths include fetuses weighing > 0.8 g, discernible digits present, no vital signs at sacrifice.

Litters with one or more nonlive implants, 110 (35%); nonlive implants include late fetal deaths and resorbed implants.

Litters with one or more malformed live fetuses, 74 (24%).

Litters with one or more affected implants, 153 (49%); affected implants include nonlive implants and malformed live fetuses.

[c] All weights expressed in grams; gd, gestation day.

[d] Maternal weight gain during gestation corrected for gravid uterine weight.

[e] Includes only litters with live fetuses.

Table II

Historical Data Summary of Malformations and Variations in CD Rats Following
Administration of Vehicle on Gestational Days 6 through 15[a]

External malformations	
No. (%) fetuses with one or more external malformations	9 (0.23)
No. (%) litters	9 (2.90)
Umbilical hernia	2
Right ear small	1
Anophthalmia (bilateral)	1
Edema (severe)	1
Edema (slight)	1
Exencephaly	1
Abnormal fusion of the face; no mouth or nose	1
Gastroschisis	1
Microdactyly (small digits)	1
Open eye (left)	1
Short tail	1
Spina bifida	1
Visceral malformations	
No. (%) fetuses with one or more visceral malformations	59 (1.50)
No. (%) litters	38 (12.26)
Hydroureter (bilateral, left or right)	45
Hydronephrosis (bilateral, left or right)	25
Situs inversus viscerum	1
Aorta behind trachea and/or esophagus	1
Dextrocardia	1
Diaphragmatic hernia	1
Right-sided aorta[b]	1
Skeletal malformations[b]	
No. (%) fetuses with one or more skeletal malformations	67 (1.70)
No. (%) litters	34 (10.97)
Short rib (XIII)	46
Missing rib(s)	9
Abnormal skull fusion (parietals, interparietal)	5
Fused sternebrae	2
Misshapen skull bone (parietals)	2
Thoracic centra off center	2
Fused arch and centra (sacral)	1
Lumbar arch(es) smaller than normal	1
Lumbar centra misaligned	1
Lumbar centra off center	1
Missing lumbar arch	1
Ribs fused to each other	1
Thoracic centra misaligned	1
Variations	
No. (%) fetuses with one or more variations	617 (15.64)
No. (%) litters	221 (71.29)
Distended ureter(s)	240
Hematoma (any location)	164

(continues)

Table II (*continued*)

Bipartite centra	134
Extra ossification site(s) on lumbar and/or sacral vertebrae[c]	60
Misaligned sternebrae	29
Frontals and parietals fused on lateral edges	16
Wavy rib	14
Enlarged nasal sinus(es)	7
Renal papillae ¼ normal size or less (right or bilateral)	5
No innominate artery	4
Incomplete ossification (parietals)	4
Red adrenal(s)	2
Clubbed limb (without bone change)	1
Globular heart	1
Kinked tail	1

[a] Vehicle is distilled water or corn oil, po. A single fetus may be represented more than once in listing individual defects. Defects are listed in order of frequency (high to low) for both vehicles combined.

Total fetuses examined, 3946; only live fetuses were examined for malformations.

Total litters examined, 310; includes only litters with live fetuses.

[b] Skeletal observations are from alizarin-stained specimens.

[c] Initial stage of ossification of the transverse process(es) of the vertebra(e).

and Japan have had requirements or recommendations for behavioral teratology testing since 1975. Such testing has not been routinely required by regulatory agencies in the United States, but studies are beginning to be required when indicated by other data (U.S. EPA, 1986b, 1988). Several comprehensive testing strategies have been proposed for behavioral evaluation (Spyker, 1975; Grant, 1976; Kimmel, 1977; Vorhees *et al.*, 1979). Recently, a standardized testing battery was evaluated for its reliability within and among laboratories (Buelke-Sam *et al.*, 1985). Results of this study showed that data from behavioral tests are extremely reliable if testing procedures are standardized and carefully controlled (Kimmel *et al.*, 1985a). Most behavioral testing batteries used have included a variety of physical developmental landmarks and tests of reflex development during the early postnatal period; evaluation of spontaneous motor activity, learning, and memory and tests of vision and audition are included. The U.S. EPA Office of Toxic Substances (U.S. EPA, 1988) has developed a guideline for developmental neurotoxicity testing that includes some evaluation of all these functions, as well as requirements for brain weights and neuropathology. A variety of other functional systems have been evaluated, including the cardiovascular, urinary, digestive, pulmonary, immune, reproductive, and endocrine

Table III

Historical Data Summary of Measures for CD-1 Mice Treated with Vehicle on Gestational Days 6 through 15[a,b]

				Range		95% confidence interval	
	N	Mean	SEM	(min.)	(max.)	(lower)	(upper)
Maternal body weight (gd 0)[c]	217	29.4	0.2	23.7	36.6	29.1	29.7
Maternal body weight (gd 6)	217	32.5	0.2	25.4	40.2	32.2	32.9
Maternal body weight (gd 11)	216	36.8	0.2	29.5	44.5	36.3	37.2
Maternal body weight (gd 15)	217	44.9	0.3	28.1	55.8	44.3	45.5
Maternal body weight (at sacrifice)	217	50.6	0.4	27.6	65.6	49.9	51.4
Maternal weight gain (gestation)	217	21.2	0.3	0.1	36.2	20.6	21.8
Maternal weight gain (treatment)	217	12.4	0.2	−2.3	20.2	12.0	12.8
Maternal weight gain (corrected)[d]	215	5.2	0.1	−2.1	13.1	4.9	5.5
Gravid uterine weight	215	16.0	0.3	0.2	25.0	15.5	16.6
Liver weight	217	2.61	0.02	1.65	3.25	2.57	2.65
Relative liver weight (% body weight)	217	5.18	0.03	3.84	6.83	5.12	5.25
Corpora lutea per dam	73	12.51	0.26	8.00	18.00	11.99	13.02
Implantation sites per dam	217	12.62	0.17	4.00	18.00	12.29	12.96
Preimplantation loss per dam (%)	73	5.28	1.19	0.00	64.29	2.90	7.65
Resorptions per litter	217	1.36	0.13	0.00	13.00	1.10	1.62
Resorptions per litter (%)	217	11.14	1.15	0.00	100.00	8.87	13.41
Late fetal deaths per litter	217	0.13	0.03	0.00	2.00	0.08	0.18
Late fetal deaths per litter (%)	217	1.03	0.20	0.00	16.67	0.63	1.43
Nonlive implants per litter	217	1.49	0.13	0.00	13.00	1.23	1.75

Nonlive implants per litter (%)	217	12.17	1.15	0.00	100.00	9.90	14.44
Affected implants per litter	217	1.60	0.13	0.00	13.00	1.34	1.87
Affected implants per litter (%)	217	13.12	1.16	0.00	100.00	10.84	15.40
Live fetuses per litter[e]	214	11.29	0.19	3.00	17.00	10.92	11.66
Male fetuses per litter[e] (%)	214	49.69	1.05	15.39	87.50	47.62	51.75
Average fetal body weight per litter[e]	214	0.974	0.006	0.657	1.280	0.961	0.987
Average female fetal body weight per litter[e]	214	0.956	0.007	0.628	1.280	0.942	0.969
Average male fetal body weight per litter[e]	214	0.991	0.007	0.680	1.280	0.977	1.004
Malformed fetuses per litter[e]	214	0.12	0.02	0.00	2.00	0.07	0.16
Malformed fetuses per litter[e] (%)	214	1.09	0.23	0.00	20.00	0.63	1.54
Malformed female fetuses per litter[e]	214	0.07	0.02	0.00	1.00	0.04	0.11
Malformed female fetuses per litter[e] (%)	214	1.12	0.29	0.00	25.00	0.54	1.69
Malformed male fetuses per litter[e]	214	0.05	0.01	0.00	1.00	0.02	0.08
Malformed male fetuses per litter[e] (%)	214	0.98	0.32	0.00	33.33	0.34	1.62

[a] Vehicle is distilled water or corn oil, po.

[b] Pregnancy rate, 87%; ratio of confirmed-pregnant dams at sacrifice to the total number of females mated × 100. The mating procedure involved "priming" (see text), pairing 1 female with 1 male overnight and checking for copulation plugs in the vagina the next morning (day 0 of gestation).

Total number of confirmed pregnant dams, 217.

Litters with live fetuses, 214; total number of live fetuses, 2416.

Litters with one or more resorptions, 121 (56%).

Litters with one or more late fetal deaths, 26 (12%); late fetal deaths include fetuses weighing > 0.3 g, discernible digits present, no vital signs at sacrifice.

Litters with one or more nonlive implants, 132 (61%); nonlive implants include late fetal deaths and resorbed implants.

Litters with one or more malformed fetuses, 23 (11%).

Litters with one or more affected implants, 142 (65%); affected implants include nonlive implants and malformed live fetuses.

[c] All weights expressed in grams; gd, gestation day.

[d] Maternal weight gain during gestation corrected for gravid uterine weight.

[e] Includes only litters with live fetuses.

Table IV
Historical Data Summary of Malformations or Variations in CD-1 Mice
Following Administration of Vehicle on Gestational Days 6 through 15[a]

External malformations	
No. (%) fetuses with one or more external malformations	4 (0.17)
No. (%) litters	4 (1.87)
Exencephaly	2
Cleft palate	1
Open eye (left)	1
Visceral malformations	
No. (%) fetuses with one or more visceral malformations	9 (0.37)
No. (%) litters	8 (3.74)
Abnormally large organ[b]	5
Displaced stomach	1
Extra vessel	1
Hydroureter (bilateral)	1
Left common carotid arises from innominate artery	1
Renal agenesis (right)	1
Agenesis of the ureters (bilateral)	1
Right-sided aorta	1
Skeletal malformations[c]	
No. (%) fetuses with one or more skeletal malformations	13 (0.54)
No. (%) litters	13 (6.07)
Fused sternebrae	4
Missing rib	4
Ribs fused to each other	2
Short rib	2
Abnormal skull fusion (frontals, parietals)	1
Fused thoracic arches	1
Thoracic centra off center	1
Variations	
No. (%) fetuses with one or more variations	233 (9.65)
No. (%) litters	101 (47.20)
Misaligned sternebrae	177
Hematoma (any location)	25
Frontals and parietals fused on lateral edges	18
Incomplete ossification[d]	5
White spots in ventricle (left)	4
Blood in amniotic sac (live fetuses only)	2
Cream colored liver lobe(s)	1
Distended ureter(s)	1
Extra ossification site between sternebrae	1
Left eye dark externally (blood internally)	1
Enlarged papillary muscle	1
Wavy rib	1

[a] Vehicle is distilled water or corn oil, po. A single fetus may be represented more than once in listing individual defects. Defects are listed in order of frequency (high to low) for both vehicles combined.

Total fetuses examined, 2415; only live fetuses were examined for malformations.

Total litters examined, 214; includes only litters with live fetuses.

[b] Enlarged organs include a kidney, a uterine horn, two epididymides, and an auricular flap.

[c] Skeletal observations are from alizarin-stained specimens.

[d] Includes frontals, parietals, ischium, pubis, thoracic centra, and lumbar and sacral arches.

Table V

Historical Data Summary of Measures for New Zealand White Rabbits Treated with Vehicle on Gestational Days 6 through 19[a,b]

	N	Mean	SEM	Range (min.)	Range (max.)	95% confidence interval (lower)	95% confidence interval (upper)
Maternal body weight (gd 0)[c]	77	4014.4	44.0	3050.0	4940.0	3926.7	4102.1
Maternal body weight (gd 6)	77	4158.2	49.0	3170.0	5220.0	4060.5	4255.9
Maternal body weight (gd 12)	77	4194.7	49.7	3180.0	5270.0	4095.8	4293.6
Maternal body weight (gd 19)	77	4240.6	48.0	3280.0	5110.0	4145.1	4336.2
Maternal body weight (at sacrifice)	77	4260.8	49.0	3230.0	5200.0	4163.1	4358.5
Maternal weight gain (gestation)	77	246.4	32.7	−230.0	900.0	181.1	311.6
Maternal weight gain (treatment)	77	82.5	22.9	−450.0	510.0	36.8	128.2
Maternal weight gain (corrected)[d]	77	−221.5	34.5	−781.7	639.4	−290.1	−152.8
Gravid uterine weight	77	467.8	17.0	26.3	805.6	434.0	501.6
Liver weight	76	110.0	2.6	70.6	187.2	104.7	115.2
Relative liver weight (% body weight)	76	2.58	0.05	1.82	3.74	2.48	2.67
Corpora lutea per dam	49	11.02	0.38	6.00	18.00	10.25	11.79
Implantation sites per dam	77	7.88	0.33	1.00	14.00	7.23	8.53
Preimplantation loss per dam (%)	49	25.98	3.66	0.00	94.44	18.62	33.34
Resorptions per litter	77	0.89	0.14	0.00	6.00	0.61	1.18
Resorptions per litter (%)	77	12.30	2.20	0.00	100.00	7.92	16.68
Late fetal deaths per litter	77	0.13	0.04	0.00	2.00	0.05	0.22
Late fetal deaths per litter (%)	77	1.30	0.44	0.00	22.22	0.42	2.17
Nonlive implants per litter	77	1.03	0.15	0.00	6.00	0.73	1.32
Nonlive implants per litter (%)	77	13.60	2.22	0.00	100.00	9.18	18.02
Affected implants per litter	77	1.47	0.17	0.00	6.00	1.13	1.81
Affected implants per litter (%)	77	19.08	2.36	0.00	100.00	14.38	23.78

(*continues*)

Table V (*continued*)

	N	Mean	SEM	Range (min.)	Range (max.)	95% confidence interval (lower)	95% confidence interval (upper)
Live fetuses per litter[e]	76	6.95	0.31	1.00	13.00	6.34	7.56
Male fetuses per litter[e] (%)	76	47.56	2.55	0.00	100.00	42.49	52.63
Average fetal body weight per litter[e]	76	46.57	0.92	26.70	64.99	44.74	48.40
Average female fetal body weight per litter[e]	72	45.55	0.93	24.09	62.00	43.70	47.40
Average male fetal body weight per litter[e]	73	46.82	0.97	29.60	65.70	44.90	48.75
Malformed fetuses per litter[e]	76	0.45	0.09	0.00	4.00	0.28	0.62
Malformed fetuses per litter[e] (%)	76	6.64	1.27	0.00	50.00	4.11	9.17
Malformed female fetuses per litter[e]	72	0.15	0.04	0.00	1.00	0.07	0.24
Malformed female fetuses per litter[e] (%)	72	5.11	1.79	0.00	100.00	1.54	8.67
Malformed male fetuses per litter[e]	73	0.32	0.08	0.00	4.00	0.16	0.48
Malformed male fetuses per litter[e] (%)	73	8.66	2.22	0.00	100.00	4.24	13.08

[a] Vehicle is distilled water or corn oil, po.

[b] Pregnancy rate, 90%; ratio of confirmed-pregnant dams at sacrifice to the total number of mated females × 100. The mating procedure involved induction of ovulation by pituitary luteinizing hormone and artificial insemination on day 0 of gestation (see text).

Total number of confirmed-pregnant dams, 77.

Litters with live fetuses, 76; total number of live fetuses, 528.

Litters with one or more resorptions, 37 (48%).

Litters with one or more late fetal deaths, 9 (12%); late fetal deaths include fetuses weighing > 10.0 g, discernible digits present, no vital signs at sacrifice.

Litters with one or more nonlive implants, 41 (53%); nonlive implants include late fetal deaths and resorbed implants.

Litters with one or more malformed live fetuses, 26 (34%).

Litters with one or more affected implants, 53 (69%); affected implants include nonlive implants and malformed live fetuses.

[c] All weights expressed in grams; gd, gestation day.

[d] Maternal weight gain during gestation corrected for gravid uterine weight.

[e] Includes only litters with live fetuses.

Table VI

Historical Data Summary of Malformations and Variations in New Zealand White Rabbits Following Administration of Vehicle on Gestational Days 6 through 19[a]

External malformations	
No. (%) fetuses with one or more external malformations	4 (0.76)
No. (%) litters	4 (5.26)
Edema	1
Exophthalmia	1
Gastroschisis	1
Umbilical hernia	1
Visceral malformations	
No. (%) fetuses with one or more visceral malformations	16 (3.03)
No. (%) litters	12 (15.79)
Convoluted retina (bilateral)	4
Abnormal cardiac papillary muscle or muscles	2
Abnormal tissue growth	2
Hydrocephaly	2
Left common carotid arises from innominate artery	2
Abnormal tricuspid valve	1
Abnormal vessel(s)	1
Abnormally large organ	1
Abnormally small organ	1
Convoluted retina (right)	1
Interventricular septal defect	1
Reversed aorta	1
Skeletal malformations[b]	
No. (%) fetuses with one or more skeletal malformations	16 (3.03)
No. (%) litters	12 (15.79)
Fused sternebrae	8
Abnormal skull fusion	7
Thoracic centra off center	1
Variations	
No. (%) fetuses with one or more variations	28 (5.30)
No. (%) litters	20 (26.32)
Hematoma (head)	12
Clubbed limb (without bone change)	3
Globular heart	3
Hematoma (back)	2
Hematoma (lower limb)	2
White spot on kidney	2
Extra ossification site(s)	1
Frontals and parietals fused on lateral edges	1
Hematoma (face)	1
Incomplete ossification	1
Misaligned sternebrae	1
Right papilla ¼ normal size or less	1

[a] Vehicle is distilled water or corn oil, po. A single fetus may be represented more than once in listing individual defects. Defects are listed in order of frequency (high to low) for all dose groups combined.

Total fetuses examined, 528; only live fetuses were examined for malformations.

Total litters examined, 76; includes only litters with live fetuses.

[b] Skeletal observations are from alizarin-stained specimens.

systems (Kavlock and Grabowoski, 1983). However, there have been few standard approaches developed because the methodologies necessary are usually very sophisticated and require highly skilled technical personnel.

VI. SHORT-TERM SCREENING SYSTEMS

Both *in vivo* and *in vitro* approaches have been proposed for the screening of chemicals for priority-setting purposes prior to further testing. Chernoff and Kavlock (1982) have reported on the use of an *in vivo* protocol in which pregnant mice were treated during organogenesis then allowed to deliver their young. The number of live pups, litter weight, survival to 3 days of age, and any obvious external defects were recorded. The assumption made was that any pups with major structural malformations would be noticeable postnatally or would die or be cannibalized by the mother, resulting in a reduced number of live pups. This protocol may be especially useful when a large number of chemicals must be screened and prioritized for more extensive testing or when the relative activity of structural analogs is of interest. The NTP has also used this protocol as part of the dose-finding studies preliminary to the standard segment II study, especially when there is the potential for conducting further evaluation of postnatal function (George *et al.*, 1986).

A number of *in vitro* test systems may also have usefulness as screening devices to set priorities for further testing (Wilson, 1978; Kimmel *et al.*, 1982; Johnson, 1984). These test systems provide alternatives to the use of intact pregnant mammals and include systems ranging from cell and organ cultures to whole organisms, such as mammalian embryos in culture. Several of these systems are undergoing validation testing, and a standard list of chemicals has been developed for this purpose (Smith *et al.*, 1983). Some systems allow the calculation of a ratio of adult to developmental toxicity (Johnson and Gabel, 1983), which may be useful in prioritizing chemicals for further testing. Because of the variety of cellular changes and interactions that must take place for normal embryological development to occur, an array of *in vitro* systems may be necessary for screening purposes in order to avoid false negatives and false positives.

Acknowledgment

This research was funded by NIEHS contract no. NO1-ES-6-2127, NCTR/NTP contract no. 222-80-2031(C), and NIEHS/NTP contract no. NO1-ES-55080 [formerly NCTR/NTP contract no. 222-83-2010(C)].

References

Abel, E. L., Bush, R., Dintcheff, B. A., and Ernst, C. A. S. (1981). Critical periods for marihuana-induced intrauterine growth retardation in the rat. *Neurobehav. Toxicol. Teratol.* **3**, 351–354.

Adams, J., and Buelke-Sam, J. (1981). Behavioral assessment of the postnatal animal: Testing and methods development. *In* "Developmental Toxicology" (C. A. Kimmel and J. Buelke-Sam, eds.), pp. 233–258. New York: Raven Press.

Aliverti, V., Bonanomi, E., Giavini, E., Leone, V. G., and Mariani, L. (1979). The extent of fetal ossification as an index of delayed development in teratogenic studies on the rat. *Teratology* **20**, 237–242.

Aliverti, V., Bonanomi, L., and Giavini, E. (1980). Hydroxyurea as a reference standard in teratological screening. Comparison of the embryotoxic and teratogenic effects following single intraperitoneal or repeated oral administration to pregnant rats. *Arch. Toxicol. Suppl.* **4**, 239–247.

Banerjee, B. N., and Durloo, R. S. (1973). Incidence of teratological anomalies in control Charles River CD-strain rats. *Toxicology* **1**, 151–154.

Blair, E. (1979). Hypothermia. *In* "Textbook of Veterinary Anesthesia" (L. Soma, ed.), pp. 555–579. Baltimore: Williams and Wilkins.

Bredderman, P. J., Foote, R. H., and Yassen, A. M. (1964). An improved artificial vagina for collecting rabbit semen. *J. Reprod. Fertil.* **7**, 401–403.

Buelke-Sam, J., Kimmel, C. A., Adams, J., Nelson, C. J., Vorhees, C. V., Wright, D. C., St. Omer, V., Korol, B. A., Butcher, R. E., Geyer, M. A., Holson, J. F., Kutscher, C. L., and Wayner, M. J. (1985). Collaborative behavioral teratology study: Results. *Neurobehav. Toxicol. Teratol.* **7**, 591–624.

Charles River Laboratories (1988). "Embryo and Fetal Developmental Toxicity (Teratology) Control Data in the Charles River Crl:CD° BR Rat". Wilmington, Massachusetts: Charles River Laboratories.

Chernoff, N., and Kavlock, R. J. (1982). An *in vivo* teratology screen utilizing pregnant mice. *J. Toxicol. Environ. Health* **10**, 541–550.

Chitlik, L. D., Bui, Q. Q., Burin, G. J., and Dapson, S. C. (1985). "Hazard Evaluation Division, Standard Evaluation Procedure, Teratology Studies" (Report 540/9-85-018). Washington, DC: U.S. Environmental Protection Agency, Office of Pesticide Programs.

Crary, D. D. (1962). Modified benzyl alcohol clearing of alizarin-stained specimens without loss of flexibility. *Stain Technol.* **37**, 124–125.

Drill, V. A., and Lazar, P., eds. (1983). "Cutaneous Toxicity." New York: Raven Press.

Fabro, S., Shull, G., and Brown, N. A. (1982). The relative teratogenic index and teratogenic potency: Proposed components of developmental toxicity risk assessment. *Teratogen. Carcinogen. Mutagen.* **2**, 61–76.

Fritz, H., and Hess, R. (1970). Ossification of the rat and mouse skeleton in the perinatal period. *Teratology* **20**, 237–242.

Gad, S. C., and Weil, C. S. (1986). Data analysis applications in toxicology. *In* "Statistics and Experimental Design for Toxicologists" (S. C. Gad and C. S. Weil, eds.), pp. 147–175. Caldwell, New Jersey: The Telford Press.

Gaylor, D. W. (1978). Methods and concepts of biometrics applied to teratology. *In* "Handbook of Teratology" (J. G. Wilson and F. C. Fraser, eds.), Vol. **4**, pp. 429–444. New York: Plenum Press.

George, J. D., Price, C. J., Marr, M. C., and Kimmel, C. A. (1986). "Teratologic evaluation of α-methyldopa (MD) (CAS No. 555-30-6) administered to CD rats on gestational days 6 through 20. Final Study Report for NCTR/NTP Contract No. 222-83-2010(C)" (National Technical Information Service Accession No. PB86-245321/AS). Research Triangle Park, North Carolina: Research Triangle Institute.

George, J. D., Price, C. J., Marr, M. C., Morrissey, R. E., and Schwetz, B. A. (1988). "Teratologic evaluation of corn oil or distilled water administered to CD-1 mice on gestational days 6 through 15. Final Study Report for NTP/NIEHS Contract No. NO1-ES-55080." Research Triangle Park, North Carolina: Research Triangle Institute.

Grant, L. D. (1976). Research strategies for behavioral teratology studies. *Environ. Health Perspect.* **18,** 85–94.

Hafez, E. S. E., ed. (1970). "Reproductive and Breeding Techniques for Laboratory Animals." Philadelphia: Lea and Febiger.

Hamm, T. E., ed. (1986). "Complications of Viral and Mycoplasma Infections in Rodents to Toxicology Testing." New York: Hemisphere.

Haseman, J. K., and Kupper, L. L. (1979). Analysis of dichotomous response data for certain toxicological experiments. *Biometrics* **35,** 281–293.

Haseman, J. K., Huff, J., and Boorman, G. A. (1984). Use of historical control data in carcinogenicity studies in rodents. *Toxicol. Pathol.* **12,** 126–135.

Jameson, C. W., and Walters, D. B., eds. (1984). "Chemistry for Toxicity Testing." Stoneham, Massachusetts: Butterworth.

Johnson, E. M., (1984). A prioritization and biological decision tree for developmental toxicity safety evaluations. *J. Am. Coll. Toxicol.* **3,** 141–147.

Johnson, E. M., and Gabel, B. E. G. (1983). An artificial embryo for detection of abnormal developmental biology. *Fund. Appl. Toxicol.* **3,** 243–249.

Kavlock, R. J., and Grabowski, C. T., eds. (1983). "Abnormal Functional Development of Heart, Lungs and Kidneys: Approaches to Functional Teratology." New York: Alan R. Liss.

Kimmel, C. A. (1977). Final Report of the Committee on Postnatal Evaluation of Animals Subjected to Insult During Development. Report available from Chairperson, U. S. Environmental Protection Agency (RD-689), Washington, DC 20460.

Kimmel, C. A., and Francis, E. Z. (1990). Proceedings of the workshop on the acceptibility and interpretation of dermal developmental toxicity studies. *Fund. Appl. Toxicol.,* in press.

Kimmel, C. A., and Trammell, C. (1981). A rapid procedure for routine double staining of cartilage and bone in fetal and adult animals. *Stain Technol.* **56,** 271–273.

Kimmel, C. A., Buelke-Sam, J., and Adams, J. (1985a). Collaborative behavioral teratology study: Implications, current applications and future directions. *Neurobehav. Toxicol. Teratol.* **7,** 669–673.

Kimmel, C. A., Price, C. J., Sadler, B. W., Tyl, R. W., and Gerling, F. S. (1985b). Comparison of distilled water (DW) and corn oil (CO) vehicle controls from historical teratology study data. *Toxicologist* **5,** 185.

Kimmel, G. L., Kimmel, C. A., and Francis, E. Z. (1987). Evaluation of maternal and developmental toxicity. *Teratog. Carcinog. Mutagen.* **7,** 203–338.

Kimmel, G. L., Smith, K., Kochhar, D. M., and Pratt, R. M. (1982). Overview of *in vitro* teratogenicity testing: Aspects of validation and application to screening. *Teratog. Carcinog. Mutagen.* **2,** 221–229.

Lumb, W. V., and Jones, E. W. (1973). "Veterinary Anesthesia," p. 452. Philadelphia: Lea and Febiger.

Marks, T. A. (1985). Animal tests employed to assess the effects of drugs and chemicals on reproduction. In "Male Fertility and Its Regulation" (T. J. Lobl and E. S. E. Hafez, eds.), pp. 245–267. Lancaster, England: MTP Press.

Marr, M. C., Myers, C. B., George, J. D., and Price, C. J. (1988). Comparison of single and double staining for evaluation of skeletal development: The effects of ethylene glycol (EG) in CD rats. Teratology 37, 476.

Morita, H., Ariyuki, F., Inomata, N., Nishimura, K., Hasegawa, Y., Miyamoto, M., and Watanabe, T. (1987). Spontaneous malformations in laboratory animals: Frequency of external, internal and skeletal malformations in rats, rabbits and mice. Cong. Anom. 27, 147–206.

National Institutes of Health (1985). "Guide for the Care and Use of Laboratory Animals" (NIH Publ. No. 86-23) Washington, DC: U.S. Department of Health and Human Services, Public Health Service.

Palmer, A. K. (1971). Sporadic malformations in laboratory animals and their influence on drug testing. In "Drugs and Fetal Development." (M. A. Klingberg, A. Abramovici, and J. Chemke, eds.), pp. 45–60. New York: Plenum Press.

Palmer, A. K. (1981). Regulatory requirements for reproductive toxicology: Theory and practice. In "Developmental Toxicology" (C. A. Kimmel and J. Buelke-Sam, eds.), pp. 259–287. New York: Raven Press.

Peltzer, M. A., and Schardein, J. L. (1966). A convenient method for processing fetuses for skeletal staining. Stain Technol. 41, 300–302.

Perraud, J. (1976). Levels of spontaneous malformations in the CD rat and the CD-1 mouse. Lab. Anim. Sci. 26, 293–300.

Phalen, R. F. (1984). "Inhalation Studies: Foundations and Techniques." Boca Raton, Florida: CRC Press.

Price, C. J., Tyl, R. W., Marr, M. C., and Kimmel, C. A. (1984a). "Teratologic evaluation of ethylene glycol (CAS No. 107-21-1) administered to CD-1 mice on gestational days 6 through 15. Final Study Report for NCTR/NTP Contract No. 222-80-2031(C)" (No. PB85-105385/GAR). Springfield, Virginia: National Technical Information Service.

Price, C. J., Tyl, R. W., Marr, M. C., and Kimmel, C. A. (1984b). "Teratologic evaluation of ethylene glycol (CAS No. 10/-21-1) administered to CD-1 mice on gestational days 6 through 15. Final Study Report No. NCTR/NTP Contract No. 222-80-2031(C)" (No. PB85-105385/GAR). Springfield, Virginia: National Technical Information Service.

Price, C. J., George, J. D., Marr, M. C., Morrissey, R. E., and Schwetz, B. A. (1988). "Teratologic evaluation of corn oil or distilled water administered to CD rats on gestational days 6 through 15. Final Study Report for NTP/NIEHS Contract NO1-ES-55080." Research Triangle Park, North Carolina: Research Triangle Institute.

Rodier, P. (1978). Postnatal functional evaluations. In "Handbook of Teratology" (J. G. Wilson and F. C. Fraser, eds.), Vol. 4, pp. 397–428. New York: Plenum Press.

SAS Institute (1985a). "SAS User's Guide: Basics," 5th Ed. Cary, North Carolina: SAS Institute.

SAS Institute (1985b). "SAS User's Guide: Statistics," 5th Ed. Cary, North Carolina: SAS Institute.

Schwetz, B. A., Nitschke, K. D., and Staples, R. E. (1977). Cleft palates in CF-1 mice after deprivation of water during pregnancy. Toxicol. Appl. Pharmacol. 40, 307–315.

Siegel, S. (1956). "Nonparametric Statistics for the Behavioral Sciences." New York: McGraw-Hill.

Smith, M. K., Kimmel, G. L., Kochhar, D. M., Shepard, T. H., Spielberg, S. P., and Wilson, J. G. (1983). A selection of candidate compounds for *in vitro* teratogenesis test validation. *Teratog. Carcinog. Mutagen.* **3**, 461–480.

Snedecor, G. W., and Cochran, W. G. (1967). "Statistical Methods," 6th Ed. Ames: Iowa State University Press.

Spyker, J. (1975). Behavioral teratology and toxicology. *In* "Behavioral Toxicology" (B. Weiss and V. G. Laties, eds.), pp. 311–349. New York: Plenum Press.

Stadler, J., Kessedjian, M.-J., and Perraud, J. (1983). Use of the New Zealand White rabbit in teratology: Incidence of spontaneous and drug-induced malformations. *Food Chem. Toxicol.* **21**, 631–636.

Staples, R. E. (1974). Detection of visceral alterations in mammalian fetuses. *Teratology* **9**, A37.

Stuckhardt, J. L., and Poppe, S. M. (1984). Fresh visceral examination of rat and rabbit fetuses used in teratogenicity testing. *Teratog. Carcinog. Mutagen.* **4**, 181–188.

Taylor, P. (1986). "Practical Teratology." New York: Academic Press.

U.S. Department of Agriculture (1970). Animal Welfare Act, Public Law 89-544, Section 6. Washington, DC: U.S. Department of Agriculture.

U.S. Department of Agriculture (1987). Animal welfare: Proposed rules. *Fed. Regist.* **52 (61)**, 10295–10322.

U.S. Environmental Protection Agency (1982). "Pesticides Assessment Guidelines. Subdivision F. Hazard Evaluation: Human and Domestic Animals" (EPA-450/98-2-025). Springfield, Virginia: National Technical Information Service.

U.S. Environmental Protection Agency (1985). Toxic substances control act test guidelines. Final rules. *Fed. Regist.* **50 (188)**, 39252–39516.

U.S. Environmental Protection Agency (1986a). Guidelines for the health assessment of suspect developmental toxicants. *Fed. Regist.* **51**, 34028–34040.

U.S. Environmental Protection Agency (1986b). Triethylene glycol monomethyl, monoethyl, and monobutyl ethers; Proposed test rule. *Fed. Regist.* **51**, 17883–17894.

U.S. Environmental Protection Agency (1988). Diethylene glycol butyl ether and diethylene glycol butyl ether acetate; Final test rule. *Fed. Regist.* **53**, 5932–5953.

U.S. Environmental Protection Agency (1989). Proposed amendments to the guidelines for the health assessment of suspect developmental toxicants; request for comments; notice. *Fed. Regist.* **54**, 9386–9403.

U.S. Food and Drug Administration (1966). "Guidelines for Reproduction and Teratology Testing of Drugs." Washington, DC: Food and Drug Administration.

U.S. Food and Drug Administration (1970). Advisory committee on protocols for safety evaluations. Panel on reproduction report on reproduction studies in the safety evaluation of food additives and pesticide residues. *Toxicol. Appl. Pharmacol.* **16**, 264–296.

U.S. Food and Drug Administration (1978). Good laboratory practice regulations for nonclinical laboratory studies. *Fed. Regist.* **43(247)**, 59985–60025.

Vorhees, C. V., and Butcher, R. E. (1982). Behavioral teratogenicity. *In* "Developmental Toxicology" (K. Snell, ed.), pp. 247–298. London: Croom-Helm Press.

Vorhees, C. V., Butcher, R. E., Brunner, R. L., and Sobotka, T. J. (1979). A developmental test battery for neurobehavioral toxicity in rats: A preliminary analysis using monosodium glutamate, calcium carrageenan and hydroxyurea. *Toxicol. Appl. Pharmacol.* **50,** 267–282.

Walker, D. G., and Wirtschafter, Z. T. (1957). "The Genesis of the Rat Skeleton. A Laboratory Atlas." Springfield, Illinois: Thomas.

Walters, D. B., and Jameson, C. W., eds. (1984). "Health and Safety for Toxicity Testing." Stoneham, Massachusetts: Butterworth.

Warkany, J. (1971). "Congenital Malformations, Notes and Comments." Chicago: Year Book Medical.

Weil, C. S. (1970). Selection of the valid number of sampling units and a consideration of their combination in toxicological studies involving reproduction, teratogenesis, and carcinogenesis. *Food Cosmet. Toxicol.* **8,** 177–182.

Whitten, A. K. (1956). Modification of the estrous cycle of the mouse by external stimuli associated with the male. *J. Endocrinol.* **13,** 399–404.

Williams, D. A. (1971). A test for differences between treatment means when several dose levels are compared with a zero dose control. *Biometrics* **27,** 103–117.

Williams, D. A. (1972). The comparison of several dose levels with a zero dose control. *Biometrics* **28,** 519–531.

Wilson, J. G. (1965). Embryological considerations in teratology. *In* "Teratology: Principles and Techniques" (J. G. Wilson and J. Warkany, eds.), pp. 215–277. Chicago: University of Chicago Press.

Wilson, J. G. (1978). Survey of *in vitro* systems: Their potential use in teratogenicity screening. *In* "Handbook of Teratology" (J. G. Wilson and F. C. Fraser, eds.), Vol. **4,** pp. 135–153. New York: Plenum Press.

Wirtschafter, Z. T. (1960). "The Genesis of the Mouse Skeleton. A Laboratory Atlas." Springfield, Illinois: Thomas.

Woo, D. C., and Hoar, R. M. (1972). "Apparent hydronephrosis" as a normal aspect of renal development in late gestation of rats: The effect of methyl salicylate. *Teratology* **6,** 191–196.

13

Pharmacokinetics: Principles, Mechanisms, and Methods

James R. Withey
Bureau of Chemical Hazards
Environmental Health Directorate
Health and Welfare Canada
Ottawa, Ontario

I. Introduction

II. Animal Models

III. Routes of Administration
   A. The Inhalation Route
   B. The Gastrointestinal Route

IV. Organ Kinetics

V. Pharmacokinetic Parameters
   A. Absorption or Uptake by the Gastrointestinal Route
   B. Uptake by the Pulmonary Route
   C. Distribution
   D. Metabolism
   E. Elimination

VI. Summary

I. INTRODUCTION

The unfolding role of toxicology as a quantitative science has led to the study of biological rate processes in an attempt to understand the complex mechanisms that accompany the administration of a xenobiotic substance to an *in vivo* biological system. Such an approach has spawned an increased interest in the subject of pharmacokinetics, as demonstrated by a number of recent books, articles, and reviews (Piotrowski, J., 1971; Wagner, J. G., 1971; Gibaldi and Perrier, 1975; Gehring *et al.*, 1976; Food Safety Council, 1978; Gehring and Young, 1978; Withey 1978; Gladtke and von Hattingberg, 1979; O'Flaherty, 1981). The semiempirical approach in toxicological testing, in which an arbitrary number of animals is dosed with or exposed to toxic substances, has also yielded to the increasing demands of biostatisticians for adequate controls, sufficient numbers of animals, and suitable numbers of dose groups (Feinstein, 1970a,b). Experimental design is now, therefore, receiving careful attention prior to the initiation of chronic toxicity testing; pharmacokinetic studies must be considered as an indispensable tool in evaluating the absorption, distribution, metabolism, and elimination of xenobiotic compounds. Information on the kinetics of these processes often allows for the rational calculation of such experimental design parameters as the interval between doses to achieve steady state blood levels (Wagner, 1971) or the prediction as to whether there will be an accumulation of the test compound in tissues (Dittert, 1977). Pharmacokinetics has also proved its usefulness in the interpretation of toxicity tests (Hammer and Bozler, 1977; Gehring, 1978) and in the interspecies extrapolation of data (Gillette, 1976; Reitz et al., 1978).

One of the important principles of the kinetic method is the description (with maximum simplification) of complex phenomena that occur in vivo by means of mathematical equations derived from biological systems that are conceived of as one or two components. Specific models are required for intravenous, intragastric, and pulmonary routes of administration. Although these simplifications allow a precise analysis of the data generated in pharmacokinetic studies, it should be remembered that they can seldom be related to the numerous simultaneous and consecutive processes that actually occur in the biological model (Withey, 1978). Many refinements to interpret specific data have been suggested, including the development of multicompartment models (Gibaldi and Perrier, 1975). Such treatments, although justifiable for specific cases, tend to intimidate the novice and require repeated demonstration of their relevance. To paraphrase Professor P. G. H. Gell, "One must be careful not to allow the sacred cow of mathematics to impede the flow of traffic" (Feinstein, 1970a).

An alternative approach, developed largely as a consequence of a need to interpret quantitative aspects of inhalation anesthesia, is to consider the body as a system of interlinked physiological compartments. These compartments are usually depicted as a series of parallel shunts connected by the systemic circulation (Fiserova-Bergerova, 1983). In variations of the physiological model, other groupings of organs and tissues should be considered or physiological processes, like metabolism, should be included as separate components (Himmelstein and Lutz, 1979; National Academy of Sciences, 1980).

Although the application of pharmacokinetics to toxicology and therapeutics is a fairly recent innovation, its origins date from more than 60 years ago when Widmark was the first to monitor blood levels after the administration of a single dose (Widmark, 1919). He was also the first to apply mathematical equations to describe the kinetics of accumulation after repeated dosing (Widmark and Tandberg, 1924). The useful parameter now known as the apparent volume of distribution was first determined in 1934 (Dominguez and Pomerene, 1934). Other milestones in the application of pharmacokinetic principles were the demonstration of a blood level–time curve that exhibited multiexponential behavior (Hemingway et al., 1935) and the use of pharmacokinetic parameters derived from a single dose to predict blood levels after multiple dosing (Boxer et al., 1948).

Nearly a century before these ventures, there were a few individuals who were keenly interested in pharmacokinetic principles and parameters. Dr. John Snow, vice president of the Westminster Medical Society, performed some remarkable experiments for that time on the pharmacodynamics of what we today call anesthetics, but he termed indifferent narcotics. Snow (1848; 1850) examined the narcotism of inhaled vapors and discovered that "the strength of narcotic vapours was in the inverse ratio of their solubility in the blood, for bromoform, bromide of ethyle and Dutch liquid". He also described the detection of ether in expired air after it had been inhaled and of alcohol in expired air "after it had been taken into the stomach".

In this chapter, the pharmacokinetic behavior of compounds after administration by intravenous (IV), intragastric (IG), and pulmonary or inhalation routes is discussed. The four principal rate processes of absorption, distribution, metabolism, and elimination and the factors that affect them are then considered. The blood is an accessible body fluid usually involved as the vehicle that conveys the administered dose to the target organs and sites; therefore, the blood is a major part of the central pharmacokinetic compartment. The majority of pharmacokinetic models developed utilize data generated by analysis of blood concentrations of the administered compound at selected time intervals following dosing. It is appropriate at this stage to consider the techniques available for blood sampling and the surgical preparation of animal models for pharmacokinetic investigations.

II. ANIMAL MODELS

There have been a number of communications that have described the surgical preparation of indwelling arterial or intravenous cannula in large and small animal models. These allow the sequential sampling of blood from a treated animal without undue stress (Van Petten et al., 1970;

Huddleston, J., 1978). Because the rat is used in the bulk of toxicological investigations, the principal steps in the cannulation of the laboratory rat are described in some detail in this section. This procedure is simple and the technique can be acquired with relatively little training, although some experience is necessary to provide an animal model that will retain a patent cannula for a period of a week or more. Up to 20 such animals can be produced per day by a competent and experienced laboratory animal technologist equipped with the proper facilities.

The initial preparation of an anesthetized rat involves shaving the skin proximate to the jugular vein. An area is similarly prepared on the dorsal surface between the scapulae. It is from this latter region that the cannula is exteriorized so as to allow facile accessibility and to inhibit animal interference with paw or mouth.

The primary incision is made after the pulse of the jugular vein is located and a portion of the right facial branch elevated. A silastic cannula of 0.030 inches (inner diameter) and 0.065 inches (outer diameter) is prepared with a chamfered end to facilitate insertion into the elevated vessel. The cannula is inserted so that the tip ultimately rests in or near the right atrium of the heart. Both ends of the exposed branch of the vein are tied off to prevent blood loss, and the cannula is held in place with a small drop of silicone adhesive on its external surface. The adhesive forms a bead at a point where the cannula rests just inside the vessel and is secured by the tie. The jugular and dorsal incisions are closed with wound clips after the proximal end of the cannula has been threaded subcutaneously to emerge between the scapulae.

This type of cannulation procedure remains viable for at least one week, provided that the cannula is flushed daily with 100 units/ml of heparinized saline. Up to thirty 0.1 ml samples of blood can be sampled from a 400 g rat over a period of a few hours to a few days postdosing without serious detriment or stress to the animal. Because the barbiturate or halogenated hydrocarbon anesthetics used in the surgical procedures perturb the usual metabolic function, animals should be given at least 48 hr after surgery to recover. In our experience, traces of halothane anesthetic can be found in the perirenal fat depots of rats or miniature swine up to 48 hr after surgery is performed.

Animals that have been surgically prepared in this way should be housed in separate cages to prevent attrition of the cannula due to aggressive interanimal grooming. Larger animals, like pigs, appear to be somewhat irritated by the short length of exteriorized cannula tubing and its plug to the extent that they will interact with the inner surface of their cage in an attempt to disrupt the surgical implant. Cages with a smooth interior surface and with externally located feed bins have been designed to inhibit this adverse activity (Withey et al., 1973).

Other methods have been proposed and used for the sequential sampling of blood (Grice, 1964). Among the more popular alternative techniques has been the "tail-clip" sampling method in which a small segment of the terminal end of the tail is severed, the cut end placed against the inside of a collecting tube, and blood "milked" from the tail with a downward motion and pressure of the hand over the tail. Great care must be taken to avoid squeezing serous fluid from the cellular tissues because this will effectively "dilute" the blood sample. In the rat, blood can also be obtained from the ventral caudal veins or artery and, in larger animals, from veins in the ear. These procedures are not difficult to perform but they usually perturb the animal somewhat, by inducing stress from handling. When these techniques are used with small animals, light anesthesia is usually administered in order to permit ready manipulation. Although this may be entirely satisfactory for obtaining samples for hematological examination, administration of an anesthetic, even in small doses, can interfere with many of the analytical methods used to determine the concentration of a test compound. The rate at which the test compound is metabolized may also be seriously affected by the effects of the anesthetic on metabolism and by the physiological parameters, such as heart rate and blood flow, which may be significantly altered by anesthesia.

Methods for obtaining blood from the orbital sinus in small animals have been described at length by Stone (1954) and Riley (1960). Restraint and careful manipulation are usually required for an unanesthetized animal. Although this method may be of occasional use for a few blood samples, it cannot be recommended for the multiple sampling necessary for good kinetic analyses.

The technique of cardiac puncture has been well described (Burhoe, 1940). Up to 4% of the body weight, as blood samples, has been withdrawn without serious effects (Farris and Griffith, 1949), although the degree of success with heart puncture is greatly enhanced by practice. Again, a serious liability of this technique is that animals should be anesthetized.

Urine can be collected with reasonable facility from animals and humans. Human subjects can be instructed to imbibe frequent and relatively large volumes of water and to follow precise procedures for the collection of urine at specific times postdosing (Van Petten et al., 1971). Animals are usually allowed water ad libitum, and their urine can be collected over a series of predetermined time intervals by means of an indwelling urethral catheter (Knipfel et al., 1975). Analysis of the sample to obtain the concentration of excreted xenobiotic, or sometimes its metabolites, includes calculations for the amounts excreted during the various time intervals. Wagner and his co-workers have developed models and solved the necessary equations for determining the rate coefficients for absorption, metabolism, and elimination of compounds from urinary excretion data (Wagner and Nelson, 1964; Wagner, 1967; Wagner, 1971). It should be remembered that measurements of excretion rates, especially when the urinary excretion of the xenobiotic *per se* is analyzed, may not concur with elimination rates measured from blood or plasma monitoring because the latter will include rates of metabolism and distribution as well as excretion by other routes.

Volatile solvents and gases that are inhaled may be largely excreted via the lung (Von Oettingen, 1964). As much as 82% of vinyl chloride is excreted by this route. In numerous studies, the vapor phase concentration of the administered material in the expired air of humans and animals has been monitored by means of a suitable mask and two-way valve (Rowe *et al.*, 1963). In the case of clinical studies with humans, the expired air is directed into a flexible bag after a subject takes several deep breaths. The contents of the sealed gas-tight container are then analyzed to provide a direct analysis of alveolar air. The proportionality of the exhaled xenobiotic concentration in expired alveolar air to that in the arterial blood is related to the Ostwald solubility coefficient (Goldstein *et al.*, 1974), and decay curves may be obtained that allow for the derivation of pharmacokinetic elimination parameters. This technique has been used extensively in industrial hygiene and toxicological studies, principally in connection with human exposure to volatile aliphatic and halogenated hydrocarbons (Soule, 1978; Stewart and Dodd, 1964).

A closed system is also useful for the study of the pharmacokinetics of uptake and metabolism (Andersen, 1983). Essentially, animals are placed in a closed chamber (such as a large desiccator or battery jar) equipped with facilities for the removal of carbon dioxide and excess water together with the replenishment of oxygen. If the chamber atmosphere is monitored for the decline in concentration of the test compound and if this is corrected for the observed loss in the absence of animals, the kinetic parameters of uptake and metabolism can be readily obtained. With this methodology, the necessity of taking samples from animals is eliminated. The closed system has been successfully used to study the pharmacokinetics of, for example, halogenated ethylenes (Filser and Bolt, 1979) and vinyl chloride (Bolt *et al.*, 1977).

The amounts of an orally administered compound excreted in feces can be useful in determining the extent of gastrointestinal uptake, but care should be taken to assess or exclude the involvement of biliary excretion and enterohepatic recycling. These mechanisms are discussed later in this chapter. Determination of amounts excreted in feces is particularly useful in the case of xenobiotics that are sequestered into fat depots, or other storage compartments, and eliminated slowly via the bile. Care must be exercised in the collection of cage droppings because contamination with urine and cage bedding may confound the analysis. Coprophageal cups can be fitted to small animals to eliminate this problem (Ruddick *et al.*, 1979).

III. ROUTES OF ADMINISTRATION

Undoubtedly, the most accessible and most useful physiological compartment of a living animal for pharmacokinetic investigations is the blood. Although urine, feces, bile, expired air, and sweat are used to study excretion of an administered substance and its metabolites, the blood represents the dynamic vehicle for the transport of toxic compounds to sites of action throughout the body. In addition, the blood has been generally recognized as the major portion of the central compartment of the pharmacokinetic model. Prior to the investigation of any other specific routes of administration of a test substance, therefore, its pharmacokinetic behavior should be studied after a bolus dose is administered directly into the bloodstream. The dynamics of the test compound after IV administration, monitored by way of the analysis of sequential blood samples taken at frequent and selected times postdosing, will be independent of any complicating factors that may influence the compound's absorption and affect its uptake and any diffusion processes that may be involved in its transfer to the bloodstream.

The shape of the elimination curve, obtained from blood concentration against time plotted on semilogarithmic paper, will determine the appropriate pharmacokinetic model that best fits the data. The mathematical approach used to decide which model best fits the data is discussed in Chapter 14 and in some recent communications (Metzler, 1969; Pedersen, 1977; Wong *et al.*, 1979). Once the model has been established, the polyexponential equation that gives the blood concentration (C_t) at any time (t) is

$$C_t = Ae^{-\alpha t} + Be^{-\beta t} + Ce^{-\gamma t} + De^{-\delta t} \ldots , \qquad (1)$$

where α, β, γ, and δ are hybrid rate coefficients and A, B, C, D . . . are the preexponential coefficients obtained directly from the semilogarithmic plot. The sum of these coefficient equals the effective blood concentration at zero time. This equation is used in predicting the blood concentration at any time after the dose is administered and in assessing the cumulative effect of multiple doses (Gibaldi and Perrier, 1975; Wagner, 1971). It should be emphasized that the hybrid rate coefficients do not relate to any specific kinetic mechanism with the physiological or pharmacokinetic rate model. In the latter case they are a complex function of those rate coefficients that describe the transfer from one pharmacokinetic model compartment to another.

The coefficients of the individual rate processes that occur between the compartments of the pharmacokinetic model are determined in terms of the coefficients and indices in the polyexponential equation (1) for the simpler systems. These are not difficult to calculate provided the assumptions, which are necessarily made in the derivation, are met or controlled by the conditions of the experiment. An inspection of these rate coefficients can yield information on the mechanisms involved and on how a test compound is handled by the animal.

Several pharmacokinetic studies have been published in which a large number of animals have been administered the same dose by the same route then killed sequentially. Although this is, perhaps, the only way to obtain data on the kinetic disposition of test compounds in the major organs, serious misinterpretations of the pharmacokinetic mechanism and of the rate coefficients can arise as a consequence of this approach (Nelson, 1963). Nevertheless, some remarkably smooth kinetic plots for the elimination of styrene monomer from organs of the rat, following IV administration, have been obtained (Withey, 1978b).

A. The Inhalation Route

There are a number of excellent reviews on the special requirements for the toxicological assessment of inhaled gases and vapors (Fraser et al., 1959; MacFarland, 1970; Silver, 1946; Leach, 1963). The methodology and equipment for the proper conduct of inhalation studies are also considered elsewhere in this book. Such studies have yielded data that have been useful in assessing the performance of anesthetic gases and in determining threshold limit values (TLVs) in industrial toxicology (American Conference of Governmental and Industrial Hygienists, 1980). It is evident from many publications that there are many artifacts, for example, the absorption of the test substance on the skin and fur of an animal subjected to whole-body exposure and the consequent erratic uptake due to the animal's natural grooming habits, that can seriously perturb pharmacokinetic studies. We have found, provided a good steady state equilibrated concentration of the gas or vapor is maintained within the chamber, that good kinetics can be obtained from a "head-only" exposure of a surgically prepared animal with an indwelling cannula. The animal model must, necessarily, be restrained. A number of restraint devices that allow the sequential sampling of blood and head-only exposure have been adopted for this purpose.

Provided that the conditions within the chamber are maintained at equilibrium throughout the exposure, the uptake, through the large surface area of the lung and its abundant blood supply, is rapid and should follow zeroth-order kinetics (Goldstein *et al.*, 1974). For small and rapidly diffusing molecules that have a high lipid solubility, the blood profile of an animal exposed to a test vapor will provide curves that rapidly reach a plateau or equilibrium level proportional to the exposure concentration. A series of such curves, obtained from rats exposed to vinyl chloride, is shown in Fig. 1 (Withey, 1976). A plot of these equilibrium blood concentrations against the chamber concentration (Fig. 2; Withey, 1976) gives a straight line, the slope of which is equivalent to the Ostwald solubility coefficient (Goldstein, *et al.*, 1974). Styrene monomer requires much longer exposure times before equilibrium is established (Fig. 3), especially at higher exposure concentrations, probably because of its molecular size and solubility characteristics (Withey and Collins, 1979).

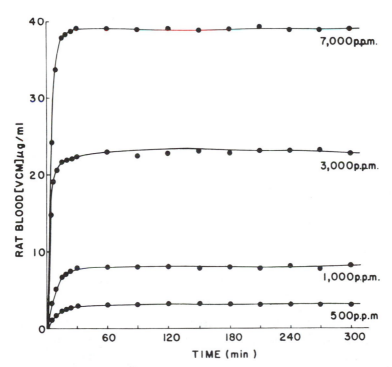

Fig. 1 Blood level curves obtained during a five-hour exposure of rats to different levels of vinyl chloride monomer.

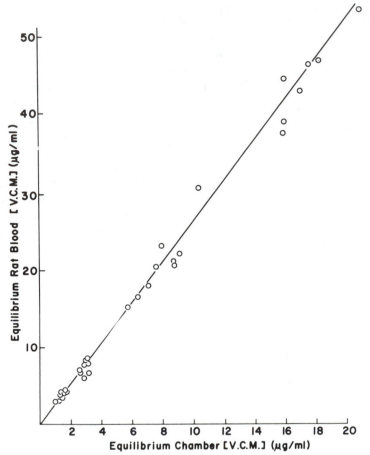

Fig. 2 Ostwald solubility curve for rats exposed to vinyl chloride monomer (From Withey, 1976).

The equation that describes the uptake kinetics in the rat during a vapor phase exposure for a two-compartment pharmacokinetic model is

$$C_1^t = \frac{k_o}{V_1}\left[\frac{k_{21}}{\alpha\beta} - \frac{(\alpha - k_{21})e^{-\alpha t}}{\alpha(\alpha - \beta)} + \frac{(\beta - k_{21})e^{-\beta t}}{\beta(\alpha - \beta)}\right] \tag{2}$$

where C_1^t is the blood concentration at any time (t) during the exposure, k_o the zeroth-order uptake rate, V_1 the volume of distribution for the central compartment, α and β the hybrid rate coefficients for the elimination process, and k_{21} the rate coefficient for the transfer from the second to the first compartment (Withey and Collins, 1979).

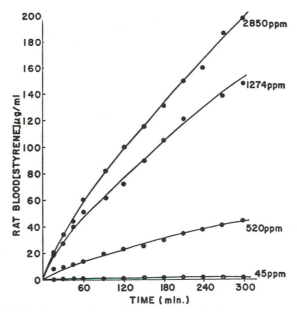

Fig. 3 Blood level curves obtained during a five-hour exposure of rats to different levels of styrene monomer (From Withey and Collins, 1979).

Elimination of a volatile test compound after an inhalation exposure will give a semilogarithmic plot of the blood level–time data that is similar to the one given after the administration of an IV bolus dose. However, remember that although the initial concentration of the test compound in the tissues will be zero when an IV dose is given, the compounds will be essentially at equilibrium with the central pharmacokinetic compartment after the steady state or plateau blood levels are reached during an inhalation exposure (Withey, 1976).

B. The Gastrointestinal Route

Uptake from the gastrointestinal (GI) tract is of major importance when humans or animals are chronically exposed to chemicals that are intentional or unintentional additives to the food supply (Food Safety Council, 1978). The fate of chemicals after oral ingestion will depend on a great many factors, some of which have been discussed previously and at length, especially in the context of the pharmacokinetics and bioavailability of drug and dosage formulations (Barr, 1968; Wagner, 1971; Gibaldi and Perrier, 1975). In view of the large number of variables involved, a discussion of some of the more important factors that affect pharmacokinetic parameters is warranted in this section. Pharmacokinetic parameters from single, oral dose studies can be used to plan and design suitable experimental protocols and may be useful to interpret the results of chronic exposures.

When a test substance enters the GI tract, its appearance in the blood compartment is regulated by (1) its physical and chemical properties (whether it is organic or inorganic, solid or liquid); (2) the vehicle in which it is administered (e.g., as an aqueous or lipid solution); and (3) the relative solubility of the compound in water and lipid solvents, which can affect diffusion and storage in the tissues. The acidic or basic nature of the substance and physiological factors, like GI transit times, metabolizing enzymes that interact with the test compound, and many more highly specific interactions that are little understood, undoubtedly play some role. The presence or absence of food in the stomach or the period for which fasting is imposed can also affect the kinetics of uptake (Linnoila et al., 1975; Doluisio et al., 1969) and are known to produce important physiological and biochemical changes that alter the absorption rate and the amount absorbed from the GI tract.

When uptake from the GI tract occurs, the total amount of test substance absorbed, in addition to some metabolites produced in the GI tract, is conveyed to the liver by way of the hepatic portal system. Consequently, all of the absorbed dose is immediately subjected to the influence of metabolizing enzymes in the liver in what has been called a "first pass effect" (Gibaldi et al., 1971; Gibaldi and Perrier, 1975). Only a fraction of a dose administered intravenously or absorbed into the systemic circulation by intraperitoneal or intramuscular routes will flow through the liver on each pass. As a result, especially for those substances that undergo extensive hepatic metabolism, the elimination rate for the same test substance given by these routes is slower than the elimination rate when the dose is given intragastrically. Thus, when the dose is given orally, it will be apparent that predictions of the pharmacokinetic elimination rate from kinetic data obtained after administration by another route (e.g., the IV route) can lead to serious misinterpretation (Loo and Riegelman, 1968).

Many chronic toxicity tests are now designed to continue throughout the lifetime of the animal. An evaluation of the pharmacokinetic parameters of absorption, distribution, metabolism, and excretion after single then repeated doses should lead to the development of an appropriate mathematical model that allows the prediction of the blood concentration throughout the duration of the study (Withey, 1978a). The pharmacokinetic studies should, at the very least, generate sufficient information to preclude the unfortunate situation of animal deaths early in the chronic study or the need to change the dose and dosing regimen as a consequence of overdosage (Burchfield *et al.,* 1975; National Cancer Institute, 1976, 1977).

The majority of studies designed to evaluate the toxicity of compounds given intragastrically have been conducted by utilizing the natural feeding habits of the test animal and mixing the test compound, in a more or less homogeneous manner, with its food supply. Although some may argue that this method does not induce stress in test animals, there can be little doubt that additional variations may be introduced as a consequence of an animal's sporadic food intake during a 24-hr period. Hence, the uncertain intake of the prescribed daily dose that results from an animal's fluctuation in food demand or, even more importantly, from the toxic effects imposed by the chemical leaves a degree of doubt that can hamper the quantitative interpretation of the results. Individually administered doses allow a much greater control over some of these variables and may pay dividends in the quantitation and interpretation of dose–toxic-response curves. It should be pointed out, however, that irritant chemicals may not be tolerated intragastrically without food and may cause artifactual forestomach lesions.

The pharmacokinetics of uptake and elimination following the administration of a single oral dose can be used to predict the blood concentration profile after multiple dosing. For illustrative purposes, it is customary to consider the repeated administration of the same dose and the same time intervals between doses. Because the dosing interval (τ) and the rate coefficients for absorption and elimination are the minimum parameters necessary to predict the accumulative effects of multiple doses for a one-compartment pharmacokinetic model, these should be obtained from single-dose studies. The time it takes the test compound to reach a steady state blood concentration, that is, the maximum (C_{max}^{∞}) and minimum (C_{min}^{∞}) fluctuations about the mean concentration (C_{mean}^{∞}) can be readily calculated from these accessible parameters (Krüger-Thiemer, 1966; Wagner, J. G., 1968). In a chronic study of some duration, it seems reasonable to assume that a rapid equilibrium or steady state of the concentration of the administered substance in the blood compartment should ultimately lead to an equilibration of levels within the body organs. If a dosing interval is chosen that differs from the half period for elimination, steady state levels will still be achieved ultimately, although the steady state blood concentration will increase with decreasing dose interval if the dose and dose interval are kept constant (Withey, 1978a).

Not all doses are handled pharmacokinetically in the one-compartment model fashion. When elimination behaves as a two-compartment
model mechanism, it is erroneous to assume that the dosing interval
should be based on the half-life of the terminal, rate-limiting step. Such
errors can lead to a relatively low "equilibrium" blood level that is
superimposed by very much higher "spikes" each time a dose is administered. Both these considerations have been discussed in recent publications (Withey, 1977b; Withey, 1978a).

IV. ORGAN KINETICS

It is, of course, seldom if ever possible to take samples of major organs in
order to monitor the kinetics of uptake and elimination. The usual
method, when such information is desired, is to expose large number of
animals to the same dose by the same route, then remove the organs after
killing one or more at selected time intervals postdosing. Kinetic parameters derived from samples obtained as a consequence of subsequent kills
are, necessarily, subject to the same limitations that are discussed in
Section III. Nevertheless, useful information can be obtained from this
method. For instance, if a lipid-soluble substance is administered intravenously to a number of animals and samples of their fat depots are
analyzed after kills at different times postdosing, it is possible to demonstrate a slow uptake followed by an even slower elimination of the
compound from the fat. This arises as a consequence of the relatively
poor vascularity and blood supply of these sites and is more likely to be
encountered with highly lipid-soluble compounds. High levels can persist
in the fat long after levels in the blood have fallen to below detectable
concentrations. Thus, a propensity for accumulation of such materials in
the lipid component of an animal body is a possibility; but determination
of the fat-loading capacity of a body may not be possible from blood or
urine samples (Järvisalo, 1978).

In some types of physiological compartment modeling, characteristics
of certain organs and tissues can be grouped to form a single physiological compartment (Andersen, 1983; Fiserova-Bergerova, 1983). The number of compartments considered in such a classification depends on the
objectives of the study. In the case of inhaled gases and vapors, tissues in
which their partial vapor pressures increase or decrease at the same rate
are treated as a single compartment.

If the tissue is considered as an isolated unit perfused by arterial blood
that contains the dissolved vapor at constant concentration, then the
partitioning rate coefficient (k) for the vapor will equal the ratio of the

perfusion (F) multiplied by the blood-to-air partition coefficient ($\lambda_{tis/air}$).

$$k = \frac{F\lambda_{bl/air}}{V\lambda_{bl/air}} \tag{3}$$

Values for each of these parameters have been evaluated for a man weighing 70 kg with a body surface area of 1.8 m^2 (Mapleson, 1963; Price, 1963).

The grouping of individual organs and tissues to yield a single physiological pharmacokinetic compartment is flexible. It is customary to consider organs with similar perfusion-volume ratios as belonging to a single group. For instance, the range of perfusion-volume ratios between 0.13 and 3.3, which comprises the adrenals, kidneys, thyroid, brain, heart, and hepatic portal system, are usually grouped into one compartment termed the vessel-rich group (VRG). The muscles and skin are termed the muscle group (MG); adipose tissue and bone marrow are the fat group (FG); whereas bones, teeth, ligaments, cartilage, and hair are usually classified as the vessel-poor group (VPG). If the solubility of the xenobiotic, administered as a dose, is similar in lean and fatty tissues, these might be combined into one compartment. Similarly, if the subject is involved in vigorous exercise during exposure, the tissues in the muscle group might be included in the vessel-rich group (Fiserova-Bergerova, 1983).

V. PHARMACOKINETIC PARAMETERS

Chapter 14 covers the mathematical analysis of raw data from which individual concentration, rate, and volume parameters of the pharmacokinetic model are determined. The usefulness of these data to the toxicologist will, of course, depend on the nature of the compound under investigation and on the nature of the application or objectives of the study. Although it is difficult to generalize and cover all aspects of each pharmacokinetic parameter, some attributes of the pharmacokinetic approach are discussed in this section.

A. Absorption or Uptake by the Gastrointestinal Route

Of the many available routes for administration of a test dose, perhaps the most common for which uptake may have an important influence on the toxicological response are the gastrointestinal and pulmonary routes. Certainly, in the assessment of human hazards, the gastrointestinal route, with respect to the hazardous products contained in the food chain, and the pulmonary route, with respect to the volatile materials in a workplace, have been extensively studied.

Some factors that can affect or perturb both the extent and rate of uptake from the gastrointestinal tract have already been considered. Others that are not easy to assess in quantitative terms may be especially important in some studies. It is well known that gastrointestinal motility can vary enormously as a consequence of stress (Wagner, 1971). Foods consumed successively are not thoroughly mixed but form layers in the stomach. The osmotic pressure of the duodenal luminal contents mainly controls the rate at which the stomach empties liquids. Fatty acids can slow stomach emptying, and lipids can stimulate the flow of bile salts (Levy, 1963; Thomas, 1963).

The presence of food in the gastrointestinal tract is known to affect the extent and rate of uptake of drugs and other xenobiotic substances (Doluisio et al., 1969; Wagner, 1966). As a consequence of this well-established phenomenon, it is customary to conduct pharmacokinetic studies involving a single oral or intragastric dosing with subjects that have fasted overnight. Remember that data collected from such studies should be used with caution when one wants to predict the effects or systemic uptake of a chronic dosing regimen in which subjects are permitted to feed ad libitum. Some substances can be recirculated by a mechanism known as enterohepatic recycling. In this recycling phenomenon, the test compound proceeds from the blood compartment, to the liver, to the bile, which is secreted into the gastrointestinal tract. Uptake into the blood from the gastrointestinal tract completes the cycle (Levine, 1978).

The physiology of the gastrointestinal tract also plays an important part in determining the rate and extent of uptake. A suitable model for the gastrointestinal lining is considered to be a bimolecular lipoid sheet covered on both sides by protein with lipoid molecules oriented perpendicularly to the cell surface (Wagner, 1971). Small, water-filled pores with a diameter of about 8 Å permit the physical passage of small molecules, but the majority of compounds are transferred by a passive diffusion process. In most cases, the membrane plays a passive role and the rate of transfer is related to the physicochemical properties of the solute and to the concentration gradient across the gastrointestinal barrier. Other more specific diffusion processes such as facilitated diffusion, active transport, pinocytosis, and convective and ion-pair absorption may be invoked (Brown and Danielli, 1964; Lifson and Hakim, 1966). Even large solid particles, relative to organic macromolecules, have been shown to pass from the gastrointestinal tract into the bloodstream, thence to be deposited at a site of action.

The pH of the gastrointestinal tract is also of some importance, particularly insofar as the absorption of completely or partially ionized molecules is concerned. In humans, the pH of the gastrointestinal tract changes along its length from a pH of 1 to 3 in the stomach, to 5 to 7 in the duodenum, and to 7 or 8 in the lower ileum. The secretion of stomach acid is subject to a diurnal effect, the fasting stomach usually being much more acidic than the postprandial stomach.

Unless special diffusion processes are invoked, molecular species that can ionize are transported across the gastrointestinal epithelium by a transport process termed the pH-partition hypothesis (Hogben et al., 1959). According to the pH-partition theory, only unionized molecules can diffuse by way of a passive mechanism across the gastrointestinal barrier; hence the lowest pK_a of an acid should be about 3 and the highest pK_a of a base about 7.8 if rapid absorption from the gastrointestinal tract is desired. It follows that acidic molecules will be preferentially absorbed from the stomach and basic molecules from the lower gastrointestinal tract. Some drugs, particularly those that have an adverse effect on the gastric epithelial lining, have been especially modified with acid-resistant coatings so as to preclude uptake prior to their transport to the lower GI tract. Others that are basic in nature, and hence ionized in the gastric contents, are preferentially absorbed from the intestines. In the latter case, a lag time, or delay period immediately following the administration of the dose during which the concentration in the blood remains zero, will be observed following oral administration. This lag time will yield a blood level–time curve in which the effective t_0 is displaced from the origin. In view of the foregoing processes, perturbation of the uptake of compounds from the gastrointestinal tract are numerous. It is important to bear this in mind when pharmacokinetic investigations of this kind are planned and data obtained from such experiments interpreted.

Very little experimental data is available to illustrate the relative importance of the many factors considered in the preceding discussion. It is surprising how many orally administered drugs follow a one-compartment open model with first-order absorption and first-order elimination (Krüger-Thiemer and Bünger, 1965, 1966; Forist and Judy, 1971). Excellent agreement has been shown between a simulated one-compartment model output from an analogue computer and blood level data obtained after the oral ingestion of amphetamines (Beckett and Tucker, 1968; Beckett et al., 1968b). Beckett and his co-workers also showed that reabsorption of this class of drug from the kidney tubules can introduce perturbations in the simple model and that fluctuations in urinary pH, and its consequent effects on excretion, further complicate the process (Beckett et al., 1968a). Nortryptyline, some lithium salts, and doxycycline hydrochloride have been cited as drugs that follow a two-compartment pharmacokinetic model (Schumacher and Weiner, 1974; Gibaldi, 1968).

In addition to those sites within the gastrointestinal trace that have already been discussed, absorption from the buccal cavity is well known and frequently used for the rapid uptake of cardiovascular drugs (Gibaldi and Kanig, 1965). Beckett and his co-workers have examined the uptake of basic drugs, including a series of amphetamines, from the buccal cavity (Beckett and Triggs, 1967; Beckett and Tucker, 1968). Other investigators have found that buccal uptake was both more rapid and efficient than GI uptake when identical doses were administered by both routes (Alkalay et al., 1973). Toxicologists should be aware of this alternative and efficient mode of uptake when designing experiments that involve a feeding study. It has been our experience to observe a dramatic increase in blood levels of test animals in the initial uptake phase after we administered a dose of a low molecular weight aliphatic chlorinated hydrocarbon in vegetable oil by gastric intubation when residual drops from the end of the cannula entered the buccal cavity upon its withdrawal. Buccal absorption can lead to significant central nervous system absorption prior to metabolism by the liver. Buccal absorption may well play an important role in the uptake of test compounds in an oral feeding study as opposed to intragastric dosing. What must be borne in mind when one conducts pharmacokinetic single-dose experiments (in order to predict the effects of multiple dosing regimens) is that many factors can perturb the pharmacokinetics of uptake during chronic studies and these factors may not be observed in single-dose studies in which the optimal control has been exercised to yield a model pharmacokinetic and animal system.

Routes of administration other than oral or gastrointestinal, such as intramuscular, intrathecal, rectal, and intraperitoneal, have been used to study absorption pharmacokinetics. These routes are, however, rarely used in toxicokinetic studies, their application being limited except in the administration of pharmaceutical preparations. The effect of route of administration on the bioavailability and pharmacokinetics of various drugs and xenobiotic compounds has been discussed in a number of publications (Burt and Beckett, 1971; Conway et al., 1973; Von Bahr et al., 1973; Gibaldi, 1975).

B. Uptake by the Pulmonary Route

A complete analysis of the factors that should be considered in the assessment of pharmacokinetic uptake is beyond the scope of this chapter. For an in-depth review of this subject, refer to Papper and Kitz

(1963) and Klaassen (1980). The uptake and steady state kinetics of anesthetic gases have received considerable attention for reasons that should be readily apparent (Goldstein et al., 1974).

It is important to note that many toxic substances enter the systemic circulation by way of the lung, either because they are gases, vapors, or aerosols, or because they are adsorbed on the surface of particulate matter lodged in the passages and extremities of the lung. A substance's rate of entry into the body via the pulmonary route is controlled by the cyclic process of respiration. In humans, inhaled vapors and gases are presented to the alveoli about 20 times per minute. The transfer of a vapor from the alveoli to the blood will be limited by the relative solubility of the vapor in blood. Transfer will continue from the alveolar air to the blood at a zeroth-order rate until a "steady state" equilibrium is achieved, and blood levels will plateau until the subject is removed from the exposure environment. Apart from the solubility of the test compound in blood, other important factors that influence its transfer to the blood are respiratory rate, tidal volume, cardiac output, and blood flow per unit volume within target tissues (Goldstein et al., 1974; Fiserova-Bergerova, 1983).

C. Distribution

A knowledge of the kinetics of distribution of a test compound from the systemic circulation to major organs and, more specifically, to target organs, is of importance to the toxicologist. How and where a compound is distributed can reveal whether organs can be involved in the toxicological assessment and in the interpretation of mechanisms of toxic action (Gillette, 1974c). It is not easy to follow the course of a drug, its concentration, and the time it takes to reach specific and vital organs within one subject. Whole-body autoradiography (Hansson and Schmiterlöw, 1961) and the subsequent determination of approximate organ concentrations by densitometry can indicate "instantaneously" which organs do and which do not take up the administered compound. Unfortunately, because both the original test compound and some or all of its metabolites will be labeled, the autoradiographic technique is somewhat nonspecific; however, indications of sequestration, accumulation, and uptake can be used to determine whether a specific compound can exert its action on the central nervous system, kidneys, liver, or some other vital organs. Use of this technique for pilot studies of pharmacokinetics in rats has been described (Liss and Kensler, 1976, Busch, 1977).

The method of administering the same dose of a test compound to a large number of animals then analyzing the major tissues at selected times after dosing can give an approximate estimate of the rates of uptake and elimination from specific organs. Such methods give only approximate rate data and may lead to false conclusions concerning the nature of the pharmacokinetic model because of those factors previously discussed in connection with the use of blood samples from sequentially sacrificed animals for pharmacokinetic evaluation. Nevertheless, in studies of this kind, it is often possible to show that well-perfused tissues, like the lung, liver, brain, and kidneys, are indistinguishable from the blood as a pharmacokinetic compartment. Therefore, they contribute to the volume of the central compartment. Indeed, as has already been pointed out, a grouping of such organs can allow an interpretation of the observed pharmacokinetics in terms of physiological compartments (Fiserova-Bergerova, 1983).

It is also possible to distinguish compounds, especially in the case of lipid-soluble substances, that are taken up slowly even after IV administration by poorly perfused tissues, such as fat. If the partition coefficient is large, these substances are slowly released back into the blood and organs that essentially compose the central compartment. In such circumstances, it is not inconceivable for fat tissue to act as a storage depot that slowly releases a compound into the blood, making its blood level concentration undetectable. Thus, the true pharmacokinetic distribution picture can be obscured if only blood concentrations of a compound are monitored. This, in turn, precludes assessment of the true body burden and propensity of the test substance to bioaccumulate. In the case of lipid-soluble compounds, it is not unusual for the ratio of concentrations in the fat to exceed those in the blood by several orders of magnitude (Shugaev, 1969; Withey, 1978b; Piotrowski, 1977).

The apparent volume of distribution (V_d) of the central compartment is a useful parameter, although it usually has no physiological reality. The volume of distribution can indicate the extent to which a substance can disperse from the blood compartment and involve other tissues within the central compartment. However, it is not unusual to find that the apparent volume of distribution is larger than the total volume of the animal. In such cases, the actual physiological model is one in which the administered compound has been distributed to other organs in equilibrium with the blood although its concentration in these tissues is higher than it is in the blood. The concept of volume of distribution and possible errors in its determination has also been discussed (Riegelman *et al.*, 1968a, 1968b).

Determination of the volume of distribution both for one-compartment and multicompartment models, has been adequately described in two excellent texts (Wagner, 1971; Gibaldi and Perrier, 1975). Reduction in the apparent volume of distribution can occur as a consequence of a number of factors, which include disease states like renal failure or cardiac and hepatic insufficiency (Gibaldi and Perrier, 1972). A similar situation arises as a consequence of the co-administration of substances that can either inhibit metabolism (e.g., phenyramidol) or reduce active renal tubule secretion (e.g., probenecid).

The fetus as a target organ has been the subject of extensive study. Special consideration of the developing fetus was accentuated in the early 1960s by the association of birth defects with the therapeutic use of thalidomide by pregnant women (McBride, 1961; Lenz, 1962a, 1962b). Most work with respect to the distribution of substances to and within the fetus and to the pharmacokinetics of such processes has been conducted with therapeutic drugs that have a potential for human use during pregnancy. Several excellent texts have been devoted to this subject (Wilson, 1973; Mirkin, 1976).

A number of important factors appear to make the developing fetus accessible to substances in the maternal systemic circulation. In the first instance, xenobiotic substances pass to the fetus through the placenta largely by a passive diffusion process. Passive diffusion imposes limits on the types of molecule that can cross the placental barrier to those with physicochemical properties that allow passage through other tissues and membranes such as the gastrointestinal tract. Lipid-soluble molecules, in an unionized state at the maternal blood pH of 7.4, will therefore have the greatest potential to transfer to the fetus (Conner and Miller, 1973). Metabolism to water-soluble products, which occurs within the uterus, will inhibit the reverse transfer of the compound to the maternal circulation and lead to its accumulation, principally in fetal tissues and the surrounding amniotic fluid. The fetus itself, with its limited capacity to metabolize those molecules that enter its tissues will, in many cases, be subjected to a greater toxicological insult than its maternal host (Wilson, 1973). Uterine fluid concentrations that are 50% greater than those in the maternal plasma, 6 hr after administration, have been demonstrated for nicotine, thiopental, isoniazid, DDT, and caffeine (Sieber and Fabro, 1971). Whether there is a major difference in the uterine secretory mechanisms of pregnancy and nonpregnant animals is an interesting question since Sieber & Fabro found that the compounds studied were transferred to uterine secretions in pregnant but not in nonpregnant animals.

Some compounds do not readily pass into fetal circulation because of their molecular size, as in the case of high molecular weight dextrans (Sieber and Fabro, 1971), or their physiological properties. Hormones like insulin, although known to cause indirect effects within the fetus, are not considered to be transferred to the fetus *per se* (Curry and Ferm, 1962).

Small lipid-soluble molecules, like chlorinated aliphatic hydrocarbons, have recently been shown to be distributed efficiently to the fetus in pregnant rats, with a linear relationship between maternal blood and fetal tissue concentrations over vapor phase exposure concentrations of up to 3,000 ppm (Withey and Karpinski, 1985a). In some cases, the relative fetal concentrations of these compounds and of styrene monomer were related to the fetal position on the uterine horn (Withey and Karpinski, 1985b).

Whole-body autoradiography is a technique that has been extensively used to study the maternal-fetal distribution phenomena of xenobiotic substances (Waddell and Marlowe, 1976). Extensive studies of fetal distribution of elemental ions, inorganic ions, central nervous system drugs, local anesthetics, agents that affect the autonomic nervous system and neuromuscular junctions, organomercury compounds, antibiotics, hormones, vitamins, and a few environmental contaminants (like DDT, dieldrin, 2,4,5,-T, and 2,4-D) have been conducted with appropriate isotopes.

A number of investigators have used animal models that have allowed direct sampling of maternal and fetal body fluids and have, therefore, been able to monitor the kinetic processes associated with the central compartment of the host and of the fetus *in utero* (Jackson and Egdahl, 1960; Willes *et al.,* 1970; Wilson *et al.,* 1983). Studies with pregnant animal models have also permitted the direct monitoring of the pharmacological effects of selected drugs (Van Petten and Willes, 1970; Conover *et al.,* 1983).

D. Metabolism

A number of factors principally related to the nature of the substance under investigation and the route by which its toxic response is elicited will affect the considerations of an appropriate pharmacokinetic investigation. Of the four major pharmacokinetic processes (absorption, distribution, metabolism, and elimination), metabolism may be the most important to examine, particularly if one or more metabolites have been established as the substance(s) responsible for the body's major toxicological response. Because metabolic pathways may be complex, with multistages and saturable processes, products and intermediates may be difficult to separate or analyze, and a complete analysis of the pharmacokinetic role of metabolism has seldom been possible.

Many compounds are converted to other molecular species and conjugates prior to their excretion from biological systems. Frequently, particularly in the case of carcinogens, the original compound may not be responsible for the evoked toxicological response. The rate of production and distribution of intermediate and ultimate metabolites is of paramount importance in assessing the mechanism of toxic action. Because the majority of biotransformations involve enzyme systems that are saturable, the associated kinetic processes may be limited in capacity to the extent that the observed data plots will be nonlinear on semilogarithmic paper, especially as the dose is increased. Such capacity-limited kinetics will give semilogarithmic plots of data that are increasingly concave to the ordinate axis as the dose increases and shows dose-dependent kinetics (Fig. 4).

In all cases in which a capacity-limited process is extensively involved in the elimination of a test compound, the so-called "Michaelis–

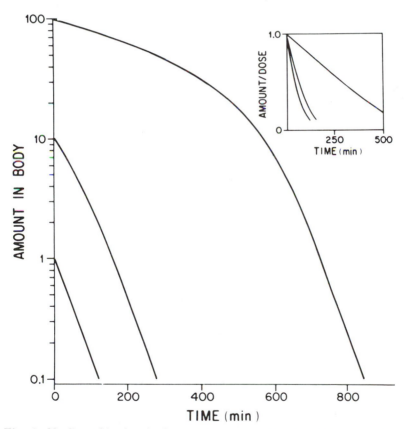

Fig. 4 Nonlinear kinetics. As the concentration of the substrate (dose) is increased, the semilogarithmic plot assumes curvature concave to the axes. The same data, plotted on a linear scale, is shown in the upper right quadrant (From Gibaldi and Perrier, 1975).

Menten" kinetics apply (Levy, 1968). In the most simple case of enzymatic metabolism, the test compound (S) will interact with active sites on the enzyme (E) to form an enzyme–test compound complex (ES). This complex will then decompose to regenerate the enzyme and to give the end product or intermediate metabolites. This process is shown in the following schematic equation.

$$E + S \overset{K_m}{\rightleftharpoons} ES \tag{4}$$
$$\downarrow$$
$$E + Products$$

The equilibrium constant (K_m) is known as the Michaelis constant, and the Michaelis–Menten kinetic equation that describes this process is

$$-\frac{dC}{dt} = \frac{V_m C}{K_m + C} \tag{5}$$

where V_m is the limiting rate of the process, C is the concentration of the substrate, and $-dC/dt$ is its rate of disappearance. In point of fact, it is readily appreciated that K_m is equal to the substrate concentration at half the maximum rate. Two limiting conditions are worthy of note. First, when K_m is very much larger than C (i.e., at low substrate concentrations)

$$-\frac{dC}{dt} = \frac{V_m C}{K_m}. \tag{6}$$

This equation has exactly the same form as a first-order rate equation. Second, when C is very much larger than K_m (i.e., at high substrate concentrations) the Michaelis–Menten equation reduces to

$$-\frac{dC}{dt} = V_m \tag{7}$$

so that the observed rate is constant. This latter situation can be readily appreciated in terms of our understanding of mechanisms of enzyme reactions in that there are a limited number of "active centers" associated with most enzyme macromolecules and these centers can become completely occupied by substrate molecules at some limiting concentration. The turnover of substrate molecules at the limiting concentration and higher will therefore be constant, hence the apparent reaction rate will be constant. Concentration and time data plotted on semilogarithmic paper will resemble the curves shown in Fig. 4. To obtain the relevant kinetic parameters, this data should be treated by some linearizing method such as a Lineweaver–Burk, Eadie, or Hofstee plot (Lineweaver and Burk, 1934; Hofstee, 1952; Laidler, 1973). Recently, nonlinear regression techniques have been introduced to fit Michaelis–Menten kinetics.

Use of radioisotope techniques, in which ^{14}C or ^3H is introduced into the molecules of the test compound, is extensive in metabolism studies. The techniques involved are usually simple and allow for identification of principal metabolites through isotope separation and dilution (Oliverio and Guarino, 1971). The various routes and the extent of elimination of a compound are also relatively easy to assess with these techniques as are its bioavailability and uptake (Watanabe et al., 1976). The advantage in using radioisotope analytical techniques is their great sensitivity. Detection of compounds that persist to levels well beyond the limits imposed by the usual physical or chemical techniques is now possible with suitable ^{14}C or ^3H counting equipment.

Because it is not possible, in most cases, to be certain of the identity of the number and proportions of different species being measured by nonspecific methods like radioisotope assays, one must be cautious in interpreting pharmacokinetic data obtained from such studies alone. At best, the hybrid rate coefficients, determined directly from a semilogarithmic plot of data obtained by a specific assay method for the compound *per se,* will be equal to or greater than the rate coefficients determined from radioisotope assay (Gibaldi and Perrier, 1975). In the measurement of the compound *per se,* this observation follows from the fact that the elimination rate will be a composite of the excretion and metabolic rates. Other tracer techniques can be extremely useful in the determination of the reaction mechanisms involved in distribution, excretion, and metabolism of a compound (Kuntzman, 1972).

A number of drugs, like diphenylhydantoin, salicylates, and ethanol, show a nonlinear relationship between the kinetics and the dose that is clearly demonstrable at relatively low doses (Lundquist and Wolthers, 1958; Levy, 1965; Gerber and Wagner, 1972; Wilkinson et al., 1977). Potential environmental contaminants like 2,4,5-T (Sauerhoff et al., 1975; Gehring et al., 1976) and dioxane (Young et al., 1978) together with industrial chemicals such as ethylene glycol (Von Wartburg et al., 1964) are also known to follow nonlinear pharmacokinetics as a consequence of the involvement of saturable metabolic pathways.

There are other saturable processes apart from metabolic pathways that can yield nonlinear pharmacokinetics. For example, renal tubule reabsorption (an active transport phenomenon) can cause urinary excretion of large doses to proceed more rapidly than the elimination of smaller doses (Jusko and Levy, 1970). Biliary excretion, sometimes leading to enterohepatic recycling, variation in tissue distribution in which tissue loading is limited, and variable binding to capacity-limited plasma proteins are other factors with a similar endpoint (Coffey et al., 1971).

There are some important toxicological implications associated with compounds that exhibit dose-dependent kinetics as a consequence of capacity-limited metabolism. In the case in which metabolism represents the principal detoxification pathway (i.e., the metabolites are relatively inactive entities), these pathways have the potential to become saturated and the dose–response curve can dramatically increase at higher dose concentrations as a consequence of the intrinsic toxicity of the text compound *per se.* Conversely, at low dose concentrations, there may well be detoxification pathways that produce innocuous metabolites. At higher concentrations, when the principal pathways have reached their limited capacity, other pathways that produce active metabolites may be invoked. Data generated in studies on the metabolism of vinyl chloride monomer (Hefner *et al.,* 1975) show that potentially toxic metabolites are conjugated to glutathione, a process that is rate limited by the hepatic production of the sulfhydryl compound and which is saturable at high doses (Gillette, 1974a, 1974b). In this case, it was suggested that the carcinogenicity of vinyl chloride monomer might have a potential threshold of effect or, at least, that regulatory limits could not be set on the basis of the extrapolation of the large amount of data on tumor yield obtained at high dose levels in rodents (Maugh, 1978). An opposing view to this argument (Hooper *et al.,* 1979) was presented based on the evidence obtained from bioassays at low doses. The animal bioassay data (Maltoni 1977; Lee *et al.,* 1978) show that tumors are produced in animals exposed to low levels of vinyl chloride (below 150 ppm). Extrapolation of the dose-response curve to higher doses of vinyl chloride predicts a higher carcinogenic response than that which is observed. This may be due to the fact that mechanisms that activate vinyl chloride to the proximate carcinogen become saturated as the dose increases (Gehring *et al.,* 1978; Watanabe *et al.,* 1978).

The importance of metabolic rate studies cannot be overemphasized. A more complete understanding of the rate processes involved in detoxification mechanisms or in production of more active metabolites, such as proximate carcinogens, is useful in the planning of realistic chronic studies and in the interpretation of data from such studies (Munro, 1977).

E. Elimination

Removal of a xenobiotic substance from the blood or the central pharmacokinetic compartment seldom occurs merely by excretion. In addition to the excretion process, metabolism and storage can account for the removal of a test compound not only from the monitored compartment but also from the site(s) of toxic action in some cases. It is, therefore, not surprising that a great deal of attention has been paid to the rates of elimination and how they can be perturbed.

Metabolism and the pharmacokinetics of detoxification and activation mechanisms have already been discussed. The removal from the systemic circulation of lipid-soluble compounds to fat depots, of colloidal substances to the reticuloendothelial system, and of heavy metals to hair and bone may be very important in terms of assessing the chronic toxicity of some compounds (Goldstein et al., 1974), particularly if those compounds are returned slowly to the central pharmacokinetic compartment at concentrations that are below the detection limits of analytical methodology.

The kidney is ideally suited to its role in the excretion of xenobiotics from the blood (Weiner, 1971). Compounds that have a low molecular weight (less than 5,000) are filtered though the glomerular membranes fairly rapidly because the kidney receives a blood supply of some 25% of the cardiac output. About 130 ml of water are filtered every minute in an adult human, of which only about 1 to 2 ml passes into the bladder as urine while the rest is reabsorbed. Reabsorption of neutral compounds, particularly those with a high lipid-water partition coefficient, occurs readily. The rate of transfer of many metabolites or ionized acidic and basic compounds from the arterial blood supply of the kidney to the urine may be limited by the pH of the system because only a neutral molecule can be transported by passive mechanisms (Milne et al., 1958). The tubular epithelium has specialized mechanisms for the transport of substances from the plasma to tubular fluid. These involve enzymes and an active secretion process. The excretion of organic cations and anions usually involves active transport by tubular excretion.

The rate of excretion of compounds from the kidney by glomerular filtration, active tubular excretion, and passive tubular reabsorption, can be determined from the ratio of the clearance of the compound to that of inulin (Cafruny, 1972). Both substances are usually infused at a constant rate, and several determinations of the inulin clearance ratio are made when plasma levels are at steady state. If the inulin clearance ratio in the presence of an xenobiotic and the inulin clearance in the absence of the xenobiotic compound are greater than 1, then the compound is probably excreted in part by a carrier-mediated transport. If the ratio is less than 1, then the compound must be reabsorbed.

VI. SUMMARY

Introduction of improved techniques in analytical methodology, such as high pressure liquid chromatography and quantitative mass spectrometry, and improvements in the sensitivity of specific analytical techniques will enhance the application of pharmacokinetic techniques to the problems of toxicology. New and improved animal models and techniques that allow access to inaccessible depots will lead to a more precise and specific analysis of the pharmacokinetics of toxic action. Certainly, we should hope that a better understanding of pharmacokinetics will prevent the repetition of situations like those described recently (Burchfield *et al.*, 1975) in which studies on a range of 20 herbicides, pesticides, and phytocides required a total of 175 changes in dose during the conduct of chronic toxicity studies on these compounds.

Single-dose pharmacokinetic studies should become an important prerequisite to long-term studies. Not only can they give important clues as to how test animals handle xenobiotic substances so that potential accumulation and overdose can be avoided, but they represent a very small fraction of the effort and expense that such experimental designs entail, particularly in lifetime studies.

References

Alkalay, D., Khemani, L., Wagner, W. E., and Bartlett, M. F. (1973) Sublingual and oral administration of methyltestosterone. A comparison of drug bioavailability. *J. Clin. Pharmacol.* **13**, 142–151.

American Converence of Governmental and Industrial Hygienists (1980). "Documentation of the Threshold Limit Values," 4th Ed., Cincinnati, Ohio: American Conference of Governmental and Industrial Hygienists.

Andersen, M. E. (1983). Flow limited clearance. *In* "Modeling of Inhalation Exposure to Vapors: Uptake, Distribution and Elimination" (V. Fiserova-Bergerova, ed.), Vol. II. Boca Raton, Florida: CRC Press.

Barr, W. H. (1968). Principles of biopharmaceutics. *Am. J. Pharm. Educ.* **32**, 958–981.

Beckett, A. H., and Triggs, E. J. (1967). Buccal absorption of basic drugs and its application to an *in vivo* model of passive drug transfer through lipid membranes. *J. Pharm. Pharmacol.* **19**, 315–415.

Beckett, A. H., Bayer, R. N., and Triggs, E. J. (1968a). Kinetics of buccal absorption of amphetamines. *J. Pharm. Pharmacol.* **20**, 92–97.

Beckett, A. H., Boyes, R. N., and Tucker, G. T. (1968b). Use of the analogue computer to predict the distribution and excretion of drugs under conditions of fluctuating urinary pH. *J. Pharm. Pharmacol.* **20**, 277–282.

Beckett, A. H., and Tucker, G. T. (1968). Application of the analogue computer to pharmacokinetic and biopharmaceutical studies with amphetamine-type compounds. *J. Pharm. Pharmacol.* **20**, 174–193.

Bolt, H. M., Laib, R. J., Kappus, H., and Buchter, A. (1977). Pharmacokinetics of vinyl chloride in the rat. *Toxicology* **7**, 179–188.

Boxer, G. E., Jelinek, V. C., Tompsett, R., DuBois, R., and Edison, A. O. (1948). Streptomycin in the blood. Chemical determinations after single and repeated intramuscular injections. *J. Pharm. Exp. Ther.* **92**, 226–235.

Brown, F., and Danielli, J. F. (1964). The cell surface and cell physiology. *In* "Cytology and Cell Physiology" (G. H. Bourne, ed.), pp. 239–310. New York: Academic Press.

Burchfield, H. P., Storrs, E. D., and Kraybill, H. F. (1975). The maximum tolerated dose in pesticide carcinogenicity studies. *Environ. Qual. Saf. Suppl.* **III,** 599–603.

Burhoe, S. O. (1940). Methods of securing blood from rats. *J. Hered.* **31,** 445–448.

Burt, R. A. P., and Beckett, A. H. (1971). The absorption and excretion of pentazocine after administration by different routes. *Br. J. Anaesth.* **43,** 427–435.

Busch, U. (1977). Whole body autoradiography (WBAR): use for pilot studies of pharmacokinetics in rats. *Acta Pharmacol. Toxicol. Suppl. 1* **41,** 28–29.

Cafruny, E. J. (1972). Renal excretion of drugs. *In* "Fundamentals of Drug Metabolism and Drug Disposition" (B. N. LaDu, H. G. Mandel, and E. L. Way, eds.), pp. 119–130. Baltimore: Williams and Wilkins.

Coffey, J. J., Bullock, F. J., and Schoenemann, P. T. (1971). Numerical solution of nonlinear pharmacokinetic equations: Effects of plasma protein binding on drug distribution and elimination. *J. Pharm. Sci.* **60,** 1623–1628.

Conner, E. A., and Miller, J. W. (1973). The distribution of selected substances into rat uterine luminal fluid. *J. Pharmacol. Exp. Ther.* **184,** 291–298.

Conover, W. B., Key, T. C., and Resnik, R. (1983). Maternal cardiovascular response to caffeine infusion in the pregnant ewe. *Am. J. Obstet. Gynecol.* **145,** 534–538.

Conway, W. D., Singhvi, S. M., Gibaldi, M., and Boyes, R. N. (1973). The effect of route of administration on the metabolic fate of terbutaline in the rat. *Xenobiotica* **3,** 813–821.

Curry, H. F., and Ferm, V. H. (1962). Blastocysts sugar concentration following maternal glucose changes. *Anat. Rec.* **142,** 21–25.

Dittert, L. W. (1977). Pharmacokinetic prediction of tissue residues. *J. Toxicol. Environ. Health* **2,** 735–756.

Doluisio, J. T., Tan, G. H., Billups, N. F., and Diamond, L. (1969). Drug absorption: Effect of fasting on intestinal drug absorption. *J. Pharm. Sci.* **58,** 1200–1202.

Dominguez, R., and Pomerene, E. (1934). Studies of the renal excretion of creatinine. *J. Biol. Chem.* **104,** 449–473.

Farris, E. J., and Griffith, P. Q. (1949). "The Rat in Laboratory Investigation," 2nd Ed. Philadelphia: Lippincott.

Feinstein, A. R. (1970a). Clinical biostatistics. I. A new name — and some other changes of the guard. *Clin. Pharm. Ther.* **11,** 135–148.

Feinstein, A. R. (1970b). Clinical biostatistics. II. Statistics versus science in the design of experiments. *Clin. Pharm. Ther.* **11,** 282–292.

Filser, J. G., and Bolt, H. M. (1979). Pharmacokinetics of halogenated ethylenes in rats. *Arch. Toxicol.* **42,** 123–136.

Fiserova-Bergerova, V. (1983). Physiological models for pulmonary administration and elimination of inert vapors and gases. *In* "Modeling of Inhalation Exposure to Vapors: Uptake, Distribution and Elimination," (V. Fiserova-Bergerova, ed.), Vol. I, pp. 73–100. Boca Raton, Florida: CRC Press.

Forist, A. A., and Judy, R. W. (1971). Comparative pharmacokinetics of chlorphenesin carbamate and methocarbamol in man. *J. Pharm. Sci.* **60,** 1686–1688.

Food Safety Council (1978). "Proposed System for Food Safety Assessment." Columbia, Maryland: Food Safety Council.

Fraser, D. A., Bales, R. E., Lippman, M. and Stokinger, H. E. (1959). Exposure chambers for research in animal inhalation. Public Health Monograph No. 57, U.S. Government Printing Office, Washington, D.C.

Gehring, P. G. (1978). Chemobiokinetics and metabolism. *In* "Principles and Methods for Evaluating the Toxicity of Chemicals," Part I. Geneva: World Health Organization.

Gehring, P. J., Blau, G. E., and Watanabe, P. G. (1976). Pharmacokinetic studies in evaluation of the toxicological and environmental hazards of chemicals. *In* "Advances in Modern Toxicology" (M. A. Mehlman, R. E. Shapiro, and H. Blumenthal, eds.) Vol. I, pp. 195–270. Washington, DC: Hemisphere.

Gehring, P. J., Watanabe, P. G., and Park, C. N. (1978). Resolution of dose-response toxicity data for chemicals requiring metabolic activation: Example—vinyl chloride. *Toxicol. Appl. Pharmacol.* **44**, 581–591.

Gehring, P. J., and Young, J. D. (1978). Application of pharmacokinetic principles in practice." Proceedings of the First International Congress on Toxicology" (G. L. Plaa and W. A. M. Duncan, eds.), pp. 119–142. New York: Academic Press.

Gerber, N., and Wagner, J. G. (1972). Exploration of dose-dependent decline of diphenyl-hydantoin plasma levels by fitting to the integrated form of the Michaelis-Menten equation. *Res. Comm. Chem. Pathol. Pharmacol.* **3**, 455–466.

Gibaldi, M. (1968). How to utilize biopharmaceutical data in drug evaluation. *Am. J. Pharm. Educ.* **32**, 929–937.

Gibaldi, M., and Kanig, J. L. (1965). The effect of body position and pH on the gastrointestinal absorption of salicylate and creatine in man. *Arch. Int. Pharmacodynam. Ther.* **161**, 343–358.

Gibaldi, M., and Perrier, D. (1972). Drug elimination and the apparent volume of distribution in multicompartment systems. *J. Pharm. Sci.* **61**, 952–954.

Gibaldi, M., and Perrier, D. (1975). "Pharmacokinetics." New York: Marcel Dekker.

Gibaldi, M., Boyer, R. N., and Feldman, S. (1971). Influence of first-pass effect on the availability of drugs on oral administration. *J. Pharm. Sci.* **60**, 1338–1342.

Gillette, J. R. (1974a). A perspective in the role of chemically reactive metabolites of foreign compounds in toxicity. I. Correlation of changes in covalent binding of reactive metabolites with changes in the incidence and severity of toxicity. *Biochem. Pharmacol.* **23**, 2785–2794.

Gillette, J. R. (1974b). A perspective on the role of chemically reactive metabolites of foreign compounds in toxicity. II. Alterations in the kinetics of covalent binding. *Biochem. Pharmacol.* **23**, 2927–2938.

Gillette, J. R. (1974c). The importance of tissue distribution in pharmacokinetics. *Pharmacol. Pharmacokinet. (Proc. Int. Conf.)* (T. Teorell, R. L. Dedrick, and P. G. Condliffe, eds.), pp. 209–231. New York: Plenum.

Gillette, J. R. (1976). Application of pharmacokintic principles in the extrapolation of animal data to humans. *Clin. Toxicol.* **9**, 709–721.

Gladtke, E., and von Hattingberg, H. (1979). "Pharmacokinetics: An Introduction." New York: Springer-Verlag.

Goldstein, A., Aronow, L., and Kalman, S. M. (1974). "Principles of Drug Action," 2nd Ed. New York: Wiley.

Grice, H. C. (1964). Methods for obtaining blood and for intravenous injections in laboratory animals. *Lab. Anim. Care* **14**, 483–493.

Hammer, R., and Bozler, G. (1977). Pharmacokinetics as an aid in the interpretation of toxicity tests. *Arzneim. Forsch.* **27**, 555–557.

Hansson, E., and Schmiterlöw, C. G. (1961). A comparison of the distribution, excretion and metabolism of a tertiary (promethazine) and a quaternary (Aprobit) phenothiazine compound labelled with S35. *Arch. Int. Pharmacodynam. Ther.* **131,** 309–324.

Hefner, R. E., Watanabe, P. G., and Gehring, P. J. (1975). Preliminary studies on the fate of inhaled vinyl chloride monomer (VCM) in rats. *Environ. Health Perspect.* **11,** 85–95.

Hemingway, A., Scott, F. H., and Wright, H. N. (1935). The kinetics of the elimination of the dye water blue from dog plasma after intravenous injection. *Am. J. Physiol.* **112,** 56–64.

Himmelstein, K. J., and Lutz, R. J. (1979). A review of the applications of physiologically based pharmacokinetic modeling. *J. Pharmacokin. Biopharm.* **7,** 127–145.

Hofstee, B. H. J. (1952). On evaluation of constants V_m and K_m in enzyme reactions. *Science* **116,** 329–331.

Hogben, C. A. M., Tocco, D. J., Brodie, B. B., and Schanker, L. S. (1959). On the mechanism of intestinal absorption of drugs. *J. Pharmacol. Exp. Ther.* **125,** 275–282.

Hooper, N. K., Harris, R. H., and Ames, B. N. (1979). Chemical carcinogens. *Science* **203,** 602–603.

Huddleston, J. (1978). Construction of indwelling cannulae and their application into various species. *Proc. Can. Assoc. Lab. Anim. Sci.* 42–47.

Jackson, B. T., and Egdahl, R. H. (1960). The performance of complex fetal operations in utero without amniotic fluid loss or other disturbances to fetal–maternal relationships. *Surgery* **48,** 564–570.

Järvisalo, J. (1978). Proceedings of the international symposium on styrene. Occupational and toxicological aspects. *Scand. J. Work Environ. Health* **4,** *Suppl. 2,* 1–264.

Jusko, W. J., and Levy, G. (1970). Pharmacokinetic evidence for saturable renal tubular reabsorption of riboflavin. *J. Pharm. Sci.* **59,** 765–772.

Klaassen, C. D. (1980). Absorption, distribution and excretion of toxicants. *In* "Casarett and Doull's Toxicology" (J. Doull, C. D. Klaassen, and M. O. Amdur, eds.), pp. 28–55. New York: MacMillan.

Knipfel, J. E., Peace, R. W., and Evans, J. A. (1975). Multiple vascular and gastric cannulation of swine for studies of gastrointestinal, liver, and peripheral tissue metabolism. *Lab. Anim. Sci.* **25,** 74–78.

Kociba, R. J., McCollister, S. B., Park, C. N., Torkelson, T. R., and Gehring, P. J. (1974). 1,4-Dioxane: I. Results of two year ingestion studies in rats. *Toxicol. Appl. Pharmacol.* **30,** 275–286.

Krüger-Thiemer, E. (1966). Formal theory of drug dosage regimens. I. *J. Theoret. Biol.* **13,** 212–235.

Krüger-Thiemer, E., and Bünger, P. (1965/66). The role of therapeutic regimen in dosage design. *Chemotherapia* **10,** 61–144.

Kuntzman, R. (1972). Applications of tracer techniques in drug metabolism studies. *In* "Fundamentals of Drug Metabolism and Drug Disposition" (B. N. LaDu, H. G. Mandel, and E. L. Way, eds.) pp. 489–504. Baltimore: Williams and Wilkins.

Laidler, K. J. (1973). "The Chemical Kinetics of Enzyme Action." Oxford: Clarendon Press.

Leach, L. T. (1963). "Inhalation chambers" (R & D Rep. U.R. 629). Washington, DC: U.S. Atomic Energy Commission.

Lee, C. C., Bhandari, J. C., Winston, M., House, W. B., Dixon, R. L., and Woods, J. J. (1978). Carcinogenicity of vinyl chloride and vinylidene chloride. *J. Toxicol. Environ. Health* **4,** 15–30.

Lenz, W. (1962a). Die Phthalidomid-embryopathie. *Dtsch. Med. Wochenschr.* **87,** 1232.

Lenz, W. (1962b). Thalidomide and congenital abnormalities. *Lancet* **1,** 45.

Levine, W. G. (1978). Biliary excretion of drugs and other xenobiotics. *Annu. Rev. Pharmacol. Toxicol.* **18,** 81–96.

Levy, G. (1963). Effect of certain tablet formulation factors on dissolution rate of the active ingredient. I. Importance of using appropriate agitation intensities for in vitro dissolution rate measurements to reflect in vivo conditions. *J. Pharm. Sci.* **52,** 1039–1046.

Levy, G. (1965). Pharmacokinetics of salicylate elimination in man. *J. Pharm. Sci.* **54,** 959.

Levy, G. (1968). Dose dependent effects in pharmacokinetics. *In* "Importance of Fundamental Principles in Drug Evaluation" (D. H. Tedeschi and R. E. Tedeschi, eds.), pp. 141–172. New York: Raven Press.

Lifson, H., and Hakim, A. A. (1966). Simple diffusion–convective model for intestinal absorption of a non-electrolyte (Urea). *Am. J. Physiol.* **211,** 1137–1146.

Linnoila, M., Korttila, K., and Mattila, M. J. (1975). Effect of food and repeated injections on serum diazepam levels. *Acta Pharmacol. Toxicol.* **36,** 181–186.

Lineweaver, H., and Burk, D. (1934). Determination of enzyme dissociation constants. *J. Am. Chem. Soc.* **56,** 658–666.

Liss, R. H., and Kensler, C. J. (1976). *In* "Advances in Modern Toxicology" (M. A. Mehlman, R. E. Shapiro, and H. Blumenthal, eds.), Vol. I, pp. 273–305. Washington, DC: Hemisphere.

Loo, J. C. K., and Riegelman, S. (1968). New method for calculating the intrinsic rate of drugs. *J. Pharm. Sci.* **57,** 918–928.

Lundquist, F., and Wolthers, H. (1958). The kinetics of alcohol elimination in man. *Acta Pharmacol. Toxicol.* **14,** 265–289.

McBride, W. G. (1961). Thalidomide and its congenital abnormalities. *Lancet* **2,** 1358.

MacFarland, H. N. (1970). Exposure chambers-design and operation. *Proc. 7th Annu. Tech. Mtg. Am. Assoc. Contam. Ctrl.* 111–115.

Maltoni, C. (1977). Vinyl chloride carcinogenicity: An experimental model for carcinogenesis studies. *In* "Origins of Human Cancer" (H. H. Hiatt, J. D. Watson, and J. A. Winsten, eds.) pp. 119–146. Cold Spring Harbor, New York: Cold Spring Harbor Laboratory.

Mapleson, W. W. (1963). Quantitative prediction of anesthetic concentrations, *In* "Uptake and Distribution of Anesthetic Agents" (E. M. Papper and R. J. Kitz, eds.). New York: McGraw-Hill.

Maugh, T. H. (1978). Chemical carcinogens: How dangerous are low doses? *Science* **202,** 37–41.

Metzler, C. M. (1969). "A user's manual for NONLIN" (Tech. Rep. 7292/9/7292/005). Kalamazoo, Michigan: Upjohn.

Milne, M. D., Scribner, B. H., and Crawford, M. A. (1958). Non-ionic diffusion and the excretion of weak acids and bases. *Am. J. Med.* **24,** 709–729.

Mirkin, B. L., (1976). "Perinatal Pharmacology and Therapeutics." New York: Academic Press.

Munro, I. C. (1977). Considerations in chronic toxicity testing: The chemical, the dose, the design. *J. Environ. Pathol. Toxicol.* **1,** 183–197.

National Academy of Sciences (1980). "Principles of Toxicological Interactions Associated with Multiple Chemical Exposures," pp. 1–20. Washington, DC: National Academy of Sciences.

National Cancer Institute (1977). "Bioassay of 1,1,1-Trichloroethane for Possible Carcinogenicity" (Publ. No. (NIH) 77-803). Bethesda: Department of Health, Education and Welfare.

National Cancer Institute (1976). "Report on Carcinogenesis Bioassay of Chloroform" (Pub. No. (NIH) 76-1279). Bethesda: Department of Health, Education and Welfare.

Nelson, E. (1963). Kinetics of drug absorption, distribution, metabolism and excretion. *Proc. Int. Congr. Chemother. 3rd, 1963* **2,** 1657–1666.

O'Flaherty, E. (1981). "Toxicants and Drugs: Kinetics and Dynamics." New York: Wiley.

Oliverio, V. T., and Guarino, A. M. (1971). Isotope dilution analysis. *In* "Concepts in Biochemical Pharmacology" (B. B. Brodie and J. R. Gillette, eds.), pp. 160–177. New York: Springer-Verlag.

Papper, E. M., and Kitz, R. J. (1963). "Uptake and Distribution of Anesthetic Agents." New York: McGraw-Hill.

Pedersen, P. V. (1977). Curve fitting and modeling in pharmacokinetics and some practical experiences with NONLIN and a new program FUNFIT. *J. Pharmacokinet. Biopharm.* **5, (5),** 513–531.

Piotrowski, J. (1971). "The Application of Metabolic and Excretion Kinetics to Problems of Industrial Toxicology." pp. 166. Bethesda: National Library of Medicine.

Piotrowski, J. (1977). "Exposure Tests for Organic Compounds in Industrial Toxicology" (NIOSH 77-144). Washington, DC: U.S. Department of Health, Education and Welfare.

Price, H. L. (1963). Circulation: General considerations. *In* "Uptake and Distribution of Anesthetic Agents" (E. M. Papper and R. J. Kitz, eds.), pp. 123–129. New York: McGraw-Hill.

Reitz, R. H., Gehring, P. J., and Park, C. N. (1978). Carcinogenic risk estimation for chloroform: An alternative to EPA's procedure. *Food Cosmet. Toxicol.* **16,** 511–514.

Riegelman, S., Loo, J. C. K., and Rowland, M. (1968a). Concept of a volume of distribution and possible errors in evaluation of this parameter. *J. Pharm. Sci.* **57,** 128–133.

Riegelman, S., Loo, J. C. K., and Rowland, M. (1968b). Shortcomings in pharmacokinetic analysis by conceiving the body to exhibit properties of a single compartment. *J. Pharm. Sci.* **57,** 117–123.

Riley, V. (1960). Adaptation of orbital bleeding technic to rapid serial blood studies. *Proc. Soc. Exp. Biol. Med.* **104,** 751–754.

Rowe, V. K., Wujkowski, T., Wolf, M. A., Sadek, S. E., and Stewart, R. D. (1963). Toxicity of a solvent mixture of 1,1,1-trichloroethylene and tetrachloroethylene as determined by laboratory animals and human subjects.

Ruddick, J. A., Craig, J., Stavric, B., Willes, R. F., and Collins, B. (1979). Uptake, distribution and metabolism of ^{14}C amaranth in the female rat. *Food Cosmet. Toxicol.* **17,** 435–442.

Sauerhoff, M. W., Blau, G. E., Braun, W. H., and Gehring, P. J. (1975). The dose dependent pharmacokinetic profile of 2,4,5-trichlorphenoxyacetic acid (2,4,5-T) following intravenous administration to rats. *Toxicol. Appl. Pharmacol.* **36,** 491–501.

Schumacher, G., and Weiner, J. (1974). Practical pharmacokinetic techniques for drug consultation and evaluation (iii) psychotherapeutic drugs as prototypes for illustrating some considerations in pharmacist-generated dosage regimens. *Am. J. Hosp. Pharm.* **31,** 59–66.

Shugaev, B. B. (1969). Concentrations of hydrocarbons in tissues as a measure of toxicity. *Arch. Environ. Health* **18,** 878–882.

Sieber, S. M., and Fabro, S. (1971). Identification of drugs in the preimplantation blasto-cyst and in the plasma, uterine secretion and urine of the pregnant rabbit. *J. Pharmacol. Exp. Ther.* **176,** 65–75.

Silver, S. D. (1946). Constant flow gassing chambers: principles influencing design and operation. *J. Lab. Clin. Med.* **31,** 1153–1161.

Snow, J. (1848). On narcotism by the inhalation of vapours. *London Med. Gazette* **42,** 330–335.

Snow, J. (1850). On narcotism by the inhalation of vapours. *London Med. Gazette* **46,** 749–754.

Soule, R. D. (1978). Sampling and analysis. *In* "Patty's Industrial Hygiene and Toxicology" (G. D. Clayton and F. E. Clayton, eds.) 3rd rev. ed., pp. 707–770. New York: Wiley.

Stewart, R. D., and Dodd, H. C. (1964). Absorption of carbon tetrachloride, trichloroethyl-ene, tetrachlorethylene, methylene chloride and 1,1,1-trichloroethane through human skin. *Am. Ind. Hyg. Assoc. J.* **25,** 439–446.

Stone, S. M. (1954). Method for obtaining venous blood from the orbital sinus of the rat or mouse. *Science* **119,** 100.

Thomas, J. E. (1963). Mechanisms and regulation of gastric emptying. *Physiol. Rev.* **37,** 453–474.

Van Petten, G. R., and Willes, R. F. (1970). β-Adrenoceptive responses in the unanesthe-tized ovine foetus. *Br. J. Pharmacol.* **38,** 572–582.

Van Petten, G. R., Becking, G. C., Withey, R. J., and Lettau, H. F. (1971). Studies on the physiological availability and metabolism of sulphonamides. II. Sulfisoxazole. *J. Clin. Pharmacol.* **11,** 35–41.

Van Petten, G. R., Evans, J. A., and Salem, F. A. (1970). A simple method for the chronic measurement of the electrocardiogram and blood pressure in the conscious rat. *J. Pharm. Pharmacol.* **22,** 467–469.

Von Bahr, C., Borga, O., Fellenius, E., and Rowland, M. (1973). Kinetics of nortryptaline in rats *in vivo* and in the isolated perfused liver. *Pharmacology* **9,** 177–186.

Von Oettingen, W. R. (1964). "The Halogenated Hydrocarbons of Industrial and Toxico-logical Importance." New York: Elsevier-North Holland.

Von Wartburg, J. P., Bethune, J. L., and Vallee, B. L. (1964). Human liver-alcohol dehy-drogenase. Kinetic and physiochemical properties. *Biochemistry* **3,** 1775–1782.

Waddell, W. J., and Marlowe, G. C. (1976). Disposition of drugs in the fetus. *In* "Perinatal Pharmacology and Therapeutics" (B. L. Mirkin, ed.), pp. 119–268. New York: Academic Press.

Wagner, J. G., and Nelson, E. (1964). Kinetic analysis of blood levels and urinary excretion in the absorptive phase after single doses of drug. *J. Pharm. Sci.* **53,** 1392–1403.

Wagner, J. G. (1966). Design and data analysis of biopharmaceutical studies in man. *Can. J. Pharm. Sci.* **1,** 55–68.

Wagner, J. G. (1967). Method for estimating rate constants for absorption, metabolism and elimination from urinary excretion data. *J. Pharm. Sci.* **56,** 489–494.

Wagner, J. G. (1968). Kinetics of pharmacologic response. I. Proposed relationships be-tween response and drug concentration in the intact animal and man. *J. Theoret. Biol.* **20,** 173–201.

Wagner, J. G. (1971). "Biopharmaceutics and relevant pharmacokinetics," 1st ed. Hamil-ton, Illinois: Drug Intelligence Publications.

Watanabe, P. G., McGowan, G. R., and Gehring, P. J. (1976). Fate of ^{14}C vinyl chloride after single oral administration in rats. *Toxicol. Appl. Pharmacol.* **37**, 49–60.

Watanabe, P. G., Zempel, D. G., Pegg, D. G., and Gehring, P. J. (1978). Hepatic macromolecular binding following exposure to vinyl chloride. *Toxicol. Appl. Pharmacol.* **44**, 571–579.

Weiner, I. M. (1971). Excretion of drugs by the kidney. *In* "Handbook of Experimental Pharmacology" (B. B. Brodie and J. R. Gillette, eds.), pp. 328–353. Berlin: Springer-Verlag.

Widmark, E. M. P. (1919). Studies on the concentration of indifferent narcotics in blood and tissues. *Acta Med. Scand.* **52**, 87–164.

Widmark, E. M. P., and Tandberg, J. (1924). The limitations for the accumulation of indifferent narcotics. Theoretical calculation. *Biochem. Z.* **147**, 358–369.

Wilkinson, P. K., Sedman, A. J., Sakmar, E., Kay, D. R., and Wagner, J. G. (1977). Pharmacokinetics of ethanol after oral administration in the fasting state. *J. Pharmacokinet. Biopharm.* **5**, 207–229.

Willes, R. F., Van Petten, G. R., and Truelove, J. F. (1970). Chronic exteriorization of vascular cannulas and ECG electrodes from the ovine foetus. *J. Appl. Physiol.* **28**, 248–250.

Wilson, J. G. (1973)., Principles of teratology. *In* "Pathology of Development" (E. V. Perrin, M. J. Finegold, and J. G. Brunson, eds.), pp. 11–30. Baltimore: Williams and Wilkins.

Wilson, S. J., Ayromlooi, J., and Errick, J. K. (1983). Pharmacokinetic and hemodynamic effects of caffeine in the pregnant sheep. *Am. J. Obstet. Gynecol.* **61**, 486–491.

Withey, J. R. (1976). Pharmacodynamics and uptake of vinyl chloride monomer administered by various routes to rats. *J. Toxicol. Environ. Health* **1**, 381–394.

Withey, J. R. (1977a). Pharmacokinetics and distribution of styrene monomer in rats after intravenous administration. *J. Toxicol. Environ. Health* **3**, 1011–1020.

Withey, J. R. (1977b). The role of pharmacokinetics in the design and conduct of chronic exposure studies. *Int. Congr. Ser. Excerpta Med.* **440**, 190–195.

Withey, J. R. (1978a). Pharmacokinetic principles. "Proceedings of the first International Congress on Toxicology" (G. L. Plaa and W. A. M. Duncan, eds.), pp. 97–118. New York: Academic Press.

Withey, J. R. (1978b). The toxicology of styrene monomer and its pharmacokinetics and distribution in the rat. *Scand. J. Work Environ. Health Suppl.* 2 **4**, 31–40.

Withey, J. R., and Collins, P. G. (1979). The distribution of styrene monomer in rats by the pulmonary route. *J. Environ. Pathol. Toxicol.* **2(6)**, 1329–1342.

Withey, J. R., and Karpinski, K. (1985a). The fetal distribution of some aliphatic chlorinated hydrocarbons in the rat after vapor phase exposure. *Biol. Res. Pregnancy* **6**, 79–88.

Withey, J. R., and Karpinski, K. (1985b). Fetal distribution of styrene in rats after vapor phase exposures. *Biol. Res. Pregnancy* **6**, 59–64.

Withey, J. R., Willes, R. F., Evans, J., and Bryce, F. R. (1973). The surgical preparation and maintenance of pigs in bioavailability studies. *Lab. Anim. Sci.* **23(1)**, 122–125.

Wong, D., Colburn, W. A., and Gibaldi, M. (1979). Fitting concentration-time data to biexponential equations. *J. Pharmacokinet. Biopharm.* **7(1)**, 97–100.

Young, J. D., Braun, W. H., and Gehring, P. J. (1978). Dose dependent fate of 1,4-dioxane in rats. *J. Toxicol. Environ. Health* **4**, 709–726.

14
Pharmacokinetic Models

B. T. Collins
Canadian Wildlife Service
Environment Canada
Ottawa, Ontario

I. INTRODUCTION

This chapter is designed to provide an introduction to the mathematics of the models used in pharmacokinetics. For ease of exposition, derivations of most mathematical solutions have not been included but outlines of these derivations are given and their source referenced where possible. The models described are those most commonly used and should be adequate to cover most applications in toxicology. Certain applications may require the use of nonstandard models for which the researcher will be required to consult other sources to derive his or her own solutions. In this chapter, the principles underlying the solutions to mathematical models and their interpretation are emphasized.

The discipline of pharmacokinetics is most closely tied by its history to drug therapy, and a substantial body of the literature is oriented toward this field (Wagner, 1971). In light of this orientation, there are many terms and procedures directed toward the understanding and control of drug therapy. Only the concepts immediately applicable to toxicology are reviewed in this chapter; the drug therapy aspects of pharmacokinetics are not. Several useful texts describing the discipline of pharmacokinetics in a much broader manner are available (Wagner, 1971; Gibaldi and Perrier, 1975; O'Flaherty, 1981; Fiserova-Bergerova, 1983). In addition, there are several overviews of pharmacokinetic principles (Cleland, 1967; Levy and Gibaldi, 1975; Carsen and Jones, 1979; Krügen-Thiemer, 1966, 1969) and a selected bibliography (Corchetto and Wargin, 1980).

The types of models that can be mathematically solved have been an area of current research (Shaw, 1976; Anderson, 1983). Much of this mathematical research is quite advanced and does not necessarily provide an understanding of basic principles. The most important concept emerging from this area is "model identifiability," which can be described as the ability of a profile of the blood concentration to uniquely identify a pharmacokinetic model over time. Statistical and mathematical ideas are also advancing many other aspects of design, analysis, and interpretation of pharmacokinetic studies (Endrenyi, 1981).

The basic one- and two-compartment models that form the basis of many pharmacokinetic studies are described in this chapter. Whenever a chemical is introduced into the bloodstream of a test animal, it distributes itself throughout the blood and to various tissues and organs. If this chemical is transferred only to tissues, which are in instantaneous equilibrium with the blood, then the pharmacokinetic properties of the chemical can be described with a one-compartment model. In this case, the rate at which the concentration in the blood changes is the same as the rate at which the concentration changes in all other tissues. Note that although the actual concentration in these tissues may vary, the entire animal can be viewed as a single unit because the concentrations in the tissues change at the same rate. If, however, the chemical is transferred to tissues that do not respond instantaneously to changes in the blood concentration, then a multicompartmental model must be used to describe the pharmacokinetic characteristics of the chemical.

Some examples of compartment models are shown in Fig. 1. The central compartment denotes the blood and tissues that are in instantaneous equilibrium with the blood, although this compartment may not have any physiological reality. The solid arrows indicate how the chemical can be transferred between compartments and out of the system. The dashed arrows denote the input to the system, which may be intravenous

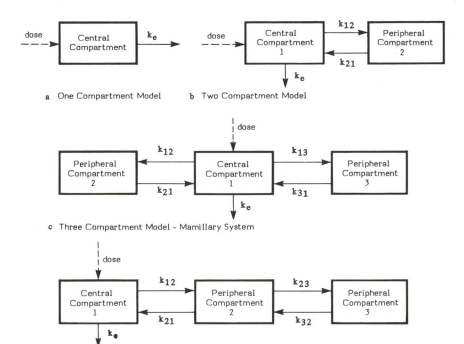

Fig. 1   Some compartment models.

bolus injection, oral dosing, or inhalation. Figure 1a is a one-compart-ment open model that was described previously. In this model, k_e is a parameter characterizing the elimination rate. For the purpose of the models presented in Fig. 1, elimination encompasses all processes that remove the administered chemical from active circulation. It includes physical elimination via urine, feces, or lungs as well as elimination via metabolism and possibly irreversible sequestration. The only character-istic of an eliminated molecule in the compartment models is that it can never reappear in systemic circulation.

In Fig. 1b, there is an additional compartment, with transfer of the chemical allowed between the two compartments. Elimination of the chemical takes place exclusively through the central compartment. In Fig. 1c and 1d, there are two peripheral compartments in addition to the central compartment. These two models are indistinguishable when the blood profile alone is examined (Shaw, 1976). The model shown in Fig. 1c is usually assumed when three-compartment pharmacokinetic models are analyzed.

The models shown in Fig. 1 are open models because the chemical is allowed to escape from the system. In a closed model, the total amount in the system is constant over time. Some researchers include an elimination compartment and sometimes the gastrointestinal tract as a source compartment to create closed models. Thus, a three-compartment model may have different meanings in some studies and publications.

Because all biological processes are first order or can be approximated by first-order processes at low doses (Gibaldi and Perrier, 1975), transfers between compartments and elimination from the central compartment are assumed to obey first-order kinetics. That is, the rate at which the process takes place is proportional to the amount or concentration of the source compartment. The proportionality constants k_e, k_{12}, k_{21}, etc. are called rate coefficients and are sufficient to characterize each transfer process. Inhalation exposure, for reasons described in Section II,C, is assumed to take place via a pseudo-zeroth-order uptake process. Often, biological processes are saturable at high doses, and a brief description of nonlinear rate processes is included in Section V.

It should be recognized that these models provide an oversimplification of the pharmacokinetic properties of the chemical within the body in that one compartment may involve several tissues with similar behavior. The techniques described in this chapter involve repeated measurements on blood or urine from a single animal and cannot be used to determine a correspondence between compartments and specific tissues and organs.

Rate coefficients are used to create a set of differential equations describing the manner in which the level in the compartment changes. These equations are best written in terms of the amounts in the compartment rather than in terms of concentrations in order to satisfy the conditions of mass balance. The equations can then be solved using the procedure of Laplace transforms (Mayersohn and Gibaldi, 1970).

In Sections II through V the mathematical models for pharmacokinetics are developed. The problems of experimental error are ignored in these sections, and it is assumed that observations fit the model exactly. The problems of working with experimental data are described in Section VI. In Section VII, the information on the models and the statistical curve fitting are brought together to give some insight into the setup of suitable pharmacokinetic studies.

II. THE ONE-COMPARTMENT MODEL

The one-compartment model shown in Fig. 1a is the simplest manner in which the conduct of a chemical in the body can be modeled. All tissues invaded by the chemical are assumed to be in instantaneous equilibrium with the blood in this model. The body is assumed to have no barriers that slow the transfer of chemical from one site to another. The behavior of the chemical in the blood compartment reflects exactly its behavior in all involved tissues. Even though the concentration may vary among tissues, note that they are assumed to change concentration instantaneously in proportion to changes in blood concentration. In the following sections, the behavior of the chemical in the blood under various dosing regimens is described.

A. Intravenous Dosing

Let $X_1(t)$ denote the amount of the chemical in the body at time t. The change in the amount in the body is given by the differential equation

$$\frac{dX_1(t)}{d(t)} = -k_e X_1(t) \tag{1}$$

where $dX_1(t)/dt$ denotes the rate of change of $X_1(t)$ with time, and k_e denotes the rate coefficient for elimination. Elimination in this context should not be confused with physical elimination from the body. Metabolism of the chemical as well as excretion through any route (urine, lungs, skin, etc.) can all contribute to the elimination of the compound.

Under intravenous dosing, the amount of chemical in the body at time 0 equals the administered dose (D). Using this side condition, equation (1) can be integrated to yield

$$X_1(t) = De^{-k_e t} \tag{2}$$

The amount in the body cannot be measured (except for radiolabeled compounds), but the concentration in the blood can. If the chemical was homogeneously and uniformly dispersed throughout a volume (V_1), then equation (2) can be divided by V_1 to give

$$C_1(t) = Ae^{-k_e t} \tag{3}$$

where $C_1(t)$ is the concentration in the central compartment and $A = D/V_1$.

Equation (3) describes an exponential decline over time. Taking logarithms on both sides of this equation yields

$$\log[C_1(t)] = \log[A] - \frac{k_e t}{2.303}, \tag{4}$$

where the factor 2.303 is introduced because common logarithms to the base 10 have been taken. From equation (4), it can be seen that a plot of the logarithm of the concentration in the blood against time will be linear

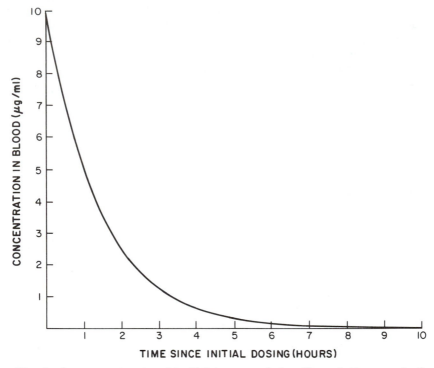

Fig. 2 One-compartment model with intravenous dosing. Change in the concentration of a chemical in the central compartment over time is shown for first-order elimination, with an elimination rate $k_e = 0.693$ hr^{-1} and an initial dose giving a concentration of 10 μg/ml of blood.

with a slope $-k_e/2.303$ and intercept log A. This is illustrated in Figs. 2 and 3. The elimination parameter k_e can be calculated from any two points on the elimination curve by

$$k_e = 2.303 \frac{\log[C(t_1)] - \log[C(t_2)]}{t_2 - t_1}, \tag{5}$$

where $C(t_1)$ and $C(t_2)$ are the concentrations at times t_1 and t_2, respectively. Alternatively, with natural logarithms, equation (5) becomes

$$k_e = \frac{\ln[C(t_1)] - \ln[C(t_2)]}{t_2 - t_1}. \tag{6}$$

In equation (3), A denotes the concentration at the time of dosing. The concentration will decline to half this value after a time $t_{\frac{1}{2}}$:

$$t_{\frac{1}{2}} = 0.693/k_e. \tag{7}$$

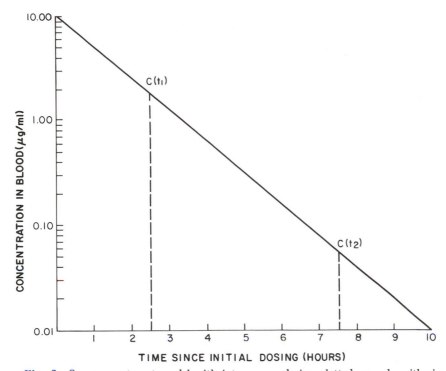

Fig. 3 One-compartment model with intravenous dosing plotted on a logarithmic scale. Changing the vertical axis of Fig. 2 to a logarithmic scale transforms the concentration curve to a straight line. The parameter k_e can be calculated from two points on the line.

This decline to half the current level will occur for every time period of length $t_{1/2}$ and provides a more readily understood method of measuring the rate with which elimination takes place. The length of time to decline by onehalf is called the apparent biological half-life.

The term V_1, which converts amounts to concentrations, is referred to as the apparent volume of distribution. At time 0, the concentration in the blood is given by A. If the administered dose (D) is known, then V_1 can be calculated as

$$V_1 = D/A. \tag{8}$$

This volume, however, may not correspond to any physiological volume within the animal because the chemical may be sequestered in tissues at levels substantially higher or lower than that in the blood. In fact, the apparent volume of distribution has in some instances been calculated as larger than the volume of the animal. The calculated value for V_1, however, when compared to an approximate blood volume can provide some insight into the extent of invasion.

An alternative method of monitoring the conduct of the chemical in the body is to measure the cumulative excretion. The rate of accumulation of the eliminated chemical is given by

$$\frac{dX_e(t)}{dt} = k_e X_1(t), \tag{9}$$

where $X_e(t)$ denotes the cumulative amount eliminated. With equation (1), equation (9) can be solved to yield

$$X_e(t) = D(1 - e^{-k_e t}). \tag{10}$$

In certain situations, elimination may take place exclusively through the urine. Measuring the cumulative amount in the urine can thus provide an estimate of the elimination rate.

B. Oral Dosing

In the previous section, it was assumed that the chemical is administered in a single intravenous bolus dose. However, in many toxicological studies, an animal is dosed orally. Under this regimen, the rate of absorption from the gastrointestinal (GI) tract must be considered in the model. Absorption can take place in several sites (buccal cavity, esophagus, stomach, and large and small intestines) and at different rates within each of these sites. In addition, factors such as GI motility and presence of food in the GI tract can affect absorption of the chemical.

Absorption is assumed to be governed by first-order kinetics in this section. As has been described, this is an extreme simplification of the actual absorption process; however, in many instances, the resulting predicted levels in the blood conform to the observed data. Several alternative models for the absorption process are available (Gladke and von Hattingberg, 1979; Gibaldi et al., 1971; Colburn, 1979) but are substantially more complex. Some procedures for examining the form of the absorption process are available (Wagner and Nelson, 1964; Loo and Riegelman, 1968).

Let $X_0(t)$ and $X_1(t)$ denote the amount of chemical in the GI tract at time (t) while k_a and k_e denote the rate coefficients for absorption and elimination, respectively. The rates of change in the amounts in the GI tract and body are given by the differential equations

$$\frac{dX_0(t)}{dt} = -k_a X_0(t) \tag{11}$$

and

$$\frac{dX_1(t)}{dt} = k_a X_0(t) - k_e X_1(t). \tag{12}$$

To solve these equations with Laplace transforms (Mayersohn and Gibaldi, 1970) yields

$$X_1(t) = \frac{Dk_a}{(k_a - k_e)} (e^{-k_e t} - e^{-k_a t}) \tag{13}$$

where D is the dose administered in the GI tract.

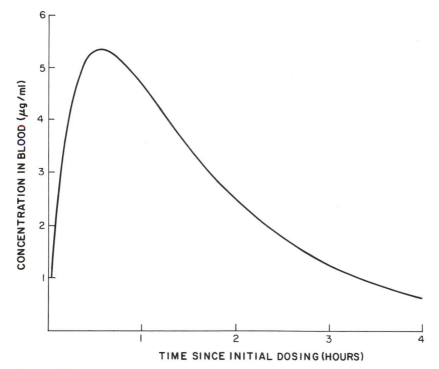

Fig. 4 One-compartment model with oral dosing. Change in the concentration of a chemical in the central compartment over time is shown for a model with first-order elimination ($k_e = 0.693$ hr^{-1}) and uptake ($k_a = 5\ k_e$) and a dose level where $fD/V_1 = 10$ μg/ml of blood.

In the previous formulation, the entire dose is absorbed. In many instances, however, only a fraction of the dose is absorbed (Wagner, 1971). Alternatively, sometimes an appreciable fraction of the dose is metabolized in the liver before reaching the systemic circulation, which is called the first pass effect (Colburn, 1979). The net result of these types of considerations is to multiply the right hand side of equation (13) by the fraction absorbed (f). If both sides of equation (13) are divided by the apparent volume of the central compartment (V_1) and the factor f is introduced, then the equation becomes

$$C_1(t) = A(e^{-\beta t} - e^{-\alpha t}) \tag{14}$$

where

$$A = fDk_a/(k_a - k_e)V_1, \; \alpha = k_a, \text{ and } \beta = k_e. \tag{15}$$

It is usually assumed that absorption has a larger rate coefficient than elimination, that is, that $k_a \geq k_e$ so that $A \geq 0$.

A graph of $C_1(t)$ as opposed to t is shown in Fig. 4. If the log concentration is plotted against time (Fig. 5), then the terminal portion of the elimination curve will be a straight line with slope $-\beta$. This phenomenon in which the slowest process comes to dominate the blood profile is typical of linear kinetic models and can be exploited to obtain graphic estimates of the parameters through a method called feathering the data (also known as curve stripping or curve peeling). This procedure is illustrated in Fig. 5. The points marked with a triangle denote points on the curve. The terminal slope β can be estimated from a straight line drawn through the final portion of the curve and from the application of equation (5). The intercept of this line is ln A. Subtracting the values on the curve prior to the terminal phase from the extrapolated terminal lines provides information on the value of α [i.e., from equation (14)].

$$Ae^{-\beta t} - C_1(t) = Ae^{-\alpha t}. \tag{16}$$

The values for the left-hand side of equation (15) are also plotted in Fig. 5 where it can be seen that these points (marked as circles) lie on a straight line with intercept ln A and negative slope $-\alpha$. In Fig. 5, the observations lie exactly on the equation for the curve. In actual experimental situations, the observations will be scattered about the true curve. Thus, in performing a curve peeling for actual data, one will have to draw a line that best fits the observations in some manner. Problems with the curve-peeling technique as a curve-fitting procedure are described in Section VI on curve fitting and model selection. Curve peeling is used to provide a quick preliminary summary of the data and should be followed with a more detailed statistical analysis as described in Section VI.

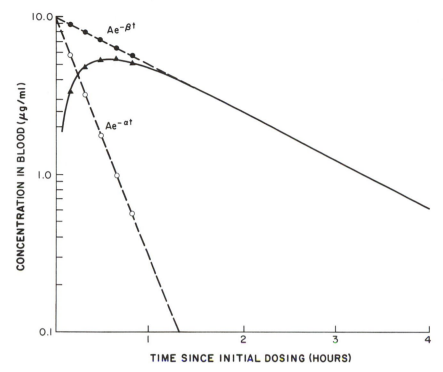

Fig. 5 One-compartment model with oral dosing plotted on a logarithmic scale. Changing the vertical axis of Fig. 4 to a logarithmic scale reveals that the terminal portion of the curve is a straight line with slope $-\beta = -k_e/2.303$. Subtracting points on the initial portion of the curve (▲) from points on the projection of the terminal straight line (●) reveals another straight line (○), with a slope $\alpha = -k_a/2.303$.

Mathematically inclined investigators will note that the solution in equation (11) requires the assumption $k_a \neq k_e$. If $k_a = k_e$, a special solution is required (Gibaldi and Perrier, 1975). If $k_a \leq k_e$, then equation (11) still gives a correct solution (with $A \leq 0$), but the terminal position of the curve provides an estimate of k_a (Gladke and von Hattingberg, 1979). Such situations are rarely encountered.

If the assumption that $k_a \geq k_e$ is considered unwarranted, then k_e can be estimated from an intravenous dosing study on a group of animals. The fitted value of k_e from intravenous dosing can be used to discriminate between the fitted values of k_e and k_a from oral dosing.

The cumulative excretion curve for oral dosing can also be derived from equation (9) if equation (13) is substituted [with the fraction absorbed (f) multiplying the right-hand side] and integrated to give

$$X_e(t) = fD \left(1 - \frac{k_a k_e}{(k_a - k_e)}\right)\left(\frac{e^{-k_e t}}{k_e} - \frac{e^{-k_a t}}{k_a}\right).$$

(17)

This equation rises from 0 at time zero to an asymptotic value of fD. The rate coefficients k_a and k_e can be estimated from the cumulative excretion data provided the elimination from all sources, including metabolites, and all routes of elimination can be collected and distinguished from the portion of the dose that is never absorbed.

The apparent volume of distribution for oral dosing cannot be estimated unless f (the fraction of the dose absorbed) and D are known. In this case, the apparent volume of distribution can be calculated from equation (15) as

$$V_1 = \frac{fD k_a}{A(k_a - k_e)}.$$

(18)

C. Inhalation Dosing

In a study in which the animal is placed in a vapor chamber and exposed to a volatile compound held at a constant concentration over time, the compound will gradually be absorbed through the lungs of the animal and enter the systemic circulation via the pulmonary capillary beds. Absorption of a chemical via inhalation is a complex function (Goldstein *et al.*, 1974) involving tidal volume, respiration rate, and rate of diffusion into the pulmonary capillaries. Absorption is based on diffusion across the surface of the alveoli and hence is a first-order process. The concentration in the alveoli, however, is continuously replenished with each breath the animal takes. Thus, if the small fluctuations in levels between breaths are ignored, the absorption takes place at a constant rate, which is referred to as a pseudo-zeroth-order process. The absorption rate is approximately constant as long as the vapor chamber concentration is held constant, but the absorption rate will increase and decrease in proportion to changes in the ambient concentration.

For the one-compartment model, the rate of change in the amount in the central compartment is given by the differential equation

$$\frac{dX_1(t)}{dt} = K_o - k_e X_1(t)$$

(19)

where K_o denotes the amount of the chemical absorbed per unit time.

Integration of equation (19) and division by the apparent volume of distribution yields

$$C_1(t) = A(1 - e^{-k_e t}) \qquad (20)$$

where

$$A = K_o / k_e V_1. \qquad (21)$$

The blood profile for this equation is shown in Fig. 6. It can be seen that the blood concentration rises to an equilibrium level A, at which the amounts absorbed and eliminated are equal. The blood will attain 50% of this equilibrium level after one half-life of the elimination rate, 90% by four half-lives, and 99% by seven half-lives.

The elimination rate coefficient k_e can be calculated by the method of feathering, provided the blood concentration is monitored until the final plateau level can be discerned. Subtracting the pre-equilibrium values from the equilibrium yields

$$A - C_1(t) = Ae^{-k_e t}. \qquad (22)$$

The right-hand side of this equation is identical to the right-hand side of equation (3), which can be analyzed as previously described.

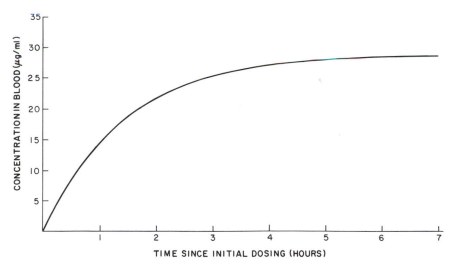

Fig. 6 One-compartment model with inhalation exposure. Accumulation of a chemical in the blood is shown for a continuous zeroth-order exposure at a rate $K_o = 20$ μg/ml/hr with a first-order elimination rate $k_e = 0.693$ hr^{-1}.

The cumulative amount eliminated can be shown from equations (9) and (19) to be

$$X_u(t) = K_o \left[t - \frac{(1 - e^{-k_e t})}{k_e} \right],$$
(23)

which increases without limit. The terminal portion is a straight line with slope K_o. If the infusion rate K_o is known, then the apparent volume of distribution V_1 can be calculated from equation (21):

$$V_1 = \frac{K_o}{k_e A}.$$
(24)

Alternate calculations of the volume of distribution are available (Chiou et al., 1978).

When exposure is terminated, the amount in the body will start to decline following equation (2). If exposure is terminated at time t, the expression

$$A(1 - e^{-k_e t})$$
(25)

is substituted for D in equation (2).

The pseudo-zeroth-order input described in this section can also be used as a model for continuous intravenous infusion (Levy and Gibaldi, 1975).

D. Multiple Dosing

Accumulation of an administered chemical and maintenance of an effective dose under a repeated dosing regimen have been central to much of pharmacokinetic research (Krüger-Thiemer, 1966, 1969). If it is assumed that equally spaced equal doses are given to an animal, then the concentration of the chemical in the blood after the nth dose can be derived from the formulas for a single dose (Gibaldi and Perrier, 1975) if each term of the form $e^{-\delta t}$ is replaced by

$$\frac{(1 - e^{-n\delta\tau})e^{-\delta s}}{(1 - e^{-\delta\tau})},$$
(26)

where τ denotes the dosing interval and s denotes the time since the last dose; that is, the time since the start of the experiment, which can be written as

$$t = (n - 1)\tau + s.$$
(27)

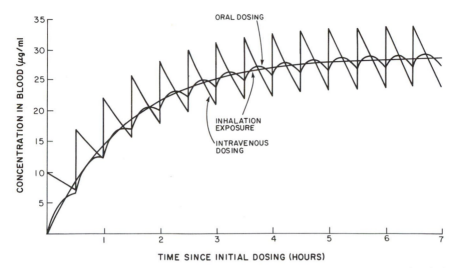

Fig. 7 One-compartment model with repeated exposure. Accumulation of a chemical in the blood is shown for three repeated exposure regimens: (1) inhalation exposure at a rate of 20 μg/ml/hr, (2) repeated intravenous dosing of 10 μg/ml of blood every half hour, and (3) repeated oral dosing with $fD/V_1 = 10$ mg/ml of blood every half hour. For all models $k_e = 0.693$ hr^{-1}, and for the oral dosing model $k_a = 5$ k_e.

In the one-compartment model for intravenous and oral dosing, formulas (3) and (14) for multiple dosing become

$$C_1(t) = \frac{A(1 - e^{-nk_e\tau})\, e^{-k_e s}}{(1 - e^{-k_e\tau})} \tag{28}$$

and

$$C_1(t) = A\left[\frac{(1 - e^{-n\beta\tau})}{(1 - e^{-\beta\tau})}\, e^{-\beta s} - \frac{(1 - e^{-n\alpha\tau})}{(1 - e^{-\alpha\tau})}\, e^{-\alpha s}\right], \tag{29}$$

respectively. The form of these two curves is shown in Fig. 7 along with the curve for inhalation exposure.

The curve for intravenous dosing, equation (28), is a sawtooth shape centered approximately on the curve for inhalation exposure. The curve has peaks corresponding to the time immediately after dosing and minimums corresponding to the dosing interval immediately prior to dosing. The levels eventually attain a stable cycle given by

$$C_1(s) = \frac{A}{(1 - e^{-k_e\tau})}\, e^{-k_e s} \tag{30}$$

Table I

Limiting Maximum and Minimum Concentrations in the
Central Compartment under Repeated Intravenous Dosing
for a One-Compartment Model[a]

Rate of elimination		Dosing interval t (days)			
k_e (day^{-1})	half-life (days)	0.5	1.0	2.0	7.0
6.93	0.1	1.032	1.001	1.000	1.000
		0.032	0.001	0.000	0.000
1.387	0.5	2.000	1.333	1.067	1.000
		1.000	0.333	0.067	0.000
0.693	1.0	3.414	2.000	1.333	1.008
		2.414	1.000	0.333	0.008
0.347	2.0	6.286	3.414	2.000	1.097
		5.286	2.414	1.000	0.097
0.0693	10.0	29.36	14.933	7.725	2.601
		28.36	13.933	6.725	1.601
0.00693	100.0	289.04	144.77	72.64	21.114
		288.04	143.77	71.64	20.114

[a] Upper entry gives limiting maximum and lower entry gives limiting
minimum with A = 1.

where s $(0 \leq s \leq \tau)$ denotes the time since the last dosing. The blood
concentration fluctuates between a maximum of

$$\frac{A}{(1 - e^{-k_e \tau})} \tag{31}$$

and a minimum of

$$\frac{Ae^{-k_e}}{(1 - e^{-k_e \tau})}. \tag{32}$$

These limiting maxima and minima are a function of the elimination
rate and dosing interval as is shown in Table I. For chemicals with a slow
elimination rate, it can be seen that concentrations in the central compartment can rise substantially before a steady rate is reached; whereas if
the elimination rate is fast, there is no appreciable accumulation.

The average level over time during this limiting stable cycle can be
calculated by integrating equation (30) between 0 and τ and dividing by τ
to give

$$\frac{A}{k_e \tau} = \frac{D}{k_e \tau V_1}. \tag{33}$$

$D/\tau V_1$ is the rate of dosing per unit volume of the central compartment.

The blood profile under repeated oral dosing is also shown in Fig. 7. The curve is similar to that for repeated intravenous dosing in that it is scalloped shaped and fluctuates around the inhalation exposure curve, eventually attaining a steady cycle. This limiting cycle is given by the equation

$$C_1(s) = A \frac{e^{-\beta s}}{(1 - e^{-\beta \tau})} - \frac{e^{-\alpha s}}{(1 - e^{-\alpha \tau})}, \tag{34}$$

where s is the time since the last dosing $0 \le s \le \tau$.

The maximum of equation (34) occurs at time

$$s_{max} = \frac{\ln[\alpha(1 - e^{-\beta \tau})/\beta(1 - e^{-\alpha \tau})]}{\alpha - \beta}, \tag{35}$$

and the maximum attained can be derived by substituting s_{max} into equation (34). The minimum occurs when $s = 0$ or $s = \tau$ equals

$$\frac{A(e^{-\beta \tau} - e^{-\alpha \tau})}{(1 - e^{-\alpha \tau})(1 - e^{-\beta \tau})}. \tag{36}$$

Finally, the average blood level during the limiting cycle is found by integrating equation (34), as was done for multiple intravenous dosing. This gives

$$\frac{A(\alpha - \beta)}{\alpha \beta \tau}, \tag{37}$$

which after substituting equation (15) yields

$$\frac{fD}{\tau k_e V_1}. \tag{38}$$

Comparison of equations (21), (33), and (38) shows that the terminal equilibrium level under inhalation exposure equals the average blood level over time for the terminal steady state under repeated intravenous or oral dosing. The terminal equilibrium level is described by two basic parameters: the elimination rate k_e and effective dosing rate reaching the systemic circulation per unit volume of the central compartment (K_o/V_1 for inhalation dosing, $D/\tau V_1$ for intravenous dosing, and $fD/\tau V_1$ for oral dosing). The terminal average blood level over time for oral dosing is independent of the absorption rate k_a.

III. THE TWO-COMPARTMENT MODEL

The one-compartment model is often inadequate to describe the conduct of an administered chemical (Riegelman *et al.*, 1968a). The body may contain various physical barriers through which the chemical compound moves slowly or becomes bound to proteins that can retard its elimination. To account for this, the two-compartment model shown in Fig. 1b was introduced (Teorell, 1937).

In this model, it is assumed that the administered compound can be transferred between a central compartment (compartment 1) and a peripheral compartment (compartment 2). The only route of elimination, however, is assumed to be from the first compartment because the main tissues involved in elimination are well perfused with blood and assumed to be included in the central compartment. The two-compartment model with elimination from both compartments is discussed elsewhere (Kodel and Matis, 1976; Shaw, 1976).

A. Intravenous Dosing

Let $X_1(t)$ and $X_2(t)$ denote the amount of a chemical in the central and peripheral tissue, respectively, at time t. The change in the amount in these two compartments is described by the set of differential equations

$$\frac{dX_1(t)}{dt} = -(k_e + k_{12})X_1(t) + k_{21}X_2(t) \tag{39}$$

and

$$\frac{dX_2(t)}{dt} = k_{12}X_1(t) - k_{21}X_2(t), \tag{40}$$

where k_e denotes the rate coefficient for elimination and k_{12} and k_{21} denote the rate coefficients for transfer from the central to the peripheral and from the peripheral to the central compartments, respectively.

When a single bolus injection (D) is given at time 0, equations (39) and (40) can be solved (Mayersohn and Gibaldi, 1971) to yield

$$X_1(t) = \frac{D}{\beta - \alpha}(k_{21} - \alpha)e^{-\alpha t} - (k_{21} - \beta)e^{-\beta t} \tag{41}$$

and

$$X_2(t) = \frac{Dk_{12}}{\beta - \alpha}(e^{-\alpha t} - e^{-\beta t}), \tag{42}$$

respectively, where α and β are described as hybrid rate coefficients that satisfy the equations

$$\alpha + \beta = k_{21} + k_{12} + k_e \tag{43}$$

and

$$\alpha\beta = k_{21}k_e. \tag{44}$$

With the division of equation (41) by V_1, the apparent volume of the first compartment gives

$$C_1(t) = Ae^{-\alpha t} + Be^{-\beta t} \tag{45}$$

where

$$A = \frac{D(k_{21} - \alpha)}{(\beta - \alpha)V_1} \tag{46}$$

and

$$B = \frac{D(k_{21} - \beta)}{(\alpha - \beta)V_1}. \tag{47}$$

The observed blood profile will appear as shown in Fig. 8. If this curve is plotted on the same graph as that for a one-compartment model with the same terminal portion of the graph, the initial portion of the curve will be much steeper. If the logarithm of the concentration is plotted against time (Fig. 9), then the terminal portion of the curve will be a straight line with slope $-\beta$ and intercept $\ln B$. This curve is sometimes described as biphasic in contrast with the curve derived from equation (3), which is called monophasic. By convention, the slower of the two hybrid rate coefficients is labeled β. The technique of curve peeling can then be used to reveal the coefficients A and α as shown in Fig. 9. Points on the original curve are marked with triangles. Extrapolation of the terminal line is subtracted from these points to give the points marked by circles. These points lie on a straight line with intercept $\ln A$ and slope $-\alpha$. If equation (45) is rearranged, this straight line can be manifested by

$$C_1(t) - Be^{-\beta t} = Ae^{-\alpha t}. \tag{48}$$

Given the values A, α, B, and β, the underlying rate coefficients k_{12}, k_{21}, and k_e can be calculated (Mayersohn and Gibaldi, 1971) by the equations

$$k_{21} = \frac{A\beta + B\alpha}{A + B}, \tag{49}$$

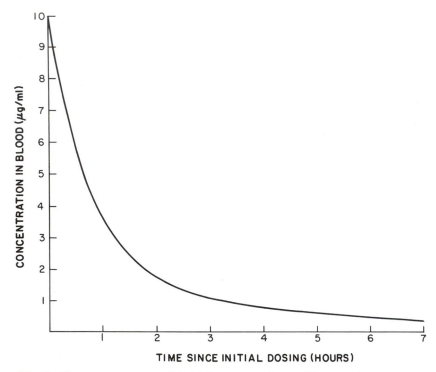

Fig. 8 Two-compartment model with intravenous dosing. Change in the concentration of a chemical in the central compartment over time is shown for a model with $k_e = 0.693\ hr^{-1}$, $k_{12} = k_{21} = 0.6\ k_e$, and an initial dose producing $10\ \mu g/ml$ of blood. The parameters of the concentration curve are $A = 8.201$, $\alpha = 1.3038$, $B = 1.799$, and $\beta = 0.221$.

$$k_e = \frac{\alpha \beta}{k_{21}}, \tag{50}$$

and

$$k_{12} = \alpha + \beta - k_e - k_{21}. \tag{51}$$

The hybrid rate coefficient β describes the terminal portion of the elimination curve. It measures the rate of clearance of the chemical from the body after a type of stable decline rate appears. For this reason, the half-life associated with β is called the biological half-life. From equation (42), it can be seen that the amount in the second compartment also has a terminal elimination with the same rate coefficient. Thus, during this portion of chemical elimination, the amounts in the two compartments attain a constant ratio; a plot of the log of the amounts in the two compartments will give parallel terminal lines. The two compartments,

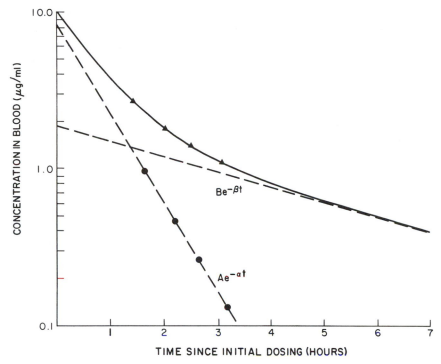

Fig. 9 Two-compartment model with intravenous dosing plotted on a logarithmic scale. Changing the vertical axis of Fig. 8 to a logarithmic scale reveals that the terminal portion of the curve is a straight line with slope $-\beta$ and intercept log (B). Subtracting the projection of this straight line from the original curve produces another straight line with slope $-\alpha$ and intercept log (A).

however, are not in equilibrium during this period (Riegelman *et al.*, 1968a) because the equilibrium condition $k_{12}X_1(t) = k_{21}X_2(t)$ is not satisfied.

Chemical concentration in the central compartment at time 0 is $A + B$ from equation (45). If the administered dose (D) is known, then the apparent volume of distribution of the central compartment can be calculated from the equation

$$\frac{D}{V_1} = A + B \tag{52}$$

or

$$V_1 = \frac{D}{A + B}. \tag{53}$$

As is the case for the one-compartment model, this volume must be interpreted carefully because it may not correspond to a physiological volume. In addition, this calculated volume does not include the volume of the peripheral compartment, hence the chemical may be distributed to a larger volume than that indicated by this calculation.

The volume of the peripheral compartment cannot be estimated from the observed concentration in the central compartment because no measurement of concentration is made in the peripheral compartment. If it is assumed that at equilibrium the two compartments had an identical concentration (Klotz, 1976), one can derive the equation

$$V_1 + V_2 = V_1\left(\frac{k_{12} + k_{21}}{k_{21}}\right). \tag{54}$$

This equation coupled with equation (50) enables a calculation of the total volume involved in the kinetics. Other investigators (O'Flaherty, 1981) suggest using D/B as a measure of volume of distribution, and other definitions exist (Riegelman et $al.$, 1968b).

The total body burden of the chemical at any point in time is given by $X_1(t) + X_2(t)$. When the administered chemical is radiolabeled and the amount remaining in the body measured with a whole-body count, the total body burden is measured. It has been shown that measuring the whole-body amount can dilute the influence of the term with faster decay in the elimination curve and make a two-compartment open model appear similar to a one-compartment model (Wagner, 1968).

The cumulative amount excreted, from equations (9) and (41), is

$$X_e(t) = D\left[1 - \frac{(\beta - k_e)}{(\beta - \alpha)}\,e^{-\alpha t} - \frac{(\alpha - k_e)}{(\alpha - \beta)}\,e^{-\beta t}\right]. \tag{55}$$

This equation is of the form

$$X_e(t) = C - A'e^{-\alpha t} - B'e^{-\beta t} \tag{56}$$

where

$$C = D, \tag{57}$$

$$A' = \frac{D(\beta - k_e)}{(\beta - \alpha)}, \tag{58}$$

and

$$B' = \frac{D(\alpha - k_e)}{(\alpha - \beta)}. \tag{59}$$

Equation (56) can be fitted by curve peeling if the curve-peeling techniques for equations (20) and (45) are combined. The model rate coefficients can then be derived from the equations

$$k_e = \frac{A'\alpha + B'\beta}{C}, \tag{60}$$

$$k_{21} = \alpha\beta/k_e, \tag{61}$$

and

$$k_{12} = \alpha + \beta - k_e - k_{21}. \tag{62}$$

Thus, estimates of the underlying rate coefficients can be made from measurements on cumulative excretion. In situations in which the urine is the exclusive vehicle of elimination, this is feasible. In this situation, it should be verified that the cumulative amount excreted equals the dose given.

B. Oral Dosing

As for the one-compartment model, the conduct of an administered chemical under a single oral dose can be derived. If the GI tract is assumed to feed the chemical into the body exclusively through the central compartment, the amounts in the GI tract and in the central and peripheral compartments are given by the differential equations

$$\frac{dX_0(t)}{dt} = -k_a X_0(t), \tag{63}$$

$$\frac{dX_1(t)}{dt} = k_a X_0(t) - (k_{12} + k_e)X_1(t) + k_{21}X_2(t), \tag{64}$$

and

$$\frac{dX_2(t)}{dt} = k_{12}X_1(t) - k_{21}X_2(t). \tag{65}$$

Solving these equations with Laplace transforms gives the amounts in each compartment at time t. Introducing the fraction of the dose absorbed (f), as is done for the one-compartment model, results in the solutions

$$X_1(t) = fD\gamma \left[\frac{(k_{21} - \alpha)}{(\gamma - \alpha)(\beta - \alpha)} e^{-\alpha t} + \frac{(k_{21} - \beta)}{(\gamma - \beta)(\alpha - \beta)} e^{-\beta t} \right.$$

$$\left. + \frac{(k_{21} - \gamma)}{(\alpha - \gamma)(\beta - \gamma)} e^{-\gamma t} \right] \tag{66}$$

and

$$X_2(t) = k_{12} k_a fD \left[\frac{e^{-\alpha t}}{(\gamma - \alpha)(\beta - \alpha)} + \frac{e^{-\beta t}}{(\alpha - \beta)(\gamma - \beta)} + \frac{e^{-\gamma t}}{(\alpha - \gamma)(\beta - \gamma)} \right]$$

$$\tag{67}$$

where α and β are the hybrid rate coefficients introduced in the solution for intravenous dosing for the two-compartment intravenous model. Thus, equations (43) and (44) also apply as well as

$$\gamma = k_a. \tag{68}$$

Mathematically inclined investigators will note that there are two assumptions implicit in the given solution to the differential equations: k_a does not equal either α or β and k_a does not equal k_{21}. These two assumptions correspond to the assumption that k_a does not equal k_e in the one-compartment model for oral dosing. If either of these two assumptions are violated, a special solution to the differential equations is required.

If equation (66) is divided by V_1, the apparent volume of the first compartment yields

$$C_1(t) = Ae^{-\alpha t} + Be^{-\beta t} - (A + B)e^{-\gamma t}, \tag{69}$$

where

$$A = \frac{fD\gamma(k_{21} - \alpha)}{V_1(\gamma - \alpha)(\beta - \alpha)} \tag{70}$$

and

$$B = \frac{fD\gamma(k_{21} - \beta)}{V_1(\alpha - \beta)(\gamma - \beta)}. \tag{71}$$

A graph of $C_1(t)$ as opposed to t is shown on a linear scale in Fig. 10 and on a logarithmic scale in Fig. 11. The coefficients A, α, B, β, and γ can be determined from this curve by curve-peeling methods similar to those described previously.

In the one-compartment model for oral dosing, it is necessary either to assume that $k_a \geq k_e$ in order to identify the two rate coefficients or to estimate k_e initially from an intravenous dosing study. Similarly, for the

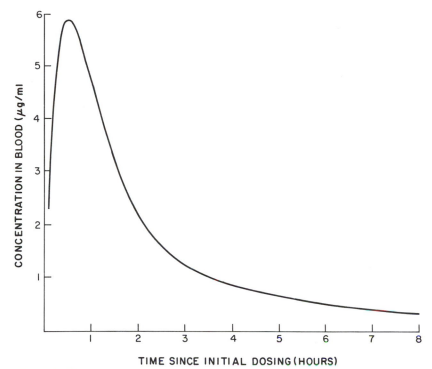

TIME SINCE INITIAL DOSING (HOURS)

Fig. 10 Two-compartment model with oral dosing. Change in the concentration of a chemical in the central compartment is shown for a model with $k_e = 0.693$ hr^{-1}, $k_{12} = k_{21} = 0.6 k_e$, $k_a = 5 k_e$, and an initial dose level $fD/V_1 = 10$ $\mu g/ml$.

two-compartment model described in this section, discriminating between k_e, α, and β cannot be done with the blood concentration curve alone. Although absorption is often considered to be the most rapid of the rate processes, it is not true that the rate coefficient for absorption k_a necessarily will be larger than the hybrid rate coefficients α and β. Calculation of the model rate coefficients should be done under each possible ordering of the coefficients α, β, and γ. This can be done if one rate coefficient (say γ) is designated equal to k_a and if the model rate coefficients are calculated from the equations

$$k_{21} = \frac{A\beta\gamma + B\alpha\gamma - (A + B)\alpha\beta}{A\alpha + B\beta - (A + B)\gamma}, \tag{72}$$

$$k_e = \frac{\alpha\beta}{k_{21}}, \tag{73}$$

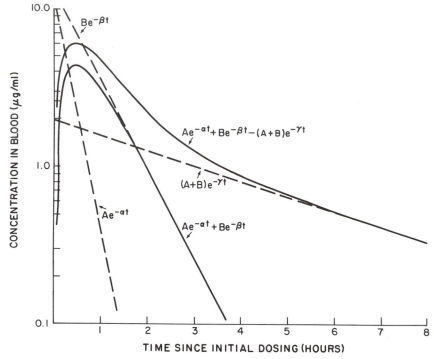

Fig. 11 Two-compartment model with oral dosing plotted on a logarithmic scale. Changing the vertical axis of Fig. 10 to a logarithmic scale reveals that the terminal portion of the curve is a straight line with slope $-\gamma$ and intercept log $(A + B)$. Subtracting the projection of this line from the initial curve reveals another curve with a straight terminal portion [slope $-\beta$ and intercept log (B)]. Finally, subtracting the second curve from the second straight line uncovers a third straight line with slope $-\alpha$ and intercept (A).

and

$$k_{12} = \alpha + \beta - k_e - k_{21}. \tag{74}$$

Examining the three sets of estimates of the rate coefficients may reveal unacceptable estimates for certain rate coefficients (i.e., negative or unrealistically large values), which will eliminate some uncertainty. Alternatively, the hybrid rate coefficients can be estimated from an intravenous dosing study, and the absorption rate coefficient k_a can be determined by elimination.

The apparent volume of the central compartment can be calculated from equation (70) or (71) if the amount absorbed (fD) is known. The total volume of the central and peripheral compartments can be calculated with equation (54), provided the assumption in this calculation is accepted.

C. Inhalation Dosing

If a pseudo-zeroth-order uptake process as described in Section II,C is assumed, the differential equations for the two-compartment model are

$$\frac{dX_1(t)}{dt} = K_o - (k_e + k_{12})\, X_1(t) + k_{21} X_2(t) \tag{75}$$

and

$$\frac{dX_2(t)}{dt} = k_{12} X_1(t) - k_{21} X_2(t), \tag{76}$$

where K_o denotes the amount absorbed per unit time. Solving equations (75) and (76) gives

$$X_1(t) = \frac{K_o(\alpha - k_{21})}{\alpha(\alpha - \beta)}\, (1 - e^{-\alpha t}) + \frac{K_o(\beta - k_{21})}{\beta(\beta - \alpha)}\, (1 - e^{-\beta t}) \tag{77}$$

and

$$X_2(t) = K_o k_{12} \left[\frac{1}{\alpha\beta} + \frac{e^{-\alpha t}}{\alpha(\alpha - \beta)} + \frac{e^{-\beta t}}{\beta(\beta - \alpha)} \right] \tag{78}$$

where α and β, which satisfy equations (43) and (44), are the same hybrid rate coefficients introduced in equation (41). Converting equation (77) to concentration in the central compartment by dividing by V_1 gives

$$C_1(t) = A(1 - e^{-\alpha t}) + B(1 - e^{-\beta t}) \tag{79}$$

where

$$A = \frac{K_o(\alpha - k_{21})}{V_1 \alpha(\alpha - \beta)} \tag{80}$$

and

$$B = \frac{K_o(\beta - k_{21})}{V_1 \beta(\beta - \alpha)}. \tag{81}$$

A graph of $C_1(t)$ against t is shown in Fig. 12. It can be seen that the concentration increases to a limiting value of

$$A + B = \frac{K_o}{V_1 k_e}. \tag{82}$$

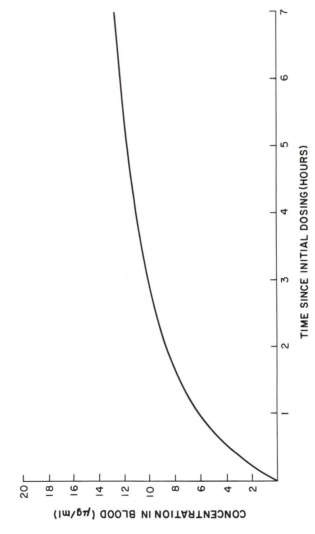

Fig. 12 Two-compartment model with inhalation exposure. Accumulation of a chemical in the blood is shown for a model with $k_e = 0.693 \text{ hr}^{-1}$, $k_{12} = k_{21} = 0.6 \, k_e$ and $k_0 = 10 \, \mu\text{g/ml}$ of blood/hr.

The rate at which this equilibrium value is reached is more difficult to calculate than that for a one-compartment model, but a lower bound can be created with the slower rate coefficient. For example, after one β half-life, the central compartment will have achieved somewhat more than 50% of the final level, and after two β half-lives somewhat more than 75%.

The parameters A, α, B, and β can be calculated from a series of points along the curve by curve peeling, provided the terminal level can be discerned. The values $C_1(t)$ are subtracted from the final value $A + B$, which, from equation (79), gives

$$A + B - C_1(t) = Ae^{-\alpha t} + Be^{-\beta t}. \tag{83}$$

The right-hand side of this equation can be fitted by the same methods of curve peeling described for equation (45).

Given the parameters A, α, B, and β, the underlying rate coefficients can be calculated with the equations

$$k_e = \frac{A\alpha + B\beta}{A + B}, \tag{84}$$

$$k_{21} = \frac{\alpha\beta}{k_e}, \tag{85}$$

and

$$k_{12} = \alpha + \beta - k_e - k_{21}. \tag{86}$$

From equation (78), it is obvious that the chemical levels in the peripheral compartment also rise to a plateau level in which the two compartments are in equilibrium, that is,

$$k_{12}X_1(t) = k_{21}X_2(t) \tag{87}$$

for a sufficiently large t. This equilibrium has been exploited (Withey and Collins, 1979) to provide another procedure to estimate rate coefficients. An animal is exposed in a vapor chamber until equilibrium of a chemical is attained. The exposure is then stopped and the blood level is monitored as it declines. Differential equations for a study of this type are the same as those for intravenous dosing, that is, equations (39) and (40). However the side condition, given in equation (87), is imposed at $t = 0$. Solving these equations and converting to concentrations gives

$$C_1(t) = A'e^{-\alpha t} + B'e^{-\beta t} \tag{88}$$

where α and β are the usual rate coefficients for the two-compartment model,

$$A' = \frac{X_1(o)(\beta - k_e)}{V_1(\alpha - \beta)}, \tag{89}$$

and

$$B' = \frac{X_1(o)(\alpha - k_e)}{V_1(\alpha - \beta)}. \tag{90}$$

Some investigators (Gladke and von Hattingberg, 1979; O'Flaherty, 1981) have stated that after equilibrium is attained, the two-compartment model behaves like a one-compartment model. Equation (88) shows that this is not true. The curve describing the elimination is not linear in the log scale, and this has been demonstrated in actual experiments (Withey and Collins, 1979). The underlying transfer rate coefficients can be derived from the A', α, B', and β in equation (88) by the equations

$$k_e = \frac{A'\alpha + B'\beta}{A' + B'}, \tag{91}$$

$$k_{21} = \frac{A' + B'}{A'/\beta + B'/\alpha}, \tag{92}$$

and

$$k_{12} = \alpha + \beta - k_e - k_{21}. \tag{93}$$

D. Multiple Dosing

As is discussed in Section III,B, it is relatively easy to develop formulas for the blood concentration of a chemical after repeated equally spaced equal doses are given intravenously or orally. Equation (26) can be substituted where appropriate. The two-compartment intravenous dosing model, equation (45), becomes

$$C_1(t) = \frac{A(1 - e^{-n\alpha\tau})}{(1 - e^{-\alpha\tau})} e^{-\alpha s} + \frac{B(1 - e^{-n\beta\tau})}{(1 - e^{-\beta\tau})} e^{-\beta s}. \tag{94}$$

A graph of $C(t)$ as opposed to t is shown in Fig. 13. The blood profile is similar to that for repeated intravenous dosing in the one-compartment model, but this curve can exhibit sharper spikes in the concentration than the curve for the one-compartment model (Withey, 1977).

As t (and n) increase, the curve eventually attains a stable cycle in

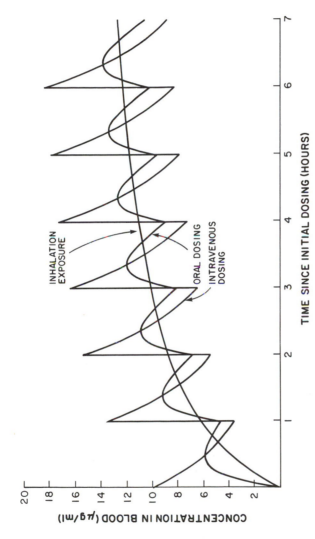

Fig. 13 Two-compartment model with repeated exposure. Accumulation of a chemical in the blood is shown for three repeated exposure regimens: (1) continuous zeroth-order exposure at a rate of 10 μg/ml/hr, (2) repeated intravenous dosing of 10 mg/ml of blood every hour, (3) repeated oral dosing with fD/V$_1$ = 10 mg/ml of blood every hour. For all models k_e = 0.693 hr^{-1}, k_{12} = k_{21} = 0.6 k_e, and for the oral dosing model k_a = 5 k_e.

which the amount of input (D) equals the amount eliminated during each dosing interval. The blood concentration during this cycle is given by

$$C_1(s) = \frac{A}{(1 - e^{-\alpha\tau})} e^{-\alpha s} + \frac{B}{(1 - e^{-\beta\tau})} e^{-\beta s} \qquad (95)$$

where s ($0 \leq s \leq \tau$) denotes the time since dosing. The blood concentration immediately after dosing achieves a maximum of

$$\frac{A}{(1 - e^{-\alpha\tau})} + \frac{B}{(1 - e^{-\beta\tau})} \qquad (96)$$

and declines to a minimum of

$$\frac{Ae^{-\alpha\tau}}{(1 - e^{-\alpha\tau})} + \frac{Be^{-\beta\tau}}{(1 - e^{-\beta\tau})} \qquad (97)$$

immediately prior to dosing.

The average level during this limiting stable cycle is calculated by integrating equation (95) between 0 and τ and dividing by τ. After simplification, equations (49) and (50) can be used to give

$$\frac{A + B}{\tau k_e}. \qquad (98)$$

Similarly, the concentration in the blood after repeated oral dosing can be derived for the two-compartment model if equation (26) is substituted in equation (69), which gives

$$C_1(t) = \frac{A(1 - e^{-n\alpha\tau})}{(1 - e^{-\alpha\tau})} e^{-\alpha s} + \frac{B(1 - e^{-n\beta\tau})}{(1 - e^{-\beta\tau})} e^{-\beta s}$$
$$- \frac{(A + B)(1 - e^{-n\gamma\tau})}{(1 - e^{-\gamma\tau})} e^{-\gamma s}. \qquad (99)$$

This curve is depicted in Fig. 13 along with the ones for repeated intravenous dosing and inhalation exposure. The blood profile increases and decreases in a scalloped curve around the inhalation exposure curve, eventually attaining a stable cycle given by

$$C_1(s) = \frac{A}{(1 - e^{-\alpha\tau})} e^{-\alpha s} + \frac{B}{(1 - e^{-\beta\tau})} e^{-\beta s} - \frac{(A + B)}{(1 - e^{-\gamma\tau})} e^{-\gamma s} \qquad (100)$$

where s denotes the time since dosing. The average level can be calculated by integration. After simplification, in which equations (44), (70), and (71) are used, the average level equals

$$\frac{fD}{V_1 k_e}. \qquad (101)$$

Equations (82), (98), and (101) give the terminal or limiting average level over time for continual dosing. It can be seen that this final level in the central compartment is independent of the rate coefficients involving the peripheral compartment and is identical to those for a one-compartment model [equations (21), (33), and (38)]. As is shown in the one-compartment model, the terminal level for inhalation exposure and limiting average level over time for intravenous or oral dosing are the same.

IV. MORE COMPLEX MODELS

Two variations of the three-compartment model are the mamillary model (Fig. 1c) and the caternary model (Fig. 1d), which is less commonly used. A closed version of the mamillary model was the first type studied (Sheppard and Householder, 1951), and the open mamillary model shown in Fig. 1c was proposed later (Matthews, 1957). With intravenous chemical dosing, both the mamillary and caternary give rise to the equation

$$C_1(t) = Ae^{-\alpha t} + Be^{-\beta t} + Ce^{-\gamma t} \tag{102}$$

where A, B, C, α, β, and γ are complicated functions of the original transfer rate coefficients. Thus, it is impossible to differentiate these two models on the basis of blood concentrations alone. It can further be shown that

$$k_e = \frac{A + B + C}{A/\alpha + B/\beta + C/\gamma} \tag{103}$$

for both models.

Thus, k_e can be estimated without knowing which of the two models is correct. The inability to determine the correct model has led to discussion of whether it is worthwhile to impose an arbitrary model (Wagner, 1975). For example, it may be sufficient to know that a three-compartment model exists without knowing the exact form of the model.

The Laplace transform technique can provide a solution to any linear compartmental model, but for more complex models, the solution can be onerous. Once an equation is solved, the fitted parameters A, α, B, β, C, γ, etc. are used to calculate the underlying rate coefficients of the model. For some models, this calculation is impossible (Shaw, 1975; Griffiths, 1979) and the model is called nonidentifiable. The Laplace transform technique can be avoided through numerical solution of the model, and computer programs that do this are available (Allen, 1982).

V. NONLINEAR PHARMACOKINETICS

Throughout this chapter, it has been assumed that all transfer processes between compartments are first order. However, as described in Chapter 13, many metabolic pathways and other processes are saturable. It can be shown (Wagner, 1969) that, when there are limited receptors for metabolism, the decline in the level of the drug is approximated by the Michaelis–Menton equation.

Consider a one-compartment model for intravenous dosing in which the elimination rate is described by the Michaelis–Menton equation. The differential equation for this model is

$$\frac{dC(t)}{dt} = -\frac{V_m C(t)}{K_m + C(t)} \tag{104}$$

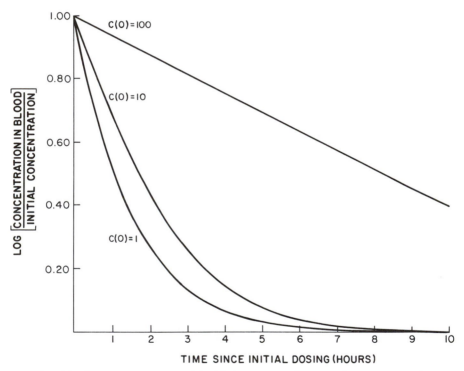

Fig. 14 One-compartment model with intravenous dosing and a Michaelis–Menton equation describing elimination. Decline in the chemical concentration in the blood after initial doses of 1, 10, and 100 μg/ml of blood are shown. The concentrations have been divided by the initial dose so that they can be shown on one graph. The parameters of elimination are $K_m = 10$ μg/ml and $V_m = 6.93$ μg/ml/hr. With an initial dose of 100 μg/ml, the initial portion of the elimination curve is linear.

where V_m and K_m are parameters describing the elimination process. Two special cases can be noted: (1) if K_m is much larger than $C(t)$, equation (104) becomes a first-order decline and (2) if K_m is much smaller than $C(t)$, equation (104) becomes a zeroth-order decline.

Integrating equation (104) gives

$$C(t) + K_m \ln[C(t)] = -V_m t + K_m \ln[C(o)] + C(o). \qquad (105)$$

This equation cannot be solved for $C(t)$ in closed form, but $C(t)$ can be calculated by iteration. Graphs of the concentration and log concentration over time are shown in Figs. 14 and 15, respectively. If the initial concentration is sufficiently high, it can be seen that a plot of concentration against time is initially linear, whereas the plot is curved over the entire range for lower starting concentrations. The logarithm of the concentration, however, always attains terminal linearity. For low doses,

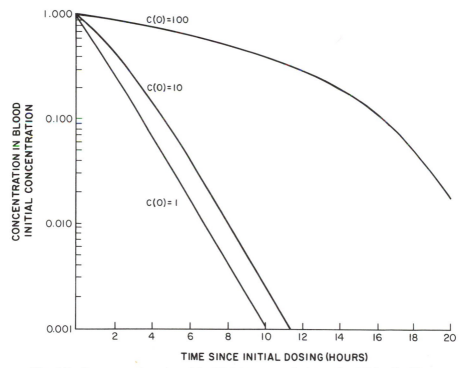

Fig. 15 One-compartment model with intravenous dosing and a Michaelis–Menton equation describing elimination shown in a logarithmic scale. Changing the scale on the vertical axis of Fig. 14 reveals that the terminal portions of the curves for the two lowest doses are linear by 6 hr after dosing, whereas the curve for the largest dose is not linear 20 hr after dosing.

the deviation from linearity is not apparent and behaves essentially like a first-order kinetic elimination curve. It is because of this change in the apparent kinetics with dose that this nonlineal situation is often referred to as dose-dependent kinetics.

In more complex models, incorporation of a saturable process of the form given by equation (104) has been done by several researchers (Wagner, 1969; Wilkinson *et al.*, 1977; Young *et al.*, 1978). These models do not have closed form solutions, and investigating the properties of the solutions is often complicated.

The most important implication of nonlinear kinetics is that concentrations of chemical in the body are no longer proportional to dose, which has serious consequences on the toxicology of the chemical (Anderson *et al.*, 1980; Krewski *et al.*, 1982). Prediction of accumulation for repeated dosing becomes complex because equation (26) is no longer valid.

VI. CURVE FITTING AND MODEL SELECTION

In the previous sections, observations were assumed to fall exactly on the blood concentration–time curve. Under actual experimental conditions, however, the observed values will not lie exactly along a curve for several reasons.

1. The model is only an approximation of the kinetic processes that take place in the animal.
2. The kinetics vary over time due to food consumption, diurnal variation, and external stimuli.
3. Although blood samples are taken, chemical concentrations may vary throughout the animal, immediately after dosing in particular.
4. Chemical analysis of the sample may be imprecise.

From a series of observations of concentrations over time either from blood or urine levels, the question as to how much data can be used to estimate the underlying pharmacokinetic model and its parameters arises. The most basic approach to answering this question is suggested in the preceding sections. The procedure of curve peeling can be used to provide estimates of the parameters of the blood profile curve for any given model. Furthermore, the extent of curve peeling necessary to provide an adequate fit estimates the number of compartments in the model.

The main advantage of curve peeling as a model-fitting technique is that it can be done easily with semilog graph paper and a hand calculator. The disadvantage is that the estimates are based on eye judgments and will vary among individuals. When a one-compartment intravenous dosing model is matched with data that fits the model well, this variation may be unimportant and each estimate of the curve parameters will be similar. However, when a multiphase model is fitted, small discrepancies in the terminal phase of the curve fitting can cause substantial differences in the estimates of the later stages in curve peeling. Therefore, it is advantageous to computerize curve fittings in multiphase models.

Because data do not exactly fit a proposed model, the model that best approximates the data should be chosen. Usually, a least-squares approach is used to fit an equation to a data set. Pharmacokinetic models are nonlinear in the parameters (despite being based on linear kinetics), and the best fitting curve must be found through iteration. Procedures for nonlinear curve fitting are presented in Chapter 24. All nonlinear curve-fitting techniques involve onerous calculations and must be done on a computer. There are several widely available general purpose programs such as BMDP3R (Dixon, 1975) and NLIN (SAS Institute, 1985), as well as several programs written especially for pharmacokinetic curve fitting (Metzler, 1969; Pedersen, 1977; D'Argenio and Schumitzky, 1979; Allen, 1982).

Curve fitting should be done separately for each animal because repeat observations on the same animal can be expected to exhibit serial correlation. Fitting a curve to several animals simultaneously does not take into account the difference within and among animal variability. Estimation of variability, produced by many of the general nonlinear curve-fitting packages, should be treated with caution and used only as a measure of the adequacy of the curve fitting within the animal. The fitted parameters obtained for each animal can be used as input for subsequent statistical analysis of data (e.g., comparisons across dose groups or confidence intervals on the group mean value) because the animal is the experimental unit for this type of study.

Most nonlinear curve-fitting programs require an initial estimate of the parameters of the curve. This can be provided by graphic (curve-peeling) estimates. The programs can then proceed to find the curve that best fits the observed data. These programs, however, are not infallible and should not be expected to provide good parameter estimates with highly variable data. Resultant curves and residuals should always be examined for adequacy of the curve-fitting process (Endrenyi and Wong, 1981). One advantage of computerized curve fitting is the ability to easily examine the effects of various weightings of the data and to discard suspect values on the resultant estimated parameters. A log transform of the fitted curve and observed data is often helpful in improving the scatter of the residuals. This log transform parallels the log transform used in the curve-peeling technique. Alternatively, automatic weighting schemes (Hollins and McCullough, 1971) have been proposed.

Another advantage of computerized curve fitting is that many programs provide estimates of the variance of the parameters. In simple models, these estimates of variance are accurate for samples as small as 12 (Metzler, 1981). In the two-compartment model, the curve can be defined either by the hybrid parameters A, α, B, and β or by the underlying model parameters D/V, k_e, k_{12}, and k_{21}. If the curve is fitted to the underlying parameters, direct estimates of their precision are available (Wong *et al.*, 1979). Otherwise, the procedure of fitting hybrid parameters then estimating underlying parameters with equations (49), (50), and (51) is interchangeable with the procedure fitting the underlying parameters directly. The procedure of fitting the parameters directly has been further studied (Jennrich and Bright, 1976; Allen, 1982) but is still not commonly used.

The appropriateness of least-squares procedures has become a topic of substantial concern to statisticians due to its susceptibility to distortion by outlying observations. Several robust methods of analysis for pharmacokinetic data have been proposed (Rodda *et al.*, 1975; Frome and Yakatan, 1980; Atkins and Nimmo, 1981). Other investigators have proposed marginal likelihood procedures (Minder and McMillan, 1977) or use of the covariance structure of data (Kodel and Matis, 1976) as alternatives to least-squares nonlinear regression for certain pharmacokinetic problems. Robust methods are popular statistical tools to guard against outliers, but some statisticians prefer a judicious discarding of outliers after a careful examination of residuals. Some of these methods can, however, provide more suitable confidence limits for the estimated parameters than least-squares procedures.

Curve fitting for nonlinear kinetic models presents other problems because the equation for the blood profile cannot be written in closed form. A procedure of double interation can be applied, but this is time-consuming and hence expensive (Metzler, 1981). Alternatively, the program NONLIN (Metzler, 1969) can fit differential equations directly, or differential equations can be approximated by difference equations and recast to allow a least-squares curve fitting (Rustagi and Singh, 1977).

The final problem discussed in this section is that of model selection. The curve-peeling procedure of determining the number of compartments is unsatisfactory because it is subjective, and minor errors in determining the terminal phases can cause substantial deviations in the assessment of the initial portion of the curve. A more objective method of estimation is provided by successive fitting of monophasic, biphasic, triphasic, etc., models to data. The improvement can be assessed at each step and compared to the appropriate F statistic. The stepwise analysis can be discontinued when a nonsignificant improvement results. This F statistic is at best approximate and is justified only through analogy to linear models.

VII. EXPERIMENTAL DESIGN

In this section, the information on the models and the statistical curve fitting are brought together to provide some insight into how the required data can best be collected. Number and placement of the times of observation are aspects of experimental design covered in this section. Other important aspects of the experimental process, such as preparing the animal and running pilot studies to obtain initial assessment of the blood profile, are described in Chapter 13.

Basic statistical theory shows that the more observations available, the more precise the results. This advice must be tempered with several realistic constraints imposed by pharmacokinetic studies. For example, the frequency of blood sampling is restricted by the physical limitations of withdrawing a sample without causing arterial collapse, whereas the number of samples collected is restricted because exsanguination will perturb the kinetics under study. Studies on the rat are generally limited to 30 samples in one day, above which physiological disturbance may occur.

The theory of optimal experimental design has been applied to pharmacokinetics (Endrenyi, 1981) but as with many other applications of this theory it has made little impact. One criteria for optimizing an experimental design is called D optimality. Under this criteria, the determinant of the design matrix is minimized. For a model that involves p parameters, D-optimal designs require observations to be taken at p well-defined points. If the sample size (n) is greater than p, then samples are evenly distributed to the p times of observation (Endrenyi and Wong, 1981).

In the one-compartment model, equation (2), for example, implies that two sampling points as widely spaced as possible be used, one immediately after dosing and the other immediately before the chemical concentration in the blood declines below detectable levels. Because the second time point can be determined only if k_e is known, the logic of the procedure is somewhat circular (i.e., one can design an optimal experiment to determine k_e only if k_e is known). An additional drawback to such a design is the lack of information on the suitability of the one-compartment model. In general, pharmacokinetic studies are conducted to provide information on the correct model as well as to fit the parameters of the selected model.

Because the terminal phase of all pharmacokinetic studies determines the biological half-life, which generally dominates all calculations of accumulation and clearance, it should be estimated accurately. It is suggested that a minimum of six points be taken during the terminal phase so that the linearity of the observations can be visually assessed on a semilog plot of the data. Premature termination of the experiment can result in overestimation (Gibaldi, 1968) or underestimation (Gibaldi and Weintraub, 1971) of the biologic half-life or even in incorrect model assignment (DiSanto and Wagner, 1972). Hence, it is recommended that the terminal phase be followed for at least four half-lives or until levels decline below detectable limits.

Multicompartmental models give rise to multiphasic blood profiles. It is well known that equations of the form (45) cannot be fitted accurately with least-squares procedures unless the rate coefficients α and β are well separated. A value of $\alpha/\beta \geq 5$ is recommended for parameter nonredundancy (Reich, 1981). A minimum of six observations is recommended for each phase of the curve to ensure a three-to-one ratio of observations to parameters, which is a reasonable guideline against overfitting curves. One consequence of this recommendation is that the points are not evenly spaced throughout the observation period. Observations are taken more frequently during the initial phases then gradually at wider and wider intervals as the trial progresses.

It has been reported that resolution of the terminal phase of elimination can be improved through repeated intravenous dosing (Gibaldi and Weintraub, 1971; Dittert, 1977). The advantages are considered to arise from attainment of a near tissue-blood equilibrium after repeated dosing, which allowed the terminal decline to manifest itself earlier than a single dosing study would permit. From this logic, it would appear that inhalation exposure until true equilibrium is reached may prove even more superior in this regard.

Monitoring of blood levels is best done separately for each individual animal because pooling of observations from several animals introduces interanimal variability in the model assessment (see Chapter 13). It is inevitable that data come from different animals when organ levels are monitored. Such studies involve sequential kills of animals after various period on test. The variance among animals contributes to the error component in the curve fitting and may substantially reduce the precision of the estimates.

Pharmacokinetic studies can also be based on urine samples. The equations for these studies are presented for several models and dosing regimes throughout this chapter. There are several problems involved in urinary studies (Boxenbaum et al., 1974), which limit their value in comparison with blood monitoring studies. For example, the excreted chemical is held in the bladder for indefinite periods, making calculations of the cumulative amount excreted to time t uncertain. Because the cumulative amount excreted is calculated through summation of all previous determinations, cumulation of all errors will result in the analysis, which violates the primary assumption of independent observations necessary to justify least-squares analysis.

References

Allen, D. M. (1982). Software for fitting linear differential equations to data. *Am. Stat. Assoc. Proc. Statist. Comput. Sect.* 1–6.

Anderson, D. H. (1983). "Compartmental Models and Tracer Kinetics." New York: Springer-Verlag.

Anderson, M. W., Hoel, D. G., and Kaplan, N. L. (1980). A general scheme for the incorporation of pharmacokinetics in low-dose risk estimation for chemical carcinogenesis: Example-vinyl chloride. *Toxicol. Appl. Pharmacol.* **55**, 154–161.

Atkins, G. L., and Nimmo, I. A. (1981). Robust alternatives to least squares curve fitting. *In* "Kinetic Data Analysis: Design and Analysis of Pharmacokinetic Experiments" (L. Endrenyi, ed.) New York: Plenum Press.

Barr, W. H. (1968). Principles of biopharmaceutics. *J. Pharm. Educ.* **32**, 958–981.

Boxenbaum, H. G., Riegelman, S., and Elashoff, R. M. (1974). Statistical estimations in pharmacokinetics. *J. Pharmacokinet. Biopharm.* **2**, 123–148.

Carsen, E. R., and Jones, E. A. (1979). Use of kinetic analysis and mathematical modeling in the study of metabolic pathways in vivo. *N. Engl. J. Med.* **300 (18)**, 1016–1086.

Chiou, W. L., Peng, G. W., and Nation, R. L. (1978). Rapid estimation of volume of distribution after a short intravenous infusion and its application to dosing adjustments. *J. Clin. Pharmacol.* **18**, 266–271.

Cleland, W. W. (1967). The statistical analysis of enzyme kinetic data. *Adv. Enzymol.* **29**, 1–33.

Colburn, W. A. (1979). A pharmacokinetic model to differentiate preabsorptive gut epithelial and hepatic first-pass metabolism. *J. Pharmacokinet. Biopharm.* **7**, 407–415.

Corchetto, D. M., and Wargin, W. A. (1980). A bibliography for selected pharmacokinetic topics. *Drug Intell. Clin. Pharm.* **14**, 769–776.

D'Argenio, D. Z., and Schumitzky, A. (1979). A program package for simulation and parameter estimation in pharmacokinetic systems. *Comput. Prog. Biomed.* **9**, 115–134.

DiSanto, A. R., and Wagner, J. G. (1972). Potential erroneous assignment of non-linear data to the classical linear two-compartment open model. *J. Pharm. Sci.* **61**, 552–555.

Dittert, L. W. (1977). Pharmacokinetic prediction of tissue residues. *J. Toxicol. Environ. Health* **2**, 735–756.

Dixon, W. J., ed. (1975). "Biomedical Computer Programs P Series." Berkeley: University of California Press.

Endrenyi, L. (1981). Design of experiments for estimating enzyme and pharmacokinetic parameters. *In* "Kinetic Data Analysis: Design and Analysis of Pharmacokinetic Experiments" (L. Endrenyi, ed.). New York: Plenum Press.

Endrenyi, L., and Wong, F. H. F. (1981). Tests for the behavior of experimental errors. *In*

"Kinetic Data Analysis: Design and Analysis of Pharmacokinetic Experiments" (L. Endrenyi, ed.). New York: Plenum Press.

Fiserova-Bergerova, V. (1983). "Modeling of Inhalation Exposure to Vapours: Uptake, Distribution and Elimination," Vol. 1 and 2. Boca Raton, Florida: CRC Press.

Frome, E. L., and Yakatan, G. J. (1980). Statistical estimation of the pharmacokinetic parameters in the one-compartment open model. *Commun. Statist.-Simula. Computa.* **B,** 202–222.

Gibaldi, M. (1968). How to utilize biopharmaceutical data in drug evaluation. *Am. J. Pharm. Educ.* **32,** 929–937.

Gibaldi, M., and Perrier, D. (1975). "Pharmacokinetics." New York: Marcel Dekker.

Gibaldi, M., and Weintraub, H. (1971). Some considerations as to the determination and significance of biologic half-life. *J. Pharm. Sci.* **60,** 624–626.

Gibaldi, M., Boyes, R. N., and Feldman, S. (1971). Influence of first pass effect on availability of drugs on oral administration. *J. Pharm. Sci.* **60,** 1338–1340.

Gladke, E., and von Hattingberg, H. M. (1979). "Pharmacokinetics: An Introduction." New York: Springer-Verlag.

Goldstein, A., Aronow, L., and Kalman, S. M. (1974). "Principles of Drug Actions," 2nd ed. New York: Wiley.

Griffiths, D. (1979). Structural identifiability for compartmental models. *Technometrics* **21,** 257–259.

Hollins, J. G., and McCullough, R. S. (1971). Radiation dosimetry of internal contamination by inorganic compounds of cobalt: An analysis of cobalt metabolism in rats. *Health Physics* **21,** 233–246.

Jenrich, R. I., and Bright, P. B. (1976). Fitting systems of linear differential equations using computer-generated exact derivatives. *Technometrics* **4,** 385–392.

Klotz, U. (1976). Pathophysiological and disease induced changes in drug distribution volume: Pharmacokinetic implications. *Clin. Pharmacokinet.* **1,** 204–218.

Kodel, R. L., and Matis, J. H. (1976). Estimating the rate constants in a two-compartment stochastic model. *Biometrics* **32,** 377–400.

Krewski, D., Clayson, D., Collins, B., and Munro, I. C. (1982). Toxicological procedures for assessing the carcinogenic potential of agricultural chemicals. *In* "Genetic Toxicity" (R. A. Fleck and A. Hollaender, eds.). New York: Plenum Press.

Krüger-Thiemer, E. (1966). Formal theory of drug dosage regimens I. *J. Theor. Biol.* **13,** 212–235.

Krüger-Thiemer, E. (1969). Formal theory of drug dosage regimens II. The exact plateau effect. *J. Theor. Biol.* **23,** 169–190.

Levy, G., and Gibaldi, M. (1975). Pharmacokinetics. *In* "Handbook of Experimental Pharmacology" (O. Eicher, A. Farah, H. Herkin, and A. D. Welch, eds.).

Loo, J. C. K., and Riegelman, S. (1968). New method for calculating the intrinsic absorption rate of drugs. *J. Pharm. Sci.* **57,** 918–928.

Matthews, C. M. E. (1957). The theory of tracer experiments with ^{131}I-labeled plasma proteins. *Phys. Med. Biol.* **2,** 36–53.

Mayersohn, M., and Gibaldi, H. (1970). Mathematical methods in pharmacokinetics, I: Use of the Laplace transform for solving differential rate equations. *Am. J. Pharm. Educ.* **34,** 608–614.

Mayersohn, M., and Gibaldi, H. (1971). Mathematical methods in pharmacokinetics, II: Solution of the two-compartment model. *Am. J. Pharm. Educ.* **35,** 19–27.

Metzler, C. M. (1969). "A User Manual for NONLIN." Kalamazoo, Michigan: Upjohn.

Metzler, C. M. (1981). Statistical properties of kinetic estimates. *In* "Kinetic Data Analysis: Design and Analysis of Pharmacokinetic Experiments" (L. Endrenyi, ed.). New York: Plenum Press.

Minder, C. E., and McMillan, I. (1977). Estimation of linear compartmental model parameters using marginal likelihood. *Biometrics* **33,** 333–341.

O'Flaherty, E. J. (1981). "Toxicants and Drugs: Kinetics and Dynamics." New York: Wiley.

Pedersen, P. V. (1977). Curve fitting and modeling in pharmacokinetics some practical experiences with NONLIN and a new program FUNFIT. *J. Pharmacokinet. Biopharm.* **5,** 513–531.

Reich, J. G. (1981). On parameter redundancy in curve fitting of enzyme data. *In* "Kinetic Data Analysis: Design and Analysis of Pharmacokinetic Experiments" (L. Endrenyi, ed.). New York: Plenum Press.

Riegelman, S., Loo, J. C. K., and Rowland, M. (1968a). Shortcomings in pharmacokinetic analysis by conceiving the body to exhibit properties of a single compartment. *J. Pharm. Sci.* **57,** 117–123.

Riegelman, S., Loo, J. C. K., and Rowland, M. (1968b). Concept of a volume of distribution and possible errors in evaluating this parameter. *J. Pharm. Sci.* **57,** 128–133.

Rodda, B. E., Sampson, C. B., and Smith, D. W. (1975). The one-compartment open model: Some statistical aspects of parameter estimation. *Appl. Statist.* **24,** 309–318.

Rustagi, J. S., and Singh, U. (1977). Statistical analysis of compartmental models with applications to pharmacokinetics and bioavailability. *In* "Applications of Statistics" (P. R. Krishnaiah, ed.). New York: North Holland.

SAS Institute (1985). "SAS User's Guide: Statistics," 5th ed. Cary, North Carolina: SAS Institute.

Shaw, B. K. (1976). Data analysis problems in the area of pharmacokinetics research. *Biometrics* **32,** 145–157.

Sheppard, C. W., and Householder, A. S. (1951). The mathematical basis of the interpretation of tracer experiments in closed steady state systems. *J. Appl. Phys.* **22,** 510–520.

Teorell, T. (1937). Kinetics of distribution of substances administered to the body. *Arch. Int. Pharmacodynam. Ther.* **57,** 205–240.

Wagner, J. G. (1968). Half-life and volume of distribution. *Drug Intell. Clin. Pharm.* **2,** 126–133.

Wagner, J. G. (1969). Aspects of pharmacokinetics and biopharmaceutics in relation to drug activity. *Am. J. Pharm.* **141,** 5–20.

Wagner, J. G. (1971). "Biopharmaceutics and Relevant Pharmacokinetics," 1st ed. Hamilton, Illinois: Drug Intelligence Publications.

Wagner, J. G. (1975). Do you need a pharmacokinetic model, and, if so which one? *J. Pharmacokinet. Biopharm.* **3,** 457–477.

Wagner, J. G., and Nelson, E. (1964). Kinetic analysis of blood levels and urinary excretion in the absorptive phase after single doses of drug. *J. Pharm. Sci.* **53,** 1392–1403.

Wilkinson, P. K., Sedman, A. J., Sakmar, E., Kay, D. R., and Wagner, J. G. (1977). Pharmacokinetics of ethanol after oral administration in the fasting state. *J. Pharmacokinet. Biopharm.* **5**, 207–224.

Withey, J. R. (1977). The role of pharmacokinetics in the design and conduct of chronic exposure studies, *Int. Congr. Ser. Excerpta Med.* **440**, 190–195.

Withey, J. R., and Collins, P. G. (1979). The distribution of styrene monomer in rats by the pulmonary route. *J. Environ. Pathol. Toxicol.* **2(6)**, 1329–1342.

Wong, D., Colburn, W. A., and Gibaldi, M. (1979). Fitting concentration-time data to biexponential equations. *J. Pharmacokinet. Biopharm.* **7**, 97–100.

Young, J. D., Braun, W. H., and Gehring, P. J. (1978). Dose dependent fate of 1,4 dioxane in rats. *J. Toxicol. Environ. Health* **4**, 709–726.

15
Principles and Procedures in Behavioral Toxicity Testing

Deborah C. Rice
Toxicology Research Division
Food Directorate
Health Protection Branch
Health and Welfare Canada
Ottawa, Ontario

I. INTRODUCTION

Toxicologists are becoming increasingly aware of the need to monitor more subtle indicators of toxicity than signs of morbidity, such as weight loss, change in food or fluid intake, and gross pathological and light microscopic findings. Attention has focused in recent years on testing of the functional output of organ systems, including the immune, endocrine, hematopoietic, and nervous systems. It has become clear that one of the most insidious functional change in humans produced by the population's exposure to toxic substances is behavioral (Table I). Many toxic substances act primarily on the nervous system, including heavy metals

Table I
Selected Examples of Neurotoxic Effects in Humans

Toxic substances	Neurotoxic effects
Metals	
Mercury (alkyl)	Sensory disturbances (visual, auditory, somatosensory), tremors, ataxia, confusion, memory loss
Lead	Peripheral neuropathy; in children encephalopathy, mental retardation, learning and attention difficulties
Cadmium	Peripheral neuropathy, anosmia
Arsenic	Paresthesia, peripheral neuropathy, anosmia
Manganese	Motor disturbances, tremor, speech disturbances, psychiatric symptoms
Solvents	
Acrylamide	Paresthesia, ataxia, tremor, psychiatric symptoms, peripheral neuropathy
Carbon disulfide	Paresthesia, anosmia, depression
Toluene	Ataxia, slurring of speech, psychiatric symptoms
Pesticides	
Organochlorine (DDT, chlordecone)	Ataxia, tremor, confusion, memory disorders, personality disorders
Organophosphorus	Sensory disturbances (auditory, visual, somatosensory), ataxia, peripheral neuropathy, memory disorders, personality disorders, psychiatric symptoms (psychoses)

such as mercury, lead, and manganese; organic solvents such as carbon disulfide and toluene; pesticides such as organophosphates; and air pollutants such as carbon monoxide. Often, changes in nervous system function result from years of exposure to these chemicals, either in the workplace or in the environment. In addition, many toxic agents that perturb other body systems and produce pain, discomfort, fatigue, or secondary effects on nervous system function affect behavior as well.

The field of behavioral toxicology arose to monitor these health effects because they are recognized as important. Methods available to the practitioner of behavioral toxicology are many and varied and can be drawn from the fields of experimental psychology, behavioral pharmacology, and the broad umbrella of the neurosciences. Indeed, an advantage in pursuing the effects of toxicants on behavior is the wide range of methodology available to determine neurotoxic effects.

Behavioral toxicology is receiving increasing recognition by various regulatory agencies around the world. Presently, the United Kingdom and Japan require neurotoxicity testing, and the U.S. Environmental

Protection Agency (EPA) has developed testing protocols to address specific aspects of behavioral toxicity testing (U.S. EPA, 1985, 1986). Several important workshops have been convened recently (U.S. Food and Drug Administration, 1986; U.S. National Research Council, 1986; World Health Organization, 1986) to characterize available behavioral methodology in detail and to make recommendations on strategies of behavioral toxicity testing. An important collaborative behavioral teratology study, organized by the U.S. National Center for Toxicological Research and performed in six independent laboratories in the United States, has demonstrated a high degree of interlaboratory reliability regarding behavioral methodology (Buelke-Sam *et al.*, 1985). Such recent developments underscore the firm foundation upon which behavioral toxicological methodology is based and the increasing recognition of its importance in toxicity testing.

II. GENERAL STRATEGY

A. Choice of Tests

Behavioral toxicity testing can easily be incorporated into traditional testing protocols, with methodologies appropriate to acute, subchronic, chronic, and reproductive phases of chemical (or drug) testing. Typically, observation of the animal is part of traditional toxicological protocols and can serve as an indicator of possible neurotoxic effects. Signs such as lethargy or hyperactivity, piloerection, convulsions, ataxia, abnormal gate, tremor, and abnormal maternal behavior may be indicative of neurotoxicity. If such signs are observed, more detailed analyses can be incorporated into further testing protocols, including chronic or reproductive studies. Animals or a subset of animals committed to other toxicity studies can often be used for behavioral testing. Thus, behavioral testing, like other specialized toxicity testing such as immune or endocrine, need not (indeed should not) be performed in isolation from the data gathered in traditional toxicity studies.

The choice of behavioral methods runs the gamut from gross, simple observation requiring no equipment to extremely sophisticated measurements of specific nervous system functions. Each level of testing has advantages and disadvantages and occupies an appropriate place in the hierarchy of toxicity testing. It has been suggested that a "tiered" approach be used in toxicity testing including behavioral testing (National Academy of Sciences, 1975; U.S. Food and Drug Administration, 1986; World Health Organization, 1986). Such a scheme can begin with simple, rapid, and inexpensive tests to determine if behavioral effects are present then progress to tests of increasing complexity, duration, and cost (Table II). For chemicals for which there are no behavioral data, testing should begin at relatively high doses during an acute exposure, for example, as part of an acute toxicity study. A number of investigators have proposed observational batteries designed to assess major overt neurotoxic effects of chemicals (Irwin, 1968; Gad, 1982). These batteries consist of a series of semiquantitative measures such as tremor, convulsions, ataxia, autonomic signs, paralysis, surface righting, and posture. Such batteries are appropriate in initial toxicity testing because they utilize semiquantitative subjective measures and are rapid and easy to implement. In addition, food and water consumption and body weight should be considered in the context of behavioral assessment.

Following the initial observational battery, there are a number of somewhat more specific tests available that may still be considered "screening procedures" because they are relatively nonspecific. A variety of such screening test batteries has been proposed (cf. Adams and Buelke-Sam, 1981; Mitchell et al., 1982; Buelke-Sam et al., 1985; Vorhees, 1986) and may include such measures as negative geotaxis and surface righting, orientation to stimuli (visual, auditory, olfactory), auditory startle habituation, locomotor activity, and simple learning. The best strategy is to choose a number of tests that assess different functions, such as motor, sensory, and "cognitive" functions. Although a well-developed battery is capable of yielding important information about "where to look next", it must be remembered that the results of screening tests are not useful for determining no-effect levels because they lack the necessary sensitivity.

If effects are observed on any of the screening tests, a more detailed behavioral analysis should be made. Testing will typically include examination of learning and memory, intermittent schedules of reinforcement, and perhaps more detailed evaluation of sensory and motor function. At this level of testing, it is necessary to evaluate toxicity carefully in other organ systems. Performance on a behavioral task may be altered by the animal being ill (e.g., from liver damage) as well as by primary changes in nervous system function. Toxicity in other organ systems must be considered in the evaluation of behavioral data. Failure to recognize nonspecific effects may result in attribution of behavioral changes to specific deficits, such as memory or motor deficits, when the findings are, in fact, the result of toxicity in organ systems other than the nervous system.

The final level of testing is designed to characterize in detail the nature of the toxic effect and to determine the lowest level at which any effect is observable. The most sensitive methodology is used with the most appropriate species. Exposure should be relevant to the human situation in

Table II
Sample Scheme for Behavioral Toxicity Testing[a]

Type of exposure	General	Screening (Tier 1)	Tier 2	Tier 3
Acute or subacute	Food/water consumption Weight Gross ataxia or abnormal posture Lethargy or excitement Convulsions Tremor	Orientation Reflex startle Habituation Hind limb splay Grip strength Locomotor activity (quantified)	Intermittent schedules Simple learning tests Avoidance procedures	
Subchronic or chronic			Intermittent schedules Modulation of reflex startle Simple learning (simple discrimination, mazes, avoidance procedures)	Psychophysical procedures (sensory) Complex learning (matching to sample, discrimination reversal, repeated acquisition) Complex motor performance
Reproduction	Teratogenicity Behavior of dam Physical milestones (tooth eruption, etc.) Food/water consumption of dam Gross ataxia or abnormal posture Lethargy or excitement Convulsions Tremor	Orientation Reflex startle Habituation Locomotor activity	Intermittent schedules Modulation of reflex startle Simple learning	Complex learning

[a] The number of tiers included in this example are arbitrary, for purposes of clarity. Numbers suggested by different *ad hoc* groups vary from two to four.

terms of level, duration, and route of chemical or drug administration. Such testing should be carried out for any agent to which large numbers of people are exposed, and for which there is good evidence of nervous system toxicity.

For many agents, some information will be available concerning behavioral effects. These data may be derived from animal studies or from human exposure. If the substance is a known neurotoxicant, there is no need to perform a screening battery. Other simple procedures may also be omitted. This will be especially true if the signs and symptoms of poisoning are known in humans. In such a case, experimental work should be focused on determining a no-effect level with tests that reflect the important effects in humans. If a toxicant is known or strongly suspected to affect a certain neurotransmitter system, then behavioral tests can be chosen that are known to affect the pathways involved. This is particularly relevant for some pesticides, for example.

The species chosen should be the most appropriate available with sensitivity to the toxicant similar to that of humans; that is, signs of toxicity in the test animal should be as similar to those observed in humans as possible and should occur at comparable body burdens. If motor or sensory systems are affected, these systems in the animal should be anatomically and functionally similar to the human. Similarly, if intellect or memory are impaired by the toxicant, characterization of subtle deficits requires a species with relatively sophisticated intellectual ability.

B. General Considerations

For screening procedures, the rat or mouse will typically be the species of choice. The number of animals should be relatively large because these techniques are relatively insensitive and often produce large between-subject and/or within-subject variability. As more sophisticated tests are used to characterize the toxic effects, the rodent may often not provide an appropriate model. Cats are a better choice for determining toxicity to the visual system, for example, although this species does not have the same acuity or color vision as humans or other primates. For some kinds of sensory and "cognitive" testing, the monkey is the only appropriate choice. This greatly increases cost and usually results in only a few animals being tested. In some instances, the more sophisticated methodology (e.g., psychophysical procedures) decreases variability to a point at which valid conclusions may be drawn only from a few test animals. For many procedures, however, testing a small number of animals significantly decreases sensitivity; therefore, it can be disadvantageous to use procedures so complicated that only a few animals may be tested.

During the initial stages of testing (such as during acute toxicity testing), doses will be high, often producing gross toxicity, for example, weight loss, changes in food and water consumption, changes in body temperature, and ataxia. Detailed behavioral testing at these doses is not warranted because behavioral effects will be due partly or totally to gross toxicity. For example, malnutrition is known to produce behavioral changes, including intellectual impairment, in rodents (Sobotka *et al.*, 1976; Peters, 1979), primates (O'Connell *et al.*, 1978), and humans (Cabak and Najdanvic, 1965). If behavioral changes are observed at high doses, more detailed behavioral testing must be done with dosing and exposure regimens relevant to human exposure levels. This will more than likely entail chronic exposure or chronic intermittant exposure, with route of administration usually being oral ingestion or inhalation, or occasionally percutaneous. At the chronic level of testing, behavioral monitoring must be carried out in conjunction with monitoring of other measures of toxicity in order for the general health status of the animal to be known concurrently. Only in this way will it be possible to determine whether the behavioral effects are the result of a chemical's primary effect on the nervous system or the result of its toxic effect on other organ systems. In addition, such monitoring is necessary to determine whether the nervous system is the most sensitive (or one of the most sensitive) system to the effects of the toxicant. Sophisticated behavioral testing is contraindicated when doses produce gross toxicity or when it is obvious that other systems are more sensitive.

Screening procedures typically require interaction of the experimenter and subject during testing. As well, observational batteries often include subjective scoring. In order to avoid bias, the experimenter must be blind to the treatment group of the animals under test. At higher levels of testing, equipment should be automated to eliminate interaction of experimenter and subject, which always produces an unknown number of unqualifiable variables even if the experimenter does not know to which treatment group the subjects belong. If at all possible, all personnel (technicians, animal handlers) should be blind to group assignments to avoid unintentional differential handling of treated and control subjects. The environment should be kept as stable as possible because factors such as change of room, handlers, or feeding and watering routine may significantly affect the behavior of the animal. This is particularly true for nonrodent species. Changes that are unavoidable should be made gradually and systematically. The time of day of testing may affect the behavior of individuals. The best strategy for keeping variability to a minimum is to test any individual at the same time each day while balancing dose groups across time. If it is of interest to test an individual at different times throughout the day (for locomotor activity, for example), such manipulations should be made according to a balanced design and analyzed accordingly.

The period of development during which an organism is exposed to a toxicant is an extremely important variable in the magnitude and type of toxicity produced. Perinatal exposure can produce functional alterations at levels insufficient to produce overtly toxic signs (cf. Adams and Buelke-Sam, 1981). Perinatal exposure can also produce toxic effects qualitatively different from those resulting from adult exposure. For example, methylmercury produces sensory and gait disturbances in the adult; but in the infant, it produces severe mental retardation, cerebral palsy, and even death at doses only slightly toxic to the mother (Weiss, 1983). The geriatric population may also be at greater risk from toxic insult. It is well known that elderly people are more sensitive to drugs, yet virtually no experimental work has focused on whether aging increases sensitivity to the effects of toxicants. Probably the most important question is whether lifetime exposure to low levels of toxicants produces intellectual impairment or psychological symptoms in the middle aged or contributes to severe deterioration of mental function in the elderly. It seems feasible that such issues can be explored in rodents that live only two or three years. For example, Spyker (1975) found that methylmercury toxicity became apparent in old mice that had appeared to be healthy when younger.

C. Experimental Design and Data Interpretation

Experimental designs fall into two broad categories, within-subjects and between-groups designs. In a within-subjects design, each subject serves as its own control. Typically, a baseline of response is established, then performance is monitored during or after toxicant exposure. In a between-groups design, the performance of groups is compared. A within-subject design is used to generate acute dose-effect functions, whereas a between-group design is frequently necessitated by longitudinal or developmental (including behavioral teratology) studies. A variant of the within-subject design may also be useful for following the course of toxicity produced by chronic exposure to a chemical as well as for determining reversibility. In this paradigm, a control group may also be included to assess changes in baseline performance across time in the absence of toxic exposure.

In behavioral toxicology, as in other areas of toxicology, it is important to include statistical considerations in the design of a study. Usually, it will be possible to estimate the number of subjects required to detect an effect (if present) from behavioral data previously gathered for the toxicant of interest and/or from the proposed behavioral methodology. For example, the relatively large variability observed in many primary tests may necessitate more subjects per group, but fewer subjects may be needed in secondary test groups. Conversely, a within-subject design in which each subject serves as its own control will typically require fewer subjects per group than a between-groups design. Psychophysical procedures for characterization of sensory deficits, in which the performance of control subjects should vary minimally from each other or in which the within-subjects design is used, will also require relatively few subjects. If a threshold calculation or a no-effect level is required, such considerations should also be included in the study design. A statistician should be consulted regarding number of treatment groups required and range and assignment of doses.

Teratological or other protocols designed to assess developmental effects present some additional issues. The statistical handling of possible litter and gender effects must be considered when the study is designed because it potentially affects the number of subjects required. In longitudinal studies, age effects must be considered in both analysis and interpretation. If the same subjects are tested on a number of behavioral endpoints in different order, it may be appropriate to consider order effect in the statistical analysis. For example, in behavioral teratology studies, screening procedures such as simple assessment of motor or sensory function may require that portions of each group be tested at different ages because large numbers of subjects cannot feasibly be tested on the same day. Similarly, a crossover design may be used such that one test is performed on day 5 and another on day 9, for example, with half the subjects receiving each test at the specified age.

A feature common to many behavioral experiments is that repeated measures of the same parameter are collected from each subject. This is often combined with small numbers of subjects in each treatment group, particularly for secondary or tertiary tests. The typical statistical method applied to such a design by psychologists is the analysis of variance (ANOVA) for repeated measures. Indeed, the ANOVA has been suggested as the procedure of choice for behavioral teratology studies (Butcher and Nelson, 1985). The ANOVA is powerful in detecting changes over the course of repeated measurement, the B effect, but has much less power to detect effects between groups, the A effect. To behavioral toxicologists, the B effect is seldom of interest; the A effect (and possibly the AB interaction) are the statistics of interest. In addition, behavioral data often violate the assumptions of normality and independence of covariance required for parametric analysis (see Chapter 16).

Another common design feature, similar to the collection of repeated data points of the same parameter, is the collection of several or even many parameters from each subject in one experiment. In lengthy chronic or longitudinal studies, the same subjects may participate in a number of behavioral tests over the course of the experiment. Typically, the number of subjects compared to the number of parameters measured is too few to allow the use of standard multivariate techniques. It is often desirable to use statistical techniques more elegant and holistic than large numbers of individual comparisons, which in any case may be too conservative if the α level is distributed over all comparisons (as in the Bonferoni procedure).

An important aspect of behavioral data often ignored is variability, both intra- and intersubject. For example, variability in the treated group(s) may often be greater than in the control group (Cory-Slechta *et al.*, 1981; Rice, 1985) due to the presence of responders and nonresponders among the treated subjects (Good, 1979; Cox, 1981) or to the fact that the treatment affects animals differentially. On the other hand, the variability in the treated group(s) may be less than that of the controls due to "ceiling" or "floor" effects in the performance of treated subjects. In either event, the differences in intersubject variability may represent a legitimate toxicological endpoint. (Performance on intermittent schedules of reinforcement illustrates these phenomena. For example, the same dose of a drug such as amphetamine may increase rates of response in some subjects and decrease it in others, depending on baseline rate of response and individual susceptibility to the psychoactive effects of amphetamine. Thus, there may be a change in between-subject variability under drug treatment even in the absence of an overall difference in the average response rate between drug and nondrug conditions.) Similarly, the intrasubject variability of performance, either within or between test sessions, may differ between control and treated subjects even after the data are normalized for absolute magnitude of response (Rice, 1983, 1984a; Rice and Gilbert, 1985). Such differences in intrasubject variability may be sensitive indicators of toxicity and deserve analysis in their own right.

If the data are to be used in risk assessment (and even if they are not), it may be desirable to determine the sensitivity of the study to detect an effect after the study is completed. The change required for an effect to be detected given the number of subjects, the variability of data, and the chosen α (usually 0.05) may be calculated by such measures as the coefficient of detection. For example, in a collaborative behavioral teratology study in which six independent laboratories participated, coefficients of detection for most measures ranged between 10 and 50%, suggesting that the studies as designed were adequate to detect a treatment effect if one existed (Buelke-Sam *et al.*, 1985). On the other hand, performance on an intermittent schedule of reinforcement by a group of lead-treated monkeys and controls (Rice *et al.*, 1979) required at least a 400% difference in performance between the groups in order to be detected (Rice, 1980), given the number of animals (four per group) and variation between animals. This is a huge difference, such that if no effect had been detected, these results would require cautious interpretation.

III. BEHAVIORAL DEFINITIONS

Behavior may be defined as anything an organism does — any move an organism makes. The behavior of an organism at any moment is the result of the external environment, the past history of the organism, and the internal environment (biochemical or electrical processes, hormonal levels, etc.) within the organism. The behaviorist studies the functional relationship between the behavior of an organism and these variables. The behavioral toxicologist includes exposure to a chemical as one of these variables. An aspect of the environment that controls behavior in a functional manner is termed a stimulus. A unit of behavior, defined by the experimenter, is termed a response. There are two types of responses: respondent and operant. In addition, either type of response may be unconditioned (unlearned) or conditioned (learned).

Respondent behaviors include such actions as smooth muscle contraction, autonomic responses, glandular secretions, and elicited motor responses such as reflexes. Unlearned respondents are used frequently in observational batteries and include such measures as orienting to stimuli or reflex startle to intense stimuli. In the Soviet Union, learned respondents are used extensively in toxicology (Pavlenko, 1975). The famous experiment of Pavlov, in which dogs learned to salivate at the sound of a bell after numerous pairings of the bell being followed by presentation of food, is an example of a conditioned respondent. Respondents are paired with an eliciting stimulus in a one-for-one relationship (i.e., bell–salivation).

Operant responses, on the other hand, have no single eliciting stimuli but occur within the context of many environmental stimuli. The consequences of a certain behavior affect the probability that this behavior will be produced again. Locomotor activity is often given as an example of an unlearned operant (Tilson and Harry, 1982) because there is no attempt on the part of the experimenter to condition a particular type of response. An extremely powerful tool at the disposal of the behavioral toxicologist is that of operant conditioning (cf. Laties, 1982). Operant conditioning takes advantage of the control that the immediate outcome of behavior has in determining the subsequent frequency of similar behavior. If the outcome of a particular behavior increases its frequency, it is termed a positive reinforcer (i.e., food). If it decreases the frequency, it is called negative reinforcer (i.e., shock). The great strength of this technique is that it may be used to teach a large variety of tasks with wide complexity. Questions can be asked about attention, learning, memory, sensory function, and general well-being of the subject. Many techniques discussed in this chapter rely on the principles of operant conditioning. Behavioral assessment would be impossible without a thorough understanding of these principles on the part of the investigator.

IV. SPECIFIC METHODS IN BEHAVIORAL TOXICOLOGY

For the purposes of discussion, the behavior of organisms can be divided into motor function, sensory function, learning and memory, and performance on intermittent schedules of reinforcement. These classes are somewhat arbitrary, and virtually all behavioral tests measure more than one of these functions. For example, motor function affects almost all testing; intact sensory function is necessary for learning; performance on intermittent schedules most certainly has a learning component, and so forth. Often, different functions are not separable by one test or type of test; therefore, it is imperative to study several types of behavior to determine the function(s) that is affected. It should be pointed out that none of the procedures described in the following sections should be examined in isolation because all are part of a comprehensive investigation of the potential behavioral effects of a toxicant.

The examples of tests presented in each section are certainly not an exhaustive list but were chosen because they are often used or because they promise to contribute substantially to the understanding of behavioral toxicity. Similarly, the references cited are representative examples and do not constitute a review of the behavioral toxicology literature.

A. Motor Function

Deficits in motor function are frequently produced in humans as a result of their toxic exposure to a chemical. Heavy metals such as mercury, lead, and manganese; insecticides such as chlordecone (Kepone) or organophosphorus compounds; and air pollutants such as carbon disulfide all produce changes in motor function. Gross assessment of motor function should be performed as part of an initial toxicity screen. Batteries that

include observational assessment of muscle tone, body posture, equilibrium, and gross coordination have been suggested (Irwin, 1968; Gad,
1982). The next level of testing includes such techniques as ability to stay
on a rotating rod or quantification of hindlimb splay. The former requires
an automated apparatus as well as animal training and practice in order
to reduce test variability to acceptable levels. The latter technique is
simpler, involving the placement of ink on the paws of rodents after
which they are dropped from a specific height (Edwards and Parker,
1977). Quantification of hindlimb splay does not require training of the
animal and is fast and easy. Gilbert and Maurissen (1982) compared
these two methods using three toxicants known to affect motor function.
They found both techniques to be approximately equal in sensitivity,
although the splay test was slightly more sensitive under certain conditions. Another screening procedure for assessment of neuromotor function requires that a rodent grasp a bar attached to a strain gauge after
which the animal is pulled on manually until it lets go (Tilson and Cabe,
1979). Assessment of swimming ability is also suitable for incorporation
into screening tests. The rodent is placed into a pool of water and such
measures as swimming movement, position in the water, and ability to
keep the head above water are assessed. These analyses may reveal motor
deficits that are not apparent during locomotion on land (Spyker et al.,
1972).

Little work has been focused on more sophisticated tests for assessing
neuromuscular function. One promising procedure employs operant techniques to train an animal to depress a lever within a specific force band
and time period (Falk, 1970), thus allowing assessment of the effects of
toxic agents on fine motor control or strength.

The test that probably is used most extensively in screening for nervous system toxicity is locomotor activity, in large part because no training is required and activity can be measured rapidly. Locomotor activity
represents the functional output of many systems of the body, including
but certainly not exclusively motor systems. In addition, although such
measurements may appear straightforward, there are many variables
that must be considered. Motor activity is not a single activity but
consists of many acts, such as horizontal and vertical movement, sniff-
ing, rearing, grooming, and scratching. With some types of measuring
devices, even tremor may be monitored. There are, therefore, many
methods of monitoring, including scoring the classes of movement by
observation, measuring horizontal movement only, measuring vertical
displacement with devices that gauge force generated against the floor,
and combinations of these measurements. Even within a class of automated devices, there is large variability in the configuration of each

apparatus and in the method of measurement. With different kinds of apparatuses, different behaviors can be measured.

When a toxicant is introduced, activity may increase, decrease, or remain unchanged depending on choice of apparatus, age of the animal, relative novelty and complexity of the environment, and many other variables (Reiter and MacPhail, 1982). Although a change in an animal's activity as the result of its exposure to a toxicant indicates a change in the function of its nervous system, interpretation is not straightforward. The change can be due to the toxicant's primary effect on nervous system function or to its effect on some other system that results in a secondary effect on nervous system function. Certainly, extrapolation from activity measurements in rodents to such phenomena as "hyperactivity" in children is unwarranted, both because of the lack of consistency in the experimental work and because such syndromes in humans do not consist exclusively, or necessarily, of increases in motor activity.

B. Sensory Function

Sensory disturbances often result from human exposure to toxic agents, both as vague symptoms reported by the patient and as clearly demonstratable deficits in sensory function. Deficits in visual, auditory, and tactile functions have been reported for a variety of toxicants, including metals (methylmercury and lead) acrylamide, solvents, and pesticides (Iwata, 1980; Spencer and Schaumberg, 1980). A variety of techniques, from very simple to extremely sophisticated, has been utilized to assess sensory function in animals exposed to toxicants. Probably the grossest of these is the orienting response (Marshall, 1975), which consists of observing whether the animal turns toward a crude stimulus (click, light, touch, etc.). Such a procedure is subjective, nonspecific, and insensitive and indicates only the possibility of gross sensory impairment. The auditory startle reflex and discrimination learning tests are often viewed as tests of sensory function. However, there are many other systems involved in these tests; therefore, sensory effects may not be discriminable from motor effects, learning and memory, and attention abilities (Evans, 1978).

An extremely promising technique for sensory system evaluation is modulation of reflex startle by presentation of a low intensity stimulus immediately prior to a high intensity stimulus that elicits the startle response (Hoffman and Ison, 1980). Such a technique may be used to estimate sensory threshold, and sensory deficits may be differentiated from nonsensory, such as motor, deficits (Fechter and Young, 1983). This technique is, therefore, specific and reasonably sensitive. It has the advantage of being inexpensive and rapid and requires no training of the animal.

Operant training of an animal allows a very detailed evaluation of sensory function. Such techniques are time-consuming and sometimes expensive, but they are useful for careful characterization of toxicant effects for which there is good evidence of sensory impairment. The species chosen for testing must have sensory function as similar to humans as possible. For visual system testing, for example, the rodent is usually not an appropriate model because its visual system differs in fundamental ways from that of humans.

Animals can be trained to report reliably and in great detail about their sensory perception. This is accomplished through "psychophysical" techniques; that is, sensory function is determined by behavioral means. Such methodology is appropriate for determination of no-effect levels and for detailed characterization of toxic effects. Conditioned suppression (Smith, 1970) is a useful technique for estimating sensory thresholds. A steady baseline rate of responding (such as a lever pressing or licking) is established by use of an intermittent schedule of reinforcement. A test stimulus is presented to an animal several times during its ongoing behavior and signals a specific latency (usually two or three minutes) to an unavoidable electric shock. The animal decreases its rate of response (suppresses) during the stimulus in anticipation of the shock, which indicates that the animal detects the stimulus. This technique can be employed to estimate threshold and to detect changes in threshold produced by a toxicant (Hendricks, 1966; Henton, 1969; Nienhuys and Clark, 1978).

Stebbins et al. (1966) characterized the thresholds for detection of sound over the range of frequencies normally detectable in the monkey, and the effect of an ototoxic agent on these thresholds. They did this by training the monkey to keep its hand in contact with a sensor until it detected the onset of a tone and to break its contact upon detection of the tone. Intensity of the tone was then varied for each frequency tested to determine the intensity at which the monkey was unable to detect the tone. The researchers were thus able to follow the development of hearing loss produced by an ototoxic antibiotic, from initial high frequency loss to later low frequency loss. These changes in hearing in the monkey were correlated with the pattern of receptor loss in the inner ear (Stebbins and Rudy, 1978).

A psychophysical procedure was also used to determine the spatial visual function of monkeys exposed chronically to methylmercury, but showed no overt signs of poisoning (Rice and Gilbert, 1982). In this experiment, the monkey faced two oscilloscopes, one blank and one displaying vertical bars. The monkey had access to two levers, one corresponding to each oscilloscope. The task was to respond on the lever corresponding to the scope on which the bars appeared. The oscilloscope displaying the bars varied randomly from trial to trial. The frequency and darkness of the bars was varied in a systematic manner, allowing a determination of the spatial visual function of each monkey. Monkeys exposed to methylmercury were found to have deficits of high but not low frequency spatial vision. Similar behavioral techniques have been used to characterize visual (Merigan *et al.*, 1982) and somatosensory (Maurissen *et al.*, 1983) impairment produced by acrylamide. Such studies demonstrate the power of operant techniques in detection of very subtle sensory deficits, which may be the only discernable effects of a toxicant at low level exposure.

C. Learning and Memory

Loss of memory and inability to concentrate are symptoms frequently reported as a result of human exposure to toxicants such as PCBs, solvents, methylmercury, and pesticides. Further, developmental exposure may produce mental retardation or learning impairment (Needleman *et al.*, 1979; Clarkson *et al.*, 1981). It is therefore of great value to test such abilities in animals as markers of toxic effect. There are many techniques available for assessment of learning and memory. Aside from gross screening procedures, this area has probably received the most attention from behavioral toxicologists. Techniques range in complexity from those appropriate for screening to characterization of specific deficits. A screening procedure that is often considered a test of learning is habituation (Cabe and Eckerman, 1982), which is a progressive decrease in reactivity to repeated presentations of a stimulus. Reactivity can be measured in terms of response of the whole organism, as in startle or orienting, or in terms of habituation of a discrete reflexive response, such as blinking. Obviously, habituation must be differentiated from motor effects, fatigue, and sensory adaptation. It is a measure of gross integration of the nervous system and may not involve the higher centers.

A learned behavior that is obviously of adaptive advantage to an animal is its ability to avoid a substance that it ingested shortly before the onset of an illness or adverse effect. This conditional taste aversion can be used to measure toxicity, for example, by pairing a novel taste (a sugar treat, for example) with administration of a toxicant. If the animal feels ill soon afterward, it will avoid the novel substance in the future. This technique has proved to be sensitive to the effects of neurotoxic agents (MacPhail, 1982).

At the next level of sophistication, avoidance procedures (utilizing negative reinforcement) are frequently used. Passive avoidance procedures require the animal (rodent) to refrain from leaving a specific area in order to avoid a shock to the feet. Active avoidance requires the animal to move from a specific area at the onset of a cue in order not to be shocked. These procedures are greatly affected by the baseline level of arousal and ongoing motor activity of the animal. It may often be the case that a toxicant produces an effect on one and not on the other of these avoidance tests, or affects the behavior in opposing ways, depending on whether the animal is more or less active than the control animal. These tests, therefore, are considered rather nonspecific.

Discrimination tasks have proved useful in detecting effects of toxicants on learning and memory. The procedure most often employed is termed a "forced choice" because the animal is presented with two or more stimuli simultaneously and must indicate its choice by some operant response. These tasks are typically one of two types: spatial and nonspatial. With spatial discrimination, the animal must respond to a certain position (i.e., left) in order to be reinforced. A nonspatial task requires responding to a specific stimulus (pattern, color, direction of a tone) regardless of position. Different operants may be utilized in discrimination testing. For rodents, mazes of various sorts are often employed, whereas for other species (as well as for rodents) operants besides locomotion are utilized.

Primates are often tested in a Wisconsin General Testing Apparatus (WGTA; Harlow and Bromer, 1938). The monkey faces a panel on which stimuli are placed. A reinforcement, such as a raisin, is placed in a recessed well under the correct stimulus. The monkey's response consists of displacing one of these stimuli; if the choice is correct the reinforcement is collected. Automated apparatuses are used with all laboratory species. Typically, the response consists of pressing one of several available levers or push buttons in order to signal the choice. Levine *et al.* (1977) have developed a technique for rodents in which a photocell beam is interrupted with the nose as an operant. The technique requires no training by the investigator and may be used with young animals.

Discrimination tasks have proved to be sensitive to impairment resulting from exposure to lead (Cory-Slechta, 1984). The difficulty of the task may be an important variable on the effects of a toxicant on performance. For example, Winneke *et al.* (1977) found that rats exposed to lead were deficient in their ability to discriminate size but not in their ability to discriminate the orientation of lines.

Once the task is learned, a discrimination reversal paradigm provides additional information on the animal's learning ability. The previously correct stimulus becomes the incorrect one, so that the animal is required to learn a response opposite from the one previously learned. The discrimination reversal paradigm may often be more sensitive to neurotoxicity than simply acquisition of discrimination tasks, as has been found in monkeys exposed to lead early in life (Bushnell and Bowman, 1979a, 1979b; Rice and Willes, 1979; Rice, 1985).

There are several other means to test spatial orientation or memory that require little or no training of the animal. An apparatus appropriate for use with rodents is the radial arm maze. Typically, this maze consists of a central arena from which radiate a number of arms like spokes of a wheel. The end of each arm is baited with a reinforcement, and the animal simply has to find all the reinforcements within a certain period of time. The most economical strategy is to enter each arm only once. There obviously need not be a memory component to this task, depending on the strategy adopted by the animal (i.e., "always turn left"). Similarly, motor impairment confounds this task because the number of reinforcements collected in a specified time is the typical dependent variable. The neurotoxicant trimethyltin has been found to disrupt a rodent's ability to perform this test (Walsh et al., 1982b). A somewhat analogous task used for primates is the Hamilton Search Task. A row of boxes, each containing a reinforcement, is presented to the monkey. The monkey can collect the reinforcement from each box by lifting the lid; again, the most economical approach is to lift each lid only once. This test differs from the radial arm maze in that a delay is instituted between responses during which the boxes are withdrawn from the monkey's reach, thus making memory more likely a component of the performance. (It is possible to institute a delay in the radial arm maze as well, but this is most often not done.) Monkeys exposed to lead postnatally required more trials to learn to perform this task than did their controls (Levin and Bowman, 1983).

There are several operant tasks that offer the opportunity to separate an animal's learning from its performance of a known task (Thompson and Moerschbaecher, 1978). Repeated acquisition is such a task and requires the animal to learn a new sequence of lever presses each session. The learning baseline may be more sensitive to disruption by a toxicant than the performance of an already acquired sequence.

A task that tests attention and short-term memory is matching to sample. Monkeys are most typically used for these tasks, although other species also are capable of learning them. In a nonspatial matching-to-sample task, for example, the animal is presented with a stimulus (color, pattern, object) that is then withdrawn. Following this, a set of stimuli are presented, and the animal indicates which of these is identical in some dimension to the sample stimulus. Delays of various durations may be instituted between the presentation of the sample and test stimuli to test short-term memory. Such tasks have been found to be sensitive to effects produced by lead in monkeys who were exposed to it in early life (Rice, 1984b).

D. Intermittent Schedules of Reinforcement

Performance generated by intermittent schedules of reinforcement has played an important role in behavioral pharmacology and is proving a useful tool in behavioral toxicology (Laties, 1982). On an intermittent schedule, an animal is not reinforced for every response but for a number of responses according to certain "rules". There are a number of excellent reviews on principles and procedures of schedules of reinforcement (Ferster and Skinner, 1957; Reynolds, 1958; Kelleher and Morse, 1968; Schoenfeld, 1970). Most intermittent schedules are based on reinforcing the organism as a function of the number of responses emitted, some temporal requirement for emission of responses, or a combination of these. For example, a fixed ratio (FR) schedule requires the animal to emit a fixed number of responses in order to be reinforced. A fixed interval (FI) schedule, on the other hand, requires that a certain fixed length of time elapse before a response is reinforced. Although only one response need be emitted at the end of the interval for reinforcement, the organism typically emits many responses during the interval. Interval schedules generally generate a lower rate of responding than do ratio schedules. The FI schedule generates a characteristic pattern of responding for which a variety of parameters may be analyzed. These parameters are potentially sensitive to disruption by psychoactive agents (Kelleher and Morse, 1968). Another schedule of some utility in behavioral toxicology is the differential reinforcement of low rate (DRL) schedule in which the animal is required to wait a specified time between responses in order to be reinforced.

Intermittent schedules may also be maintained by negative reinforcement, usually by a brief mild electric shock. The most popular of these is continuous or "Sidman" avoidance in which each response postpones a shock by a fixed amount of time. By spacing its successive responses within this time interval, the animal may postpone shock indefinitely. This schedule is particularly useful as a comparison to behavior generated by positive reinforcement if a toxicant is suspected of producing anorexia. Simple intermittent schedules such as these have been used fairly widely in behavioral toxicology, and have proved to be sensitive to the effects of a number of industrial and environmental toxicants (Padich and Zenick, 1977; Dietz et al., 1978; Geller et al., 1979; Zenick et al., 1979; Shigeta et al., 1980; Alfano and Petit, 1981; MacPhail and Leander, 1981; McMillan, 1982; Walsh et al., 1982a; Rice, 1984a; Rice and Gilbert, 1985).

Intermittent schedules of reinforcement can be combined to form more complicated schedules such as multiple schedules of reinforcement. For example, if fixed ratio and fixed interval schedules are presented to an animal in succession during a single test session, the resulting multiple schedule is termed a multiple FR-FI schedule. Each component of the multiple schedule is independent and occurs in the presence of a different external discrimination stimulus that signals the schedule component in effect. Schedule components are typically presented in an alternating fashion, first one schedule and then the other; this allows the investigator to collect data on both types of behavior almost simultaneously. This schedule in particular has proved to be useful in detecting behavioral toxicity (Levine, 1976; Dews and Wenger, 1979; Leander and MacPhail, 1980; McMillan, 1982).

Multiple schedules offer the investigator an opportunity to study behavior controlled by different variables, which may be differentially sensitive to the effects of a toxicant. For example, toluene produced a decrease in test animals' response rate in the FR component and an increase in their response rate in the DRL component of a multiple schedule (Colotla et al., 1979); further, the relative sensitivity of the two components was different. Similarly, the animals' response in the FI component of a multiple FR-FI was sensitive to disruption by methyl n-amyl ketone (Anger et al., 1979), whereas their response in the FR component was not. The FI component of the multiple FI-FR schedule was more sensitive to disruption in both monkeys (Rice, 1984a) and rodents (Angell and Weiss, 1982) who sustained developmental lead exposure.

Schedules of reinforcement may be used to monitor toxic effects other than or in addition to direct effects on the central nervous system. These may include peripheral nervous system toxicity, or damage to some other organ systems resulting in general malaise or the animal's feeling "sick" (Laties, 1982). For example, acrylamide, an organic solvent that produces a "dying back" axonopathy, produced decreases in animals' FR response rate (Tilson et al., 1980). The FR schedule typically produces high response rates and thus may be sensitive to impaired motor function. Rats exposed to ozone decreased their responding on an FI schedule, which was interpreted as a decrease in their motivation as a result of the general discomfort produced by ozone (Weiss et al., 1981).

E. Social Behaviors

Animals, particularly mammals, engage in a wide variety of social, sexual, and maternal (or paternal) behaviors that are multidimensional and extremely complex. Despite the obvious importance of social behavior in humans, very little research has been focused on the effects of toxicants on social interactions, and the utility of such interactions in behavioral toxicology is unknown. The reason for this may be the enormous number of variables, which necessitates focusing on only a few parameters to the exclusion of all others. Moreover, many of these behaviors are specific to certain species (for example, grooming, pup retrieval, submissive gestures, etc.), raising the question of the validity of extrapolation to human behavior.

V. CONCLUSIONS

Behavior is the functional output of the nervous system and, as such, represents the most reliable and easily interpretable indicator of nervous system toxicity. It is becoming increasingly apparent that xenobiotically induced damage to the nervous system represents a significant hazard to humans, especially as a result of chronic and/or developmental exposure. Behavioral testing will play a significant part in toxicity testing in the future and should be integrated into other toxicity testing, especially in chronic studies.

If little is known about an agent, screening tests are the appropriate starting point. It must be remembered that these tests are both insensitive and nonspecific. If positive results are obtained, specific testing must be carried out at lower dose levels and/or for longer duration. Agents known to be neurotoxic from episodes of human poisoning need to be evaluated carefully with sophisticated methodology. Careful evaluation may also be appropriate for chemicals dispersed throughout the environment to which large segments of the population are exposed.

References

Adams, J., and Buelke-Sam, J. (1981). Behavioral assessment of the postnatal animal: Testing and methods development. *In* "Developmental Toxicology" (C. A. Kimmel and J. Buelke-Sam, ed.), pp. 233–257. New York: Raven Press.

Alfano, D. P., and Petit, T. L. (1981). Behavioral effects of postnatal lead exposure: Possible relationship to hippocampal dysfunction. *Behav. Neural. Biol.* **32,** 319–333.

Angell, F., and Weiss, B. (1982). Operant behavior of rats exposed to lead before or after weaning. *Toxicol. Appl. Pharmacol.* **63,** 62–71.

Anger, W. K., Jordan, M. K., and Lynch, D. W. (1979). Effects of inhalation exposure and intraperitoneal injections of methyl n-amyl ketone on multiple fixed-ratio, fixed-interval response rates in rats. *Toxicol. Appl. Pharmacol.* **49,** 407–416.

Buelke-Sam, J., Kimmel, C. A., and Adams, J., eds. (1985). Design considerations in screening for behavioral teratogens: Results of the collaborative behavioral teratology study. *Neurobehav. Toxicol. Teratol.* **7(6).**

Bushnell, P. J., and Bowman, R. E. (1979a). Reversal learning deficits in young monkeys exposed to lead. *Pharmacol. Biochem. Behav.* **10**, 733–742.

Bushnell, P. J., and Bowman, R. E. (1979b). Persistence of impaired reversal learning in young monkeys exposed to low levels of dietary lead. *J. Toxicol. Environ. Health* **5**, 1015–1023.

Butcher, R. E., and Nelson, C. J. (1985). Design and analysis issues in behavioral teratology testing. *Neurobehav. Toxicol. Teratol.* **7**, 659.

Cabak, V., and Najdanvic, R. (1965). Effects of undernutrition in early life on physical and mental development. *Arch. Dis. Child.* **40**, 532–534.

Cabe, P. A., and Eckerman, D. A. (1982). Assessment of learning and memory dysfunction in agent-exposed animals. *In* "Nervous System Toxicology" (D. L. Mitchell, ed.), pp. 133–198. New York: Raven Press.

Clarkson, T. W., Cox, C., Marsh, D. O., Myers, G. J., Al-Tikriti, S. K., Amin-Zaki, S., and Dabbagh, A. R. (1981). Dose-response relationships for adult and prenatal exposures to methylmercury. *In* "Measurement of Risk" (G. G. Berg and H. B. Maillie, eds.), pp. 56–77. New York: Plenum Press.

Colotla, A., Bautista, M., Lorenzana-Jimenez, M., and Rodriguez, R. (1979). Effects of solvents on schedule-controlled behavior. *Neurobehav. Toxicol. Suppl. 1* **1**, 113–118.

Cory-Slechta, D. A. (1984). The behavioral toxicity of lead: problems and perspectives. *In* "Advances in Behavioral Pharmacology" (T. Thompson and P. Dews, eds.), Vol. IV, pp. 211–255. New York: Academic Press.

Cory-Slechta, D. A., and Thompson, T. (1979). Behavioral toxicity of chronic postweaning lead exposure in the rat. *Toxicol. Appl. Pharmacol.* **47**, 151–159.

Cory-Slechta, D. A., Bissen, T., Young, M., and Thompson, T. (1981). Chronic postweaning lead exposure and response duration performance. *Toxicol. Appl. Pharmacol.* **60**, 78–84.

Cox, C. (1981). Detection of a treatment effect when only a portion of subjects respond. *In* "Nutrition and Behavior" (S. A. Millar, ed.), pp. 285–289. Philadelphia: The Franklin Institute Press.

Dews, P. (1982). Epistemology of screening for behavioral toxicity. *In* "Nervous System Toxicology" (C. L. Mitchell, ed.), pp. 229–236. New York: Raven Press.

Dews, P. B., and Wenger, G. R. (1979). Testing for behavioral effects of agents. *Neurobehav. Toxicol. (Suppl. 1)* **1**, 119–127.

Dietz, D. D., McMillan, D. E., Grant, L. D., and Kimmel, C. A. (1978). Effects of lead on temporally-spaced responding in rats. *Drug Chem. Toxicol.* **1**(4), 401–419.

Edwards, P. M., and Parker, V. H. (1977). A simple, sensitive and objective method for early assessment of acrylamide neuropathy in rats. *Toxicol. Appl. Pharmacol.* **40**, 589–591.

Evans, H. Y. (1978). Behavioral assessment of visual toxicity. *Environ. Health Perspect.* **26**, 53–57.

Falk, J. L. (1970). The behavioral measurement of fine motor control: Effects of pharmacological agents. *In* "Readings in Behavioral Pharmacology" (T. Thompson, R. Pickens, and R. A. Meich, eds.), pp. 223–236. New York: Appleton-Century-Croft.

Fechter, L. D., and Young, J. S. (1983). Discrimination of auditory from non-auditory toxicity by reflex modulation audiometry: Effects of triethyltin. *Toxicol. Appl. Pharmacol.* **70**, 216–227.

Ferster, C. B., and Skinner, B. F. (1957). "Schedules of reinforcement." New York: Appleton-Century-Crofts.

Gad, S. C. (1982). A neuromuscular screen for use in industrial toxicology. *J. Toxicol. Environ. Health* **9,** 691–704.

Geller, I., Mendez, V., Hamilton, M., Hartmann, R. J., and Gause, E. (1979). Effects of carbon monoxide on operant behavior of laboratory rats and baboons. *Neurobehav. Toxicol. (Suppl. 1)* **1,** 179–184.

Gilbert, S. G., and Maurissen, J. P. (1982). Assessment of the effects of acrylamide, methylmercury and 2,5-hexanedione on motor function in mice. *J. Toxicol. Environ. Health* **10,** 31–41.

Good, P. (1979). Detection of a treatment effect when not all experimental subjects will respond to treatment. *Biometrics* **35,** 483–489.

Harlow, H. F. and Bromer, J. A. (1938). A test apparatus for monkeys. *Psychol. Rec.* **19,** 434–438.

Hendricks, J. (1966). Flicker thresholds as determined by a modified conditioned suppression procedure. *J. Exp. Anal. Behav.* **9,** 501–506.

Henton, W. W. (1969). Conditioned suppression to odorous stimuli in pigeons. *J. Exp. Anal. Behav.* **12,** 175–185.

Hoffman, H. S., and Ison, J. R. (1980). Reflex modulation in the domain of startle. *Psychol. Rev.* **87,** 175–189.

Irwin, S. (1968). Comprehensive observational assessment. In: A systematic quantitative procedure for assessing the behavioral and physiological state of the mouse. *Psychopharmacology* **13,** 222–257.

Iwata, K. (1980). Neuroophthalmologic indices of Minamata disease in Niigata. *In* "Neurotoxicity of the Visual System" (W. H. Merigan and B. Weiss, eds.), pp. 165–185. New York: Raven Press.

Kelleher, R. T., and Morse, W. H. (1968). Determinants of the specificity of behavioral effects of drugs. *Ergeb. Physiol.* **60,** 1–56.

Laties, V. G. (1982). Contributions of operant conditioning to behavioral toxicology. *In* "Nervous System Toxicology" (C. L. Mitchell, ed.), pp. 67–80. New York: Raven Press.

Leander, J. D., and MacPhail, R. C. (1980). Effect of chlordimeform (a formamidine pesticide) on schedule-controlled responding of pigeons. *Neurobehav. Toxicol.* **2,** 315–321.

Levin, E. D., and Bowman, R. E. (1983). The effect of pre- or postnatal lead exposure on Hamilton Search Task in monkeys. *Neurobehav. Toxicol. Teratol.* **5,** 391–394.

Levine, T. E. (1976). Effects of carbon disulfide and FLA-63 on operant behavior in pigeons. *J. Pharmacol. Exp. Ther.* **199,** 669–678.

Levine, T. E., Bornschein, R. L., and Michaelson, I. A. (1977). Technique for assessing visual discrimination learning in mice. *Pharmacol. Biochem. Behav.* **7,** 567–570.

McMillan, D. E. (1982). Effects of chronic administration of pesticides on schedule-controlled responding by rats and pigeons. *In* "Effects of Chronic Exposures to Pesticides on Animal Systems" (J. E. Chambers and J. D. Yarbrough, eds.), pp. 211–226. New York: Raven Press.

MacPhail, R. C., and Leander, J. (1981). Chlordimeform effects on schedule-controlled behavior in rats. *Neurobehav. Toxicol. Teratol.* **3,** 19–26.

MacPhail, R. C. (1982). Studies on the flavor aversions induced by trialkyltin compounds. *Neurobehav. Toxicol. Teratol.* **4,** 225–230.

Marshall, J. F. (1975). Increased orientation to sensory stimuli following medial hypothalamic damage in rats. *Brain Res.* **86,** 373–387.

Maurissen, J. P., Weiss, B., and Davis, H. T. (1983). Somatosensory thresholds in monkeys exposed to acrylamide. *Toxicol. Appl. Pharmacol.* **71**, 266–279.

Merigan, W. H., Barkdoll, E., and Maurissen, J. P. (1982). Acrylamide-induced visual impairment in primates. *Toxicol. Appl. Pharmacol.* **62**, 342–345.

Mitchell, C. L., Tilson, H. A., and Cabe, P. A. (1982). Screening for neurobehavioral toxicology: Factors to consider. *In* "Nervous System Toxicology" (C. L. Mitchell, ed.), pp. 237–245. New York: Raven Press.

National Academy of Sciences (1975). "Principles for evaluating chemicals in the environment." Washington, DC: National Academy of Sciences.

Needleman, H. L., Gunroe, C., Leviton, A., Reed, R., Peresie, H., Maker, C., and Barrett, P. (1979). Deficits in psychologic and classroom performance of children with elevated dentine lead levels. *N. Eng. J. Med.* **300**, 59–65.

Nienhuys, T. G., and Clark, G. M. (1978). Frequency discrimination following selective destruction of cochlear inner and outer hair cells. *Science* **199**, 1356–1357.

O'Connell, M., Yeaton, S. P., and Stroebel, D. A. (1978). Visual discrimination in the protein malnourished rhesus. *Physiol. Biochem. Behav.* **20**, 251–256.

Padich, R., and Zenick, H. (1977). The effects of developmental and/or direct lead exposure on FR behavior in the rat. *Pharmacol. Biochem. Behav.* **6**, 371–375.

Pavlenko, S. M. (1975). Methods for the study of the central nervous system in toxicological tests. *In* "Methods Used in the USSR for Establishing Biologically Safe Levels of Toxic Substances", pp. 86–108. Geneva: World Health Organization.

Peters, D. P. (1979). Effects of prenatal nutrition on learning and motivation in rats. *Physiol. Behav.* **22**, 1067–1071.

Reiter, L. W., and MacPhail, R. C. (1982). Factors influencing motor activity measurements in neurotoxicology. *In* "Nervous System Toxicology" (C. L. Mitchell, ed.), pp. 45–65. New York: Raven Press.

Reynolds, G. S. (1958). "A Primer of Operant Conditioning." Glenview, Illinois: Scott, Foresman.

Rice, D. C. (1980). Neurotoxicity and behavior — Behavioral aberrations. *Toxicol. Forum*, 183–197.

Rice, D. C. (1983). Central nervous system effects of perinatal exposure to lead or methylmercury in the monkey. *In* "Reproductive and Developmental Toxicity of Metals" (T. W. Clarkson, G. Nordberg, and D. Sager, eds.), pp. 517–540. New York: Plenum Press.

Rice, D. C. (1984a). Effect of lead on schedule-controlled behavior in monkeys. *In* "Behavioral Pharmacology: The Current Status" (L. S. Seiden and R. L. Balster, eds.), pp. 473–486. New York: Alan R. Liss.

Rice, D. C. (1984b). Behavioral deficit (delayed matching to sample) in monkeys exposed from birth to low levels of lead. *Toxicol. Appl. Pharmacol.* **75**, 337–345.

Rice, D. C. (1985). Chronic low lead exposure from birth produces deficits in discrimination reversal in monkeys. *Toxicol. Appl. Pharmacol.* **77**, 201–210.

Rice, D. C., and Gilbert, S. G. (1982). Early chronic low-level methylmercury poisoning in monkeys impairs spatial vision. *Science* **216**, 759–761.

Rice, D. C., and Gilbert, S. G. (1985). Low-level lead exposure from birth produces behavioral toxicity (DRL) in monkeys. *Toxicol. Appl. Pharmacol.* **80**, 421–426.

Rice, D. C., and Willes, R. F. (1979). Neonatal low-level lead exposure in monkeys (Macaca fascicularis): Effect on two-choice non-spatial form discrimination. *J. Environ. Pathol. Toxicol.* **2**, 1195–1203.

Rice, D. C., Gilbert, S. G., and Willes, R. F. (1979). Neonatal low-level lead exposure in monkeys: Locomotor activity, schedule-controlled behavior, and the effects of amphetamine. *Toxicol. Appl. Pharmacol.* **51**, 503–513.

Schoenfeld, W. N. ed. (1970). "The Theory of Reinforcement Schedules." New York: Appleton-Century-Croft.

Shigeta, S., Misawa, T., Aikawa, H., and Yokoyama, M. (1980). Effects of learning schedules on operant behavior in lead administered rats. *Jpn. J. Hyg.* **35**, 752–760.

Smith, J. (1970). Conditioned suppression as an animal psychophysical technique. *In* "Animal Psychophysics: The Design and Conduct of Sensory Experiments" (W. C. Stebbins, ed.), pp. 125–160. New York: Appleton-Century-Croft.

Sobotka, T. J., Cook, M. P., and Brodie, R. E. (1976). Effects of neonatal malnutrition and perinatal exposure to various pesticides. *Mater. Med. Pol. (Eng. Ed.)* **8**, 152–155.

Spencer, P. S., and Schaumberg, H. H. (1980). "Experimental and Clinical Neurotoxicology." Baltimore: Williams and Wilkins.

Spyker, J. M. (1975). Assessing the impact of low level chemicals on development: behavior and latent effects. *Fed. Proc., Fed. Am. Soc. Exp. Biol.* **34**, 1835–1844.

Spyker, J. M., Sparber, S. B., and Goldberg, A. M. (1972). Subtle consequences of methylmercury exposure: Behavioral deviations in offspring of treated mothers. *Science* **177**, 621–623.

Stebbins, W. C., Green, S., and Miller, F. L. (1966). Auditory sensitivity in the monkey. *Science* **153**, 1646–1647.

Stebbins, W. C., and Rudy, M. C. (1978). Behavioral ototoxicity. *Environ. Health Perspect.* **26**, 43–51.

Thompson, P. M., and Moerschbaecher, J. M. (1978). Operant methodology in the study of learning. *Environ. Health Perspect.* **26**, 77–87.

Tilson, H. A., and Cabe, P. A. (1979). The effects of acrylamide given acutely or in repeated doses on fore- and hindlimb function in rats. *Toxicol. Appl. Pharmacol.* **47**, 253–260.

Tilson, H. A., and Harry, G. J. (1982). Behavioral principles for use in behavioral toxicology and pharmacology. *In* "Nervous System Toxicology" (C. L. Mitchell, ed.), pp. 1–28. New York: Raven Press.

Tilson, H. A., Cabe, P. A., and Burne, T. A. (1980). Behavioral procedures for the assessment of neurotoxicity. *In* "Experimental and Clinical Neurotoxicity" (P. S. Spencer and H. H. Schaumburg, eds.), pp. 758–766. Baltimore: Williams and Wilkins.

U.S. Food and Drug Administration (1986). "Predicting Neurotoxic and Behavioral Dysfunction from Preclinical Toxicologic Data." Bethesda: Life Sciences Research Office.

U.S. Environmental Protection Agency, Office of Toxic Substances (1985). Toxic substances control act test guidelines: Final rule. 40 CFR part 798: Health effect test guidelines. Subpart G — Neurotoxicity. *Fed. Regist.* **50**, 39458–39470.

U.S. Environmental Protection Agency, Office of Toxic Substances (1986). Triethylene glycol monomethyl, monoethyl, and monobutyl ethers: proposed test rule. Developmental neurotoxicity screen. *Fed. Regist.* **51**, 17890–17892.

U.S. National Research Council, Safe Drinking Water Committee (1986). "Drinking Water and Health," Vol. 6, pp. 312. Washington, DC: National Academy Press.

Vorhees, C. V. (1986). Methods for assessing the adverse effects of foods and other chemicals on animal behavior. *In* "Nutrition Reviews, Diet and Behavior: A Multidisciplinary Evaluation" (R. E. Olson, ed.), Vol. 44, pp. 185–192. Washington, DC: Nutrition Foundation.

Walsh, J. M., Curley, M. D., Burch, L. S., and Kurlansik, L. (1982a). The behavioral toxicity of a tributyltin ester in the rat. *Neurobehav. Toxicol. Teratol.* **4,** 241–246.

Walsh, T. J., Miller, D. B., and Dyer, R. S. (1982b). Trimethyltin, a selective limbic system neurotoxicant, impairs radial-arm maze performances. *Neurobehav. Toxicol. Teratol.* **4,** 177–184.

Weiss, B. (1983). Behavioral toxicity of heavy metals. *In* "Neurobiology of the Trace Elements," (I. Dreosti and R. Smith, eds.), Vol. 1, pp. 1–50. Clifton, New Jersey: Humana Press.

Weiss, B., Ferin, J., Merigan, W., Stern, S., and Cox, C. (1981). Modification of rat operant behavior by ozone exposure. *Toxicol. Appl. Pharmacol.* **58,** 244–251.

Winneke, G., Brockhaus, A., and Baltissen, R. (1977). Neurobehavioral and systemic effects of long-term blood lead elevation in rats. I. Discrimination learning and open field behavior. *Arch. Toxicol.* **37,** 247–263.

World Health Organization (1986). "Environmental Health Criteria 60, Principles and Methods for the Assessment of Neurotoxicity Associated with Exposure to Chemicals." Geneva: World Health Organization.

Zenick, H., Rodriguez, W., Ward, J., and Elkington, B. (1979). Deficits in fixed-interval performance following prenatal and postnatal lead exposure. *Dev. Psychobiol.* **12(5),** 509–514.

16
Assessment of Immunotoxicity

Kenneth C. Norbury
Johnson & Johnson Patient Care
North Brunswick, New Jersey

Peter T. Thomas
IIT Research Institute
Chicago, Illinois

I. Introduction

II. Anatomical Considerations of the Immune System
   A. Bone Marrow
   B. Phagocytic Cell Series
   C. Lymphocytes

III. Function of the Immune System: The Immune Response

IV. Potential Effects of Xenobiotics on the Immune System
   A. Overview
   B. Immunosuppression
   C. Immunostimulation
   D. Hypersensitivity

V. Rationale for and Relevance of Immunotoxicity Testing

VI. Study Design and Conduct
   A. Evaluation of Standard Protocols
   B. Selection of Immune Function Tests
   C. The Integrated Phased Approach to Immunotoxicity Testing Developed
      by the National Toxicology Program
   D. Selection of Species
   E. Administration of Test Material and Antigen
   F. Miscellaneous Factors

VII. Interpretation of Data

VIII. Prediction of Risk

IX. Conclusion

I. INTRODUCTION

There is currently a growing concern among toxicologists, health specialists, and regulatory agencies about the link between human disease and chemically induced alterations of the immune system (Descotes, 1986). In recent years, there have been increasing numbers of reports documenting immune dysfunction in humans accidentally exposed to xenobiotics (Bekesi et al., 1978; Kammuller et al., 1984; Kalland, 1985; Hoffman et al., 1986). Such incidents are significant in light of the association between therapeutic use of immunosuppressive agents and increased incidence of infectious disease (Allen, 1976) and neoplastic transformation (Penn, 1985). In addition, it is well recognized that allergic reactions can be induced by a variety of chemicals and drugs (see Amos and Park, 1985). Collectively, such associations are often referred to as immunotoxic; hence. the field known as immunotoxicology evolved.

Many definitions of immunotoxicity have been proposed. The inadvertent modification of the immune response by foods, drugs, and environmental contaminants is a general definition (Mosher, 1978). Crucial to this definition are the words "immune response" because it is widely recognized that the immune system is a dynamic organization of many specialized cell types intertwined in a complex, regulated network (Bick, 1982, 1985). Davies (1983) has expressed another viewpoint in describing immunotoxicity as an undesirable effect caused by an inappropriate immune response. For example, drugs that cause immunosuppression may be useful in preventing acute graft rejection (desirable effect), but they may also decrease host resistance to infection (undesirable effect). Conversely, agents that enhance immunity in patients with an immunodeficiency or cancer (desirable effect) may predispose patients to autoimmune disease or hypersensitivity reactions (undesirable effect). Of course, any drug or chemical, regardless of its primary pharmacological action, may have the potential to alter the immune response.

Much attention has been increasingly focused on the possible adverse effects of many drugs and chemicals on the immune competence of exposed individuals (Descotes, 1985a). Use of experimental animals to evaluate immunotoxicity was sparked by Vos (1977) in a comprehensive review of environmental chemicals known to cause immune suppression. Since then, considerable effort has been expended, largely through the National Toxicology Program (NTP), to develop and validate selected immunological tests in rodents (Moore et al., 1982; Thomas et al., 1985a; Luster et al., 1988). At the same time, government regulatory agencies (Spiers et al., 1978; Spiers and Spiers, 1979; Roberts and Chapman, 1981; Benson and Roberts, 1982) as well as the pharmaceutical (Norbury, 1982a,

1982b, 1985) and chemical industries (Dean *et al.,* 1983) have requested assessment of immunotoxic risks in prospective epidemiological studies in humans (Bekesi *et al.,* 1978; Hoffman *et al.,* 1986).

Current procedures for assessing toxicity to the immune system include hematological evaluation and determination of lymphoid organ weight and microscopic architecture. However, in an increasing number of cases, it has become necessary to include a more specific evaluation of immune function because of the growing realization that the immune system is a target organ for toxicity and plays a crucial role in the maintenance of health (International Seminar, 1984). In this chapter, we deal specifically with the issues concerning the design, conduct, and interpretation of studies to assess immunotoxicity. Our goal is to provide a balanced viewpoint that is relevant to industry and regulatory agencies in assessment of immunotoxic risk. For a more thorough consideration of hematological and pathological procedures for monitoring routine toxicity studies, refer to Chapters 18 and 20.

II. ANATOMICAL CONSIDERATIONS OF THE IMMUNE SYSTEM

A. Bone Marrow

When considering the anatomy of the immune system, one must include as primary lymphoid organs the bone marrow and thymus (and the bursa of Fabricius in avian species). Secondary lymphoid organs include the spleen, lymph nodes, gut-associated lymphoid tissue (GALT) such as the appendix and Peyer's patches, and bronchial-associated lymphoid tissue (BALT). Obviously, any one of these organs may be the target of toxic chemicals. For example, benzene, antimetabolites, mustards, arsenic, chloramphenicol, gold, hydantoin derivatives, and phenylbutazone are known to cause pancytopenia, a decrease in the circulating numbers of all formed elements of the bone marrow (Harris and Kellermeyer, 1970). If severe enough, such changes may alter either host resistance to infection or, possibly, tumor surveillance.

It must be emphasized that the bone marrow is a critical target organ for immunotoxicity because of the pluripotent stem cells present there (Irons, 1985a). Stem cells are precursors to all cell types that comprise the immune apparatus, including lymphocytes, natural killer cells, and null cells as well as macrophages, granulocytes and polymorphonuclear leukocytes (PMNs). The most common manifestation of chemically induced bone marrow damage is granulocytopenia, a reduction in circulating granulocytes induced by alkylating agents, antimetabolites, phenothiazines, nonsteroidal anti-inflammatory drugs, antithyroid drugs, and some anticonvulsants (Pisciotta, 1973). Conversely, granulocytosis, or an increased number of granulocytes, occurs after the administration of epinephrine and cortisone, but its physiological significance is unknown. Benzene, chloramphenicol, and phenylbutazone have also been associated with acute myelogenous leukemia, which is a malignant form of granulocytosis.

B. Phagocytic Cell Series

Primary host defense mechanisms against infectious agents initially involve nonspecific natural barriers such as the skin and the linings of the intestinal tract and lung. The immune system is the second line of defense against foreign organisms or extraneous materials. Immunological defenses generally involve phagocytosis, cell-mediated immunity (CMI), and/or humoral immunity (HI). Phagocytic cells are part of the reticuloendothelial system (RES) and include PMNs (neutrophils, eosinophils, and basophils) and cells of the monocyte/macrophage series. These latter cell types include both circulating cells and cells fixed in various tissues such as type II alveolar macrophages (lung) and Kupffer cells (liver). In addition, for experimental purposes, macrophages can be recruited into the peritoneal cavity by inflammatory agents like thioglycollate, mineral oil, starch, and sodium caseinate. These cells can be readily distinguished microscopically from lymphocytes or PMNs by the presence of certain characteristic enzymes (esterase). One of the most common characteristics of macrophages is their ability to phagocytize particles (colloidal carbon and latex beads), microbes, and other cells such as sheep erythrocytes (SRBC). Other functions of macrophages are described later in Section III.

Among the wide variety of agents toxic to the phagocytic cell series are certain airborne pollutants and glucocorticoids. Inhalation of metals and complex metallic mixtures alters alveolar macrophage function and renders the host more susceptible to airborne infections (Aranyi et al., 1979, 1981, 1985). On the other hand, pharmacological doses of glucocorticoids decrease the number (but not the rate of production) of granulocytes that undergo diapedesis and enter an inflammatory exudate, thus presumably accounting for the increased susceptibility to infections of patients on steroidal therapy.

C. Lymphocytes

In simple terms, lymphocytes derived from and educated in the thymus are referred to as T cells and are primarily responsible for CMI. Mature

T cells are widely distributed and can be found in the splenic periarteriolar sheath and paracortex of lymph nodes. On the other hand, HI is mediated by lymphocytes that produce antibodies (immunoglobulins) and are termed B cells because they are derived from the bursa of Fabricius in avian species. An organ equivalent to this bursa has not been found in mammals. B cells reside primarily in the bone marrow, splenic follicles, and lymph node cortex. Of course, lymphocytes, like PMNs and monocytes, can also be found in circulating blood, GALT, and BALT. Less is known about GALT and BALT, but it is believed that they are intimately involved in host defense against antigenic material that is either ingested (Newby and Stokes, 1984) or inhaled (Bice, 1985).

III. FUNCTION OF THE IMMUNE SYSTEM: THE IMMUNE RESPONSE

Although the general role of the immune system has long been known, the exact functions and interactions of each of its components and cell types are still being elucidated. The numerous and highly specialized amplification and feedback steps involved in immune regulation complicate this process. For example, the development of monoclonal antibodies has made possible the identification, in different species, of T-cell subpopulations that help (T helper/inducer) or suppress (T suppressor/cytotoxic) the immune response. T cells can modulate the immune response by releasing soluble, biologically active chemical substances called lymphokines. T cells can be further characterized into subsets that mediate delayed hypersensitivity, affect rejection of allogenic tissue grafts, and mediate immunity against infectious agents and transformed cells. Certain of these cell types may be differentiated and their localization in tissue pinpointed with the use of specific immunological and fluorometric reagents.

With respect to humoral immunity, B cells differentiate into plasma cells following antigenic stimulation and produce immunoglobulin molecules of different classes (IgG, IgM, IgE, IgD, and IgA) termed antibodies. These molecules specifically interact with the antigen (bacteria, virus, fungus, parasite, protein, cell, etc.) that initially triggered the response (see Fig. 1). As alluded to earlier, the immune response is highly regulated. Macrophages process and present antigen during the course of antibody production (Fig. 1); during the course of cellular interactions, they produce prostaglandins, monokines, interferons, and ectoenzymes. One such macrophage product, interleukin-1 (IL-1), activates T-helper cells. In addition to their central role in immunoregulation, macrophages are also capable of effector functions, namely, phagocytosis, as well as microbicidal and tumoricidal activities.

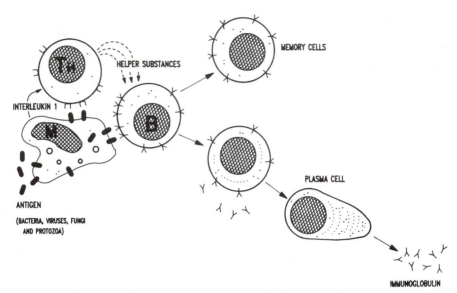

Fig. 1   Schematic diagram of immune response leading to antibody production (Norbury, 1985). Reprinted by permission of *J. Am. Coll. Toxicol.*

Two other important cell populations are the natural killer (NK) cell and the null (K) cell. NK cells are large granular lymphocytes that appear to mediate resistance against microbes, certain viruses, and tumors in the absence of prior exposure (Herberman, 1980; Hoshino *et al.*, 1984). Finally, K cells are active in antibody-dependent cell-mediated cytotoxicity (ADCC; Perlmann *et al.*, 1972).

The complement system is another aspect of the immune system that is important in host resistance to infection. In addition, complement is also involved in certain drug-induced immunotoxic reactions, as discussed in Section IV. The activation of complement can initiate a series of interactions that lead to cell lysis. Alternatively, certain by-products of the process are created that can stimulate cell migration (chemotaxis) and the release of many pharmacologically active compounds.

All these constituents interact to provide the host with an evolutionarily advanced and dynamic system that can specifically respond in a variety of ways to protect the body from environmental exposure to pathogens. Furthermore, the immune system has memory and can respond more vigorously upon reexposure to antigen. Recent research indicates that the functioning immune system is intimately related to, and may be regulated by, the neuroendocrine system of the host (Ader, 1981; Spector, 1983; Hadden, 1987).

IV. POTENTIAL EFFECTS OF XENOBIOTICS ON THE IMMUNE SYSTEM

A. Overview

The immune system is critically important to host resistance against a variety of pathogens as well as against cancer cells. Figure 2 illustrates some potential interactions and effects of chemicals and other substances with immune function. Depending on the nature of the substance (i.e., protein or low molecular weight chemical) or the route of exposure (e.g., local or systemic), a variety of possible effects exist. The potential adverse effects on the immune system may be manifested by an increased incidence of infectious disease, neoplasia, allergy, hypersensitivity, or autoimmune disease, all of which are potentially life threatening. Each of these adverse conditions is discussed under three broad categories: immunosuppression, immunostimulation, and hypersensitivity.

B. Immunosuppression

Immunosuppression (immunodepression), one of the most obvious manifestations of toxicity to the immune system, may be the result of direct or

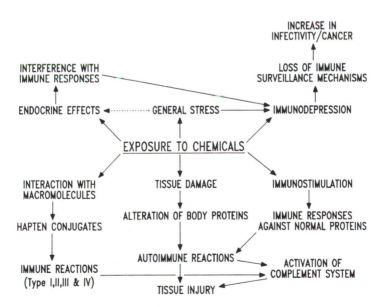

Fig. 2 Potential effects on immune function following host exposure to any drug or xenobiotic (Norbury, 1985). Reprinted by permission of *J. Am. Coll. Toxicol.*

indirect effects from exposure to xenobiotics. CMI is suppressed directly by a variety of chemicals, such as cyclosporin A (CsA), phorbol diesters, and organotins, whereas HI seems to be the target of low doses of cyclophosphamide and of metals like cadmium and mercury. Exposure to lead, polycyclic aromatic hydrocarbons, polychlorinated biphenyls, and 2,3,7,8-tetrachlorodibenzo-p-dioxin (TCDD) results in severe immunotoxicity to both CMI and HI. For recent reviews of immunosuppression caused by a wide variety of agents, refer to Koller (1985), Dean et al. (1986), and Thomas (1989).

The effects of immunosuppression include increases in the incidence of infection and cancer. For example, infections are more common among patients undergoing long-term corticosteroid treatment, anticancer therapy, or treatment with immunosuppressive drugs following kidney transplantation (Descotes, 1985a). Incidence of cancer is also higher in patients following organ transplantation, again associated with immunosuppressive treatment (Penn, 1985). Secondary malignancies have been described in patients cured of their initial neoplasm by (immunosuppressive) chemotherapeutic agents (Descotes, 1985b). In fact, several experimental studies in rodents have shown that a number of carcinogens (i.e., diethylstilbestrol, benzidine, benzo(a)pyrene, and dimethylnitrosamine) are also immunosuppressive (Dean et al., 1982b; Holsapple, et al., 1984; Luster et al., 1984; Thomas et al., 1985a). Whether these findings relate to the epigenetic factors in carcinogenesis remains to be shown.

Mechanisms that may result in direct immunosuppression include interference with cell surface receptors or soluble factors required for antigen recognition and cell-cell cooperation, decreased T-helper cell number or function, activation of T-suppressor cell activity, production of prostaglandins, and/or biochemical alterations such as inhibition of DNA/RNA and protein synthesis. Indirect immunosuppression may occur secondarily to nutritional deficiency, to generalized toxicity (so-called stress factors), or to stimulation and release of adrenal glucocorticosteroids.

Autoimmune disorders have also been associated with immunodepression. Methyldopa may cause autoimmune hemolytic anemia in which a selective inhibition of suppressor T cells occurs (Russel, 1981). Finally, myasthenia gravis or systemic lupus erythematosus (SLE) is more prevalent in patients with certain types of immune dysregulation.

C. Immunostimulation

In this day and age when a new generation of compounds is being developed for the immunotherapeutic treatment of immunodeficiency and cancer, one might not consider such compounds as possible immunotoxicants. Just because immunosuppression is recognized as a potentially detrimental health risk does not imply that drug-induced immunostimulation or immunopotentiation is always beneficial. For example, the immunostimulatory properties of penicillamine may account for the occurrence of myasthenia gravis or other autoimmune-like conditions (Descotes, 1986).

Some mechanisms that may lead to immunostimulation include increased T-helper cell number or function and/or inhibition of suppressor T-cell activity, resulting in stimulation of B-cell activity and production of tissue-specific cytotoxic autoantibodies that can produce autoimmunity. For example, induction of B-cell proliferation in thymectomized (T-cell deficient) mice can change an otherwise normal mouse into one with autoimmune disease (Smith *et al.,* 1982); the disease is characterized by antibodies circulating to cellular material, most commonly to nucleic acids. It is also possible that excessive and prolonged stimulation of lymphocyte DNA synthesis may eventually result in lymphoproliferative disorders such as leukemia.

D. Hypersensitivity

Another common effect that chemicals and drugs elicit is hypersensitivity involving antibodies, immune complexes (often involving complement), or sensitized lymphocytes. Table I outlines the four general categories of allergic responses according to the Coombs and Gell (1975) classification. In contrast to situations in which a drug or chemical exerts its adverse effect(s) directly or indirectly upon the immune apparatus, a hypersensitive reaction of the immune response system is actually triggered against a xenobiotic or its biotransformed product, resulting in cell injury. The compound (hapten) covalently binds to tissue macromolecules (protein) to form a hapten-protein conjugate, thus altering these macromolecules phenotypically to express new "determinants" recognized as different from "self" by the host immune system. B lymphocytes can then respond by producing antibodies of the IgE, IgG, or IgM classes that react with mast cells or other PMNs, K cells, or complement. Cell injury can result from the release of mediators that induce an inflammatory response or from complement-mediated cell membrane damage (cytolysis). Finally, T lymphocytes also can respond to altered self-determinants and mediate a delayed-type hypersensitivity (DTH) response by releasing lymphokines that induce inflammatory reaction. These lymphokines activate and attract PMNs and later attract activated macrophages.

Table I

Examples of the Four Types of Hypersensitivity Reactions[a]

Agents: clinical manifestations	Hypersensitive reaction	Cells involved	Antibody	Mechanism of cell injury
Food additives: GI allergy Penicillin: urticaria and dermatitis	Type I (anaphylactic)	Mast cell	IgE (and others)	Degranulation and release of inflammatory mediators such as histamine, proteolytic enzymes, chemotactic factors, prostaglandins, and leukotrienes
Cephalosporins: hemolytic anemia Aminopyrine: leukopenia Quinidine, gold: thrombocytopenia	Type II (cytotoxic)	Null (K) cells[b]	IgG, IgM	Antibody-dependent cellular cytotoxicity, opsonization, or complement-mediated lysis
Hydralazine: systemic lupus erythematosis Methicillin: chronic glomerulonephritis	Type III (immune complex)	PMNs[c]	IgG, IgM	Immune complex deposition in various tissues activates complement, which attracts PMNs causing local damage by release of inflammatory mediators
Nickel, penicillin, dinitrochlorobenzene, phenothiazines: contact dermatitis	Type IV (delayed hypersensitivity)	T cells (sensitized); macrophages	None	Release of lymphokines activates and attracts macrophages, which release mediators that induce inflammatory reaction

[a] Defined by Coombs and Gell (1975).

[b] Also T cells, monocyte/macrophages, platelets, neutrophils, and eosinophils.

[c] Polymorphonuclear leukocytes.

Allergic and hypersensitivity reactions to drugs have been the focus of considerable research (de Weck and Bundgaard, 1983). The exact frequency of occurrence is not known but may be as high as 20–30% of reported adverse drug reactions (Griffin, 1983). The fact that only a small fraction of the population may demonstrate immunologically mediated injury has hampered progress toward the development of predictive tests and animal models, except possibly for contact sensitization. Furthermore, such reactions are not characteristically dose dependent, making detection and statistical evaluation difficult.

Drugs are the most common cause of thrombocytopenia (Smith, 1980). Autoimmune thrombocytopenia is caused by quinidine and phenacetin, leading to increased peripheral platelet destruction. Aminopyrine, phenylbutazone, and methyluracil can act as haptens and bind to peripheral granulocytes, creating a hapten conjugate (see Fig. 2). When a specific antibody subsequently reacts with the cell to form an antigen-antibody complex, the granulocyte is destroyed by the reticuloendothelial system. Other examples of agents reportedly associated with autoimmune diseases are hydralazine and procainamide (SLE-like syndrome), methyldopa (hemolytic anemia), and gold and mercury (glomerulonephritis).

V. RATIONALE FOR AND RELEVANCE OF IMMUNOTOXICITY TESTING

Because of the critical role of the immune system in host defense, survival, and, indeed, the quality of life, there typically exist several mechanisms for controlling infection and for surveillance of cancer. For example, immunity to the bacterium *Listeria monocytogenes* and to herpes simplex virus type 2 is mediated primarily by T cells and macrophages (North, 1973; Newborg and North, 1980; Morahan, 1983); whereas pulmonary elimination of B16F10 melanoma, a transplantable tumor cell line in mice, depends on NK cells and macrophages (Murray *et al.*, 1985). Therefore, some believe that host-resistance models such as these are the most relevant measures of overall immunocompetence (Thomas *et al.*, 1985b; Kerkvliet, 1986).

When discussing the relevance of immunotoxicity testing and extrapolating the results of laboratory animal studies to humans, one must consider the concept of immune reserve. The evolutionary development of immunity, with all its checks and balances, has resulted in a system quite refractory to external insult. Therefore, the population in general exhibits a certain range of immune reactivity, as conceptually illustrated in Fig. 3. The range of "normal" function can be defined by any one of a number of functional criteria. For example, among normal humans, T-

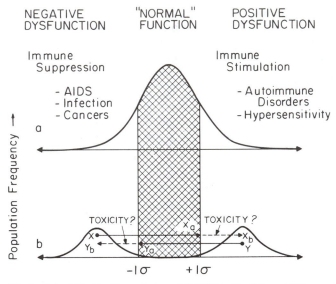

Fig. 3 Diagram depicting immune status as distributed in the population. a. Hypothetical distribution of normal immune function. b. Hypothetical distribution of positive and negative dysfunction and potential effects of immunomodulation.

lymphocyte blastogenesis to specific mitogens, antigens, or allogenic leukocytes displays a wide range of reactivity. These data will exhibit a normal distribution if appropriately transformed. Responses outside the normal range are associated with and are diagnostic tools for certain immune disorders (Fig. 3a).

Negative dysfunction in a population includes immunosuppression as exemplified by AIDS, increased susceptibility to infection, or increased incidence of cancer. On the other hand, positive dysfunction includes immunostimulation characterized by hypersensitivity, autoimmunity, or possibly cancer. For the sake of argument, any xenobiotic is potentially capable of causing a shift in the curve away from "normal" to either negative or positive dysfunction.

Figure 3b conceptualizes the relationship between the distributions of those people suffering from immune disorders and those with "normal" immune function. Pharmaceutical companies are interested in developing drugs that will modulate the immune system in such a way as to shift function into the normal range ($X \rightarrow X_a$ and $Y \rightarrow Y_a$). However, unwanted toxicity or adverse effects can occur in either direction if the immunomodulatory effects go beyond those that are considered normal ($X_a' \rightarrow X_b$ and $Y_a \rightarrow Y_b$).

Whether or not exposure to chemicals present in the environment affects the immunocompetence of the general population has not been determined and remains a critical issue for immunotoxicologists. Although environmental immunotoxicologists are concerned about inadvertent modification of immunity in the general population, those involved in new drug development in general and in immunotherapeutic drug development in particular must consider the immunological status of the patient population to be targeted. For example, knowing the potential immunological side effects of a potent new compound may be more important if the compound is destined for use in patients with AIDS or with an autoimmune disease such as SLE than if it is to be used in patients who are not previously immunocompromised.

Although the literature is replete with evidence of the relationship between an increased susceptibility to infection and cancer in animals and humans treated with immunosuppressive drugs, many other therapeutic substances also have demonstrable effects on immune response (i.e., enhancement or suppression; Lewis *et al.*, 1982). Most recently, the withdrawal of the drugs Zomax and Merital from the market because of apparent immune-mediated reactions further demonstrates the need to develop reliable methods for predicting adverse immunological reactions in humans.

VI. STUDY DESIGN AND CONDUCT

A. Evaluation of Standard Protocols

Current standard protocols for conventional toxicity studies having a duration of two weeks or more typically include certain basic parameters that offer some insight into potential immunotoxic effects, as shown in Table II. Clinical signs, including mortality, morbidity, decreased body weight, etc., may provide clues to possible depression of immune competence or to a shift toward negative dysfunction (Fig. 3). However, measurement of these changes alone may be too subjective and nonspecific to be reliable and sensitive indicators of immunotoxicity.

Current practices in routine hematological evaluation include, among other measurements, quantitation of circulating lymphocytes. However, as mentioned in Section II,C, lymphocytes are a heterogeneous cell population. With the availability of specific reagents, such as monoclonal antibodies, and techniques, such as flow cytometry, it is now possible to quantitate these lymphocyte subpopulations (Hudson *et al.*, 1985). However, as with any new technology, one must exercise caution in data interpretation. For example, although it may at first be tempting to determine the ratio of T-helper (inducer) cells to T-cytotoxic/suppressor

Table II

Examples of Antemortem and Postmortem Findings That May Include Potential
Immunotoxicity if Treatment Related

Parameter	Possible observation (cause)	Possible state of immune competence
Antemortem		
Mortality	Increased (infection)	Depressed
Body weight	Decreased (infection)	Depressed
Clinical signs	Rales, nasal discharge, (respiratory infection)	Depressed
	Swollen cervical area (Sialodacryoadenitis virus)	Depressed
Physical examinations	Enlarged tonsils (infection)	Depressed
Hematology	Leukopenia/lymphopenia	Depressed
	Leukocytosis (infection/ cancer)	Enhanced/depressed
	Thrombocytopenia	Hypersensitivity
	Neutropenia	Hypersensitivity
Protein electrophoresis	Hypogammaglobulinemia	Depressed
	Hypergammaglobulinemia (ongoing immune response or infection)	Enhanced/activated
Postmortem		
Organ weights		
Thymus	Decreased	Depressed
Histopathology		
Adrenal glands	Cortical hypertrophy (stress)	Depressed (secondary)
Bone marrow	Hypoplasia	Depressed
Kidney	Amyloidosis	Autoimmunity
	Glomerulonephritis (immune complex)	Hypersensitivity
Lung	Pneumonitis (infection)	Depressed
Lymph node (see also spleen)	Atrophy	Depressed
Spleen	Hypertrophy/hyperplasia	Enhanced/activated
	Depletion of follicles	Depressed B cells
	Hypocellularity of periarteriolar sheath	Depressed T cells
	Active germinal centers	Enhanced/activated
Thymus	Atrophy	Depressed
Thyroid	Inflammation	Autoimmunity

cells, which is highly reduced in AIDS patients, considerable lowering of this ratio also occurs in other diseases that may present symptoms of lymphadenopathy, weight loss, and fever (Herrmann, 1984). Such findings should deter investigators from placing too much emphasis on changes in this ratio. Furthermore, such an enumeration may not always correlate with immune function, because antigen-responsive cells constitute a relatively small percentage of the total circulating pool.

Subtle changes in lymphocyte number may not be detected due to the wide range of values considered normal. Functional changes may be evident in the absence of detectable changes in numbers, as in the case of CsA (Shevach, 1985). In contrast to other immunosuppressive agents like azothiaprine, CsA appears to be relatively free of toxicity and does not impair the number or proliferative capacity of hematopoietic stem cells. However, other immunological changes were observed during toxicity studies of CsA, namely, atrophy of lymphoid tissue, thrombocytopenia, and nephrotoxicity believed to be autoimmune-mediated (Ryffel *et al.*, 1983).

It has been suggested by Wong *et al.* (1984) that lymphoid organs such as the thymus be weighed during necropsy of animals even in acute toxicity studies; however, thymic atrophy may also be caused by stress or general toxicity. Although histopathological diagnosis is useful in demonstrating frank toxicity of potent immunotoxic compounds such as TCDD (Vos, 1977), lack of pathological changes does not necessarily mean that the compound in question cannot alter immune function. In other words, immune function may be affected at dose levels at which pathological changes are not readily evident.

There is general agreement among immunotoxicologists that the direct effect of most immune modulators on the immune system may not be detected from hematological and pathological parameters alone, particularly in studies of longer duration (90 days or more) in which dose levels are lower than those in acute or short-term studies. Histopathology is definitive only when at least a twofold difference is noted by other methods, such as tissue cellularity, particularly in bone marrow (Irons, 1985b). Pathologists, it is true, can determine changes associated with altered cell morphology, tissue organization, or growth (e.g., hypoplasia or neoplasia) that may not be readily determined with standard immune function tests. However, one must recognize the fact that cellularity and morphology *per se* are not measures of immune function. Bone marrow can have normal cellularity or even hypercellularity and still fail to produce normal formed elements or normal numbers of formed elements. Pathological parameters can be extended to include immunopathological procedures, such as immunofluorescence and histochemical techniques

(Hinton *et al.*, 1987) with specific antibodies directed against T and B cells.

B. Selection of Immune Function Tests

A diagram that shows the relationship of some routine toxicological categories to more specific immune function tests is depicted in Fig. 4. This scheme can be helpful in identifying an appropriate immune function test and its association to hematological, pathological, and/or serum biochemical parameters. It should be emphasized that, for many reasons given earlier, our preference is not to limit the initial toxicity study strictly to standard toxicopathological parameters but to select judiciously one or more immune function tests to supplement the toxicity study.

The existence of complementary and compensatory mechanisms imparts functional reserve to the host but complicates immunotoxicity studies. Consequently, there exists many *in vivo* and *in vitro* functional tests used by clinicians to measure immune competence in humans (Golub *et al.*, 1974). In order for functional tests to serve as a tool for the clinician, they must meet strict requirements for reproducibility and

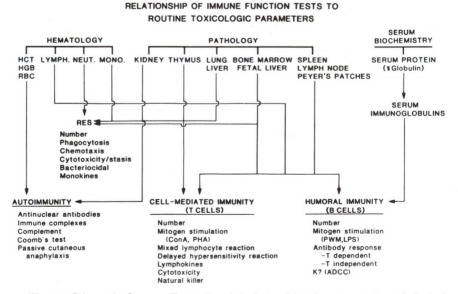

Fig. 4 Schematic diagram illustrating the relationship of routine toxicopathological parameters to selected immune function tests.

relevance to a disease state (Batty and Torrigiani, 1976). The same criteria must be met if a battery of immune function tests are to be developed in experimental animals for purposes of risk assessment, whether it be for unknown environmental compounds or for development of new immunotherapeutic drugs.

When appropriate immune function tests are being developed, the particular assays desired should be practical in terms of expense, simplicity, and reproducibility. They also should be readily applicable to routine practices in the conventional toxicology laboratory. The number of possible assays is great, therefore it is necessary to exercise wisdom in the selection of tests while delineating the appropriate approach to evaluate potential immunotoxicity. Because no single assay is fully able to assess potential immunotoxicity, a panel of assays is usually necessary. Such panels can be either quite comprehensive (Dean et al., 1982a) or deliberately abbreviated (Norbury, 1985), depending on the needs of the particular laboratory.

A few representative tests that measure the activity of different aspects and cells of the immune system are listed in Fig. 4. One is generally free to select the appropriate panel of immune function tests based on preliminary pharmacotoxicological data, structure–activity relationships, experience with particular tests, and, hopefully, discussions among scientists from all relevant fields. Although there is considerable overlap, we briefly discuss some representative immune function tests under five categories: RES, autoimmunity/hypersensitivity, CMI, HI, and host resistance.

1. Reticuloendothelial System

As stated earlier in Sections II,B and III, cells of the RES are not only phagocytic but also are capable of certain other effector functions. When cocultured in vitro with virally infected or neoplastically transformed cells, activated macrophages can either inhibit growth of the transformed cells (cytostasis) or directly kill them (cytolysis). RES clearance and killing in vivo may be measured by uptake of colloidal carbon in tissues (liver) or by vascular clearance of microorganisms. Granulocyte function can be measured by phagocytosis, chemotaxis, and bactericidal activity, but the nitroblue tetrazolium (NBT) dye reduction procedure has been widely used clinically to diagnose persons with chronic granulomatous disease (Baehner and Nathan, 1968). The number of granulocytes reducing dye is quantitated histochemically and correlates with enzymatic ability to kill phagocytosed bacteria. For details on these various methodologies and approaches to studying the effects of xenobiotics on macrophages and PMNs, refer to several references (Norbury and Fidler, 1975; Luster et al., 1982; Lewis and Adams, 1985; Kerkvliet, 1986).

2. Autoimmunity/Hypersensitivity

In spite of efforts to define and characterize autoimmunity as part of the Coombs and Gell (1975) classification, detection of potential autoimmunity induced by xenobiotics remains obscure. It is generally agreed that the immune system, which is delicately balanced, may become sensitized to its own self-antigens on the cell membrane. If a highly reactive low molecular weight (< 1000 daltons) compound (hapten) is capable of forming a covalent bond with protein amino groups or other nucleophiles, then there is the potential to generate immunogenic macromolecules against which (auto-) antibodies can be produced. If the macromolecule happens to be a normal cellular component, that particular cell can be destroyed by cytotoxic antibodies, sensitized T cells, or activated macrophages.

Recent studies have provided evidence of the immune system's role in the pathogenesis of halothane-induced hepatotoxicity (Callis et al., 1986). Exposure to halothane results in the production of antibody against a covalently bound oxidative intermediate of halothane in both experimental animals and humans. This intermediate has been shown to essentially alter the surface structure of hepatocytes into a nonself immunogen, thereby inducing antibody-dependent cell-mediated cytotoxicity (Vergani et al., 1980) and senstitized lymphocytes (Vergani et al., 1978; Mieli-Vergani et al., 1980). Such findings raise the possibility of development of a more general immunochemical approach to identify substances that may potentially cause systemic hypersensitivity reactions. In addition, antinuclear antibodies, positive Coombs' test, immune complex deposition, elevated complement levels, and in vitro proliferation of T cells in response to a drug linked to the relevant immunizing macromolecule (i.e., protein or DNA) are possible indicators of autoimmune disease (Russel, 1981).

Assays that measure Type IV cell-mediated hypersensitivity reactions are somewhat easier to perform and are classically characterized by skin test reactivity to extracts of Mycobacterium tuberculosis. Contact sensitivity reactions can be assessed in one of several different ways (Draize et al., 1944; Buehler, 1965; Magnusson and Kligman, 1969; Gad et al., 1986).

3. Cell-Mediated Immunity

One can assess T-cell and NK cell functions by measuring proliferation, production of lymphokines, and cytotoxicity in vitro and by performing certain *in vivo* procedures. Proliferation, or blastogenesis, can be performed on rodent spleen cells (Luster *et al.*, 1982; Thomas *et al.*, 1985a; Kerkvliet, 1986) or on lymphocytes from whole blood (Norbury, 1985). These cells will respond *in vitro* by undergoing mitogenesis when exposed to plant lectins, such as phytohemagglutinin or concanavalin A, or to lymphocytes from allogeneic animal strains. In the latter case, allogeneic stimulator cells in the mixed lymphocyte culture (MLC) are prevented from undergoing DNA synthesis by pretreatment with irradiation or mitomycin C. In both cases, the responding lymphocytes synthesize DNA, which is quantitated by the uptake of radiolabeled thymidine. Both the MLC and mitogenesis assays are widely used to evaluate human immunocompetence in the diagnosis of disease, as well as to type for allograft transplantation and monitor the course of chemotherapy.

Methodologies for measuring cytotoxicity of T cells (Cerottini and Brunner, 1974; Kerkvliet, 1986) and NK cells (Herberman, 1974; Herberman *et al.*, 1975) are similar. Target cells, usually tumor cells, are prelabeled with chromium-51 and cocultured for up to six hours with lymphocytes from spleen at various lymphocyte/target cell ratios. The amount of radiolabel released above the spontaneous background indicates the level of cytotoxicity, which may vary depending on the lymphocyte/target cell ratio.

The steps necessary for any acquired cell-mediated immune reaction, namely, antigen recognition and processing, blastogenesis and clonal proliferation, migration of committed (memory) T cells to the site of challenge, and production and release of inflammatory mediators and lymphokines, can be assessed by delayed hypersensitivity (Luster *et al.*, 1982; Lefford, 1974) or popliteal lymph node enlargement (Noble and Norbury, 1986). The antigen may be injected either in the pinna of the ear or in the footpad. Endpoints include weight of these tissues or *in vivo* uptake of radiolabeled thymidine into the site of antigen challenge. The DTH also involves presensitization of the animal to the antigen, which may be used as a measure of memory T-cell effector function. Lymphokine production can also be evaluated directly *in vitro* (Luster *et al.*, 1982; Exon *et al.*, 1984).

4. Humoral Immunity

B cells, like T cells, can also be stimulated to undergo blastogenesis *in vitro*. Certain bacterial cell wall products such as lipopolysaccharide (LPS), *Salmonella typhimurium* mitogen (Stunz and Feldbush, 1986), and pokeweed mitogen (which can also stimulate T cells; Luster *et al.*, 1982; Kerkvliet, 1986) are commonly used. Antibody responses to antigens that require T-cell help (so-called T-dependent antigens like SRBC, keyhole limpet hemocyanin, and bovine serum albumin) and those that do not (T-independent antigens such as LPS, DNP-Ficoll, and type III pneumococcal polysaccharide) represent important measures of the holistic immune response. Defective humoral immune responses to the former antigens but not to the latter suggest that T-helper cell function may be altered. If the immune response to both types of antigens show perturbations following administration of a xenobiotic, then macrophages and/or B-cell function may be altered. Additional studies would, therefore, be necessary to elucidate whether one or the other or both were affected.

Humoral immunity is measured most commonly by two different methods: serum antibody titers by enzyme-linked immunosorbent assay (ELISA), radioimmunoassay, hemagglutination, etc., or determination of the number of antibody-forming cells (AFCs) in the spleen. To elicit a humoral immune response for measurement of serum antibody, the antigen is injected one or more times with or without adjuvant. Blood from immunized animals is collected at various intervals and sera stored frozen until evaluation of antigen-specific antibody of the IgM and IgG types can be made (Vos et al., 1982; Koller et al., 1983). The AFCs can be determined according to Cunningham's modification of the Jerne hemolytic plaque assay (Jerne and Nordin, 1963; Cunningham and Szenberg, 1968). Spleen cell suspensions containing antibody-secreting plasma cells are mixed with the antigen and complement and placed in a chamber formed between two microscope slides. The antigen most commonly used is SRBC. However, it is possible to quantitate specific AFCs to other antigens (e.g., ovalbumin) by attaching the protein to SRBC indicator cells. Specific antibody secreted by plasma cells binds to the SRBC directly or to the protein attached to the indicator cells. In the presence of complement, SRBC lysis occurs, creating a clear area ("plaque") on the slide. Antibody of the IgM class is most easily measured by this technique. Measurement of IgG antibody is possible with the use of a facilitating antiserum. Because each plaque is thought to represent one plasma cell, the enumeration of plaques correlates well with the number of antibody-forming cells. There are many modifications of this assay, some of which can eliminate the subjective counting of individual plaque forming cells (PFCs; Sedgwick and Holt, 1983; Kerkvliet, 1986).

Finally, even though K cells require antibody to mediate antibody-dependent cellular cytotoxicity (ADCC), they appear to lack the unique marker conventionally attributed to T and B cells, hence, they are called null cells. Measurement of ADCC in vitro is described in detail by Brier et al. (1975), but its biological relevance has yet to be fully resolved.

5. Host Resistance

Increased susceptibility to infection or tumor cell challenge can be an *in vivo* manifestation of immunotoxicity. The ability to resist the challenge of an infectious agent can be determined in rodents by a variety of methods, including a change in mortality following challenge. To document impaired host resistance, the agent is usually administered at a concentration that will produce a lethality of 20% in control animals. After a defined period (i.e., 14 days), the number of deaths are recorded. Various agents (viruses, bacteria, parasites, and tumors) have been used, each carefully characterized with respect to the primary host defense mechanism mediating the immune response against the infectious agent. For further details, refer to a number of representative studies in this area (Bradley and Morahan, 1982; Dean *et al.,* 1982a; Thomas *et al.,* 1985a; Luster *et al.,* 1988).

C. The Integrated Phased Approach to Immunotoxicity Testing Developed by the National Toxicology Program

One particular approach to assessing immunomodulation was developed by the NTP (Luster *et al.,* 1988). The goal of this interlaboratory validation study was to determine, from a wide variety of host-resistance and immune function tests performed with mice, which assays would be most reproducible and predictive of immunotoxicity. Particular emphasis was placed on documenting reproducibility of the model systems within and among laboratories and on establishing correlations between altered immune function and impairment of host defenses. Considerations were made for screening tests that could routinely be part of 14-, 30-, or 90-day toxicity studies.

Due to the wide variety of tests available for screening compounds for immunomodulation and to the large number of compounds that potentially can be evaluated, a phased approach for immunotoxicity assessment in the mouse was developed by the NTP. An example of the types of assays used in the NTP testing scheme is shown in Table III. Phase I involves a relatively minimal effort and includes assays for both CMI and HI, integrated with the more traditional assays for clinical pathology and histopathology. Phase II, which represents a more in-depth investigation, includes additional assays for CMI, HI, nonspecific immunity, and host resistance.

Depending on the results of the phase I assays, a more in-depth evaluation of immune function can be pursued according to the scheme described as phase II. The phase II *in vitro* assays were selected because

Table III

Example of a Phased Approach to Determine Immunotoxicity[a]

Parameter	Procedures
Screen (phase I)	
Immunopathology	Hematology — complete blood count and differential
	Weights — body, spleen, thymus, kidney, liver
	Cellularity — Spleen
	Histopathology — spleen, thymus, lymph node
Humoral-mediated immunity	IgM antibody plaque-forming cells to sheep erythrocytes (SRBC); lipopolysaccharide (LPS) mitogen response
Cell-mediated immunity	T-cell response to mitogens and allogenic (foreign) cells
Nonspecific immunity	Natural killer cell activity
Comprehensive (phase II)	
Immunopathology	Quantitation of splenic B and T cell numbers
Humoral-mediated immunity	Enumeration of IgG antibody response to SRBCs
Cell-mediated immunity	Cytotoxic T-cell lysis of tumor cells; delayed-type hypersensitivity response
Nonspecific immunity	Macrophage function
Host resistance challenge models[b]	Tumor cell models
	PYB6 sarcoma
	B16F10 melanoma
	Bacterial models
	Listeria monocytogenes
	Streptococcus species
	Viral models
	Influenza
	Parasite models
	Plasmodium yoelii

[a] Adapted from Luster *et al.* (1988). The testing panel was developed with young adult B6C3F1 female mice.

[b] For any particular chemical tested, only two or three host-resistance models are selected for examination.

they are sensitive, reproducible, can measure relatively well-defined portions of the immune response, and can serve to probe more specific effector cell function. The *in vivo* challenge assays evaluate, in a holistic manner, the overall state of immunity. Not all assays listed in phase II need to be performed, but they should be selected depending in large part on the results from the phase I studies. Evidence of immunomodulation at relevant dose levels and a dose-response relationship are important prerequisites for proceeding from phase I into phase II. For drugs, these prerequisites relate to the therapeutic dose anticipated in humans, and, for chemicals of occupational or environmental significance, to the anticipated (or documented) human exposure levels.

It should be stressed that the phased testing scheme outlined represents only one approach in one animal species. The functional heterogeneity of the immune response permits a flexible approach to immune profile development of unknown compounds. For instance, one may choose to substitute determination of serum antibody titers for measurement of AFCs. Regardless of the approach or the animal model used, the tests used to evaluate immune function must be well characterized, reproducible, and relevant to appropriate disease states. It is critical that the assay of choice yield similar results among different laboratories. Furthermore, variability must also be documented. When an immunomodulatory profile of an unknown compound is being determined, intralaboratory historical data make it possible to compare the magnitude of present control responses with those of the past to determine if the assay is working within proper limits. Circannual variations in responses also should be documented. Incorporation of positive controls into each assay is important because controls document if the system is functioning normally and provide a basis of comparison to the effects of the test compound. Finally, it also helps to automate whenever possible in order to reduce the burden upon manpower and resources and to facilitate data collection, monitoring, and storage.

When making decisions concerning risk assessment or continued development of a particular drug, one must know the relationship between altered immune function and changes in host resistance. The main disadvantages to whole-animal challenge studies are the costs associated with housing and caring for the large number of animals needed and the specialized laboratory facilities often required for handling potentially pathogenic organisms. In short, *in vitro* immune function endpoints provide a relatively inexpensive and sensitive measurement of immunity. However, *in vivo* infectious and tumor challenge models may provide a more relevant measurement of immune competence, which is particularly useful in risk assessment.

D. Selection of Species

The species is an important consideration if immunological findings are to be correlated effectively with other toxicopathological changes. The mouse is widely used in immunotoxicological studies (Kerkvliet, 1986;

Thomas *et al.*, 1985a, 1985b; Luster *et al.*, 1988) for several reasons. First and foremost is the fact that, aside from humans, the murine immune system is the best characterized. Indeed, many immune function assays currently used in humans were developed and characterized in the mouse. Immunological assays either are under development or routinely used in other species, such as dogs, chickens, goats, horses, pigs, sheep, cattle, cats, fish, and rabbits (Kende *et al.*, 1984), which does permit the direct evaluation of domestic species exposed to immunotoxicants. However, it must be emphasized that immunological reagents for many of the larger species are not as readily available as those for rodent species (Schultz and Yang, 1984). Furthermore, a majority of the reproducible bacterial, viral, and tumor challenge models are not available in species other than the mouse. Economic factors such as animal and housing costs also need to be considered. For the most part, with the exception of host resistance, many of the same model systems currently used in mice have been or are being adapted to the rat (Koller and Exon, 1985; Norbury, 1985), the traditional species used in subchronic and chronic toxicity studies.

It is well recognized that B and T cells, NK cells, and macrophages of rodents compare favorably to humans with respect to similarities in function. Furthermore, the assays in the experimental and clinical laboratories are virtually identical. Because the rat, dog, and monkey are commonly used by the pharmaceutical industry to evaluate potential toxicity, it stands to reason that these same species should be used to assess immunotoxicity at the same dosage levels, routes, and duration of exposure as proposed for clinical use. A similar maxim applies to the evaluation of environmental chemicals: use the standard species predictive of risk and mimic natural exposure.

E. Administration of Test Material and Antigen

Route of administration and duration of exposure are also important considerations. The route of exposure can be selected either to maximize the probability of observing an effect or to simulate the exposure condition of humans. Duration of exposure is the same as that used for conventional acute, subchronic, or chronic toxicity studies. Immune function tests are easily integrated into these studies, without necessarily increasing the number of animals on the study (Exon *et al.*, 1984).

Understanding the relationship between administration of the test article and the antigen used to measure the immune response is critical when designing immunotoxicology studies. The effects seen following chemical exposure may be directly related to the timing between chemical exposure and antigen challenge. When antigen sensitization and chemical exposure is concurrent, it is important to consider possible interaction. Therefore, it may be necessary to employ different routes of exposure for antigen sensitization and chemical administration.

F. Miscellaneous Factors

A number of factors are commonly recognized for their potential influence on the immune system particularly hormonal and nutritional status, age, and exposure conditions (refer to Dean et al., 1982a; Luster et al., 1982). We have described others previously in this chapter and elsewhere (Norbury, 1982a). One of the most important considerations is selection of appropriate dose levels. The dosages used in rodent studies to elicit immunomodulating effects should be reasonable multiples of the common or anticipated clinical dose. Thus, it has been recommended that both drug sponsors and regulatory agencies attempt to determine if experimentally observed adverse immunologic effects are of actual clinical significance (Robens, 1984).

VII. INTERPRETATION OF DATA

During the elicitation of an immune response, at least four steps must occur: recognition (receptors), cell proliferation (clonal expansion involving DNA synthesis), differentiation, and production of an end product or effect (effector cell generation). An understanding of chemical- or drug-induced effects requires a knowledge of the potential site of action, that is, the step that may be blocked or otherwise altered by the toxicant. For example, the alkylating agent cyclophosphamide and the folic acid antagonist methotrexate interfere with cell proliferation by inhibiting DNA synthesis.

With the current state-of-the-art methodology meeting many of the rigorous demands to be simple, automated, reproducible, relevant to the concerns of the toxicologist, and adaptable to good laboratory practices, toxicologists are beginning to appreciate the potential immune function assays can have in helping them to answer questions of immunotoxic importance. In the past, serum immunoglobulin levels were considered adequate for assessing HI, and mitogen stimulation perhaps may have been a sufficient indicator of CMI. Today, however, quantitating serum immunoglobulin levels is less sensitive than measuring specific antibody titers following antigenic challenge. Furthermore, lymphocyte blastogenesis induced by mitogens is considered by some to be an inadequate measure of CMI. This is because mitogens are polyclonal stimulators, not specific antigens. Therefore, it is not possible to use them to measure specific immunocompetence (Schultz and Yang, 1984).

The hallmark of a reliable *in vitro* immune function test is determined by how well it correlates to an appropriate *in vivo* animal challenge model. Although host resistance is multifaceted, generally involving more than a single arm of the immune system, it is possible to show an *in vivo – in vitro* correlation. For example, resistance to influenza viral infection in its early stages depends on NK cells (Stein-Streilein *et al.*, 1985). Later, adequate HI and CMI responses are important (Virelizier, 1975; Hoshino *et al.*, 1983; Stein-Streilein *et al.*, 1985). There is significant correlation between reduced CMI, reduced AFC responses (suggesting impaired HI), and increased susceptibility to influenza viral infection with several xenobiotics tested (Luster *et al.*, 1988).

In the interpretation of immunological data, changes of 20–30% on either side of normal may be real and reproducible, but their biological significance may not be easily identified due to the immunological reserve referred to previously. Perhaps their biological importance will become more evident when other factors, such as stress, advanced age, malnutrition, or exposure to pathogens that deplete certain immunological reserves are considered. In general, the preliminary data being generated by several laboratories (Luster *et al.*, 1988) suggest that the clinical-biological effects of altered host resistance do not become apparent until a threshold of approximately 50% or greater is reached in a relevant *in vitro* immune function test. This presumably is due to immune reserve.

At the present time, elucidation of mechanisms of xenobiotic-induced immunotoxicity remains primarily an academic pursuit. One particularly exciting example of a possible mechanism involves the relationship among the expression of an aromatic hydrocarbon (AH) gene complex, the molecular conformation of certain halogenated aromatic hydrocarbons, and immunotoxicity. Studies in C57BL/6 (AH+) mice and DBA/2 (AH-) mice suggest that certain toxic effects of TCDD (teratogenesis and thymic involution) segregate with the AH locus (Poland and Glover, 1980). The immunotoxic effects of TCDD appear to be associated with those AH+ mouse strains having a cytosolic receptor responsible for mediating aryl hydrocarbon hydroxylase activity (Silkworth and Grabstein, 1982). In addition, C57BL/6 mice exhibit thymic atrophy, decreased relative spleen weights, and reduced humoral immune responses when treated with the planar compound 3,4,3′,4′-tetrachlorobiphenyl (TCB). These effects are not seen in similarly treated DBA/2 mice or in either strain treated with the nonplanar but closely related compound 2,5,2′,5′-TCB (Vecchi *et al.*, 1983).

The mouse model of the AH locus is perhaps the best characterized mechanism of xenobiotic-induced immunotoxicity for halogenated hydrocarbons. However, it may not be relevant for other classes of compounds or species. When elucidating mechanisms of immunomodulation, one must understand the relationship among the different cell types in the particular tests being evaluated. In addition, the possible role other factors play in immune regulation must be considered. Such factors include alpha and beta adrenoceptors, cyclic nucleotides, prostaglandins, histamine, adrenal corticosteroids, insulin, and the cholinergic system (Hadden, 1971; Sanders and Munson, 1985). Although this may at first seem confusing due to the apparent complexity of the interactions involved, one should be reminded of the multiplicity of receptors for many of these substances present on cells of the immune system. For a more comprehensive treatment of how immunity is modulated, refer to Mitchell (1985) and others (Hadden *et al.*, 1983; Cruse and Lewis, 1986).

Although experimental, another promising procedure for elucidating mechanisms of action and identifying target cell types involves *in vitro* immunization of spleen cell cultures (Mishell and Dutton, 1966). Murine spleen cells are most commonly used and are obtained from naive (or in some cases antigenically "primed") animals. The cells are exposed *in vitro* to specific antigen (commonly SRBC) for several days in the presence of the test xenobiotic. If the culture conditions are correct, the generation of specific AFCs (the endpoint measured) occurs much the same way it does *in vivo*. This approach allows great flexibility in determining which target cell types are affected by exposure to a given xenobiotic. This assay has the added advantage in that it can be coupled with metabolic activation systems (Tucker and Munson, 1981). It is also possible to separate the macrophages that readily adhere to plastic from the nonadherent T and B cells, treat the respective populations *in vitro* with a xenobiotic, then reconstitute the cultures prior to the introduction of antigen. This approach was used to determine that the macrophage, not the lymphocyte, was functionally altered following asbestos exposure (White and Munson, 1986).

One final feature to consider when interpreting data is the relative sensitivity of the immune system at various stages of development. Exposure of test animals to compounds during gestation (*in utero*) or the neonatal period has been shown to produce immunological changes in their offspring (Roberts and Chapman, 1981; Schmidt, 1984; Thomas and Faith, 1985). It is also well documented that the immune system undergoes an "aging" process (natural senescence) that is associated with reduced immune function (Kay, 1978) and increased preponderance of neoplasia and autoimmune disease. Such background findings, including stress-related phenomena, can be confusing if not adequately ruled out.

VIII. PREDICTION OF RISK

Obviously, the future of immunotoxicity testing depends on the ability of selected immune function tests to predict risk. Even a small change in the ability to deal with infectious agents may not be tolerable under certain conditions (Robens, 1984). Although preliminary studies have suggested that immune function tests seem to correlate with clinical instances of immunological incompetence (for review, see Dean et al., 1982a; Dean et al., 1985), more work is necessary. It should be emphasized that the majority of experimental data have focused solely on evaluating the immunosuppressive effect of xenobiotics. Yet, even cyclophosphamide, a well-known potent immunosuppressive drug, can exhibit stimulatory action depending on the dose employed (Turk and Parker, 1979; Norbury and Noble, 1978; Noble and Norbury, 1983). Additional studies are needed to evaluate the potential effects of immunostimulants on the immune system and to determine whether any disruption occurs in the delicately balanced immunoregulatory network. Furthermore, more attention should be focused on developing better models for predicting allergic potential in humans.

Although it is possible experimentally to demonstrate drug- or chemical-induced immune suppression (Dean et al., 1982b), it is difficult to prove that immune suppression induced by environmental chemicals is a national health problem. The critical immunotoxicological issue to be resolved is whether or not the general population is at risk because of its continuous "low level" exposure to environmental toxicants or drugs. If marginal immunotoxic effects are seen in animal studies, the only reasonable way to extrapolate to humans is to perform an epidemiological survey of an exposed group, keying in on the incidence of infections, neoplasia, and, if necessary, even sick days (Dean et al., 1979).

Host resistance to infection currently is the most relevant endpoint for assessing chemical-induced immunotoxicity. The advantages for whole-animal challenge experiments is that they provide an overall holistic approach to the in vivo state of immune competence. Furthermore, data from several laboratories have shown that these assays are quite reproducible over time (Luster et al., 1988). The endpoints measured include mortality and survival. However, quantitation of the organism or virus during infection in target organs important in pathogenesis would provide information concerning the kinetics of host resistance and immune reserve. With these data, meaningful risk-benefit analyses can be made concerning the immunomodulatory affects of a novel drug or environmental toxicant.

A discussion of immunotoxicity is not complete without some reference to the current status of regulatory guidelines for immunotoxicity testing. The European Economic Community first proposed guidelines in 1977. Groups within the U.S. Food and Drug Administration are proposing immunological testing guidelines for certain new antiviral drugs (P. Hoyle, personal communication). At the present time, the U.S. Environmental Protection Agency (1982) has incorporated immunotoxicology testing guidelines into biochemical pest control registration. It should be further noted that immunotoxicity studies have been conducted by the National Center for Toxicologic Research (Roberts and Chapman, 1981; Spiers et al., 1978; Spiers and Spiers, 1979; Benson and Roberts, 1982) and by the NTP (Moore et al., 1982; Luster et al., 1988). Thus, considerable effort has been made in immunotoxicology by scientists from various regulatory agencies, which indicates more than a passive involvement in this area.

IX. CONCLUSION

It is becoming increasingly clear that the immune system is extremely important in the maintenance of health. It is also recognized that drugs and compounds encountered in the environment (Haber and Pfitzer, 1982) have the potential to modulate host defense mechanisms and immunity. Certain population groups may be at risk from even mild immune dysfunction caused by xenobiotics. The most important question is: How much immune modulation does, in fact, occur following deliberate or inadvertent exposure to xenobiotics before measurable changes in host resistance to infections and neoplasia are apparent?

We have presented an integrated approach to assessing immunomodulation using measures of immune function during the course of conventional toxicity studies. The immune system should not be viewed in isolation from other organ systems. Substances from a variety of different therapeutic classes, whether of synthetic, natural, or biological origin, may affect the immune response resulting in suppression, stimulation, hypersensitivity, or autoimmunity. This fact, along with the realization that the immune system is a truly dynamic, functional system, supports the position that all chemicals and drugs deserve more careful scrutiny for possible immunotoxicity. Assessment of changes in the morphology of particular cell types is simply not enough. The advantage of immunotoxicity testing is that the methodology described, which is designed to assess immunotoxic effects of unknown compounds, can also be used in the biotechnology sector and elsewhere for development of new immunotherapeutic drugs.

More effort is needed in the future to further characterize the immunological profiles of species like the rat, dog, and monkey that are routinely used in toxicity testing. A broader data base needs to be validated with several reference compounds. More studies are needed to test the effects on immune function after (low dose) chronic administration of drugs and other xenobiotics to animals. Areas requiring further basic research include hypersensitivity and autoimmunity induced systemically by routes of exposure other than dermal. In addition, the role of the various lymphocyte subsets, the mechanisms involved in disrupting the delicately balanced immunological network, and the point at which an immunological change is considered toxic need to be further defined. To be successful, a multidisciplinary approach involving toxicologists, pathologists, immunologists, and epidemiologists is essential.

References

Ader, R. (ed.) (1981). "Psychoneuroimmunology." New York: Academic Press.

Allen, J. C. (1976). Infection compromising neoplastic disease and cytotoxic therapy. In "Infection and the Compromised Host" (J. C. Allen, ed.), pp. 151–171. Baltimore. Williams and Wilkins.

Amos, H. E., and Park, B. K. (1985). Understanding immunotoxic drug reactions. In "Immunotoxicology and Immunopharmacology" (J. H. Dean, M. I. Luster, A. E. Munson, and H. Amos, eds.), pp. 207–228. New York: Raven Press.

Aranyi, C., Miller, F. J., Andres, S., Ehrlich, R., Fenters, J., Gardner, D., and Waters, M. (1979). Cytotoxicity to alveolar macrophages of trace metals absorbed on fly ash. Environ. Res. 20, 14–23.

Aranyi, C., Gardner, D. E., and Huisingh, J. L. (1981). "Evaluation of potential inhalation hazard of particulate silicous compounds by in vitro alveolar macrophage test: Application of industrial particulates containing hazardous impurities" (D. D. Dunnam, ed.). Philadelphia: American Society For Testing Materials.

Aranyi, C., Bradof, J., O'Shea, W., Graham, J., and Miller, F. (1985). Effects of arsenic trioxide inhalation exposure on pulmonary antibacterial defenses in mice. J. Toxicol. Environ. Health 15, 163–172.

Baehner, R. L., and Nathan, D. G. (1968). Quantitative nitroblue tetrazolium in chronic granulomatous disease. N. Eng. J. Med. 278, 971–976.

Batty, I., and Torrigiani, G. (1976). Standardization of reagents and methodology in immunology. In "Manual of Clinical Immunology" (N. Ross and H. Friedman, eds.), pp. 911–917. Washington, DC: American Society for Microbiology.

Bekesi, J. G., Holland, J. F., Anderson, H. A., Fischbein, A. S., Rom, W., Wolff, M. S., and

Selikoff, I. J. (1978). Lymphocyte function of Michigan dairy farmers exposed to poly-brominated biphenyls. *Science* **199,** 1207–1209.

Benson, R. W., and Roberts, D. W. (1982). Evaluation of the immune response to type III pneumococcal polysaccharide as a means to evaluate T-independent immune function in the rat. *J. Toxicol. Environ. Health* **10,** 859–870.

Bice, D. E. (1985). Methods and approaches for assessing immunotoxicity of the lower respiratory tract. *In* "Immunotoxicology and Immunopharmacology" (J. H. Dean, M. I. Luster, A. E. Munson, and H. Amos, eds.), pp. 145–157. New York: Raven Press.

Bick, P. (1982). Immune system as a target organ for toxicity. *Environ. Health Perspect.* **43,** 3–7.

Bick, P. (1985). The immune system: Organization and function. *In* "Immunotoxicology and Immunopharmacology" (J. H. Dean, M. I. Luster, A. E. Munson, and H. Amos, eds.), pp. 1–10. New York: Raven Press.

Bradley, S. G., and Morahan, P. S. (1982). Approaches to assessing host resistance. *Environ. Health Perspect.* **43,** 51–69.

Brier, A. M., Chess, L., and Schlossman, S. F. (1975). Human antibody dependent cellular cytotoxicity: Isolation and identification of a subpopulation of peripheral blood lympho-cytes which kill antibody coated autologous target cells. *J. Clin. Invest.* **56,** 1580–1586.

Buehler, E. V. (1965). Delayed contact hypersensitivity in the guinea pig. *Arch. Dermatol.* **91,** 171–177.

Callis, A. H., Brooks, S. D., Waters, S. J., Lucas, D. O., Gandolfi, A. J., Sipes, I. G., Satoh, H., and Pohl, L. R. (1986). Evidence of a role of the immune system in the pathogenesis of halothane hepatitis. *In* "Molecular and Cellular Mechanisms of Anesthetics" (S. H. Roth and K. W. Miller, eds.), pp. 443–453. New York: Plenum.

Cerottini, J-C., and Brunner, K. T. (1974). Cell-mediated cytotoxicity, allograft rejection, and tumor immunity. *In* "Advances in Immunology" (F. J. Dixon and H. G. Kunkel, eds.), pp. 67–132. New York: Academic Press.

Coombs, R. R. A., and Gell, P. G. H. (1975). Classification of allergic reactions responsible for clinical hypersensitivity and disease. *In* "Clinical Aspects of Immunology" (P. G. H. Gell, R. R. A. Coombs, and P. J. Lachman, eds.), p. 761. Oxford: Blackwell Scientific Publications.

Cruse, J. M., and Lewis, R. E. (eds.) (1986). "Immunoregulation and Autoimmunity." New York: Karger.

Cunningham, A. G., and Szenberg, A. (1968). Further improvements in the plaqueing technique for detecting single antibody-forming cells. *Immunology.* **14,** 599–600.

Davies, G. E. (1983). Immunotoxicology-A viewpoint from industry. *In* "Immunotoxico-logy" (G. G. Gibson, R. Hubbard, and D. V. Parke, eds.), pp. 413–417. New York: Academic Press.

Dean, J. M., Padarathsingh, M. L., and Jerrells, J. R. (1979). Assessment of immunobiolo-gical effects induced by chemicals, drugs or food additives. I. Tier testing and screening approach. *Drug Chem. Toxicol.* **2,** 5–17.

Dean, J. H., Luster, M. I., and Boorman, G. A. (1982a). Immunotoxicology. *In* "Immuno-pharmacology" (P. Sirois and M. Rola-Pleszczynski, eds.), pp. 349–397. New York: Elsevier Biomedical Press.

Dean, J. H., Luster, M. I., Boorman, G. A., and Lauer, L. D. (1982b). Approaches and procedures available to examine the immunotoxicity of chemicals and drugs. *Pharmacol. Rev.* **34,** 137–148.

Dean, J. H., Luster, M. I., Murray, M. J., and Lauer, L. D. (1983). Approaches and methodology for examining the immunological effects of xenobiotics. *In* "Immunotoxicology" (G. G. Gibson, R. Hubbard, and D. V. Parke, eds.), pp. 205–218. New York: Academic Press.

Dean, J. H., Luster, M. I., Munson, A. E., and Amos, H. (eds.) (1985). "Immunotoxicology and Immunopharmacology." New York: Raven Press.

Dean, J. H., Murray, M. J., and Ward, E. C. (1986). Toxic responses of the immune system. *In* "Toxicology: The Basic Science of Poisons" (C. D. Klassen, M. O. Amdur, and J. Doull, eds.), 3rd ed., pp. 245–285. New York: MacMillan.

Descotes, J. (1985a). "Immunotoxicology of Drugs and Chemicals." Amsterdam: Elsevier Science Publishers.

Descotes, J. (1985b). Adverse consequences of chemical immunomodulation. *Clin. Res. Pract. Drug Regul. Aff.* **3,** 45–52.

Descotes, J. (1986). Immunotoxicology: Health aspects and regulatory issues. *Trends Pharm. Sci.* **7,** 1–3.

de Weck, A. L., and Bundgaard, H. (eds.) (1983). "Allergic Reactions to Drugs." New York: Springer-Verlag.

Draize, J. H., Woodard, G., and Calvery, H. O. (1944). Methods for the study of irritation and toxicity of substances applied topically to the skin and mucous membranes. *J. Pharm. Exp. Ther.* **82,** 377–390.

Exon, J. H., Koller, L. D., Henningsen, G. M., and Osborne, C. A. (1984). Multiple immunoassay in a single animal: A practical approach to immunotoxicologic testing. *Fund. Appl. Toxicol.* **4,** 278–283.

Gad, S. C., Dunn, B. J., Dobbs, D. W., Reilly, C., and Walsh, R. D. (1986). Development and validation of an alternative dermal sensitization test: The mouse ear swelling test (MEST). *Toxicol. Appl. Pharmacol.* **84,** 93–114.

Golub, S. H., O'Connell, T., and Morton, D. L. (1974). Correlation of *in vivo* and *in vitro* assays of immunocompetence in cancer patients. *Cancer Res.* **34,** 1833–1837.

Griffin, J. P. (1983). Drug-induced allergic and hypersensitivity reactions. *Practitioner* **227,** 1283–1297.

Haber, E., and Pfitzer, E. A. (1982). Immunological aspects of toxicology: A workshop. *Regul. Toxicol. Pharmacol.* **2,** 247–265.

Hadden, J. W. (1971). Sympathetic modulation of immune response. *N. Eng. J. Med.* **285,** 178.

Hadden, J. W., Chedid, L., Dukor, P., Spreafico, F., and Willoughby, D. (eds.) (1983). "Advances in Immunopharmacology 2." New York: Pergamon Press.

Hadden, J. W. (1987). Neuroendocrine modulation of the thymus-dependent immune system: agonists and mechanisms. *Ann. N.Y. Acad. Sci.* **496,** 39–48.

Harris, J. W., and Kellermeyer, R. W. (1970). "The Red Cell Production, Metabolism, Destruction: Normal and Abnormal." Cambridge: Harvard University Press.

Herberman, R. B. (1974). Cell-mediated immunity to tumor cells. *Adv. Cancer Res.* **19,** 207–263.

Herberman, R. B. (ed.) (1980). "Natural Cell-Mediated Immunity Against Tumors." New York: Academic Press.

Herberman, R. B., Nunn, M. E., and Larvin, D. H. (1975). Natural cytotoxic reactivity of mouse lymphoid cells against syngeneic and allogeneic tumors. I. Distribution of reactivity and specificity. *Int. J. Cancer* **16,** 216–225.

Herrmann, F. (1984). Lymphocyte phenotypes in patients with highly reduced T inducer to T cytotoxic/suppressor ratio. *Clin. Exp. Immunol.* **56**, 476–478.

Hinton, D. M., Jessop, J. J., Arnold, A., Albert, R. H., and Hines, F. A. (1987). Evaluation of immunotoxicity in a subchronic feeding study of triphenyl phosphate. *Toxicol. Ind. Health* **3**, 71–89.

Hoffman, R. E., Stehr-Green, P. A., Webb, K. B., Evans, G., Knutsen, A. P., Schramm, W. F., Staake, J. L., Gibson, B. B., and Steinberg, K. K. (1986). Health effects of long-term exposure to 2,3,7,8-tetrachlorodibenzo-p-dioxin. *J. Am. Med. Assoc.* **255**, 2031–2038.

Holsapple, M. P., Tucker, A. T., McNerney, P. J., and White, K. L. (1984). Effects of N-nitrosodimethylamine on humoral immunity. *J. Pharmacol. Exp. Ther.* **229**, 493.

Hoshino, A., Takenaka, H., Mizukoski, P., Imanishi, J., Kishida, T., and Tovey, M. (1983). Effect of anti-interferon serum on influenza virus infection in mice. *Antiviral Res.* **3**, 59–65.

Hoshino, T., Karen, H. S., and Uchida, A. (eds.) (1984). "Natural Killer Activity and Its Regulations." Princeton. Excerpt Medica.

Hudson, J. L., Duque, R. E., and Lovett, E. J. (1985). Applications of flow cytometry in immunotoxicology. *In* "Immunotoxicology and Immunopharmacology" (J. H. Dean, M. I. Luster, A. E. Munson, and H. Amos, eds.), pp. 159–177. New York: Raven Press.

International Seminar on the Immunological System as a Target for Toxic Damage (1984). Luxembourg.

Irons, R. D. (ed.) (1985a). "Toxicology of the Blood and Bone Marrow," (Target Organ Toxicology Series). New York: Raven Press.

Irons, R. D. (1985b). Histology of the immune system: Structure and function. *In* "Immunotoxicology and Immunopharmacology" (J. H. Dean, M. I. Luster, A. E. Munson, and H. Amos, eds.), pp. 11–22. New York: Raven Press.

Jerne, N. K., and Nordin, A. A. (1963). Plaque formation in agar by single antibody producing cells. *Science* **140**, 405.

Kalland, T. (1985). Immunotoxicology of diethylstilbestrol in man. *In* "Immunotoxicology and Immunopharmacology" (J. H. Dean, M. I. Luster, A. E. Munson, and H. Amos, eds.), pp. 407–414. New York: Raven Press.

Kammuller, M. E., Penninks, A. H., and Seinen, W. (1984). Spanish toxic oil syndrome is a chemically induced GVHD-like epidemic. *Lancet* **i**, 1174–1175.

Kay, M. M. B. (1978). Effect of age on T cell differentiation. *Fed. Proc. Fed. Am. Soc. Exp. Biol.* **37**, 1241–1244.

Kende, M., Gainer, J., and Chirigos, M. (eds.) (1984). "Chemical Regulation of Immunity in Veterinary Medicine." New York: Alan R. Liss.

Kerkvliet, N. I. (1986). Measurements of immunity and modifications by toxicants. *In* "Safety Evaluation of Drugs and Chemicals" (W. E. Lloyd, ed.), pp. 235–256. New York: Hemisphere Publishing.

Koller, L. D. (1985). Effect of chemical sensitivity on the immune system. *Immunol. Allergy Pract.* **7**, 13–25.

Koller, L. D., and Exon, J. H. (1985). The rat as a model for immunotoxicity assessment. *In* "Immunotoxicology and Immunopharmacology" (J. H. Dean, M. I. Luster, A. E. Munson, and H. Amos, eds.), pp. 99–111. New York: Raven Press.

Koller, L. D., Exon, J. H., and Norbury, K. C. (1983). Induction of humoral immunity to protein antigen without adjuvant in rats exposed to immunosuppressive chemicals. *J. Toxicol. Environ. Health* **12**, 173–181.

Lefford, M. J. (1974). The measurement of tubercular hypersensitivity in rats. *Int. Arch. Allergy Appl. Immunol.* **47**, 570–585.

Lewis, A. J., Carlson, R. P., and Chang, J. (1982). Therapeutic modulation of cellular mediated immunity. *Annu. Rep. Med. Chem.* **17**, 191–202.

Lewis, J. G., and Adams, D. O. (1985). The mononuclear phagocyte system and its interactions with xenobiotics. In "Immunotoxicology and Immunopharmacology" (J. H. Dean, M. I. Luster, A. E. Munson, and H. Amos, eds.), pp. 23–44. New York: Raven Press.

Luster, M. I., Dean, J. H., and Moore, J. A. (1982). Evaluation of immune functions in toxicology. In "Principle and Methods of Toxicology" (W. W. Hayes, ed.), pp. 561–586. New York: Raven Press.

Luster, M. I., Hayes, H. T., Korach, K., Tucker, A. N., Dean, J. H., Greenlee, W. F., and Boorman, G. A. (1984). Estrogen immunosuppression is regulated through estrogenic responses in the thymus. *J. Immunol.* **133**, 110–116.

Luster, M. I., Munson, A. E., Thomas, P., Holsapple, M. P., Fenters, J. D., White, K. L., Lauer, L. D., and Dean, J. D. (1988). Development of a testing battery to assess chemical-induced immunotoxicity. *Fund. Appl. Toxicol.* **10**, 2–19.

Magnusson, B., and Kligman, A. M. (1969). The identification of contact allergens by animal assay. The guinea pig maximization test. *J. Invest. Dermatol.* **52**, 268–276.

Mieli-Vergani, G., Vergani, D., Tredger, J. M., Eddleston, A. L. W. F., Davis, M., and Williams, R. (1980). Lymphocyte cytotoxicity to halothane altered hepatocytes in patients with severe hepatic necrosis following halthane anesthesia. *J. Clin. Lab. Immunol.* **4**, 49–51.

Mishell, R. I., and Dutton, R. W. (1966). Immunization of normal spleen cell suspensions *in vitro. Science* **153**, 1004.

Mitchell, M. S. (ed.) (1985). "The Modulation of Immunity." New York: Pergamon Press.

Moore, J. A., Huff, J. E., and Dean, J. H. (1982). The national toxicology program and immunological toxicology. *Pharmacol. Rev.* **34**, 13–16.

Morahan, P. S. (1983). Interactions of herpes viruses with mononuclear phagocytes. In "Immunobiology of Herpes Simplex Virus Infection" (B. Rouse and C. Lopez, eds.), pp. 71–84. Boca Raton, Florida: CRC Press.

Mosher, I. M. (ed.) (1978). Inadvertent modification of the immune response. *Proc. Fourth FDA Sci. Symp.*

Murray, M. J., Lauer, L. D., Luster, M. I., Leubke, R. W., Adams, D. O., and Dean, J. H. (1985). Correlation of murine susceptibility to tumor, parasite and bacterial challenge with altered cell-mediated immunity following systemic exposure to the tumor promotor phorbol myristate acetate. *Int. J. Immunopharmacol.* **7**, 491–501.

Newby, T. J., and Stokes, C. R. (eds.) (1984). "Local Immune Response of the Gut." Boca Raton, Florida: CRC Press.

Newborg, M., and North, R. (1980). On the mechanisms of T-cell independent anti-Listeria resistance in nude mice. *J. Immunol.* **124**, 571–576.

Noble, C., and Norbury, K. C. (1983). The differential sensitivity of rat peripheral blood T cells to immunosuppressants: Cyclophosphamide and dexamethasone. *J. Immunopharmacol.* **5**, 341–358.

Noble, C., and Norbury, K. C. (1986). Use of the popliteal lymph node enlargement assay to measure rat T-cell function in immunotoxicologic testing. *Int. J. Immunopharmacol.* **8**, 449–453.

Norbury, K. C. (1982a). Immunotoxicology in the pharmaceutical industry. *Environ. Health Perspect.* **43,** 53–59.

Norbury, K. C. (1982b). Methods currently used in the pharmaceutical industry for evaluating immunotoxic effects. *Pharmacol. Rev.* **34,** 131–136.

Norbury, K. C. (1985). Immunotoxicological evaluation: An overview. *J. Am. Coll. Toxicol.* **4,** 279–290.

Norbury, K. C., and Fidler, I. J. (1975). *In vitro* tumor cell destruction by syngeneic mouse macrophages: Methods for assaying cytotoxicity. *J. Immunol. Methods* **7,** 109–122.

Norbury, K. C., and Noble, C. (1978). Routine assessment of immunocompetence in rats: The effect of cyclophosphamide. *In* "Inadvertent Modification of the Immune Response" (I. M. Mosher, ed.). Washington, DC: U.S. Food and Drug Administration, Office of Health Affairs.

North, R. J. (1973). Importance of thymus-derived lymphocytes in cell-mediated immunity to infection. *Cell. Immunol.* **7,** 166–176.

Penn, I. (1985). Neoplastic consequences of immunosuppression. *In* "Immunotoxicology and Immunopharmacology" (J. H. Dean, M. I. Luster, A. E. Munson, and H. Amos, eds.), pp. 79–89. New York: Raven Press.

Perlmann, P., Perlmann, H., and Wigzell, H. (1972). Lymphocyte mediated cytotoxicity *in vitro*. Induction and inhibition by humoral antibody and natural effector cells. *Transplant. Rev.* **13,** 521–523.

Pisciotta, A. V. (1973). Immune and toxic mechanisms in drug-induced agranulocytosis. *Semin. Hematol.* **10,** 279–310.

Poland, A., and Glover, E. (1980). 2,3,7,8-Tetrachlorodibenzo-dioxin: Segregation of toxicity with the AH locus. *Mol. Pharmacol.* **13,** 924–934.

Robens, J. F. (1984). Drugs as inadvertent immune modulators. *In* "Chemical Regulations of Immunity in Veterinary Medicine" (M. Keude, J. Gainer, and M. Chirigos, eds.), pp. 337–346. New York: Alan R. Liss.

Roberts, D. W., and Chapman, J. R. (1981). Concepts essential to the assessment of toxicity to the developing immune system. *In* "Developmental Toxicology" (D. A. Kimmel and J. Buelke-Sam, eds.), pp. 167–190. New York: Raven Press.

Russel, A. S. (1981). Drug-induced autoimmune disease. *Clin. Immunol. Allergy* **1,** 57–76.

Ryffel, B., Donatsch, P., Madorin, M., Matter, B. E., Ruttimann, G., Schon, H., Stoll, R., and Wilson, J. (1983). Toxicological evaluation of cyclosporin A. *Arch. Toxicol.* **53,** 107–141.

Sanders, V. M., and Munson, A. E. (1985). Norepinephrine and the antibody response. *Pharm. Rev.* **37,** 229–248.

Schmidt, R. R. (1984). Altered development of immunocompetence following prenatal or combined prenatal-postnatal insult: A timely review. *J. Am. Coll. Toxicol.* **3,** 57–72.

Schultz, R. D., and Yang, W. C. (1984). Immunologic methods to assess immune competence in domesticated animals. *In* "Chemical Regulation of Immunity in Veterinary Medicine" (M. Kende, J. Gainer, and M. Chirigos, eds.), pp. 127–149. New York: Alan R. Liss.

Sedgwick, J. D., and Holt, P. G. (1983). A solid phase immunoenzymatic technique for the enumeration of specific antibody-forming cells. *J. Immunol. Methods* **57,** 301–309.

Shevach, E. M. (1985). The effects of cyclosporin A on the immune system. *Annu. Rev. Immunol.* **3,** 397–423.

Silkworth, J., and Grabstein, E. (1982). Polychlorinated biphenyl immunotoxicity dependence on isomer planarity and the AH gene complex. *Toxicol. Appl. Pharmacol.* **65**, 109–115.

Smith, H. R., Green, D. R., Raveche, E. S., Smathers, P. A., Gershon, R. K., and Steinberg, A. D. (1982). Studies of the induction of anti-DNA in normal mice. *J. Immunol.* **129**, 2332–2334.

Smith, R. D. (1980). Toxic responses of the blood. *In* "Toxicology, The Basic Science of Poisons" (J. Doull, C. D. Klaassen, and M. O. Amdur, eds.), 2nd ed. pp. 311–331. New York: MacMillan.

Spector, N. H. (1983). Neuroimmunomodulation: The evidence. *In* "Advances in Immunopharmacology 2" (J. W. Hadden, L. Chedid, P. Dukor, F. Spreafico, and D. Willoughby, eds.), pp. 451–456. New York: Pergamon Press.

Spiers, R. S., Benson, R. W., and Schiffman, G. J. (1978). Models for assessing the affect of toxicants on immunocompetence in mice. I. The effect of diphtheria, pertussis and tetanus vaccine on antibody responses to type pheumococcal polysaccharide. *J. Environ. Pathol. Toxicol.* **1**, 689–699.

Spiers, R. S., and Spiers, E. E. (1979). An *in vivo* model for assessing effects of drugs and toxicants on immunocompetence. *Drug Chem. Toxicol.* **2**, 19–33.

Stein-Streilein, J., and Guffee, J. (1986). *In vivo* treatment of mice and hamsters with antibodies to asialo GMI increases morbidity and mortality to pulmonary influenza infection. *J. Immunol.* **136**, 1435–1441.

Stein-Streilein, J., Whitte, P. L., Streilein, J. W., and Guffee, J. (1985). Local cellular defenses in influenza-infected lungs. *Cell. Immunol.* **95**, 234–245.

Stunz, L. L., and Feldbush, T. L. (1986). Polyclonal activation of rat B cells. I. A single mitogenic signal can stimulate proliferation, but three signals are required for differentiation. *J. Immunol.* **136**, 4006–4012.

Thomas, P. T. (1989). Approaches used to assess chemically induced impairment of host resistance and immune function. *In* "Hazard Assessment of Chemicals" (J. Saxena, ed.), Vol. 6, pp. 49–83. New York: Hemisphere.

Thomas, P. T., and Faith, R. E. (1985). Adult and perinatal immunotoxicity induced by halogenated aromatic hydrocarbons. *In* "Immunotoxicology and Immunopharmacology" (J. H. Dean, M. I. Luster, A. E. Munson, and H. Amos, eds.), pp. 305–313. New York: Raven Press.

Thomas, P. T., Fugmann, R. A., Aranyi, C., and Fenters, J. D. (1985a). Development and validation of a panel of host resistance and immune function assays designed to detect chemical-induced immunomodulation. *In* "New Approaches in Toxicity Testing and their Application in Human Risk Assessment" (A. P. Li, ed.), pp. 213–222. New York: Raven Press.

Thomas, P. T., Ratajczak, H., Aranyi, C., Gibbons, R., and Fenters, J. (1985b). Evaluation of host resistance and immune function in cadmium-exposed mice. *Toxicol. Appl. Pharmacol.* **80**, 446–456.

Tucker, A. N., and Munson, A. E. (1981). *In vitro* inhibition of the primary antibody response to sheep erythrocytes by cyclophosphamide. *Toxicol. Appl. Pharmacol.* **59**, 617–619.

Turk, J. L., and Parker, D. (1979). The effect of cyclophosphamide on the immune response. *J. Immunopharmacol.* **1**, 127–137.

U.S. Environmental Protection Agency (1982). "Pesticide Assessment Guidelines Subdivision M: Biorational Pesticides." Washington, DC: Office of Pesticides and Toxic Substances.

Vecchi, A., Sironi, A., Canegrati, M., Recchia, M., and Garattini, S. (1983). Immunosuppressive effects of 2,3,7,8-tetrachlorodibenzo-p-dioxin in strains of mice with different susceptibilities to induction of aryl hydrocarbon hydroxylase. *Toxicol. Appl. Pharmacol.* **68,** 434–441.

Vergani, D., Mieli-Vergani, G., Alberti, A., Neuberger, J., Eddleston, A. L. W. F., Davis, M., and Williams, R. (1980). Antibodies to the surface of halothane-altered rabbit hepatocytes in patients with severe halothane-associated hepatitis. *N. Eng. J. Med.* **303,** 66–71.

Vergani, D., Tsantoulas, D., Eddleston, A. L. W. F., Davis, M., and Williams, R. (1978). Sensitization to halothane-altered liver components in severe hepatic necrosis after halothane anesthesia. *Lancet* **2,** 801–803.

Virelizier, J. (1975). Host defenses against influenza virus: The role of anti-hemagglutinin antibody. *J. Immunol.* **115,** 434–439.

Vos, J. G. (1977). Immune suppression as related to toxicology. *CRC Crit. Rev. Toxicol.* **5,** 67–101.

Vos, J. G., Krajnc, E. I., and Beekhof, P. (1982). Use of the enzyme-linked immunosorbent assay (ELISA) in immunotoxicity testing. *Environ. Health Perspect.* **43,** 115–121.

White, K. L., Jr., and Munson, A. E. (1986). Suppression of the *in vitro* humoral immune response by chrysotile asbestos. *Toxicol. Appl. Pharmacol.* **82,** 493–504.

Wong, S., Dean, J. H., Norbury, K. C., and Munson, A. E. (1984). Immunotoxicology symposium highlights. *J. Am. Coll. Toxicol.* **3,** 115–120.

Part VI
Monitoring the Study

17
Health Monitoring and Clinical Examination

Douglas L. Arnold
Toxicology Research Division
Bureau of Chemical Safety
Food Directorate
Health Protection Branch
Health and Welfare Canada
Ottawa, Ontario

Harold C. Grice
CANTOX, Inc.
Nepean, Ontario

I. Introduction

II. Background

III. Caging and Animal Health Monitoring

IV. Daily and Weekly Monitoring Procedures

V. Chronic Study Objectives
   A. Monitoring Animals with Serious Clinical Findings
   B. Developing Criteria for Euthanasia
   C. The Challenge: Difficult Diagnoses

VI. Training of Personnel

I. INTRODUCTION

In most toxicological studies used for regulatory purposes, each test group contains 50 animals or less; therefore, each animal may be viewed as a surrogate for millions of people. One major exception to this generality are potential pharmaceutical agents required to undergo further clinical testing in humans. However, due to the small sample size in most toxicological studies, it is essential that the maximum amount of valid information be obtained from each animal.

Few toxicological testing facilities have the capability to monitor study animals periodically during an entire 24-hour period. Consequently, it is to be expected that some test animals will die unattended. This situation is of particular concern in chronic studies in which an animal is stressed by the test substance and/or commonly occuring diseases, such as amyloidosis in mice and chronic progressive nephropathy in rats. When a chronic study is being conducted, it is advisable to maintain animals on test for as long as possible to allow latent toxicological manifestations to be expressed, but this time must be balanced against the fact that advanced disease processes may obscure toxicological events (Arnold et al., 1980). When animals in any toxicology test die unattended, specimens are unavailable for electron microscopy, terminal hematology (see Chapter 18), serum chemistry (see Chapter 19), tissue analyses for the test substance and its metabolites, and autolysis that may preclude histopathological evaluation.

The loss of such data means a lower return on the research investment and can dramatically alter the interpretation and extrapolation of study data, or possibly invalidate the study. The science of toxicology is evolving toward the use of more subtle toxic parameters relative to immunological and behavioral alterations as opposed to death, tumors, or birth defects. In an effort to ensure that valuable specimens are not lost, quality control (see Chapter 8) and a health monitoring program are necessary (Arnold et al., 1977; Fox, 1977).

II. BACKGROUND

The initiation of a health monitoring, clinical examination program is often a coordinated effort involving the principle investigator, the study pathologist, the veterinarian, and the animal care specialist (see Chapters 2 and 3). The success of the program is obviously dependent on the motivation of the technical staff monitoring the test animals on a daily basis. Our experience indicates that the motivation of the technical staff working with the animals is directly related to their knowledge of the study objectives. Their ability to document each animal's clinical history thoroughly together with the various laboratory findings, and the gross and microscopic assessment is essential for the proper understanding and evaluation of toxic and/or disease states.

For practical purposes, the health monitoring procedures discussed in this chapter are primarily for small laboratory animals and are based on principles derived from veterinary clinical medicine. These procedures were originally developed to assess the health status of animals during a chronic study, but many of the concepts and principles are applicable to all *in vivo* toxicological tests including those conducted with larger species.

III. CAGING AND ANIMAL HEALTH MONITORING

Although small laboratory animals in their natural habitat are communal creatures, for many toxicological studies it is necessary to house test animals individually so that individual animal data can be attained. It is well recognized that housing animals individually, versus various types of group housing (Andervont, 1944; Fare, 1965; Hatch *et al.*, 1965; Sigg *et al.*, 1966; Welch and Welch, 1966), will effect growth rate, organ weight, behavior, and other parameters monitored during toxicity tests. Some of these effects may be due to competition for feed, laboratory environment, or strain differences. Consequently, there is no ideal caging procedure, only alternatives from which the toxicologist must choose to meet the particular requirements of the experiment (Fox *et al.*, 1979).

When attempts are made to ascertain whether clinical observations in the test population are treatment related and statistically different from the control group, it is important to remember that the cage is the unit of statistical analysis, not the animal. Housing of several animals per cage decreases the statistical sensitivity of the data analyses. Therefore, when several animals are housed in each cage, more animals are required to attain a statistical sensitivity similar to individually caged animals.

In a chronic rodent study in which some animals were housed in pairs and others individually, the individually housed animals tended to be more aggressive, although both sets of animals were handled and manipulated in the same way and with a similar frequency. The animals housed in pairs were always better groomed and, as they become older, they appeared healthier and more vigorous. One disadvantage of paired housing was that the more dominant animal tended to move about the cage when the technician was visually examining the animals, making it difficult for the technician to observe and evaluate the health status of its cage mate, who might be more submissive, retiring, or possibly ill (Arnold *et al.*, 1985).

For animals that do not adjust suitably to group housing, or for species like the mouse that tend to fight, the use of group cages may result in premature "deaths" and specimen losses. In taking all factors into account, it is our view that individual caging is preferable.

IV. DAILY AND WEEKLY MONITORING PROCEDURES

An experienced technician is responsible for the daily monitoring and initial clinical examination of the animals. This individual has the major responsibility for minimizing the number of animals that die unattended. It is important to ensure that the technician undertakes these duties conscientiously throughout the study, particularly in chronic studies when geriatric diseases begin to appear.

The daily routine starts and ends with a visual examination of each test animal. The basic twice-daily observations are performed primarily to ascertain if the animal is drinking, eating, defecating, urinating, and moving freely about its cage. These normal habits are good indicators that the animal is probably in relatively good health and that death is not imminent. Each animal's cage is opened to facilitate observation of the animal's general behavior (i.e., normal, hyper-, or hypoactive). Because each animal may respond differently, it is necessary that the same technician be involved, preferably for the duration of the study, to become familiar with each animal's eccentricities. Such a procedure often provides early detection of behavioral changes, indicative of a toxicological response or a disease condition. Items observed during the twice-daily check include:

1. Condition of the animals' coat for texture and cleanliness: the coat should be sleek and shiny. A dull coat that is poorly groomed suggests ill-health. The coat of a dehydrated animal does not fall smoothly into place when picked up and released. Hair soiled with urine may indicate urinary tract problems. Alopecia may be indicative of nutritional deficiencies, parasitic disease, or toxic effects.
2. Signs and source of bleeding: external or bleeding from an orifice is usually readily apparent. The only sign of internal bleeding may be pale mucous membranes or a possible change in fecal coloration.
3. Signs of normal elimination: is the animal urinating and defecating? Is the quantity, consistency, and coloration normal? Geriatric male rats should be removed from their cage two or three times a week and examined for the presence of a "penis plug". This plug can block urination and/or increase the possibility of urinary tract infection.
4. Discoloration of the ears and mucous membranes: if yellow, the animal is jaundiced and if paler than normal, it may be anemic.
5. Signs of respiratory distress or disease: is the animal's breathing labored or abnormal? Is a raspy sound audible when the animal breathes? Is a nasal or ocular discharge present? Does the animal respond atypically when it is held or palpated in the rib cage area? Is the rib cage distended?
6. Feed and water consumption: it should be determined if the automatic watering device is functioning properly. If a bottle is used, it should be ascertained whether any water was consumed. If no water was apparently drunk, the water bottle should be checked for an air lock, which may have prevented the animal from obtaining water. Occasionally, a

change in the animal room temperature and/or humidity will alter an animal's dietary habits. Assessment of feed consumption is expedited by feed containers that can be visually inspected. Although the use of spill-proof feeders hinders a rapid assessment of feed consumption, they enhance the accuracy of consumption data. The lack of feed consumption can be due to malocclusion of or fractured/broken jaw if wire mesh cages are used. For geriatric animals, anorexia often indicates a more serious health problem, and every effort should be made to determine its cause.

Initial observations concerning individual animals may be recorded in the daily log book maintained in each animal room; however, it is preferable that observations be recorded in the animal's individual clinical file. Each recording is dated and initialed by the technician in compliance with good laboratory practice requirements (U.S. Food and Drug Administration, 1978; U.S. Environmental Protection Agency, 1983a, 1983b; see Chapter 22). All clinical observations may be described either in technical or lay terms; however, the terms should be standardized, understood, and employed similarly by all staff involved in monitoring the animals. Serious conditions, such as anorexia, for which a cause is not readily apparent, suspected disease, or treatment-related consequences should be brought to the attention of a more senior technician. This individual then performs a more detailed examination, which is somewhat more extensive than the scheduled weekly examination on each test animal. The detailed exam should include holding the animal and palpating it for evidence of disease or toxic responses such as subcutaneous nodules; enlargements of the liver, kidney, spleen, or other visceral organs; areas of tenderness or tenseness; enlargement of joints; or decreased mobility.

Regardless of the animal's perceived health status, technicians should be encouraged to handle the animals frequently during the conduct of all toxicological studies. In addition to "getting to know" the animal, the frequent handling of animals results in a more manageable animal and allows the technician to examine it for prolonged periods if necessary without the need for a light anesthesia. This is especially important in a geriatric population in which the difference between an anesthetic and lethal dosage may be small due to alterations in the liver or lung physiology (Grice and Burek, 1984).

Abdominal palpation of test animals should be performed early in the morning to avoid undetected animal loss during the night. For example, if an animal has polyarteritis nodosa (Yang, 1965), a large liver tumor, or other disease conditions in which the visceral blood vessels are fragile, then internal hemorrhaging due to palpation may lead to the demise of the animal within a few hours. If the abdomen is palpated in the afternoon, the animal might die overnight and the tissues could be extensively autolyzed. Another reason to palpate the abdomen in the morning is to identify moribund or distressed animals that may require euthanasia, which is more efficiently conducted when a full complement of staff is present.

Other aspects of the examination might be:

1. Assessment of muscle tone, general strength (i.e., will it "climb" back into its cage), and gait and posture reflexes if changes are suggestive of muscular deficit.
2. Determination of body temperature: readings of less than 100°F are usually not seen unless the animal is moribund; over 102°F may be suggestive of an infectious processes.[1]
3. Auscultation with a stethoscope for heart and respiratory irregularities.[1]
4. Evaluation of a blood sample for hematological (see Chapter 18) and/ or clinical chemical abnormalities (see Chapter 19); a urine sample for cytology or chemical abnormalities; a fecal sample for the presence of occult blood; or a swab for the presence of bacteria.[1]
5. Assessment of neurological responses such as ocular reaction to light and reflexes exhibited by toe or tail pinch.
6. Assessment of food and water consumption as well as recent body weight changes. (Decreased feed consumption may be due to lengthy incisors that should be cut with a pair of bone cutters. Due to their brittle nature, they may splinter and affect the animals' feed consumption for a few days.)

The results of this examination should provide a positive diagnosis or a strong tentative diagnosis as to whether the clinical signs observed are toxic manifestations of a test compound or an unrelated disease condition. In the latter situation, the colony veterinarian should be consulted, and additional clinical laboratory or bacteriological evaluation tests may be required to confirm preliminary diagnosis. Experienced, competent technicians can diagnose many diseases or toxic states, for example, the signs commonly associated with pituitary tumors. This disease occurs at a high incidence in aging Sprague Dawley rats as a progressive debilitation which results in an initial semimoribund state, wherein the animal becomes anorexic and listless. This phase is usually followed by a two-week period wherein the animal temporarily regains its usual demeanor,

---

[1] Steps 2, 3, and 4 are not usually undertaken for the scheduled weekly examination.

eats better, appears more alert, and moves freely about its cage. The animal then degenerates to a moribund state. When these events are observed, euthanasia is appropriate. In addition, due apparently to increased pressures within the skull, the animal's eyelids are partially closed.

After rodents have been on test for 10–12 months, more emphasis is placed on the weekly examination outlined in this section. This is particularly important in a chronic study when the animals are affected by geriatric diseases. In some situations, it may be necessary to conduct clinical examinations more frequently. Need for close observation is dictated by the general state of the animals' health. As morbibity starts to increase, so should the frequency of clinical examinations. The study director should review each animal's clinical file at frequent intervals in an attempt to determine possible trends in disease or toxic states.

Examination of weekly computer printouts (see Chapter 23), which give variations in body weight (a gain or loss from the previous week) and feed consumption, in addition to the perfunctory and weekly clinical examination, may indicate more subtle health problems. For example, a mature rat that has lost weight for two consecutive weeks, has lost more than 10 g in one week, or has consumed less than 120 g of feed in a week should be examined in detail in an attempt to ascertain the apparent cause. As rats get older, they tend to eat less and lose weight. In geriatric Sprague Dawley rats, it is not uncommon for animals to lose up to 25% of their maximum body weight over a 2–4 month period with little if any change in demeanor or general state of health.

V. CHRONIC STUDY OBJECTIVES

It is essential in the conduct of toxicological studies that tissues from all animals be available for histopathological evaluation. Loss of specimens from the data base because sick animals died unexpectantly may seriously affect the validity of a study because these animals may be those most affected by the test agent. It is also important that euthanasia not be premature because a well-designed and judiciously conducted euthanasia program helps to focus on the early development of lesions. A euthanasia program can provide valuable information on the nature and course of toxic or disease states.

There is some concern about an overly aggressive euthanasia program that can obscure findings, particularly if animals are killed before tumors and other chronic effects have had time to develop. If a euthanasia program is properly conducted, this is unlikely to happen because only animals that are expected to die within a few days are euthanized.

Tumors or chronic toxic effects do not develop suddenly within a few days.

In an attempt to encourage quality animal care, a group of experts convened by the International Agency for Research on Cancer (1980) have stated that "an experiment is not really a satisfactory long-term carcinogenicity study if the mortality in the control or low dose group is higher than 50% before the end of [test] week 104 of age for rats, [test] week 96 for mice and [test] week 80 for hamsters". In an attempt to meet this criteria, we have developed a program for the intensive monitoring of sick animals as well as criteria for euthanasia.

A. Monitoring Animals with Serious Clinical Findings

To carry out such a monitoring program successfully requires that animals with serious or life-threatening health problems be closely monitored. The procedure we have adopted is to establish a separate rack in the animal test room for the exclusive housing of animals with a serious health problem. The rack is designated as the intensive care unit (ICU). Animals are usually assigned to this rack by the study director or the veterinarian.

The ICU has shoe box-type cages made of polycarbonate with a filter top so that animals can be frequently observed without being unduly disturbed. Body weight and feed consumption of every animal in this rack is determined on a daily basis and findings recorded in the daily log book. An experienced technician reviews the findings with the study director before deciding whether to return an animal to its original cage, maintain it in ICU, or have it euthanized.

Although many research facilities put a special label on a cage containing a very sick animal, it is our experience that the ICU achieves the same objectives more effectively because particular focus is placed on the sick or debilitated animals. In addition, the ICU keeps these animals away from the remaining animals, somewhat reducing the chance for aersolization of potential pathogenic organisms; however, it does not dramatically alter the animal's macroenvironment since they are still maintained in the same animal room.

B. Developing Criteria for Euthanasia

The final step in the health monitoring program is the decision as to when an animal should be killed rather than allowed to die unattended. The personnel often appointed to make this decision are either the attending veterinarian, the study director, or the pathologist in conjunction with the technician who is responsible for the day-to-day monitoring of the ICU. In making a decision to euthanize an animal, one must use good clinical judgment. Studying the clinical history of the animal, making a clinical examination, including use of diagnostic aids, and arriving at a diagnosis and prognosis regarding the animal's health status are all part of the process. Each case should be well documented so that it is clearly evident why an animal was euthanized. In addition, such documentation may assist the pathologist in selection of tissue samples as well as facilitate study review and audits.

A number of clinical signs indicate that an animal's prognosis is unfavorable and that euthanasia is probably advisable. The following signs and descriptions are intended to serve as guidelines inasmuch as they provide a degree of uniformity regarding any decisions for euthanasia.

1. Anorexia

a. Complete

Mature rats that do not eat or drink can lose up to 40 g in body weight each day and will not survive for long. The decision regarding euthanasia for such cases can be made on a daily basis.

b. Partial and Sustained

This anorexic state is usually accompanied by a linear decline in body weight and a corresponding reduction in feed consumption (for example, 5–15 g/day weight loss and approximately 5–10 g of feed/day). Sustained anorexia may be the initial clinical indication of a serious disease problem or may suggest malocclusion. The final decision to euthanize may be delayed for a few days to ascertain whether an animal is able to attain better health status.

c. Secondary Anorexia

A gradual loss in appetite and body weight that can be observed over several weeks or months requires special observation. In mature animals, a total body weight loss, amounting to 20% to 25% of the animals' maximum attained body weight, can accumulate over several months. Severe anorexia and adipsia are terminal signs of severe conditions for which the animal should be euthanized.

2. Debility

The persistent impairment of body functions such as urination, defecation, or mobility may be clinically associated with a loss or lack of strength. In some cases, this is a direct result of either organ dysfunction (necrosis, nephrosis, etc.) or benign/malignant tumors (sarcomas, transitional cell tumors of the bladder, etc.). Anorexia or adipsia, whether completely or partially sustained, are symptomatic of the associated debility. Extent of the impairment dictates the time frame within which a final decision regarding euthanasia must be made.

Similar observations are indirectly precipitated in secondary complications when tumor growth impedes proper organ function. For example, the growth of a pituitary tumor may result in partial displacement and pressure on the brain. As the tumor enlarges, symptoms will vary according to the degree of brain involvement. An enlarging tumor, which presses on a nerve, can produce a localized paralysis. A large thymus tumor will impair respiratory function. Any loss of appetite associated with indirectly caused impairments is termed "secondary anorexia". Secondary anorexia and its accompanying body weight loss is generally gradual and observed over several weeks or months. The severity of the impairment will proceed to the point at which termination should be considered.

3. Cachexia

Signs of general ill-health and malnutrition are characteristic of various disease conditions frequently associated with variable weight loss. Weight loss not associated with a viral or bacterial disease can be handled in the manner previously discussed in the section on anorexia. For rodent studies, it is inappropriate to treat any animal with a disease condition during a toxicological study; consequently, confirmation of a viral or bacterial disease state in a significant number of animals may require termination of the study. For larger animals, such as dogs and nonhuman primates, it may be appropriate to treat a diseased condition, but such a decision may result in a confounding factor regarding data evaluation.

4. Pain

Because treatment during a toxicological study is inappropriate, animals in obvious pain associated with accident or illness, which is likely to be protracted, should be euthanized.

5. Respiratory Distress

A sudden onset of respiratory distress is usually indicative of an acute respiratory disease and is likely to involve several animals. Chronic respiratory disease (CRD) is accompanied by a slow, progressive weight loss and a characteristic chest "rattle" with obvious respiratory distress. Animals should be isolated when this condition is first suspected in an attempt to limit the exposure of healthy animals. Any animal diagnosed as having CRD is immediately euthanized. The continuation of the study may be in question, depending on the incidence and control of the disease.

Respiratory distress may be a secondary effect of tumor growth that impinges upon the thoracic cavity or respiratory tree. Respiratory distress also is seen with tumor growth within the abdominal cavity when normal movement of the diaphragm is affected. Because tumor-related respiratory distress is nontransmittable, euthanasia is solely dependent on the animal's prognosis. Even though prognosis may indicate a lengthy illness, secondary respiratory distress should be of critical concern.

6. Blood Dyscrasias

When clinical signs indicate anemia and the cause is not readily apparent (for example, with internal bleeding), hematological testing should be conducted to define the type of anemia. Suspected leukemias should be confirmed by hematological examination (see Chapter 18).

C. The Challenge: Difficult Diagnoses

Implementation and conduct of a successful health monitoring program require experience and dedication. It is a continuous challenge to improve diagnostic techniques, particularly for those conditions that are difficult to diagnose successfully. One such condition, as indicated previously, is mesenteric periarteritis nodosa (Yang, 1965), which occurs in about 2% of our Sprague–Dawley rats used in chronic feeding studies. Such animals often die suddenly from rupture of one of the aneurysmal dilations of the arteries. Another 3 to 5% of the Sprague–Dawley rats in our chronic studies die suddenly, often without any history of anorexia or weight loss or any apparent reason for their demise. The only gross pathological findings at necropsy may be a slight enlargement of the liver or kidney. Upon microscopic examination, the cause of the demise is often found to be interstitial pneumonitis or membranous glomerular nephritis.

VI. TRAINING OF PERSONNEL

The training of personnel for a clinical monitoring program is essentially an informal on-the-job program that builds on the formal education and experience of the animal technician, the veterinarian, the pathologist, and the toxicologist. The toxicologist should review the appropriate literature prior to the development of a study protocol. Based upon such a review, he or she has to develop some concepts of what toxicological signs may be expected. The pathologist or veterinarian may suggest the periodic utilization of various test animal specimens for evaluation by hematological and/or clinical laboratories. The veterinarian may have special requirements regarding tissue samples, for example, to aid in the differentiation of toxicological and disease entities or to maintain the desired level of quality control (Fox et al., 1979).

The animal health technician needs to develop a "cage-side manner" that allows for the appropriate handling of an animal to facilitate general examination and palpation procedures. Animal technicians are the cornerstone of a successful clinical examination program. A major component of the technicians' training in our facility involves their attendance at necropsies and their assistance to the pathologist in the conduct of the necropsy. The reality of the clinical signs are forcefully registered when gross lesions are examined. Keen animal technicians usually request to attend a necropsy when they have been following an animal whose disease status has proved difficult to diagnose.

Training of animal technicians also involves their participation in discussions, wherein data from the hematology and clinical chemistry laboratory and other ancillary studies (pharmacokinetics, immunology etc.) are reviewed in conjunction with the pathological findings. The professional outlines how all data are used to explain disease processes. In this way, the technicians' diagnostic skills are enriched and they acquire an appreciation of their contribution to the successful conduct of the study.

Acknowledgments

The comments of Drs. C. Chappel and J. Emerson on specific portions of this text are gratefully acknowledged.

References

Andervont, H. B. (1944) Influence of environment on mammary cancer in mice. J. Natl. Cancer Inst. (US) 4, 579–581.

Arnold, D. L., Charbonneau, S. M., Zawidzka, Z. Z., and Grice, H. C. (1977). Monitoring animal health during chronic toxicity studies. J. Environ. Pathol. Toxicol. 1, 227–239.

Arnold, D. L., Moodie, C. A., Charbonneau, S. M., Grice, H. C., McGuire, P. F., Bryce, F. R., Collins, B. T., Zawidzka, Z. Z., Krewski, D. R., Nera, E. A., and Munro, I. C. (1985). Long-term toxicity of hexachlorobenzene in the rat and the effect of dietary vitamin A. Food Chem. Toxicol. 23, 779–793.

Arnold, D. L., Moodie, C. A., Grice, H. C., Charbonneau, S. M., Stavric, B., Collins, B. T., McGuire, P. F., Zawidzka, Z. Z., and Munro, I. C. (1980). Long-term toxicity of ortho-toluenesulfonamide and sodium saccharin in the rat. *Toxicol. Appl. Pharmacol.* **52,** 113–152.

Fare, G. (1965). The influence of number of mice in a box on experimental skin tumour production. *Br. J. Cancer* **19,** 871–877.

Fox, J. G. (1977). Clinical assessment of laboratory rodents in long-term bioassay studies. *J. Environ. Pathol. Toxicol.* **1,** 199–226.

Fox, J. G., Thibert, P., Arnold, D. L., Krewski, D. R., and Grice, H. C. (1979). Toxicology studies. Part II. The laboratory animal. *Food Cosmet. Toxicol.* **17,** 661–676.

Grice, H. C., and Burek, J. D. (1984). Age-Associated (Geriatric) Pathology: Its Impact on Long-Term Toxicity Studies. *In* "Current Issues in Toxicology" (H. C. Grice, ed.) pp. 57–107. New York: Springer-Verlag.

Hatch, A., Wiberg, G., Zawidzka, Z., Cann, M., Airth, J., and Grice, H. (1965). Isolation syndrome in the rat. *Toxicol. Appl. Pharmacol.* **7,** 737–745.

International Agency for Research on Cancer (1980). Basic requirements for long-term assays for carcinogenicity. *IARC Monogr. Suppl. 2,* 23–83.

Sigg, E., Day, C., and Colombo, C. (1966). Endocrine factors in isolation-induced aggressiveness in rodents. *Endocrinology* **78,** 679–684.

U.S. Environmental Protection Agency (1983a). Part III, toxic substance control; Good laboratory practice standards; Final rule. *Fed. Regist.* **48,** 53922–53944.

U.S. Environmental Protection Agency (1983b). Part IV, pesticide program; Good laboratory practice standards; Final rule. *Fed. Regist.* **48,** 53946–53969.

U.S. Food and Drug Administration (1978). Department of Health, Education, and Welfare, nonclinical laboratory studies, good laboratory practice regulations. *Fed. Regist.* **43,** 59986–060020.

Welch, B. L., and Welch, A. S. (1966). Graded effect of social stimulation upon d-amphetamine toxicity, agressiveness and heart and adrenal weight. *J. Pharmacol. Exp. Ther.* **151,** 331–338.

Yang, Y. H. (1965). Polyarteritis nodosa in laboratory rats. *Lab. Invest.* **14,** 81–85.

18
Hematological Evaluation

Zofia Z. Zawidzka
Toxicology Research Division
Bureau of Chemical Safety
Food Directorate
Health Protection Branch
Health and Welfare Canada
Ottawa, Ontario

I. INTRODUCTION

Why is hematological assessment, as part of toxicological studies, important? The fact that hematotoxic effects may be life threatening has been generally recognized and described as "most feared and respected" (Saslaw and Carlisle, 1969). The toxic substance may affect circulating blood cells (erythrocytes, leukocytes, and platelets) or those developing in the blood-forming organs involving various stages of hematopoietic activity such as cell division, maturation, release, and destruction, as well as cell function (e.g., granulocyte phagocytic properties). In addition, host exposure to certain chemicals and/or drugs may directly or indirectly induce disturbances in hemostatic mechanisms and result in a bleeding diathesis.

Because hematological alterations observed in the experimental animal may also be caused by physiological or pathological changes not related to treatment, there is a need for a battery of screening tests to help the investigator correctly assess and interpret hematotoxic findings. The basic hematological profile, consisting of relatively simple tests, can provide accurate and pertinent diagnostic information. Moreover, these tests can readily be adapted to small laboratory animals and limited volumes of blood.

Several aspects of hematological screening procedures are considered in this chapter because they may substantially influence reliability of the tests selected and/or validity of the results obtained. These are:

routine, special, and terminal evaluation (purpose and type)
requisites for valid hematological procedures
selection of practical tests
evaluation of cellular elements in differential diagnosis
evaluation of hemostasis and differential diagnosis of hemostatic defects

II. ROUTINE, SPECIAL, AND TERMINAL EVALUATION: PURPOSE AND TYPE

Routine hematological assessment is used as a guide to detect occult disease, to select suitable animals for study, and to monitor their health status. Assessment involves blood examination before, during, and at the end of a study on all or selected groups of animals. Periodic screenings are useful in confirming diagnoses and in predicting the course of disease (e.g., prognosis or progression of the animal's response to therapeutic or experimental treatments). In addition, routine blood examination is also helpful in differential diagnosis of secondary hematological manifestations of disease. For example, anemia can be associated with malignancy or chronic infections, leukocytosis with infections, and hemoconcentration with hypoxia or dehydration.

Routine screening commonly consists of hemoglobin (Hb) and packed cell volume (PCV) measurements, mean corpuscular hemoglobin concentration (MCHC), total and differential leukocyte count, as well as evaluation of erythrocytes, leukocytes, and platelets from blood smears. If semiautomatic counters or multichannel cell analyzers are used, several additional parameters may be obtained on the same sample. If hematological effects of treatment based on routine examination values are observed, further tests may be needed. For example, in cases of anemia, reticulocyte counts are useful for evaluating erythropoietic activity; if a bleeding tendency is suspected, platelet count and hemostatic function should be evaluated. Specific platelet function tests have been recommended for toxicological screening (Hawkins, 1972), but these require relatively large quantities of blood (unavailable in rodents) and expensive instrumentation; consequently, they may not be practical. However, for toxicological studies, minimum screening procedures for the detection of abnormalities of coagulation and platelets have been recommended by the Workshop Group on Clotting and Platelets (Vargaftig *et al.*, 1979) and by Theus and Zbinden (1984).

Specialized hematological assessment is required when evidence of blood dyscrasias occur in any experimental animal. Examples include enlarged lymph nodes and/or spleen, unexplained anemia, and evidence of hemorrhagic episodes.

Terminal hematological studies, including examination of blood and hematopoietic organs, are necessary on animals requiring euthanasia before the conclusion of the study and on all or designated groups of animals at the termination of the study in order to characterize hematotoxic changes, if present, or to exclude treatment-related effects. All animals with signs of hematological complications should be thoroughly investigated to confirm tentative diagnoses and/or to define the extent of disease. This becomes possible at the time of necropsy when larger quantities of blood and tissue samples are readily available. These procedures are basic and well established; however, newer approaches applicable to detecting early hematotoxic damage are also available (Irons, 1985). The importance of studying blood and bone marrow toxicity to assess risks involved in human exposure to toxic substances and using current sophisticated methods (e.g., flow cytofluorometric and cytogenetic analyses), which increase the sensitivity of hematological evaluation, has been excellently emphasized (Irons, 1985).

A. Requisites for Valid Hematological Procedures

Valid hematological assessment requires knowledge of normal morphology of blood cells and their precursors and familiarity with species-specific morphological differences in both mature and immature blood cells. A working knowledge of atypical or pathological blood cells and a general knowledge of the mechanisms of hemostasis including platelet function, coagulation, and fibrinolysis, as well as recognition of the importance of species-specific differences is also required. The efficiency and effectiveness of hematological assessment as a diagnostic aid is directly proportional to the specificity, sensitivity, precision, and reproducibility of the methods. Unavoidable technical errors can be minimized by assuring correct performance of the test, that is, by using standard operation procedures (SOPs; see Chapter 22). Also important is knowledge of the principles underlying these procedures and the sources of potential error; sound judgment in test selection and technical skill in performance; and correct evaluation and interpretation of results obtained.

There are several excellent books dealing with the different aspects of hematology that are useful for differential diagnostic purposes. A suggested reading list is included at the end of this chapter.

Quality control is essential to good laboratory performance (Wintrobe et al., 1974). This includes proper blood collection (Wintrobe *et al.,* 1974); strict calibration and maintenance of instruments (Gilmer *et al.,* 1977; Koepke, 1977); meticulous adherence to technical details of selected methods (Hawkey, 1975); control of reagents; daily testing of commercially available standards and cellular preparations (Wintrobe *et al.,* 1974); plasma standards for coagulation tests (Dodds, 1980) and biological controls. Methods and instrumentation have been designed and developed primarily for analyzing human blood. When these are used for animal blood, necessary modifications may be introduced. It is desirable, however, to periodically check the performance of the instrument used on animal blood cells outside the size range of human red cells. This can be accomplished by running a set of tests, similar to those required for commercial cell control preparations, on healthy animals maintained specifically for this purpose. The possibility of hematological changes being induced by frequent sampling should always be considered and avoided, particularly in smaller species.

All hematological procedures begin with blood procurement, which plays an important role in subsequent evaluations. Tests of hemostatic function may be profoundly influenced by inadequate or careless sampling (Table I).

1. Equipment for Drawing Blood

All equipment used for drawing blood samples should be clean and dry. Needles should be short beveled and sharp. Needle size depends on the species, the quantity of blood required, and the intended procedure. Coverslips require a special cleaning procedure (Cartwright, 1968), and glassware used for coagulation tests should be either disposable or suitably prepared (Bowie *et al.,* 1971). Plastic tubes can be substituted when siliconized glassware is required.

2. Anticoagulants

The type and quantity of anticoagulant needed depend on the test involved. The mode of action of the anticoagulant should not alter or

Table I

Common Errors Related to Sampling and Specimen Handling

Problems encountered during sampling and/or specimen handling	Evaluation of affected cellular elements	Evaluation of affected hemostatic function
Animals		
a. Stress, rough handling, fear, struggle, and pain	Mild to gross changes in cellular constituents, with unpredictable results (a)[a]	Increased clotting activity (a)[a].
Equipment		
b. Improperly washed glassware	Loss of isotonicity with escape of intracellular substances from ruptured erythrocytes (hemolysis) (i)	Release of erythrocyte and platelet phospholipids which have coagulant activity (i, l)
c. Scratched or rough surface		Activation and consumption of clotting factors (b, c, e, h, j, k)
Anticoagulants		
d. Unsuitable anticoagulant	Erythrocyte size and shape changes (b, d, f, g, n)	Loss of clotting activity (b, m, n)
e. Inadequate amount of anticoagulant	Mechanical lysis (hemolysis) (l)	Alterations in the optimal quantity of calcium ions required for clot formation (e, f, g)
f. Excess anticoagulant	Chemically-induced hemolysis (b)	Unsuitable anticoagulation (d)
g. Incorrect concentration of anticoagulant	All or some erythrocyte values unacceptable	
Blood collection and handling		
h. Difficult blood taking	Loss of leukocyte morphologic characteristics and ability to stain properly (d,m)	Irreversible changes in platelet function (b, c, d, e, f, g, h, k, l, m, n)
i. Sample contamination with water	Leukocyte evaluation unreliable	Results are invalidated if one or more of the above problems occur while evaluating hemostasis
j. Sample contamination with tissue juice	Platelet clumping precludes accurate counting (d, h, k, l)	
k. Poor or delayed mixing	Partial or complete clotting of the sample causes utilization of platelets and trapping of other blood cells in the fibrin meshwork (e, g, h, j, k), counts are unacceptable	
l. Excessive manipulation of the sample (e.g., vigorous shaking)		
m. Excessive delay between sampling and test performance		
n. Samples kept at an incorrect temperature		
o. Errors in sample labeling	Errors in reporting of hematologic results (o)	

[a] These letters refer to letters in column on left of table.

interact with the substance being investigated. Two most suitable and commonly used anticoagulants in hematological procedures are sodium or tripotassium salt of ethylenediaminetetraacetic acid (EDTA) for cellular assessment (1.0–1.5 mg/ml of blood) and trisodium citrate[1] for coagulation and platelet studies at a concentration of 1 volume of anticoagulant to 9 volumes of blood, assuming the PCV is 0.45 liter/liter. Trisodium citrate is not commonly used for cellular assessment because of the dilution factor introduced into the sample.

3. Blood Sampling

Stress must be minimized because it profoundly influences blood constituents and may rapidly cause marked alteration in cellular values (Hawkey, 1975; Schalm et al., 1975; Payne et al., 1976; Archer, 1977). Improper restraint, housing of animals in the same room as those being killed or in noisy or busy areas should be avoided or minimized. Ether-induced anesthesia, although widely accepted in the past but greatly curtailed in recent years because of safety concerns, has been replaced frequently with carbon dioxide (Fowler et al., 1980). At present its use is limited to relatively few procedures. It should be noted that, when used, it produces splenic contraction and marked increase in blood cell constituents (Schalm et al., 1975). When it is used for short periods (up to 2 min) to collect samples, hematological values are not significantly affected in the rat (Cann et al., 1965). On the other hand, some tranquilizers and anesthetics such as barbital compounds reduce cellular blood levels by causing splenic sequestration (Schalm et al., 1975). Halothane has a similar effect although other mechanisms may be involved (Steffey et al., 1976). Ketamine hydrochloride produces minimal effects when combined with acepromazine (Porter, 1982). Anesthetics are rarely used in dogs or larger animals because physical restraint is usually sufficient.

During chronic studies, samples may be obtained directly from the earflap marginal vein in guinea pigs (Bullock, 1983) and rabbits (Grice, 1964); the orbital sinus (provided fluid contamination is avoided), clipped toe nail, or tail tip in small rodents (Grice, 1964) including mice (Stoltz and Bendall, 1975); and the superficial tail artery or vein (Hurwitz, 1971; Stearns and Lee, 1984) and the jugular vein in rats (Archer and Riley, 1981). Serial tail amputations are not recommended, especially in older rats, because of a high probability of sample contamination with body fluids. In addition, undesirable side effects such as infection, prolonged bleeding, and tail mutilation can occur from amputations in

---

[1] 0.13–0.14 M w/v (Dodds, 1980) and 0.106 M (Chart and Sanderson, 1979) have been suggested for most laboratory animals, with the exception of rabbit blood, which requires a higher concentration (0.2 M) of anticoagulant (Bjoraker and Ketcham, 1981).

rats. Venous blood is usually taken from the radial vein of the forelimbs in dogs and cats (Grice, 1964; Archer, 1977), the femoral vein in monkeys (Martin *et al.*, 1973), the brachial vein (Grice, 1964) or venous occipital sinus in birds (Vuillaume, 1983), and several venipuncture sites in armadillos (Moore, 1983). In pigs, the anterior vena cava or posterior jugular vein is often used although tail and ear veins are sometimes employed (Archer, 1977). Cardiac puncture should be considered only as a last resort in larger laboratory animals because it requires anesthesia and is hazardous. Anesthesia is also recommended for cardiac puncture in rodents (Archer, 1965). Additional information on sampling sites and methods may be found in Bivin and Smith (1984) and Smith *et al.*(1986).

The skin over the sampling site should be dry. A small amount of vaseline may be used to flatten hair, help expose the vein, and prevent blood drops from spreading when direct samples are taken. Bleeding is usually stopped by gentle pressure with gauze over the puncture. A special "hemostat" made from a rubber stopper is an excellent device to stop tail bleeding (Stoltz and Bendall, 1975). Terminal blood samples may be obtained from the abdominal aorta of anesthetized animals (Grice, 1964) or from the inferior vena cava of mice (Adeghe and Cohen, 1986).

All sampling must be accomplished as quickly as possible. In cases of failure, a fresh needle should be used on any new attempt to avoid activation of coagulation. Anticoagulants prevent coagulation but cannot arrest the sequence of events leading to clot formation once it has been triggered. The minimal amount of blood necessary for obtaining the required information should be drawn (Archer, 1977).

4. Sampling of Hematopoietic Organs

If required, bone marrow may be aspirated from a live animal or obtained at necropsy. Several considerations are warranted for bone marrow aspiration. Aseptic techniques should be employed and animals properly restrained. General anesthesia is recommended, but local anesthesia of the skin and highly sensitive periosteum may be used in larger animals. The best sample site should be selected, and samples should not be excessively diluted with blood.

The richest material usually comes from the needle content. Smears are made immediately and preferably with no anticoagulant. Detailed description of the procedure can be found in Gilmore *et al.* (1964), Lewis (1967), Switzer (1967), Valli *et al.* (1969), Schalm and Switzer (1972), Schalm *et al.* (1975), and Archer (1977). Terminal assessment is advisable for elaboration of disease manifestations observed in the peripheral blood.

At necropsy, marrow samples should be obtained and smears made not later than 15 minutes after cardiac arrest. In most laboratory animals, the femur is an excellent source of marrow. It should be removed, dissected, and split longitudinally. The best marrow is found in the proximal end of the bone in the subendosteal area where relatively few fat cells occur. In the dog, the richest hematopoietic activity is found in the rib (Calvo *et al.*, 1975). The marrow is scooped onto a clean coverslip and smears made either by a touch method or by gentle pulling of a marrow particle adhering to the coverslip across another coverslip or slide. "Squashing" the marrow results in rupturing and/or distorting cells.

Samples can also be obtained at biopsy or necropsy from lymph nodes, thymus, and spleen. The organ is cut with a dry and sharp scalpel, and the cut surface is lightly imprinted on coverslips or slides. All preparations should be quickly air dried to avoid possible cellular distortion.

B. Selection of Practical Tests

When selecting tests for hematological evaluation, one should consider the following points.

1. Type of information required
2. Routine health monitoring
3. Special evaluation necessitated by presence of clinical signs indicating hematopoietic disturbance and/or hemostatic impairment
4. Basic attributes of the method (specificity, sensitivity, accuracy, and reproducibility)
5. Feasibility of performing tests on large numbers of animals particularly if the delay between sampling and performance is likely to alter results
6. Limitations in blood procurement (number and type of tests in small rodents tailored to quantity of blood that can be safely obtained without influencing the resting hematological state)

As a rule, the simplest most valid test or combination of tests should be chosen (see also Chapter 19). The following description of tests commonly used in hematological evaluation is limited to the principles involved and their applicability to animal blood.

1. Packed Red Cell Volume liter/liter

a. Macromethod

Amount of blood required: 1.0 ml
Recommended anticoagulant: EDTA

Packed red cell volume (PCV) is the single most reliable test of all erythroid measurements of red cell concentration (Linman, 1966). It involves optimal packing of erythrocytes in a special tube with a minimal amount of trapped plasma and with no distortion or loss of red cell content. This is achieved by centrifugation of the tube at a strictly controlled relative centrifugal force (2260 g for 30 min; Wintrobe et al., 1974).

Additional information may be derived from observation of the centrifuged specimen (Arnold et al., 1977). Altered color or opacity of plasma may indicate hemolysis, jaundice, or lipemia. A thick buffy coat layer (which consists of leukocytes and platelets) indicates leukocytosis or leukemia. A reduced volume of sedimented red cells signals anemia, and the reverse indicates polycythemia.

b. Micromethod

Amount of blood required: approximately 50 μl
Recommended anticoagulant: EDTA or heparin

If the microcapillary tubes are pretreated with heparin, direct samples may be taken. The tube is filled to about 3/4 of its length with blood, sealed at one end, and centrifuged in a special microcentrifuge at about 12,500 g for 3–5 minutes depending on the centrifuge model and tube size. Results are read on a special scale or with a reading device. The small amount of blood required and the short processing time are advantages of this method.

c. Automated Hematocrit

Amount of blood required: see erythrocyte enumeration

Hematocrit (HCT) computed values can be estimated by multiparameter electronic counters or counters with special accessories. Values obtained by automated methods appear to be more reliable than those derived from manual methods (Fairbanks, 1980).

d. Comments

Most laboratory animal erythrocytes are smaller than their human counterparts and are proportionally more numerous. Furthermore, their shape tends to become more spherical as size decreases. Erythrocyte shape is also related to the ability of the cell to expand and resist rupture. Spherically shaped cells rupture more readily even in a normal environment; therefore, PCV or HCT assays should be made as soon as possible after blood collection. Excess EDTA, if used, affects erythrocyte sizes and renders values inaccurate. Stress, excitement (Schalm et al., 1975), and feeding (Reece and Wahlstrom, 1970; Greenwood, 1977) may increase erythrocytic values although species variations in such responses exist. Altitude as well as seasonal (Thomas and Kittrell, 1966) and diurnal (Hawkey, 1975; Hodges, 1977) variations also influence erythrocyte concentrations. Some of these factors, such as diurnal variation and stress, point out the need for random sampling among all treatment groups.

2. Erythrocyte Enumeration $N \times 10^{12}$/liter

Amount of blood required: $20-40$ μl
Recommended anticoagulant: EDTA or none for direct counts

The reliability of the erythrocyte enumeration (RBC) value depends largely on the method used. The count is necessary for the calculation of mean corpuscular indices.

a. Manual Method

Although manual RBC counting has been almost totally replaced by semiautomated or automated methods, in some pathological cases visual counting may be necessary. Two basic points should be observed in visual counting: the specimen must be properly handled when dilutions are made; preparation and counting must be done carefully and correctly (Cartwright, 1968).

b. Automatic Cell Enumeration

Two important steps are required to achieve accuracy and reproducibility in RBC enumeration.

Step 1. Preparation of the Instrument Calibrate and select suitable settings for the given species so that all erythrocytes are counted and noise signals excluded (Weide *et al.,* 1962; Wisecup and Crouch, 1963; Schalm *et al.,* 1975). Check for instability of electronic components, electrical interference, air bubbles, leaks, and obstructions. Use particle-free diluents maintained at the correct temperature. Test quality control standard preparations daily under the same experimental conditions as the test bloods.

Step 2. Preparation of the Sample Properly collect blood. If required, carefully prepare erythrocyte predilutions and count immediately. Perform counting according to the manufacturer's instructions. Correctly record results.

c. Comments

Automatic counting is superior in accuracy and precision to manual counting, provided that both the instrument and specimens are handled correctly and the operator has a good working knowledge of the principles, operation, and malfunctions of the instrument. Animal erythrocytes, because of their variety in size, numbers, and stability, require special attention. Counts expected to exceed 5×10^{12}/liter should be diluted to an acceptable concentration in order to minimize coincidental loss. Smaller aperture tubes have been recommended as well as higher cell dilutions for erythrocytes of very small volume (< 40 fl; Winter, 1965). In some multiparameter cell analyzers, readjustment of aperture current allows for placing the particle pulses in the proper range location to accommodate counting of small erythrocytes (Weiser, 1987). Performing counts within one hour after collection safeguards against the loss of the more fragile cells and reduces the variability of any time-dependent anticoagulant affect on cell volume. In pathological conditions that result in cell clumping, spuriously low counts and high mean cell volume may be obtained; therefore, manual counts are more reliable in these cases. False results are also caused by extremely high leukocyte counts (Cartwright, 1968) and platelet clumps (Schalm *et al.,* 1975).

3. Mean Corpuscular Indices

Mean corpuscular indices are measurements derived from erythrocyte values (RBC, PCV or HCT, and hemoglobin concentration). Their validity depends on the accuracy of the test results from which they are calculated. The indices are useful and sensitive parameters of erythrocyte evaluation.

a. Mean Corpuscular Volume

MCV, expressed in femtoliters (fl), is the volume of the average red cell calculated from the number of red cells and PCV.

$$\text{MCV (fl)} = \frac{\text{PCV liter/liter} \times 1000}{\text{RBC} \times 10^{12}/\text{liter}} \tag{1}$$

MCV may also be measured directly with some electronic counters.

b. Mean Corpuscular Hemoglobin Concentration

MCHC, expressed in grams of hemoglobin per liter of packed red cells (g/liter), is the ratio of hemoglobin weight to the average red cell volume in which it is contained. It is calculated from the hemoglobin value and PCV or HCT.

$$\text{MCHC(g/liter)} = \frac{\text{Hb g/liter}}{\text{PCV liter/liter}} \tag{2}$$

c. Mean Corpuscular Hemoglobin

MCH, expressed in picograms (pg), is the amount of hemoglobin by weight per the average red cell calculated from the hemoglobin value and RBC.

$$\text{MCH (pg)} = \frac{\text{Hb g/liter}}{\text{RBC} \times 10^{12}/\text{liter}} \tag{3}$$

d. Comments

MCV, when measured electronically or derived by a computerized size distribution analysis, is precise and not influenced by such physiological variables as excitement. It can be an excellent indicator of certain types of anemia (Payne et al., 1976; Fehr, 1987). The measurement is influenced by improper instrument calibration, changes in temperature, plasma osmotic imbalance, traces of detergent, pH and tonicity of the diluent, as well as by excessive amounts of EDTA. The rat erythrocyte is particularly susceptible to size alterations (Legge and Shortman, 1968). Presence of cold agglutinins in the blood causes red cell clumping that results in spurious MCV, MCHC, and MCH (de Lange et al., 1972).

MCHC is an indirect measurement, and its accuracy depends on the validity of hemoglobin and PCV or HCT values. It is considered the most constant and precise index whether derived from manual or automated methods. In vertebrates, the amount of hemoglobin capable of supplying a required amount of oxygen to tissues is amazingly constant (Hawkey, 1977). MCHC therefore differs little between species and only rarely exceeds 370 g/liter value. In relatively recent studies, however, flow cytometry analysis of the density-fractionated red cells demonstrated substantial density differences between light and heavier red cell fractions (Fehr, 1987). Furthermore, dispersions of the red cell volume and hemoglobin concentration were observed to vary independently and be species specific, revealing a lower hemoglobin concentration dispersion in some mammalian species red cells, that is, lower in canine and murine erythrocytes than in the human erythrocytes (Groner et al., 1986). According to Fehr (1987), higher MCHC values of some red cell fractions, obtained by sophisticated morphometry methods, invalidate the view that the solubility of hemoglobin in living red cells is limited to 370-380 g/liter, which is generally accepted as the maximal value of MCHC. It has also been suggested that the hemoglobin solubility limit in human and rat red cells is 419 g/liter and 379 g/liter respectively (Groner et al., 1986). Thus, the validity of nonhuman MCHC 380 g/liter is questionable and may indicate a technical error, especially when obtained from electronic counters and sizing instruments. Consequently, it is possible that hemoglobin concentration histograms, if available, may be even more sensitive and informative than volume histograms (see red cell volume distribution width following) alone or volume histograms coupled with other erythrocyte indices (Fehr, 1987).

MCH depends on the size of the erythrocyte and the weight of hemoglobin present in the cell. It adds little to the information provided by MCV and MCHC indices (Payne *et al.*, 1976).

4. Red Cell Volume Distribution Width

Red cell volume distribution width (RDW) is calculated as the coefficient of variation of the red cell volume distribution histogram and is expressed as a percentage. It is obtained as part of the report displayed and printed by some multichannel cell analyzers or from a suitable channelyzer with an automated cell counter.

Comments

RDW is an accurate method of red cell sizing (quantitative evaluation of anisocytosis). When used in conjunction with MCV and included in the hematological evaluation, it is helpful in detecting and identifying early red cell changes (e.g., nutritional deficiencies) and in providing an initial differential diagnosis of the existing abnormality in humans (Bessman *et al.*, 1983).

In animal blood, the erythrogram sensitivity in response to erythrocyte volume disturbances has been observed (Weiser and Kociba, 1982, 1983a, 1983b; Weiser and O'Grady, 1983) and normal species-specific ranges reported (Weiser, 1982).

5. Hemoglobin Concentration g/liter

Amount of blood required: 20–40 μl
Recommended anticoagulant: EDTA or none if taken directly

a. Cyanmethemoglobin Method

The cyanmethemoglobin method for hemoglobin measurement has been recommended by the International Committee for Standardization in Hematology and is most widely used. In this method, all hemoglobin derivatives except sulfhemoglobin are converted by ferricyanide to methemoglobin, which combines with cyanide to form the stable pigment cyanmethemoglobin. The reaction is stoichiometric; stable and accurate standards are commercially available.

b. Comments

Several factors can alter the optical density of diluted hemoglobin preparations and yield spurious results. Marked leukocytosis (white cells above
50×10^9/liter; Wintrobe *et al.*, 1974) and presence of Heinz bodies
(Schmauch bodies in cats; Schalm *et al.*, 1975) will alter optical density
reading. To obtain more accurate values, the diluted hemoglobin should
be centrifuged at approximately 1,150 *g* for 10 min, the supernatant carefully transferred to a clean tube and the hemoglobin determined in the
usual manner.

Lipemia also affects results. To obtain a fairly accurate estimation, a
dilution free of red cells is set up with a corresponding amount of autologous plasma. The diluent and its value is subtracted from that of the
whole blood dilution.

6. Methemoglobin Concentration

**Amount of blood required: 0.2 ml of whole blood or 0.15 ml
washed erythrocytes
Recommended anticoagulant: none if taken directly, heparin,
or EDTA**

Methemoglobin (MetHb) concentration is reported as a percentage of
Hb concentration or in g/liter. MetHb forms when the iron of Hb is
oxidized from the ferrous to ferric state. The latter is unable to bind
reversibly and release oxygen. MetHb forms continuously in normal
erythrocytes but is reduced by a specific MetHb reductase enzyme system. Methemoglobinemia may be produced by excessive exposure to
oxidant substances and/or by intraerythrocytic abnormalities.

a. Quantitative Method (Tönz, 1968)

The Hb present in a portion of stroma-free, hemolysed sample is converted to MetHb by an oxidizing agent and measured. Another portion of
the hemolysate is left intact and measured for MetHb content. MetHb
present in both portions is then transformed to cyanmethemoglobin by
the addition of potassium cyanide. The percentage of MetHb in the
sample is calculated from the extinction difference in each portion of the
hemolysate. If absolute MetHb values are required, they are calculated
from the Hb content of the samples and expressed in g/liter.

b. Comments

Because normal intraerythrocytic mechanisms will reduce MetHb within
5–12 hrs, the samples should be processed shortly after sampling, or

suitable measures should be taken to prevent spontaneous MetHb reduction (Sleight and Sinha, 1968). Species differences in MetHb formation exist (Clark and de la Garza, 1967) and should be considered whenever MetHb estimation is undertaken in laboratory animals.

7. Reticulocyte Count

Amount of blood required: approximately 20 μl
Recommended anticoagulant: EDTA or none if taken directly

Reticulocyte count is reported in percent of erythrocytes. A semiquantitative estimation may be obtained by multiplying the percentage of reticulocytes by the red cell count, expressed as $N \times 10^9$/liter.

Reticulocytes are young erythrocytes in the final stage of maturation. Reticulocyte assessment is an important aspect of hematological evaluation and a sensitive index of bone marrow erythropoietic activity. A supravital staining technique is used to demonstrate the characteristic residual RNA-containing material. The use of new methylene blue is generally accepted and satisfactory. Blood is mixed with the dye and incubated prior to the making of smears. Air-dried smears may be counterstained with a Romanowsky-type stain. Smears are examined microscopically under oil immersion lens.

Comments

Marrow erythropoietic activity in most mammals is reflected by the number and maturation stage of circulating reticulocytes. There are some exceptions (e.g., the horse; Schalm et al., 1975; Jeffcott, 1977). Young reticulocytes contain heavy aggregates of reticula that become gradually finer and fewer as the cell matures. Eventually, only scant punctate foci of reticula are left. Manner of drying the smear, concentration of the dye, and pH of the staining solution may also influence the shape and density of reticula (Wintrobe et al., 1974). The feline reticulocyte is noteworthy because it matures slowly and, in a healthy cat, most circulating reticulocytes have only a few discrete granules. There is no general agreement as to whether "old" feline reticulocytes should be included in the count (Cramer and Lewis, 1972; Schalm et al., 1975; Alsaker et al., 1977; Mackey, 1977). Age-related variations in the number of circulating reticulocytes occur in many animals, and seasonal variations have been reported in rabbits (Pintor and Grassini, 1957) and frogs (Schermer, 1967). In rodents, circulating reticulocytes may appear in clusters (Hawkey, 1975).

8. Demonstration of Heinz Bodies

Amount of blood required: approximately 50 μl
Recommended anticoagulant: EDTA or none if taken directly
and processed immediately

Heinz bodies are small refractile intraerythrocytic bodies resulting from
Hb oxidative injury. They may be demonstrated by supravital stains,
such as crystal violet (Cartwright, 1968) and new methylene blue, or
observed in unstained wet preparations under phase-contrast microscopy. For toxicological studies, permanent preparations with supravital
stains may be desirable.

9. Leukocyte Enumeration N × 10⁹/liter

Amount of blood required: 20−40 μl
Recommended anticoagulant: EDTA or none if taken directly

Erythrocytes are lysed prior to counting leukocytes or white blood cells
(WBCs). All remarks including instrument modifications (Weiser, 1987),
and pertaining to manual and automatic methods for erythrocyte enumeration also apply to WBC enumeration.

Comments

In automated methods, the same dilution of blood or whole blood sample
can be used for leukocyte and erythrocyte enumeration, hemoglobin
determination, and other hematological parameters.

Regardless of the method, nucleated red cells cannot be distinguished
from leukocytes and are included in the count. The number of nucleated
erythrocytes should be determined from the differential leukocyte count
and subtracted from the total WBC count, provided all nucleated red
cells are included in the total count. The choice of the stromatolysing
agent used in automated counting is important. It should be sufficiently
potent to lyse all erythrocytes but leave leukocytes intact. Incomplete red
cell lysis may result in spuriously high WBC counts because stroma and
debris will be included in the count. Once suspended in the stromatolysing solution, leukocytes should be counted within 15−20 minutes to
prevent any loss due to the cytolytic properties of the agent. The leukocytes of some species, for example, the mouse, are highly susceptible to
lysis. Bovine preleukemic and leukemic lymphocytes appear to be excep-
tionally fragile (Schalm *et al.*, 1975). Platelet clumps, if present, may
produce false high counts. Abnormally low counts should be verified by a
manual method.

10. Platelet Enumeration N × 10⁹/liter

Amount of blood required: approximately 20 µl for manual count; up to 1 ml for automated methods; cell analyzers providing whole blood platelet counts require only a fixed amount of blood for all parameters (e.g., 100 µl).
Recommended anticoagulant: EDTA

a. Manual Methods

Phase-contrast method (Brecher and Cronkite, 1950), light microscopy method (Schalm *et al.*, 1975; Archer, 1977), and quantitative peripheral smear estimation of platelets (Schalm *et al.*, 1975; Nosanchuk *et al.*, 1978) are rapid and reasonably accurate indirect counting methods.

b. Automated Methods Requiring Platelet Rich Plasma

Platelet rich plasma (PRP) can be obtained either by sedimentation or centrifugation. Special platelet counters and a centrifuge designed for this purpose are available. Counters used primarily for RBC and WBC but calibrated for platelet counting and equipped with a suitable aperture are also satisfactory. To take full advantage of automated methods, manufacturer's instructions should be closely followed.

c. Automated Whole Blood Platelet Counting and Sizing

A whole blood sample is automatically diluted within the instrument, platelets are counted and sized, and a histogram is produced. The results are printed, including mean platelet volume (MPV) and platelet distribution width (PDW).

d. Comments

Of the manual methods, the phase-contrast method is considered superior to light microscopy because it permits better discrimination between platelets and debris (Cartwright, 1968). This difficulty is partly overcome when commercial diluent systems are used (Wertz and Koepke, 1977).

The advantages of automated platelet counting in PRP over manual methods have been generally acknowledged (Cartwright, 1968; Gottfried *et al.*, 1976). In animals with poor erythrocyte sedimentation (e.g., bovine), a modified sedimentation method for diluted whole blood has been suggested (Maxie, 1977).

Whole blood platelet enumeration appears to be both rapid and reliable (Bessman, 1980; Ross *et al.*, 1980). The whole procedure is simplified and the accuracy of the count significantly improved (Wertz and Triplett, 1980; Cornbleet and Kessinger, 1985). Technical difficulties asso-

ciated with PRP preparation and excessive handling are avoided (Dumoulin-Lagrange and Capelle, 1983). This is an important advantage
when dealing with animal platelets that are often prone to spontaneous
clumping (e.g., cat), even if blood is properly sampled and handled.

With increased availability of routine platelet counting and sizing, the
usefulness of these parameters for experimental studies becomes obvious
(Eason et al., 1986). A platelet histogram provides a sensitive and accurate quantitative assessment of platelet volume heterogeneity and is
superior to qualitative evaluation of the smear alone. The smear check,
however, is always indicated, especially if counts and/or histograms are
abnormal, to exclude spurious results caused by the presence of platelet
clumps, debris, and particles other than platelets (Dumoulin-Lagrange
and Capelle, 1983; Mayer et al., 1985).

Platelet clumping precludes a meaningful count by any method. Hemolysis, introducing red cell fragments, and high WBC counts also contribute to erratic or false high counts when automated methods are used.
Very high platelet counts (e.g., rat) may require sample dilution, whereas
thrombocytopenic blood samples should be less diluted to increase the
accuracy of counting if manual or PRP counting methods are used.

EDTA, a commonly used anticoagulant for routine hematological testing, requires particular attention because it causes platelet swelling.
Changes in platelet size induced by EDTA are time dependent, thus
creating difficulties in establishing normal ranges for MPV. Moreover,
changes produced by EDTA appear to differ between normal and abnormal platelets (Corash, 1983). A combination of acid-citrate-dextrose
(ACD) and Na_2EDTA has been suggested as the anticoagulant of choice
for the counting and sizing of human platelets (Thompson et al., 1983).

Recent studies for establishing reference techniques for animal bloods
were based on EDTA anticoagulated samples in accordance with requirements for multiparameter counting systems (Weiser and Kociba, 1984).
It should be emphasized that when EDTA is used, the time interval
between blood sampling and stabilization of platelet volume is critical for
consistent interpretation of MPV changes (Dumoulin-Lagrange and Capelle, 1983).

11. Preparation and Examination of Blood Smear

Amount of blood required: approximately 10 – 15 μl
**Recommended anticoagulant: EDTA or preferably smears
made without anticoagulant**

The correct interpretation of a well-made and -stained blood film is one
of the most important aspects of a hematological evaluation (Archer,

1977; Cartwright, 1968; Linman, 1966; Wintrobe *et al.,* 1981). Poor preparation and/or staining can result in misleading information and consequent misinterpretation.

a. Preparation Method

Smears are made on clean coverslips or slides and should be quickly air-dried to prevent cell distortion. A correctly made smear is characterized by an evenly distributed single cell layer with clear background.

b. Staining

The International Committee for Standardization in Haematology (1984) recently published a reference method for staining blood and bone marrow films with azure B and eosin Y (Romanowsky-type stain such as Wrights, Leishman, Giemsa, or Jenner). Optimal staining time differs from species to species and from batch to batch of stain. Automatic staining devices are now available, and those with adjustable timing are very useful.

A well-stained smear appears pink-lavender to the naked eye and has the following microscopic characteristics:

Erythrocytes	Pink
Leukocytes	
Nuclei	Purplish-blue with clearly differentiated chromatin detail
Cytoplasm	Various shades of blue depending on the cell line
Cytoplasmic granules	Violet-pink in neutrophils, red-orange in eosinophils, purple-blue in basophils, azurophilic in lymphocytes, pinkish in monocytes
Platelets	
Granulomere (granular portion)	Appears azurophilic
Hyalomere (cytoplasmic portion)	Appears hyaline, light blue

c. Microscopic Examination

Systematic examination of the smear first with the high dry objective, then under oil immersion, provides information regarding morphology of the individual cell. Substantiation of quantitative values of various cellular elements and morphological assessment are made of:

  1. Erythrocytes: size, color (hemoglobin content), shape including

fragmentation (Rebar *et al.,* 1981), presence of cellular inclusion bodies which may be observed in the Romanowsky type stain such as basophilic stippling, Howell-Jolly bodies (quite common in cats), siderocytes, and presence of nucleated erythrocytes.

2. Leukocytes: leukocytosis or leukopenia should be confirmed; morphologically cells may be normal, atypical, or characterized by degenerative and toxic changes. Presence of immature and malignant cells should be reported.

3. Platelets: thrombocytopenia should be confirmed, presence or absence of platelet clumps as well as abnormal size and staining characteristics should be noted.

The smear is also screened for the presence of intra- and extracellular parasites such as anaplasma (Schalm *et al.,* 1975), bartonella, babesia, ehrlichia (Glenn, 1970), histoplasma (Glenn, 1970; Schalm *et al.,* 1975), microfilaria in dogs (Glenn, 1970; Schalm *et al.,* 1975) and monkeys (Tada *et al.,* 1983), and malaria in monkeys (Ruch, 1967; Donovan *et al.,* 1983; Schofield *et al.,* 1985).

Differential count of leukocytes consists of consecutive count and classification of 200 cells. The results may be reported as a percentage but have to include absolute values for a realistic assessment of each cell line. Absolute values are calculated from the total and differential WBC counts.

d. Comments

Both coverslip and slide methods are acceptable. Smears should be made as soon as possible after sampling if anticoagulated blood is used. Direct smears are recommended in cases of cellular aberrations and when the classification of questionable cells is critical to the ultimate diagnosis, because all anticoagulants affect cell morphology (Linman, 1966). It has been suggested that morphological evaluation of lymphocytes from anticoagulated blood is useless in the nonhuman primate (Huser, 1970). It is essential to be familiar with the species-specific morphology of all normal cell lines before any meaningful evaluation can be undertaken. With most disease processes, dramatic changes and deviations from normal quantitative and qualitative characteristics may be observed.

12. Evaluation of Hematopoietic Organs

Smears and imprint preparations of the hematopoietic organs are stained with modified Romanowsky-type stains.

a. Gross Assessment of the Bone Marrow

Observations should be made on gross appearance of a bone marrow specimen. Color, texture, and excessive fatty infiltration are noted while smears are being made.

b. Microscopic Assessment

Under low magnification, the preparation is scanned thoroughly for smear cellularity, fatty patterns, degree of necrosis, and presence of unusual or markedly abnormal cells. Areas of best cellular distribution, morphological clarity, and adequate staining quality are selected for the differential count. A minimum of 500 cells are examined under oil immersion, preferably on two separate slides, and classified according to cell line and maturation stage. Results of the counts are reported as a percentage; the myeloid/erythroid (M:E) ratio as well as the subjective frequency of mitotic figures are included. Results of the morphological examination in descriptive terms and a narrative interpretation of the marrow observations are given. Lymph node and spleen imprints are examined for cellularity, cytological detail, and cellular aberrations and similarly reported.

c. Comments

Knowledge of species-specific normal blood cell precursors is essential. Any deviation from normal should be described and the preparation referred to an experienced hematologist. Smears and touch imprints made at necropsy are more reliable than aspirates from live animals. In necropsied preparations, there is no or little blood infiltration, multiple sites of the marrow cylinder are sampled, marrow pattern is usually well preserved, and cell population of the imprint is usually representative of the marrow.

The M:E ratio is a valid indicator of marrow activity provided that one cell system is unimpaired (Wintrobe et al., 1981). Therefore, marrow should be interpreted only in conjunction with the hematological examination (Hoff et al., 1985). For example, if the granulocytic series is assumed to be normal, an increased M:E ratio implies depressed erythroid production and, conversely, a decreased M:E ratio implies intensified erythropoietic activity.

Histological sections of hematopoietic organs are normally prepared at necropsy to complete the hematological evaluation (Valli et al., 1969; Bushby, 1970).

13. Coagulation Tests

a. One-Stage Prothrombin Time

Amount of blood required: 0.5 – 1 ml
Recommended anticoagulant: trisodium citrate

Prothrombin time (PT) is a nonspecific test measuring the functional ability of the extrinsic coagulation system involving factors I, II, V, VII, and X. Plasma clotting time is determined in seconds after addition of tissue thromboplastin (factor III) and calcium chloride at 37°C. The test is performed in duplicate by manual or automated methods. The difference between the duplicate determinations must not exceed 5%.

Rabbit brain commercial reagents produce very short coagulation endpoints in most animal plasmas. To detect slight impairments, the reagent may be diluted until the homologous control PT endpoint of 12 – 15 seconds is obtained. With this adjustment, mild deficiencies, producing 3 – 6 seconds longer PT than matched controls, may be identified (Dodds, 1980).

b. Activated Partial Thromboplastin Time

Amount of blood required: 0.5 – 1 ml
Recommended anticoagulant: trisodium citrate

Activated partial thromboplastin time (APTT) is a nonspecific test measuring the functional ability of the intrinsic system. It is prolonged when factors I, II, V, VIII, IX, X, XI, and XII are impaired. Platelet-poor plasma (PPP) is incubated with a partial thromboplastin and a factor XII activator (e.g., kaolin, celite, ellagic acid). The mixture is subsequently recalcified at 37°C and the clotting time observed. The test is performed in duplicate either manually or with automated clot timers.

c. Thrombin Time

Amount of blood required: 0.5 – 1 ml
Recommended anticoagulant: trisodium citrate

Thrombin time (TT) is an easy, accurate, and rapid test that estimates the quantity of functionally active fibrinogen (Jespersen and Sidelmann, 1982). Prolonged TT indicates reduced functional fibrinogen or presence of an inhibitor of the thrombin-fibrinogen reaction. The test is performed in duplicate at 37°C and results are reported in seconds.

d. Serial Thrombin Time

Amount of blood required: sufficient to yield 2 ml plasma
Recommended anticoagulant: 0.1 M sodium oxalate

Serial thrombin time (STT) has been described as the only known test available for fibrinolysis that offers a combination of specificity, differentiation of pathological from physiological fibrinolysin activity, speed of reaction, and quantitative assay capacity. A series of plasma aliquots are incubated for various time intervals. TT is performed in duplicate on each incubated portion of the sample. Interpretation of the test depends on the degree of TT increase in each portion of the incubated sample (Reid et al., 1984).

e. Euglobulin Lysis Time

Amount of blood required: approximately 1 ml
Recommended anticoagulant: trisodium citrate

Euglobulin lysis time (ELT) is a sensitive measure of fibrinolytic activity. Because fibrinolysis is a relatively slow process, it is necessary to reduce and delay fibrinolytic inhibitor activity with a refrigerated centrifuge for preparation of plasma followed by dilution and refrigeration of plasma for 30 min.

The euglobulin portion of the sample is precipitated at pH 5.2–5.9 and then reconstituted. Major fibrinolytic inhibitors are either labile at this pH or eliminated in the supernatant. The reconstituted precipitate is clotted with thrombin, placed at 37°C, and observed for clot lysis.

f. Fibrinogen Fibrin Degradation Products Test

Amount of blood required: 0.5–1 ml
Recommended anticoagulant: none

The Thrombo-Wellcotest[2] design used to detect the presence of fibrinogen fibrin degradation products (FDP) in the human blood can also be used for several animal species including the dog (Dodds, 1980; Chen et al., 1981) and rat. It is a sensitive latex-agglutination method, very useful as a screening aid in the diagnosis of disseminated intravascular coagulation (DIC). Latex suspension is mixed with the diluted test serum on the reaction slide and observed for macroscopic agglutination. Negative and positive controls are provided.

g. Comments

One should not be mislead by the apparent technical simplicity of coagulation tests. A slight deviation from established procedures causes marked changes in results and may render them meaningless. Several rules should be adhered to at all times (See Chapter 19).

---

[2] Thrombo-Wellcotest, Burroughs-Wellcome, Research Triangle Park, North Carolina.

1. Blood sampling is of the utmost importance (Chart and Sanderson, 1979). A difficult venipuncture or slow blood flow produces unacceptable specimens. Presence of hemolysis also precludes further examination because released erythrocytic phospholipids enhance coagulation.

2. The ratio of plasma to anticoagulant must be exact. Excess anticoagulant affects the available calcium ion concentration during recalcification and results in spuriously prolonged clotting times. (Koepke et al., 1975; Ingram and Hills, 1976).

3. Plastic or other noncontact activation equipment must be used, except when glass is specifically required.

4. Blood samples should be centrifuged as soon as possible after collection.

5. Plasma should be stoppered or capped with plastic film to prevent alterations in pH and placed at 4-10°C.

6. Tests should be performed within two hours of blood collection, if possible. If they cannot be done within four hours, small aliquots of plasma may be quick frozen and kept at -70°C until assayed. Control plasmas should be stored in the same manner as test samples.

7. Reagent-grade deionized water should be used for solution preparation.

8. The temperature of the reaction should be $37.5° \pm 1$°C, and the pH of the reaction mixture should be 7.2-7.4.

9. Incubation times of plasma-reagent mixtures, their respective amounts, and mixing technique must be exact and constant. Optimal incubation time has to be established for each species (Greene et al., 1981), method, and/or instrument.

10. The coagulation endpoints obtained with optical devices may be shorter than those obtained with electrical clot timers. Some instruments with optical systems cannot accurately test turbid (lipemic) plasmas or use cloudy (particulate) reagents. Furthermore, when clotting is prolonged, the endpoint forms fibrin strands that may not be detected at all and the test must be repeated manually.

11. The coagulation endpoints of animal plasma are usually shorter than those obtained on human plasma. It is important, therefore, to ascertain that a built-in lag phase in the clot-sensing instrument used is properly adjusted to accommodate specific needs required for animal coagulation studies.

12. Monitoring of the test system at the beginning and end of the working day is mandatory. This is done with suitable control material within the normal and abnormal ranges of the test. A pool of species-specific plasma from appropriate numbers of healthy animals must be analyzed along with the test samples being investigated.

13. Normal limits should be established for each test and each species under the same experimental conditions. They cannot be based on normal limits quoted in the literature. Test results for plasma from approximately 95% of the healthy control animals should fall within 2 SD of the mean. Test results from normal and abnormal commercially prepared control material should be within 2 SD of the accumulated mean derived from data of the previous seven or more days.

When using commercial preparations of tissue extracts and plasma substrates, one should remember that clotting factors are known to be affected significantly by species differences (Hawkey, 1975; Archer, 1977; Mifsud, 1979; Janson *et al.*, 1984). Although the use of species-specific material has been recommended (Archer, 1977), commercially prepared human or rabbit brain thromboplastins can be used for the PT test provided normal control values are included in the test report (Schalm *et al.*, 1975; Dodds, 1980). The activity of clotting factors present in all mammals and measured by conventional methods is often greatly increased when compared to human values (Hawkey, 1975).

The two tests commonly employed when a bleeding tendency is suspected, namely, bleeding time and whole blood clotting time, have been intentionally omitted for several reasons. Bleeding time is a direct measurement of the time between incision and cessation of bleeding. It is the only test that directly assesses the hemostatic function of platelets (Weiss, 1976). Standardized procedures including size and depth of incision (which must be controlled), undisturbed bleeding, and blood collection at intervals (without the incision site being touched) are required for the test to be meaningful; consequently, it is of limited use in animals. Choice of site and standardization of the incision are difficult (Dodds, 1980). Keeping the animal still is almost impossible. Simple scalpel or lancet wounds made on depilatated skin areas have not been considered satisfactory (Archer, 1977). The whole blood clotting time method is a crude way of measuring the coagulation process. There are numerous variables that influence the test, such as size and surface of the tube, temperature, and volume of blood. At best, only severe hemostatic disturbances can be detected by this method (Bowie *et al.*, 1971).

III. HEMATOLOGICAL EVALUATION OF CELLULAR ELEMENTS

A. Erythrocyte Evaluation

Normal erythrocyte function depends on the delicate balance of red cell production and destruction. If this stability is altered, two significant nonspecific conditions may occur: anemia or polycythemia.

1. Anemia

Anemia can be classified into several types (Table II). Laboratory findings essential for differential diagnosis are summarized in Table III.

In conjunction with anemia, other cellular abnormalities that may be observed in the blood are:

1. Increased polychromatophilia, nucleated red cells, and Howell–Jolly bodies in accelerated erythropoiesis
2. Spherocytes, fragmented red cells, Heinz bodies, basophilic stippling, MetHb, blood parasites, erythrophagocytosis, and increased erythrocyte osmotic fragility in disorders characterized by excessive erythrocyte destruction
3. Target cells in anemias of inflammation
4. Large hypersegmented neutrophils in megaloblastic anemia
5. Siderocytes in sideroblastic anemia

In conjunction with anemia, other cellular abnormalities that may be observed in the bone marrow are:

1. Prominent megaloblastic changes in red cell precursors and giant metamyelocytes in megaloblastic anemia
2. Nuclear budding, karyorrhexis, and intercellular bridging in severe iron-deficiency anemia
3. Ring sideroblasts in sideroblastic anemia

Table II
Etiological Classification of Anemia

Blood loss	Increased erythrocyte destruction	Impaired erythrocyte production (ineffective erythropoiesis, hypoplasia, pure red cell aplasia)
Acute hemorrhage	Congenital or acquired hemolytic disorders	Deficiencies of essential nutrients
Subacute hemorrhage	Drug or chemical toxicity	Chemical toxicity
Chronic hemorrhage	Immunological disease	Immunological problems
	Mechanical cell destruction	Endocrine abnormalities
	Infection	Chronic renal disease
	Associated with malignancy	Liver disease
		Marrow displacement associated with malignancy
		Idiopathic

Table III

Morphological Classification of Anemia

Morphological Type of anemia	Cause	Typical Findings								
		PCV	Hb	RBC	MCV	MCHC	RETIC	WBC	PLT	Bone Marrow
Normocytic Normochromic	Hemorrhage (recent)	↓ᵃ	↓	↓	Nᵇ	N	N	N or ↑ᶜ	N	N
	Hemolytic disease	↓	↓	↓	N	N	N	↑	↑	Hyperactive
	Idiopathic; chemical injury; chronic disorders; bone marrow infiltration	↓	↓	↓	N	N	N or ↓	Vᵈ	Uᵉ N	V
Macrocytic nonmegalobastic	Associated with accelerated erythropoiesis (hemorrhage-later stage, hemolytic anemia)	↓	↓	↓	↑	N	↑	↑	↑	Hyperactive with ↑ erythropoiesis
	Hepatic disease, hypo- or pure-red-cell aplasia	↓	↓	↓	↑	N	N or ↓	V	U N	V
Macrocytic megaloblastic	Folate and vitamin B_{12} deficiency; drug induced; associated with myelodysplastic disorders involving red cell series	↓	↓	↓	↑	N	↓↓↓	↓ or ↑	N or ↑	Hypo- or hyperactive
Microcytic hypochromic	Iron deficiency; disorders of iron metabolism; disorders of Hb synthesis	↓↓	↓↓	↓	↓	↓	N or ↓	N or V	V or ↑	N to mildly hyperactive

ᵃ Decreased.
ᵇ Normal.
ᶜ Increased.
ᵈ Variable.
ᵉ Usually.

4. Giant multinuclear cells and other degenerative changes in early erythroid precursors in serious erythropoietic disturbances

2. Polycythemia or Erythrocytosis

The term *polycythemia* itself means an increase in the number of red cells and hemoglobin concentration per unit volume of blood above the level established as normal for a given species. The term does not refer to other cellular elements. Erythrocytosis is categorized as relative and absolute.

Relative erythrocytosis means loss of fluid with the total red cells mass remaining unchanged. It is usually transient and commonly caused by dehydration or the stress syndrome. PCV, Hb, and RBC are elevated. Relative erythrocytosis is of particular importance in the hematological assessment of the small laboratory animal because normal values obtained from a dehydrated (water deprivation for a few hours) or stressed (inappropriate handling) rat may mask an existing anemia, and thus yield misleading information.

Absolute erythrocytosis means an increase in the red cell mass. The condition is further subdivided into secondary and primary polycythemia. Secondary polycythemia results from a normal bone marrow response to hypoxia or abnormal erythropoietin production. Primary polycythemia (polycythemia rubra vera, primary erythremia) is a disorder of unknown etiology involving abnormality of the regulatory mechanism of cell production. It is characterized by an absolute and marked increase in red cell mass, plasma volume, and total blood volume and is associated with leukocytosis and thrombocytosis. Immature neutrophils are often encountered.

B. Leukocyte Evaluation

The term *leukocyte* pertains to all types of white cells and their precursors. Each type has distinct morphological and functional features. There are three types seen in peripheral blood: granulocytes, lymphocytes, and monocytes. *Granulocytes* are further subdivided into neutrophils, eosinophils and basophils. *Lymphocytes* include two morphologically similar but functionally distinct groups. Thymus derived or T-cells are concerned with direct cell-mediated immunity and bursa equivalent derived or B-cells are involved in antibody production. *Monocytes* are phagocytic cells associated with removing of bacteria and cellular debris (e.g., antibody-coated erythrocytes).

The comparative aspect of leukocyte evaluation is of paramount importance. Neutrophil/lymphocyte ratio as well as the numerical and morphological responses to stimuli are greatly variable and interdependent.

1. Numerical Responses

a. Leukocytosis

Leukocytosis obtained under the same experimental conditions refers to an increased WBC count above the normal level of a given species-matched controls with respect to age, sex, and strain. Leukocytosis is usually due to neutrophilia and/or lymphocytosis. It is rarely caused by eosinophilia.

Conditions producing absolute neutrophilia include a variety of causes: infections; hormonal influence; metabolic, drug, and chemical intoxications; acute blood loss; myeloproliferative disorders (some types of leukemia); and rapidly growing neoplasms. Physiological neutrophilia follows severe emotional stress, fear, strenuous exercise, and epinephrine administration (Schalm et al., 1975).

Leukemoid reaction is a massive leukocyte response resulting from causes other than leukemia.

Absolute eosinophilia is associated with parasitic infections, allergic states, and other chronic diseases that involve continuous mast cell degranulation (Schalm et al., 1975). It is also observed in some hematological disorders including eosinophilic leukemia.

Basophils are rarely elevated above normal levels in animals. Absolute basophilia is seen in basophilic leukemia (MacEwen et al., 1975) and in sensitization to an antigen or allergen (Schalm et al., 1975).

Absolute lymphocytosis occurs mainly in certain viral infections and in some lymphoproliferative disorders, lymphatic leukemia being the most prominent. Absolute monocytosis is usually related to chronic bacterial infections, some parasitic infections, some lymphoproliferative disorders, neoplastic disease, and monocytic leukemia.

b. Leukopenia

Leukopenia refers to a reduction in the WBC count below the normal limit established for a given species. It is usually effected by the depression of one or more cell lines. Some common causes are viral diseases, overwhelming infections, and drug or chemical toxicity.

Absolute neutropenia may result from an increased cell destruction, as in conditions connected with hypersplenism, from an abnormality in granulopoiesis, or from unknown etiological factors.

Absolute lymphopenia is seen in some viral diseases, in severe infections (persistent lymphopenia warrants poor prognosis), in toxemias, and in initial stages of lymphoproliferative neoplasia. Moreover, lymphopenia has been attributed to administration of adrenal steroids or heightened chronic cortical activity, X-irradiation, chemotherapeutic agents, and neonatal thymectomy (Schalm et al., 1975).

Absolute eosinopenia is associated with emotional and physical stress and adrenal corticoid activity. Absolute basopenia has been observed in pregnant rabbits (Schalm et al., 1975).

2. Morphological Responses

a. Neutrophils

Appearance of immature neutrophils in the peripheral blood is described as a "shift to the left." When neutrophilia is present, it is called a regenerative left shift; with normal neutrophil number or neutropenia it is a degenerative left shift. Immature cells may even outnumber mature cells. In monkeys, a slight increase in band neutrophils (about 5%) is considered a shift to the left because normal adult neutrophils are markedly segmented (Hawkey, 1977).

Degenerative and toxic changes associated with toxic states appear in the order of severity:

Döhle bodies
basophilic granulation
cytoplasmic basophilia
cytoplasmic vacuolization

b. Lymphocytes

Atypical lymphocytes are characterized by size and position of the nucleus; nuclear folding, indentations, clefts, and lobulation; very fine reticular or pyknotic nuclear chromatin; and deeply basophilic or pale finely vacuolated cytoplasm. Atypical lymphocytes may be occasionally seen in a healthy animal, but they frequently occur in a number of bacterial and viral infections, disease stress, autoimmune disorders, malignancies, and drug and chemical reactions.

Normal rat lymphocytes have some atypical features and are often difficult to differentiate from monocytes (Godwin et al., 1964). Primate lymphocytes also include some or many atypical cells depending on the species (Huser, 1970).

c. Blasts, Undifferentiated, and Poorly Differentiated Cells

These cells appear in a number of myelo- or lymphoproliferative disorders including leukemias.

IV. EVALUATION OF HEMOSTASIS

Hemostatic equilibrium means maintenance of blood fluidity and prevention of hemorrhage. Its efficiency depends on vascular integrity, qualitatively and quantitatively normal platelets, and adequate function of coagulation mechanisms. Fibrinolysis (dissolution of fibrin clot) also participates, indirectly, in the hemostatic balance because disturbances in the fibrinolytic system may cause bleeding or potentiate an already existing hemorrhagic tendency. A comprehensive description of comparative hemostasis and fundamental hemostatic mechanisms in humans and other animals may be found in the proceedings of a symposium held at the Zoological Society of London (Macfarlane, 1970) and in Dodds (1980).

A. Platelet Evaluation

Mammalian platelets are small nonnucleated "cells" derived from megakaryocytes by cytoplasmic fragmentation. Avian thrombocytes are nucleated and seem to be similar to lymphoid cells (Janzarik and Morgenstern, 1979).

Although both mammalian and nonmammalian thrombocytes are involved in the maintenance of vascular integrity as well as in several phases of hemostasis, there are considerable species-specific differences related to platelet function (Dodds, 1979), numbers, volume heterogeneity, and induced changes (Eason et al., 1986).

1. Quantitative Platelet Abnormalities

a. Thrombocytopenia

Thrombocytopenia means a decrease in platelet count below the normal limits established for a given species. Reduction of circulating platelets with concurrent changes in megakaryocytes may be caused by the following (Wintrobe et al., 1981; Coller, 1984; Meyers, 1985):

1. Increased platelet removal associated with increased number of megakaryocytes; platelet removal as in disseminated intravascular coagulation; platelet destruction as in autoimmune thrombocytopenic purpura.

2. Impaired platelet production, decreased platelet production associated with decreased numbers of megakaryocytes due to injury by drugs, toxic chemicals, X-irradiation, viruses, marrow replacement with neoplastic cells; ineffective production characterized by an abnormality in platelet production and often associated with greatly increased numbers of megakaryocytes as seen in megaloblastic hematopoiesis; abnormal platelet distribution associated with disorders characterized by splenomegaly and variably increased number of megakaryocytes.

Severe thrombocytopenia is accompanied by petechial or ecchymotic hemorrhage. In animals, bleeding usually does not occur unless platelet count is reduced to $< 100 \times 10^9$/liter (Dodds, 1974).

b. Thrombocytosis

Thrombocytosis means an increase in platelet count above the upper limit established for a given species due to secondary causes, such as some myeloproliferative disorders, various inflammatory diseases, infections, and some neoplasms. Thrombocytosis may also be physiologically induced. Thrombocytosis due to the primary abnormality of the bone marrow is characterized by a marked increase in marrow megakaryocytes and circulating platelets. Hemorrhagic and thromboembolic episodes may occur when platelet counts are extremely elevated (Payne *et al.*, 1976).

c. Changes in Platelet MPV and PDW

Extensive studies of platelet heterogeneity both in humans and in experimental animals have provided us with a better understanding of the relationship between platelet size and various primary and secondary hematological disorders.

A high MPV has been observed in thrombocytopenias due to increased destruction and enhanced or abnormal production, as well as in thrombocytosis related to myeloproliferative diseases. Normal or low MPV, on the other hand, appears to be associated with platelet production failure, which occurs in bone marrow injury, myelosuppression, and hypersplenism.

Many studies suggest an inverse relationship between platelet volume and platelet number; therefore, the circulating platelet biomass may be a more meaningful reflection of platelet hemostatic function than either volume or count alone (Corash, 1983; Dumoulin-Lagrange and Capelle, 1983; Thompson *et al.*, 1983; Weiser and Kociba, 1984).

2. Qualitative Platelet Abnormalities

a. Thrombopathy

Thrombopathy means platelet dysfunction due to a variety of acquired and hereditary causes.

b. Thrombasthenia

Thrombasthenia is a specific, inherited platelet disorder characterized by defective clot retraction and ADP-mediated platelet aggregation. Characterization of qualitative platelet abnormalities requires more sophisticated tests, such as platelet retention in a glass bead column and bleeding time, and detailed studies of platelet aggregation and release reaction.

B. Evaluation of Coagulation and Fibrinolysis

Coagulation disorders may be hereditary or acquired (Dodds, 1980; Feldman, 1981). Hereditary coagulation disorders recognized in animals include canine factor VII deficiency (Poller et al., 1971); canine, equine, and feline factor VIII deficiency (hemophilia A; Dodds, 1980); canine and feline factor IX deficiency (Christmas disease, hemophilia B; Dodds, 1980); canine factor X deficiency (Dodds, 1980); feline (Feldman et al., 1983), canine, and bovine (Dodds, 1980) factor XI deficiency; feline (Green and White, 1977), canine (Randolph et al., 1986), and rhesus monkey (Zawidzka and Arnold, 1986) factor XII deficiency; canine and caprine fibrinogen (factor I) deficiency (Dodds, 1980); and canine, lapine, and porcine von Willebrand's disease (Dodds, 1980). Von Willebrand's disease (VWD) is an autosomal incompletely dominant bleeding disorder in which there is reduced or abnormal von Willebrand factor activity that is measured by bleeding time, platelet retention, platelet agglutination, and plasma factor VIII-related antigen. Plasma factor VIII coagulant activity is usually but not always reduced. VWD occurs in humans, swine, and many purebreds and mongrel dogs (Dodds, 1980).

Acquired syndromes have many causes such as severe liver disease; DIC; abnormalities of the naturally occurring inhibitors, for example, antithrombin III (Green and Kabel, 1982), protein C and S (Taylor, 1983; Colucci et al., 1984), and warfarin toxicosis (Dodds, 1980); and age-related changes in hemostatic function (Urizar et al., 1984). Acquired causes of bleeding are particularly important in toxicological studies because the experimental animal is at risk for induced hemostatic disturbances that may complicate the intended or expected toxic changes.

Table IV

Typical Laboratory Findings in Various Hemorrhagic Disorders with Basic Hemostatic Screening Tests

Cause	Platelet count	APTT[a]	PT[a]	Bleeding time[b]	Suggested specialized tests
Thrombocytopenia	Reduced	Normal	Normal	Usually prolonged	
Platelet dysfunction	Normal or increased	Normal	Normal	Usually prolonged	Clot retraction; platelet retention, aggregation, and release
Deficiency of factors VIII, IX, XI, and XII	Normal	Prolonged	Normal	Normal	Factor studies[c]
Deficiency of factor VII	Normal	Normal	Prolonged	Normal	Factor studies[c]
Deficiency of factors I, II, V, X; presence of circulating inhibitors	Normal	Prolonged	Prolonged	Normal	Factor studies[c]
von Willebrand's disease	Normal	Usually normal	Normal	Usually prolonged	Plasma and platelet assays for von Willebrand factor

[a] APTT and PT are prolonged significantly only when factors drop below 30% of normal activity. Mild deficiencies usually result in values at the upper limit of normal range or slightly prolonged.

[b] Bleeding time is included for exceptional cases when this procedure can meet necessary requirements of correct performance.

[c] Factor identifications, correction studies, and specific factor assays.

DIC is a hemorrhagic disorder characterized by intravascular coagulation, platelet consumption, and accelerated fibrinolysis. Protracted oozing from venipuncture and surgical incisions, bruising, and bleeding from mucous membranes are frequently observed. The hemostatic profile varies in the course of the disease, therefore, serial screening tests as well as more sophisticated assays (Feldman *et al.*, 1981) may be needed for accurate detection. DIC can be induced by a host of diseases and miscellaneous conditions: obstetrical complications, malignancy, systemic infections, necrosis, amyloidosis, platelet disorders (Dodds, 1980), and nephrotic syndrome (Green and Kabel, 1982). Administration of certain drugs (e.g., meprobamate and diatrizoate sodium) has also been implicated in inducing the syndrome (Dodds, 1974). Occurrence of DIC in animals is probably more frequent than the relatively few reported and documented cases suggest (Dodds, 1974).

Excessive fibrinolytic activity, not related to any other hemostatic defect, is a rare hemorrhagic diathesis (pathological primary fibrinolysis) characterized by primary activation of the fibrinolytic system in the circulating blood and by digestion of fibrinogen and other proteins. It may be caused by complications from the use of thrombolytic agents (Bennet and Ogston, 1984) or occur in association with a variety of neoplastic disease, severe hepatic disease, and amyloidosis (Feldman, 1981). Secondary fibrinolysis is secondary to intravascular fibrin deposition and is associated with intravascular clotting. Unless the presence of clear-cut evidence of intravascular clotting is established, it may not be always possible to distinguish between primary and secondary fibrinolysis with routine laboratory tests (Bennet and Ogston, 1984).

Typical laboratory findings in various hemorrhagic disorders are listed in Table IV.

V. CONCLUSION

The necessity of hematological assessment in toxicological studies and the importance of observing quality control principles during hematological investigations has been emphasized in this chapter. Guidelines for valid hematological procedures and correct test selections that are applicable to experimental animals have been presented. Evaluation of cellular elements, hemostasis, and fibrinolysis as well as the role of hematological findings in differential diagnosis have been briefly discussed.

For convenience, pertinent factors to consider in hematological evaluation and reporting of results have been recapitulated in Table V.

Table V

Pertinent Factors in Hematological Evaluation and Reporting

Factors to consider	Comments
Testing	
Pretreatment testing	
Age of the animals should be provided	If adult animals are used, pretreatment testing is very useful since each animal can serve as its own control and variations between individual animals do not interfere with subtle changes or trends. When weanlings are used, testing is of limited value since hematological profile changes dramatically as the animal matures. Testing may be useful to exclude animals with hematological abnormalities.
Interim testing	
It should be clearly indicated if the same animals or satellite groups are sampled	Preferably, the same group of animals should be tested for more meaningful interpretation of the effects and exclusion of spurious results. Interim data are also useful for comparison with terminal results.
Terminal testing	
It is very important and should include tests necessary for complete hematological assessment	Sampling is easier; larger quantities of blood as well as hematopoietic organs are available. In combination with interim data transient changes, patterns of changes may be detected, and unexpected changes, previously observed in a single animal or group of animals, may be confirmed with certainty.
Methodology	
Blood sampling	Excitement, fear, use of anesthetic, and sampling site may influence results.
Type of anticoagulants used	Anticoagulant used should not interfere with or alter substance being measured.
Sample handling	Excessive manipulation of the sample, time lapse between sampling and performance of the test, and incorrect sample storage temperature may alter results (see also Table I).
Methods and instruments	Modification of methods and adjustments of instruments to accommodate species-specific requirements are important components of quality control and contribute to the validity of the tests.

Cellular assessment

Erythrocytes

In addition to basic assessment tests (RBC, HCT, Hb), the following parameters, derived from the above tests, should be included

Red cell indices: MCV and MCHC

These are extremely helpful in assessing the validity and/or abnormality of the basic red-cell parameters.

A brief assessment of cellular morphology (e.g., cells are normocytic and normochromic). If abnormalities are present, the extent of anisocytosis, hypochromasia, polychromasia, poikilocytosis, and schistocytosis should be specified, as well as the presence of Howell-Jolly bodies, nucleated red cells/100 leukocytes and/or parasites.

An accurate morphological assessment confirms preceding results (if they are correct) and permits better understanding of the induced blood dyscrasias.

Leukocytes

In addition to total WBC counts, differential counts are included when required

White cell differentials should be expressed in absolute numbers

Absolute values are more informative of the true state of a given cell line in the peripheral blood. Percentage values may be included but usually are not essential.

Number of leukocytes counted should be specified

Number of cells examined and the variability of the differential count are inversely proportional.

Morphological assessment of leukocytes, if an abnormality is observed, should be specific (e.g., presence of toxic granules, cytoplasmic basophilia, vacuolation, or intra- or extracellular parasites and presence of immature or leukemic cells).

This information permits better assessment of the degree of toxicity.

Smear should be always examined when WBC count is abnormal

To confirm count abnormality

Platelets

Counts should be confirmed by smear examination; extensive clumping, red cell fragments or debris should be reported

Platelet clumps indicate that counts may be spuriously decreased. Red cell fragments and/or debris may produce higher than true counts regardless of method used.

(continues)

Table V (*continued*)

Pertinent Factors in Hematological Evaluation and Reporting

Factors to consider	Comments
Platelet size, abnormal for a given species, should be included in the report, particularly if the counts are abnormal	Significant changes in size may be helpful in assessing count abnormality and hemostatic potential since platelet biomass determines hemostatic ability, provided platelet function is not impaired.
Coagulation studies	
Screening tests	Two different pathways are screened, therefore, the tests are not interchangeable.
One-stage prothrombin time	To screen the extrinsic system
Partial thromboplastin time (activated)	To screen the intrinsic system
If only one is performed (e.g., PT) reasons should be given for the selection of the test.	A serious hemostatic impairment involving the other mechanism could be missed unless the defect involves the final common pathway or factors participating in both mechanisms.
The following additional information should be provided	
Whether fresh or frozen and thawed plasma of both treated and control groups was assayed	Both are acceptable; however, both control and treated plasma should be either fresh or frozen and thawed.
Statement of acceptable difference between duplicate determinations of screening tests	All coagulation tests should be performed in duplicates with a limit of 5% difference between the two determinations.

Bone marrow assessment — Contributes to diagnosing blood disorders and/or explaining disease processes

Differential count — Helps to assess cell differentiation maturation and hematopoietic activity

Number of nucleated cells counted — Minimum of 500 nucleated cells should be counted

A brief description of abnormal morphologic changes such as presence of micronuclei, multinuclearity, intercellular bridging — Helps to assess the degree of erythroid (or other cell lines) derangement

Myeloid/erythroid ratio — Helps to assess granulopoiesis and/or erythropoiesis, provided that one cell system is unimpaired

Number of mitoses observed in each cell line — Helps to assess hematopoietic activity, the degree of ineffective hematopoiesis and/or activity of abnormal cells

Assessment of cellularity — Should be confirmed by a histological section examination

Abnormal results — If an abnormality is suspected and/or observed in cellular elements, coagulation studies, or bone marrow assessment

This information is very useful in interpretation and often essential for the correct evaluation of hematotoxic effects of the substance under investigation

Historical controls (ranges and means) of the animals used in a study should be provided — This greatly facilitates the review and evaluation of the data on an individual animal basis and aids in overall study assessment

All abnormal findings should be accompanied by clinical and pathological assessment of the individual animal, preferably displayed alongside the results

A list of proposed follow-up tests or assays should be prepared in advance to confirm or elucidate hematotoxic effects should they occur at any phase of the study — A well-prepared list of follow-up tests helps to avoid problems for the investigator, particularly when time is critical and blood samples limited. It may also preclude the necessity for additional studies.

Suggested Reading

Bessis, M. (1977). "Blood Smears Reinterpreted." (G. Brecher, trans.). New York: Springer International.

Donati, M. B., Davidson, J. F., and Garattini, S., eds. (1981). "Malignancy and the Hemostatic System." New York: Raven Press.

Hall, D. E. (1972). "Blood Coagulation and its Disorders in the Dog." London: Bailliere Tindall.

Miller, E. V., Ben, M., and Cass, J. S., eds. (1969). Comparative anesthesia in laboratory animals. Fed. Proc., *Fed. Am. Soc. Exp. Biol.* **28,** 1369–1586.

Olsen, R. G., ed. (1981). "Feline Leukemia." Boca Raton, Florida: CRC Press.

Owen, C. A., Jr., Bowie, E. J. W., Didisheim, P., and Thompson, J. H., eds. (1975). "The Diagnosis of Bleeding Disorders," 2d ed. Boston: Little, Brown.

Schmidt, R. M., ed. (1980). "Clinical Laboratory Science, Section I Hematology," Vol. 2. Boca Raton, Florida: CRC Press.

van Assendeleft, O. W., and England, J. M., eds. (1982). "Advances in Hematological Methods: The Blood Count." Boca Raton, Florida: CRC Press.

References

Adeghe, A. J. H., and Cohen, J. (1986). A better method for terminal bleeding of mice. *Lab. Anim.* **20,** 70–72.

Alsaker, R. D., Laber, J., Stevens, J., and Perman, V. (1977). A comparison of polychromasia and reticulocyte counts in assessing erythrocytic regenerative response in the cat. *J. Am. Vet. Med. Assoc.* **170,** 39–41.

Archer, R. K. (1965). "Haematological Techniques for Use on Animals." Oxford: Blackwell Scientific Publications.

Archer, R. K. (1977). Technical methods. *In* "Comparative Clinical Haematology" (R. K. Archer and L. B. Jeffcott, eds), pp. 537–610. Oxford: Blackwell Scientific Publications.

Archer, R. K., and Riley, J. (1981). Standardized method for bleeding rats. *Lab. Anim.* **15,** 25–28.

Arnold, D. L., Charbonneau, S. M., Zawidzka, Z. Z., and Grice, H. C. (1977). Monitoring animal health during chronic toxicity studies. *J. Environ. Pathol. Toxicol.* **1,** 227–239.

Bennet, B., and Ogston, D. (1984). Fibrinolytic bleeding syndromes. *In* "Disorders of Hemostasis" (O. D. Ratnoff and C. D. Forbes, eds.), pp. 321–349. Orlando, Florida: Grune & Stratton.

Bessman, J. D. (1980). Evaluation of automated whole-blood platelet counts and particle sizing. *Am. J. Clin. Pathol.* **74,** 157–162.

Bessman, J. D., Gilmer, P. R., and Gardner, F. H. (1983). Improved classification of anemias by MCV and RDW. *Am. J. Clin. Pathol.* **80,** 322–326.

Bivin, W. S., and Smith, G. D. (1984). Techniques of experimentation. *In* "Laboratory Animal Medicine" (J. G. Fox, B. J. Cohen, and F. M. Loew, eds.), pp. 564–569. Orlando, Florida: Academic Press.

Bjoraker, D. G., and Ketcham, T. R. (1981). 3.8% Sodium citrate (1:9) is an inadequate anticoagulant for rabbit blood with high calcium. *Thromb. Res.* **24,** 505–508.

Bowie, E. J. W., Thompson, J. H., Jr., Didisheim, P., and Owen, C. A., Jr. (1971). "Mayo Clinic Laboratory Manual of Hemostasis." Philadelphia: Saunders.

Brecher, G., and Cronkite, E. P. (1950). Morphology and enumeration of blood platelets. *J. Appl. Physiol.* **3,** 365–377.

Bullock, L. P. (1983). Repetitive blood sampling from guinea pigs *(cavia porcellus). Lab. Anim. Sci.* **33,** 70–71.

Bushby, S. R. M. (1970). Haematological studies during toxicity tests. *In* "Methods in Toxicology" (G. E. Paget, ed.), pp. 338–371. Oxford: Blackwell Scientific Publications.

Calvo, W., Fliedner, T. M., Herbst, E. W., and Fache, I. (1975). Regeneration of blood-forming organs after autologous leukocyte transfusion in lethally irradiated dogs. I. Distribution and cellularity of the bone marrow in normal dogs. *Blood* **46,** 453–457.

Cann, M. C., Zawidzka, Z. Z., Airth, J. M., and Grice, H. C. (1965). The effect of ether anesthesia on plasma corticosteroids and hematologic responses. *Can. J. Physiol. Pharmacol.* **43,** 463–468.

Cartwright, G. E. (1968). "Diagnostic Laboratory Hematology," 4th ed. New York: Grune & Stratton.

Chart, I. S., and Sanderson, J. H. (1979). Methodology of investigations on coagulation in drug-safety evaluation. *Pharmacol. Ther.* **5,** 243–246.

Chen, J. P., Williams, T. K., and Legendre, A. M. (1981). Comparisons of hemagglutination inhibition, staphylococcal clumping, and latex agglutination tests for canine fibrinolytic degradation products. *Am. J. Vet. Res.* **42,** 2049–2052.

Clark, D. A., and de la Garza, M. (1967). Species differences in methemoglobin levels produced by administration of monomethylhydrazine. *Proc. Soc. Exp. Biol. Med.* **125,** 912–916.

Coller, B. S. (1984). Platelets and their disorders. *In* "Disorders of Hemostasis" (O. D. Ratnoff and C. D. Forbes, eds.), pp. 73–176. Orlando, Florida: Grune & Stratton.

Colucci, M., Stassen, J. M., and Collen, D. (1984). Influence of protein C activation of blood coagulation and fibrinolysis in squirrel monkeys. *J. Clin. Invest.* **74,** 200–204.

Corash, L. (1983). Platelet sizing: Techniques, biological significance, and clinical applications. *Curr. Top. Hematol.* **4,** 99–122.

Cornbleet, P. J., and Kessinger, S. (1985) Accuracy of low platelet counts on the Coulter S-Plus IV. *Am. J. Clin. Pathol.* **83,**78–80.

Cramer, D. V., and Lewis, R. M. (1972). Reticulocyte response in the cat. *J. Am. Vet. Med. Assoc.* **160,** 61–67.

de Lange, J. A., Earnisse, G. J., and Veltkamp, J. J. (1972). Cold agglutinins and the Coulter counter model S. *Am. J. Clin. Pathol.* **58,** 599–600.

Dodds, W. J. (1974). Blood coagulation: Hemostasis and thrombosis. *In* "Handbook of Laboratory Animal Science" (E. C. Melby, Jr., and N. H. Altman, eds.), Vol. 2, pp. 85–116. Boca Raton, Florida: CRC Press.

Dodds, W. J. (1978). Platelet function in animals: Species specificities. *In* "Platelets: A Multidisciplinary Approach" (G. DeGaetano and S. Garattini, eds.), pp. 45–59. New York: Raven Press.

Dodds, W. J. (1980). Hemostasis and coagulation. *In* "Clinical Biochemistry of Domestic Animals" (J. J. Kaneko, ed.), 3rd ed., pp. 671–718. New York: Academic Press.

Donovan, J. C., Stokes, W. S., Montrey, R. D., and Rozmiarek, H. (1983). Hematologic characterization of naturally occurring malaria *(Plasmodium inui)* in cynomolgus monkey *(Macaca fascicularis). Lab. Anim. Sci.* **33,** 86–89.

Dumoulin-Lagrange, M., and Capelle, C. (1983). Evaluation of automated platelet counters for the enumeration and sizing of platelets in the diagnosis and management of hemostatic problems. *Semin. Thromb. Hemostasis* **9**, 235–244.

Eason, C. T., Pattison, A., Howells, D. D., Mitcheson, J., and Bonner, F. W. (1986). Platelet population profiles: Significance of species variation and drug-induced changes. *J. Appl. Toxicol.* **6**, 437–441.

Fairbanks, V. F. (1980). Nonequivalence of automated and manual hematocrit and erythrocytic indices. *Am. J. Clin. Pathol.* **73**, 55–62.

Fehr, J. (1987). New wave of automation. *Blut* **59**, 321–324.

Feldman, B. F. (1981). Coagulopathies in small animals. *J. Am. Vet. Med. Assoc.* **179**, 559–563.

Feldman, B. F., Madewell, B. R., and O'Neill, S. (1981). Disseminated intravascular coagulation: antithrombin, plasminogen, and coagulation abnormalities in 41 dogs. *J. Am. Vet. Med. Assoc.* **179**, 151–154.

Feldman, B. F., Soares, C. J., Kitchell, B. E., Brown, C. C., and O'Neill, S. (1983). Hemorrhage in a cat caused by inhibition of factor XI (plasma thromboplastin antecedent). *J. Am. Vet. Med. Assoc.* **182**, 589–591.

Fowler, J. S. L., Brown, J. S., and Flower, E. W. (1980). Comparison between ether and carbon dioxide anaesthesia for removal of small blood samples from rats. *Lab. Anim.* **14**, 275–278.

Gilmer, P. R. Jr., Williams, L. J., Koepke, J. A., and Bull, B. S. (1977). Calibration methods for automated hematology instruments. *Am. J. Clin. Pathol. Suppl.* **68**, 185–190.

Gilmore, C. E., Gilmore, V. H., and Jones, T. C. (1964). Bone marrow and peripheral blood of cats: Technique and normal values. *Pathol. Vet.* **1**, 18–40.

Glenn, B. L. (1970). Diagnosis of parasitic disease in blood of small animals. *J. Am. Vet. Med. Assoc.* **157**, 1681–1685.

Godwin, K. O., Fraser, F. J., and Ibbotson, R. N. (1964). Haematological observations on healthy (SPF) rats. *Br. J. Exp. Pathol.* **45**, 514–524.

Gottfried, E. L., Wehman, J., and Wall, B. (1976). Electronic platelet counts with the Coulter counter. *Am. J. Clin. Pathol.* **66**, 506–511.

Green, R. A., and Kabel, A. L. (1982). Hypercoagulable state in three dogs with nephrotic syndrome: role of acquired antithrombin III deficiency. *J. Am. Vet. Med. Assoc.* **181**, 914–917.

Green, R. A., and White, F. (1977). Feline factor XII (Hageman) deficiency. *Am. J. Vet. Res.* **38**, 893–895.

Greene, C. E., Tsang, V. C. W., Prestwood, A. K., and Meriwether, E. A. (1981). Coagulation studies of plasmas from healthy domesticated animals and persons. *Am. J. Vet. Res.* **42**, 2170–2177.

Greenwood, B. (1977). Haematology of the sheep and goat. *In* "Comparative Clinical Haematology" (R. K. Archer and L. B. Jeffcott, eds.), pp. 305–344. Oxford: Blackwell Scientific Publications.

Grice, H. C. (1964). Methods for obtaining blood and for intravenous injections in laboratory animals. *Lab. Anim. Care* **14**, 483–493.

Groner, W., Boyett, J., Johnson, A., and Scountlebury, M. (1986). Variability of erythrocyte size and hemoglobin content observed in man and four selected mammals. *Blood Cells* **12**, 65–80.

Hawkey, C. M. (1975). "Comparative Mammalian Haematology." London: Heinemann Medical Books.

Hawkey, C. (1977). The haematology of exotic mammals. *In* "Comparative Clinical Haematology" (R. K. Archer and L. B. Jeffcott, eds.), pp. 103–160. Oxford: Blackwell Scientific Publications.

Hawkins, R. I. (1972). The importance of platelet function tests in toxicological screening using laboratory animals. *Lab. Anim.* **6,** 155–167.

Hodges, R. D. (1977). Avian haematology. *In* "Comparative Clinical Haematology" (R. K. Archer and L. B. Jeffcott, eds.), pp. 483–517. Oxford: Blackwell Scientific Publications.

Hoff, B., Lumsden, J. H., and Valli, V. E. O. (1985). An appraisal of bone marrow biopsy of sick dogs. *Can. J. Comp. Med.* **49,** 34–42.

Hurwitz, A. (1971). A simple method for obtaining blood samples from rats. *J. Lab. Clin. Med.* **78,** 172–174.

Huser, H. J. (1970). "Atlas of Comparative Primate Hematology." New York: Academic Press.

Ingram, G. I. C., and Hills, M. (1976). The prothrombin time test: effect of varying citrate concentration. *Thromb. Haemostasis.* **36,** 230–236.

International Committee for Standardization in Haematology (1984). ICSH reference method for staining of blood and bone marrow films by azure B and eosin Y (Romanowsky stain). *Br. J. Haematol.* **57,** 707–710.

Irons, R. D. (ed.), (1985). "Toxicology of the Blood and Bone Marrow. Target Organ Toxicology Series." New York: Raven Press.

Janson, T. L., Stormorken, H., and Prydz, H. (1984). Species specificity of tissue thromboplastin. *Haemostasis* **14,** 440–444.

Janzarik, H., and Morgenstern, E. (1979). The nucleated thrombocytoid cells. I. Electron microscopic studies on chicken blood cells. *Thromb. Haemostasis* **41,** 608–621.

Jeffcott, L. B. (1977). Clinical haematology of the horse. *In* "Comparative Clinical Haematology" (R. K. Archer and L. B. Jeffcott, eds.), pp. 161–213. Oxford: Blackwell Scientific Publications.

Jespersen, J., and Sidelmann, J. (1982). A study of the conditions and accuracy of the thrombin time assay of plasma fibrinogen. *Acta Haematol.* **67,** 2–7.

Koepke, J. A., Rodgers, J. L., and Ollivier, M. J. (1975). Pre-instrumental variables in coagulation testing. *Am. J. Clin. Pathol.* **64,** 591–596.

Koepke, J. A. (1977). The calibration of automated instruments for accuracy in hemoglobinometry. *Am. J. Clin. Pathol. Suppl.* **68,** 180–184.

Legge, D. G., and Shortman, K. (1968). The effect of pH on the volume, density and shape of erythrocytes and thymic lymphocytes. *Br. J. Haematol.* **14,** 323–335.

Lewis, H. G. (1967). Bone marrow biopsy in cattle. *Vet. Rec.* **80,** 452.

Linman, J. W. (1966). "Principles of Hematology." New York: MacMillan.

MacEwen, E. G., Drazner, F. H., McClelland, A. J., and Wilkins, R. J. (1975). Treatment of basophilic leukemia in a dog. *J. Am. Vet. Med. Assoc.* **166,** 376–380.

Macfarlane, R. G. (ed.) (1970). "The Haemostatic Mechanism in Man and Other Animals." London: Academic Press.

Mackey, L. (1977). Haematology of the cat. *In* "Comparative Clinical Haematology" (R. K. Archer and L. B. Jeffcott, eds.), pp. 441–482. Oxford: Blackwell Scientific Publications.

Martin, D. P., McGowan, M. J., and Loeb, W. F. (1973). Age related changes of hematologic values in infant *Macaca mulatta*. *Lab. Anim. Sci.* **23**, 194–200.

Maxie, M. G. (1977). Evaluation of techniques for counting bovine platelets. *Can. J. Comp. Med.* **41**, 409–415.

Mayer, K., Chin, B., and Baisley, A. (1985). Evaluation of the S-Plus IV. *Am. J. Clin. Pathol.* **83**, 40–46.

Meyers, K. M. (1985). Pathobiology of animal platelets. *Adv. Vet. Sci. Comp. Med.* **30**, 131–165.

Mifsud, C. V. (1979). The sensitivity of various thromboplastins in different animal species. *Pharmacol. Ther.* **5**, 251–256.

Moore, D. M. (1983). Venipuncture sites in armadillos *(Dasypus novemcinctus)*. *Lab. Anim. Sci.* **33**, 384–385.

Nosanchuk, J. S., Chang, J., and Bennett, J. M. (1978). The analytic basis for the use of platelet estimates from peripheral blood smears. Laboratory and clinical applications. *Am. J. Clin. Pathol.* **69**, 383–387.

Payne, B. J., Lewis, H. B., Murchison, T. E., and Hart, E. A. (1976). Hematology of laboratory animals. *In* "Handbook of Laboratory Animal Science" (E. C. Melby, Jr., and N. H. Altman, eds.), Vol. 3, pp. 382–461. Boca Raton, Florida: CRC Press.

Pintor, P. P., and Grassini, V. (1957). Individual and seasonal spontaneous variations of haematological values in normal male rabbits. Statistical survey. *Acta Haematol.* **17**, 122–128.

Poller, L., Thomson, J. M., Sear, C. H. J., and Thomas, W. (1971). Identification of a congenital defect of factor VII in a colony of beagle dogs: The clinical use of the plasma. *J. Clin. Pathol.* **24**, 626–632.

Porter, W. P. (1982). Hematologic and other effects of ketamine and ketamine-acepromazine in rhesus monkeys *(Macaca mulatta)*. *Lab. Anim. Sci.* **32**, 373–375.

Randolph, J. F., Center, S. A., and Dodds, W. J. (1986). Factor XII deficiency and von Willebrand's disease in a family of miniature poodle dogs. *Cornell Vet.* **76**, 3–10.

Rebar, A. H., Lewis, H. B., DeNicola, D. B., Halliwell, W. H., and Boon, G. D. (1981). Red cell fragmentation in the dog: An editorial review. *Vet. Pathol.* **18**, 415–426.

Reece, W. O., and Wahlstrom, J. D. (1970). Effect of feeding and excitement on the packed cell volume of dogs. *Lab. Anim. Care* **20**, 1114–1117.

Reid, W. O., Henry, R. L., MacPherson, B., Hellerman, D. V., and Urwiller, K. L. (1984). Hemostasis: The balance concept of procoagulant and inhibitor systems and use of the serial thrombin time (STT). *Med. Hypotheses* **15**, 169–183.

Ross, D. W., Ayscue, L., and Gulley, M. (1980). Automated platelet counts. *Am. J. Clin. Pathol.* **74**, 151–156.

Ruch, T. C. (1967). "Diseases of Laboratory Primates." Philadelphia: Saunders.

Saslow, S., and Carlisle, H. N. (1969). Nonhuman primates in evaluation of hematoxicity. *Ann. N.Y. Acad. Sci.* **162**, 646–658.

Schalm, O. W., and Switzer, J. A. (1972). Bone marrow aspiration in the cat. *Feline Practice* Nov.–Dec.

Schalm, O. W., Jain, N. C., and Carroll, E. J. (1975). "Veterinary Hematology," 3rd ed. Philadelphia: Lea & Febiger.

Schermer, S. (1967). "The Blood Morphology of Laboratory Animals," 3rd ed. Philadelphia: Davis.

Schofield, L. D., Bennett, B. T., Collins, W. E., and Beluhan, F. Z. (1985). An outbreak of *Plasmodium inui* malaria in a colony of diabetic *Rhesus Monkeys. Lab. Anim. Sci.* **35,** 167–168.

Sleight, S. D., and Sinha, D. P. (1968). Prevention of methemoglobin reduction in blood samples. *J. Am. Vet. Med. Assoc.* **152,** 1521–1525.

Smith, C. N., Neptun, D. A., and Irons, R. D. (1986). Effect of sampling site and collection method on variations in baseline clinical pathology parameters in Fischer-344 rats. *Fundam. Appl. Toxicol.* **7,** 658–663.

Stearns, S. M., and Lee, P.W. (1984). A rapid method for repeated collection of blood from the tail of rats. *Lab. Anim. Sci.* **34,** 395–396.

Steffey, E. P., Gillespie, J. R., Berry, J. D., Eger II, E. I., and Schalm, O. W. (1976). Effect of halothane and halothane-nitrous oxide on hematocrit and plasma protein concentration in dog and monkey. *Am. J. Vet. Res.* **37,** 959–962.

Stoltz, D. R., and Bendall, R. E. (1975). A simple technic for repeated collection of blood samples from mice. *Lab. Anim. Sci.* **25,** 353–354.

Switzer, J. W. (1967). A new technique for sampling bone marrow in monkeys. *Lab. Anim. Care* **17,** 255–260.

Tada, M., Sugitani, T., Orita, S., Akita, T., Miyajima, H., and Imai, A. (1983). Identification of *Edesonfilaria malayensis* from cynomolgus monkeys *(Macaca fascicularis),* and description of the microfilariae. *Jpn. J. Parasitol.* **32,** 509–515.

Taylor, F. B., Jr. (1983). Survey and new description of the hemostasis system. *Surv. Synth. Pathol. Res.* **1,** 251–273.

Theus, R., and Zbinden, G. (1984). Toxicological assessment of the hemostatic system, regulatory requirements, and industry practice. *Regul. Toxicol. Pharmacol.* **4,** 74–95.

Thomas, R. E., and Kittrell, J. E. (1966). Effect of altitude and season on the canine hemogram. *J. Am. Vet. Med. Assoc.* **148,** 1163–1167.

Thompson, C. B., Diaz, D. D., Quinn, P. G., Lapins, M., Kurtz, S. R., and Valeri, C. R. (1983). The role of anticoagulation in the measurement of platelet volumes. *Am. J. Clin. Pathol.* **80,** 327–332.

Toñz, O. (1968). The congenital methemoglobinemias. *Bibliotheca Haematologica* **28.**

Urizar, R. E., Cerda, J., Dodds, W. J., Raymond, S. L., Largent, J. A., Simon, R., and Gilboa, N. (1984). Age-related renal, hematologic, and hemostatic abnormalities in FH/Wjd rats. *Am. J. Vet. Res.* **45,** 1624–1631.

Valli, V. E., McSherry, B. J., and Hulland, T. J. (1969). A review of bone marrow handling techniques and description of a new method. *Can. J. Comp. Med.* **33,** 68–71.

Vargaftig, B. B., Conard, J., and Samama, M. (1979). Blood coagulation and platelet function: Introduction. *Pharmacol. Ther.* **5,** 225–227.

Vuillaume, A. (1983). A new technique for taking blood samples from ducks and geese. *Avian Pathol.* **12,** 389–391.

Weide, K. D., Trapp, A. L., Weaver, C. R., and Lagace, A. (1962). Blood cell counting in animals by electronic means. I. Erythrocyte enumeration of porcine, ovine, and bovine blood. *Am. J. Vet. Res.* **23,** 632–640.

Weiser, M. G. (1982). Erythrocyte volume distribution analysis in healthy dogs, cats, horses, and dairy cows. *Am. J. Vet. Res.* **43,** 163–166.

Weiser, M. G. (1987). Modification and evaluation of a multichannel blood cell counting system for blood analysis in veterinary hematology. *J. Am. Vet. Med. Assoc.* **190,** 411–415.

Weiser, M. G., and Kociba, G. J. (1982). Persistent macrocytosis assessed by erythrocyte subpopulation analysis following erythrocyte regeneration in cats. *Blood* **60,** 295–303.

Weiser, M. G., and Kociba, G. J. (1983a). Sequential changes in erythrocyte volume distribution and microcytosis associated with iron deficiency in kittens. *Vet. Pathol.* **20,** 1–12.

Weiser, M. G., and Kociba, B. J. (1983b). Erythrocyte macrocytosis in feline leukemia virus associated anemia. *Vet. Pathol.* **20,** 687–697.

Weiser, M. G., and Kociba, G. J. (1984). Platelet concentration and platelet volume distribution in healthy cats. *Am. J. Vet. Res.* **45,** 518–522.

Weiser, M. G., and O'Grady, M. (1983). Erythrocyte volume distribution analysis and hematologic changes in dogs with iron deficiency anemia. *Vet. Pathol.* **20,** 230–241.

Weiss, H. J. (1976). Platelet function tests and their interpretation. *J. Lab. Clin. Med.* **87,** 909–912.

Wertz, R. K., and Koepke, J. A. (1977). A critical analysis of platelet counting methods. *Am. J. Clin. Pathol. Suppl.* **68,** 195–201.

Wertz, R. K., and Triplett, D. (1980). A review of platelet counting performance in the United States. *Am. J. Clin. Pathol.* **74,** 575–580.

Winter, H. (1965). Automatic red cell counting in sheep. *J. Comp. Pathol.* **75,** 205–214.

Wintrobe, M. M., Lee, G. R., Boggs, D. R., Bithell, T. C., Athens, J. W., and Foerster, J. (1974). "Clinical Hematology," 7th ed. Philadelphia: Lee & Febiger.

Wintrobe, M. M., Lee, G. R., Boggs, D. R., Bithell, T. C., Foerster, J., Athens, J. W., and Lukens, J. N. (1981). "Clinical Hematology," 8th ed. Philadelphia: Lee & Febiger.

Wisecup, W. G., and Crouch, B. G. (1963). Evaluation and calibration of an electronic particle counter for enumeration of multispecies blood cells. *Am. J. Clin. Pathol.* **39,** 349–354.

19
Clinical Chemistry

D. L. Basel
Staff Consultant
Southwest Veterinary Diagnostic Laboratory
Phoenix, Arizona

D. C. Villeneuve
Environmental Health Directorate
Health Protection Branch
Health and Welfare Canada
Ottawa, Ontario

A. P. Yagminas
Environmental Health Directorate
Health Protection Branch
Health and Welfare Canada
Ottawa, Ontario

I. INTRODUCTION

The term *clinical chemistry* refers to the measurement of analytes in blood, serum, plasma, and occasionally urine and other tissues or secretions. Analytes may be enzymes, ions, nonenzymatic proteins, or other organic or inorganic molecules. In toxicological studies, clinical chemistry is used to help assess the toxic effects of compounds given to animals by clarifying the nature, severity, and sometimes reversibility of pathological lesions and also by identifying the "no-effect" level. Biochemical data are also useful in determining the health status of test animals prior to the start of an experiment and in monitoring the health of these animals during the study. Note that the term *clinical* as used in this chapter is not related to the term *clinical study* and does not imply that tests or studies are being done on humans.

In this chapter, the reader should become familiar with some basic logistic aspects of conducting the clinical chemistry portion of *in vivo* toxicity studies. It is not the intent to instruct regarding interpretation of results. This chapter has been written primarily, for professionals who conduct *in vivo* toxicity studies although their area of expertise is not clinical chemistry or pathology.

Excluding the introduction, this chapter is divided into eight sections. Section II involves a brief discussion of general mechanisms that cause changes in the levels of some analytes. The utility and nomenclature of the more common analytes are outlined. Section III addresses the principles and guidelines used in the selection of analytes to be measured during a study. The fourth section on instrumentation presents some basic terminology and aspects of laboratory automation that pertain to its use in toxicity studies. In the fifth section, the influence of sample collection, sample quality, and miscellaneous factors on test results is briefly discussed. Relatively detailed sections on study protocols, standard operating procedures, quality assurance, and data handling follow. They emphasize certain aspects of good laboratory practice (GLP) that are discussed in more general terms in Chapters 22 and 23.

II. COMMONLY MEASURED ANALYTES AND THEIR UTILITY

It is not our purpose to discuss all analytes capable of being measured in modern, well-equipped, clinical pathology laboratories. Nor is it feasible to discuss all available methods for each analyte. The following paragraphs describe the tests most often used, with emphasis on those used to assess the status of the liver, the kidneys, and the skeletal and cardiac muscles.

As mentioned previously, clinical chemistry tests may be performed on blood, plasma, serum, or other biological fluids. Blood can be divided into two components: the particulate elements (i.e., leukocytes, erythrocytes, and platelets) and the fluid component known as plasma. Plasma is, therefore, blood from which the particulate elements have been removed. Serum is essentially plasma from which fibrinogen (a soluble plasma protein) has been removed by the process of clotting. There are distinct differences among blood, plasma, and serum, therefore, it is important to specify which is to be used as the specimen. Not all tests designed for measuring analytes in serum will work adequately if plasma or blood is substituted (and vice versa). Furthermore, there are often subtle differences between plasma and serum concentrations of some analytes that may not be outside reference limits, but these differences may be statistically significant in highly controlled laboratory studies with a well-defined population. In toxicological studies, serum is the specimen most frequently submitted for clinical chemistry analysis. In this chapter, references to the level of any analyte is to its concentration in serum unless stated otherwise.

Prior to any discussion of serum analytes, it must first be noted that a change in concentration of a given analyte is seldom, if ever, specific for a given disease or pathological mechanism. When interpreting a change in concentration of any analyte, one must consider that change in the context of the changes in other analytes; the general health and age of the animal; the quality, handling, and storage of the serum specimen; the clinical signs observed; and any gross or microscopic pathology noted.

A. Liver

Numerous tests have been developed or employed to evaluate liver function or disease. There are several pathological mechanisms on which these tests are based. Damaged hepatocytes or biliary epithelium may release cell constituents (e.g., enzymes) into the blood resulting in increased levels of these analytes. Certain metabolites normally occurring in blood are removed by the liver, and impaired function of this organ may result in elevated serum concentrations of those metabolites. Many plasma constituents are produced by the liver, and impaired function of this organ may result in decreased levels of some analytes. Alternatively, under appropriate conditions, hepatocytes or biliary epithelium may be stimulated to synthesize certain analytes resulting in increased serum levels.

The more commonly measured "liver" enzymes are alanine aminotransferase (ALT; formerly SGPT), aspartate aminotransferase (AST; formerly SGOT), sorbitol dehydrogenase (SDH), alkaline phosphatase (AP), and gamma-glutamyl transferase (GGT). Others such as ornithine carbamyl transferase, isocitrate dehydrogenase, and arginase are measured less frequently. Increased levels of ALT, AST, and SDH are usually associated with damage to hepatocytes (Van Veet and Alberts, 1968; Korsrud, et al., 1973; Dooley, 1984a, 1984b); however, AST is the least liver specific in that skeletal and cardiac muscles contain significant concentrations of this enzyme and damage to these cell types will also increase serum levels (Cornelius, 1980). Increased levels of AP (Kaplan and Righetti, 1970) and GGT (Leonard, et al., 1984) are associated with biliary disease, although AP is also elevated during pathological or physiological increases in bone remodeling activity (Rogers, 1976). In some species, such as dogs, AP and GGT levels are increased in response to elevated glucocorticoid levels (Badylak and Van Vleet 1981a).

Metabolites such as bilirubin are normally removed by the liver. Liver dysfunction often results in elevated bilirubin levels due to inadequate clearance or conjugation. Exogenous dyes such as sulfobromophthalein (Center, et al., 1983) or indocyanine green (Prasse, et al., 1983) are sometimes administered intravenously to animals to assess liver function. Because such dyes are normally removed rapidly by the liver, delayed clearance from the blood is suggestive of impaired liver function.

Most proteins found in serum (or plasma) are produced by the liver, the principle exception being immunoglobulins. Severe liver damage has been associated with decreased production of various proteins resulting in reduced serum levels of total protein, albumin, and/or globulin (Alper, 1974; Killingsworth, 1981). Decreased protein production may render other abnormal test values. For example, depletion of various coagulation factors (all are globulins) may result in prolonged prothrombin or activated partial thromboplastin times (Badylak and Van Vleet, 1981b). Other individual protein levels may also be reduced because decreased production does not necessarily affect all proteins uniformly. Note that increased loss of protein via urine or feces due to renal or gastrointestinal disease will also reduce serum protein levels. Inflammation anywhere within the body often results in increased production of specific globulin proteins by the liver (Alper, 1974). Immunoglobulin levels may also increase if there is sufficient antigenic stimulation; that is, there may be a qualitative change in the proteins produced that will not be detected solely by measuring total protein, albumin, or globulin levels. Another substance synthesized only by the liver is urea, and severe liver dysfunction has been associated with reduced urea levels (Ewing, et al., 1974).

B. Kidneys

The kidneys play a central role in regulating acid-base balance, electrolyte concentration, hydration, and excretion of various waste products and other metabolites. Abnormalities in the concentration of analytes that are primarily regulated by the kidneys result from either their reduced removal from the blood or their increased loss in the urine.

Acid-base status is seldom thoroughly investigated in most toxicological studies. Occasionally bicarbonate (or total carbon dioxide) concentration is measured to give some indication of acid-base balance. However, unless the specimens can be assayed promptly following collection, there is little value in measuring bicarbonate. The lungs also play an important role in regulating carbon dioxide concentration, thus dysfunction of the respiratory system also influences acid-base balance.

Electrolytes such as sodium, potassium, and chloride are normally excreted and/or reabsorbed by the kidneys, the process being regulated by a variety of hormones. Hence, either endocrine or kidney dysfunction may result in elevated or lowered electrolyte levels depending on the specific hormone(s) involved or portion(s) of the kidneys affected. Phosphorus and calcium levels are also regulated in part by the kidneys; therefore, any renal dysfunction may affect levels of these analytes.

Blood urea nitrogen (BUN) and creatinine are normal metabolites removed in most species primarily by the kidneys. Decreased effective kidney function results in reduced removal of these metabolites and consequent increase in their serum concentration (Osborne, et al., 1972). Substantial kidney function is usually lost, often as much as three fourths, before increases in BUN or creatinine are noted; hence, neither is a particularly sensitive indicator of kidney pathology. Alternative routes of excretion or metabolism of urea or creatinine may complicate interpretation in some species. For example, colonic bacterial flora in rats can be induced to catabolize a significant amount of creatinine (Jones and Burnett, 1972).

Most of the more common procedures used to analyze urine (urinalysis) are qualitative or semiquantitative and are not discussed in this chapter. Quantitative measurement of certain analytes (e.g. creatinine, sodium, phosphorus) in both serum and urine and calculation of fraction excretion or clearance ratios may be a useful adjunct in evaluating kidney function (Bovee and Joyce, 1979). Urine may be collected at random or all urine produced during a 24-hour period may be pooled and analyzed. Analysis of 24-hour urine specimens is considered more definitive, though random specimens (usually collected over an 8- to 16-hour period) are more practical and usually suffice. For some analytes, such as urine protein (White, *et al.,* 1984), detection of increased protein loss is simplified if urine concentrations of protein and creatinine are expressed as a ratio (protein/creatinine). Furthermore, random (non-24-hour) urine collections may be used because results correlate fairly well with those obtained by quantitative 24-hour urine collections. Although urine analyte/creatinine ratios are useful, quantitation of an analyte in a 24-hour urine specimen is still considered more definitive.

Measurement of urine enzyme levels has been advocated by some investigators as a means of detecting kidney pathology. The enzymes measured may be derived from plasma or kidney tissue itself (usually from tubular epithelium). If the enzymes are of plasma origin, increases are attributed to leakage through damaged glomeruli or tubules. Enzymes present in kidney tubular epithelium may be passed in the urine following tubular damage. The increase in urine enzyme activity may be quite marked albeit transient.

C. Muscles

Skeletal and cardiac muscle pathology may at times result in leakage of cell contents (e.g., enzymes) into blood in sufficient quantities to elevate their levels. The most commonly measured enzymes are creatine kinase (CK), lactate dehydrogenase (LD), and aspartate aminotransferase (AST). Serum level of these enzymes tends to vary a fair amount between animals of the same species; that is, the reference or normal ranges are broad (Mitruka and Rawnsley, 1981). Tissue trauma or hemolysis incurred during venipuncture contributes in part to this interanimal variation due to release of enzymes from these cells. A significant quantity of enzyme, for example LD, may also be released from platelets of some species, especially of rats (Friedel and Mattenheimer, 1970), and this also contributes to interanimal variations. Caution must therefore be used in interpreting levels of these enzymes because sampling technique, sample quality, and interspecies differences in tissue, erythrocyte, or platelet (and possibly leukocyte) enzyme content can markedly influence the levels measured.

Distinction between cardiac and skeletal muscle pathology is not possible simply by measuring CK, LD, or AST total activities. Evaluation of electrophoretic isoenzyme patterns may prove of benefit in distinguishing cardiac from skeletal muscle involvement. However, because of species differences in isoenzyme content of various tissues (Boyd, 1983), findings in one species cannot be directly extrapolated to another. The isoenzyme content of the tissues in question must be known for the animal species being tested, and the electrophoretic procedure must be tightly monitored to obtain usable information. Although in some circumstances isoenzyme determination may contribute to estimation of no-effect levels, in most instances, if animals are scheduled for sacrifice, a thorough necropsy and histopathological evaluation are probably adequate.

D. Digestive System

Intestinal tract pathology or function is not directly evaluated with most chemistry profiles. However, serum levels of many of the analytes mentioned previously may be affected by intestinal tract dysfunction. For example, loss of protein via the intestinal tract may deplete serum levels and ultimately lead to protein deficiency and emaciation. Impaired absorption of protein or other nutrients, such as calcium or iron, may have wide ranging systemic effects as well as result in decreased serum levels of these substances. Intestinal absorption studies utilizing D-xylose can be done but are cumbersome, time-consuming, and too expensive for most studies.

Evaluation of exocrine pancreatic dysfunction is probably more reliably done by gross examination and histopathology. Although serum amylase and lipase activity may be measured, levels of these enzymes are affected by factors other than pancreatic disease. For example, renal failure in dogs may elevate amylase or lipase levels (Polzin, et al., 1983). Isoenzyme analysis of amylase might prove beneficial in some species. Digestive function tests such as those measuring liberation and absorption of p-aminobenzoic acid (PABA) may be done, but again they are time-consuming and expensive.

E. Nervous System

In toxicological studies, neurological dysfunction is usually assessed by clinical signs and gross and microscopic examination of tissues. Clinical chemistry has rarely been employed. Although cerebrospinal fluid may be collected and assayed for various analytes such as glucose, protein, or chloride, this is seldom done for two reasons. First, collection of cerebrospinal fluid is a fairly involved procedure that requires proper anesthetizing, positioning, and preparation of the animals as well as individuals who are skilled in performing spinal taps. Second, the volume of fluid obtained is quite limited even in larger animals such as dogs. Occasionally cholinesterase activity is measured in homogenized brain samples (it may also be measured in serum or erythrocytes) to monitor the effects of organophosphate or carbamate compounds (Buck, *et al.*, 1976).

F. Miscellaneous

Some analytes measured and proved to be diagnostically useful in humans are not necessarily as useful in other species. One such analyte is uric acid, which is commonly utilized in humans to aid in the diagnosis of gout although other conditions such as leukemia or renal disease affect uric acid levels also (Woo and Cannon, 1984). Uric acid is the end product of purine metabolism in humans and anthropoid apes; however, most other mammalian species carry the metabolic process further to form allantoin. Consequently, uric acid levels are very low in most non-primate mammals, and measuring its concentration is of limited utility. For example, it has been reported that uric acid may increase in dogs during severe liver disease (synthesis of allantoin is impaired), but the sensitivity of this test in detecting liver disease is questionable (Hoe and Harvey, 1961) therefore other tests are used instead.

Other analytes, most notably serum enzymes such as alanine aminotransferase, gamma-glutamyl transferase, or creatine kinase, do not necessarily have the same tissue distributions or concentrations in animals as they do in humans (Boyd, 1983). For example, gamma-glutamyl transferase is present in the blood and biliary epithelium of rats although in much lower concentrations than in most other species. This has caused some individuals to question the usefulness of measuring gamma-glutamyl transferase for detecting biliary disease in rats.

The age of the animals being tested must also be considered because this will affect the levels of various analytes (Laird, 1977) such as alkaline phosphatase. If animals are placed on study while still in their growth phase, age-related changes in analytes may obscure subtle effects on some parameters or complicate interpretation when data obtained at different time intervals are compared. Appropriate statistical procedures or graphic analysis of data should minimize this problem.

There are significant sex-related differences in the levels of some analytes. For some analytes, the sex-related differences are present only in certain strains or breeds, other strains exhibiting no or insignificant differences between males and females. Because gender affects levels of some analytes, it is preferable to analyze data from each sex separately. Combining data from both sexes may obscure treatment-related changes in analytes for either or both sexes.

Strain- or breed-related differences also occur for some analytes. Knowledge of these differences is mainly required for proper assessment of baseline or control group data.

III. CHOOSING THE ANALYTES TO BE MEASURED: CHEMISTRY PROFILES

The term *chemistry profile,* as used in toxicological studies, refers to a defined set of tests performed on each specimen received. The profile must be defined prior to initiation of the study, although with proper documentation and justification it may be modified during the study. There are several factors to consider in the design of a chemistry profile for a study. These are purpose, specimen volume, test sample volume, economics, and prioritization of samples. Above all, there is a need for very careful planning and close cooperation between the involved scientists to ensure that the most appropriate tests are performed.

The primary consideration in the design of a chemistry profile should be to define its purpose. If the toxic effects of the compound are unknown, a screening or general purpose profile such as that suggested by Organization for Economic Co-operation and Development (1981) may be desirable to aid in identifying the organ(s) affected. If the target organs are known or if there is one of particular concern, the profile should be expanded or focused to include measurement of additional analytes that will aid in assessing the damage to or the function of the organ(s) in question. For example, additional tests to monitor liver function may be warranted (Davidson *et al.,* 1979).

The specimen volume that can be realistically obtained from the animals being tested should be estimated. The volume obtained will depend on several factors, most notably the species of animal being tested. Obviously a dog can spare a greater volume of blood than a mouse. Young or underweight animals cannot spare as much blood as normal weight adults. As a study progresses, animals receiving a compound, especially those in high dose groups, may be less capable than animals in the control group of replacing blood lost due to sampling; for example, they may have a reduced ability to synthesize erythrocytes. Females of most species are smaller and have a somewhat lower total blood volume than males. Occasionally, this is of practical significance in obtaining adequate specimen volume.

The volume of specimen required for each test of the contemplated profile should be calculated. This is a relatively straightforward exercise; however, sufficient volume must also be obtained to cover repeat tests and sample wastage (small losses due to coating of pipettes or containers are unavoidable). Although the sample volume required for many analytical procedures has declined remarkably over the past decade, the need for additional tests has increased and the constraints of total available specimen volume are therefore still applicable. It is important to know the sample volume requirements for each test procedure. Although requirements constantly change as new methods and sample-handling systems are developed or adopted, many procedures, especially the manual ones, still require a considerable volume of specimen. The methodology and, consequently, test sample volume requirements will vary for each laboratory but should be listed in the standard operating procedure (SOP) for that test.

The blood volume available for the chemistry profile will also be influenced by demands for other test procedures including hematology, coagulation studies, bioavailability assays, and endocrinology assays. Each of these procedures require specific amounts of blood collected in separate containers that usually contain an anticoagulant, which often makes the sample unsuitable for chemistry analysis depending on the analyte and anticoagulant in question. An example is sodium fluoride, which can cause a 20% reduction in values of total protein, inorganic phosphorus, and glucose in rabbit plasma (Bartosek and Guaitani, 1982). The number and frequency of bleeding intervals also have an impact on the amount of blood drawn at each interval because iatrogenic anemia must be avoided or minimized.

Cost per test has declined dramatically as automated and semiautomated chemistry analyzers have evolved. However, the number of tests performed per animal and the number of animals per study have also tended to increase over the past decade, hence economics is still a very real concern. In most instances, automation or semiautomation reduces costs per test substantially. Some tests, however, may require the specimen to be specially handled or prepared (e.g., erythrocyte cholinesterase). Assays that cannot be readily automated (at least with the equipment available to the laboratory) must be performed manually, thereby increasing unit cost per test. Either special handling or manual test procedures add considerable cost to the test profile.

Once these considerations have been addressed, priorities must be set that may involve some compromises. The purpose of the study and profile should be the predominant factors dictating which tests should be included in the profile. Frequently, there will be an insufficient volume of specimen attainable from each animal for all tests desired. There are several means of circumventing this, including pooling of specimens, increasing the number of animals per test, and ranking the tests in order of importance.

Pooling of specimens from all animals in a treatment group (or by sex within a group) has been proposed as one manner to obtain greater volumes for assays. This is not preferable in most circumstances because a good deal of information on responses of individual animals is lost. An average value is obtained, but the individual animal variance is not.

Increasing the number of animals per treatment is a viable alternative in some instances. Part of the group (half, for example) may then be bled for hematological or other studies, the remainder of the group may be bled and their blood used solely for chemistry analysis. This does not increase the net number of specimens analyzed for clinical chemistry purposes, but the volume available per specimen is greater, which allows a wider variety of tests to be performed.

Explicit instructions as to which tests must be obtained are at times necessary. Often, about half the analytes to be measured are designated as priority; these are assayed first and repeated if necessary. Once adequate results are obtained for priority analytes, the remaining analytes may be measured in decreasing order of importance. If sample volume is adequate for all tests, then test order should reflect whatever is most efficient for the analyst and/or instrumentation being used.

IV. INSTRUMENTATION

Technically, any laboratory equipped with a spectrophotometer has the capability to undertake the analysis of the majority of tests required in a toxicological study. In most studies, a large number of analyses are required, and the only practical way to process them is to use automated or semiautomated chemistry analyzers. Technological advances in automated instrumentation during the past 20 years have greatly improved the reliability, precision, and capacity of clinical chemistry machines. A number of sample and reagent delivery systems, techniques for mixing sample and reagents, and arrangements for monitoring reactions are available in a variety of combinations. The type of instrumentation chosen or used by a laboratory is largely dependent on its needs and resources; that is, on technician preference, laboratory test volume, types of tests required, cost, availability of service or reagents, and instrument reliability, accuracy, and precision.

Automated instruments can be placed into two broad categories based on the manner in which specimens and reagents are handled. These are termed "continuous flow" and "discrete" analyzers. Continuous flow instruments measure analytes by mixing specimen and reagents in a coiled tube. The mixture flows through the tubing continuously, one specimen following another but separated by air bubbles. Each set of tubing is dedicated to measuring a specific analyte. Larger instruments have multiple sets of tubing (channels), each measuring a different analyte. A portion of every specimen is run through each channel generating a battery of test results or "profile" for each specimen. Discrete analyzers aspirate a sample and deliver it and the reagents into a separate cup or reaction well; therefore, each sample–reagent mixture is reacted individually. Most discrete analyzers can be easily (relative to continuous flow analyzers) programmed or instructed to perform a unique set of tests on each specimen. This is an advantage in situations in which different profiles are required for different toxicological studies.

Continuous flow analyzers usually measure endpoint (or modified endpoint) chemical reactions, whereas discrete analyzers can monitor either endpoint or kinetic assays and are somewhat more versatile. Endpoint assays measure the amount of reaction product formed or substrate consumed after a given amount of time. Kinetic assays measure reaction rates such as enzyme activity; that is, they continuously measure the rate of product formation or substrate disappearance while the reaction is proceeding. Kinetic assays are often more sensitive than endpoint methods.

Microvolume test requirements are a definite advantage in chemistry analyzers used for toxicological studies. Specimen volumes than can be obtained from rodents and other small animals are usually quite limited. Thus, the smaller the volume of sample required for each test the greater the number of analytes that can be measured per profile. A high quality, accurate, reliable pipetting system in a chemistry analyzer is essential if very small quantities of sample are to be aspirated. Chemistry analyzers in which reagents or instrument settings can be "adjusted" are preferable to those in which reagents and settings are "fixed". This is because technique modifications may be required to analyze specimens other than serum. Also, new techniques may be more easily developed or adapted as needed. The main advantages of the more fixed systems are that technician variability is reduced and less skilled operators can be used with no diminution in the quality of data generated. The precision of fixed systems is often better than that of more adjustable systems, although results are not necessarily more accurate. A disadvantage of fixed systems is their inability to modify methods. An investigator is limited to those tests that the manufacturer supplies and the relatively high reagent/disposables costs per test.

Requirements for data storage and handling in most hospitals are slightly different from those in most toxicological laboratories. In human clinical medicine, it is sufficient to sort data by patient (or specimen) only. However, toxicological studies usually require that the animals and data be further sorted by dose group and sex. Most chemistry analyzers are incapable of manipulating data in this manner, consequently, it must be transmitted to a second computer for collation by group and sex. Because virtually all chemistry analyzers today have RS232 or IEEE ports, the transfer of data to ancillary computers has been simplified. For equipment without these ports, linkup to a central computer may be more cumbersome; therefore, this factor should be considered prior to acquisition of a new instrument. It is advisable to retain a programming specialist to ascertain how readily linkup and data transfer can be accomplished and how current in-house software and hardware can be meshed with the instrument in question.

A word of advice is due here. When contemplating acquisition of a new instrument, one should remember that many manufacturer representatives are unfamiliar with the needs of researchers conducting toxicological studies. It is wise to check their claims concerning instrument capabilities. If a representative blithely states that the company's instrument can do whatever you ask, we recommend you reply with the Missouri slogan "Show Me". A summary of the various types of analytical methods and instrumentation can be found in Maclin and Young (1986) or Werner (1982).

V. INFLUENCE OF SAMPLE COLLECTION, SAMPLE QUALITY, AND MISCELLANEOUS FACTORS ON TEST RESULTS

Several factors pertaining to the collection of blood specimens may affect clinical chemistry results. Such factors include sample identification, venipuncture site, anesthesia, diurnal variations, fasting as opposed to nonfasting state prior to collection, stress, and collection and analysis order of samples. Factors affecting collection of urine are also briefly discussed. Several of these (venipuncture site, anticoagulants, and stress) are discussed in Chapter 18, Section II on the requisites for valid hematological procedures. This section deals with a few additional items pertaining to serum chemistry results.

Perhaps the most important aspect of sample collection is the proper labeling and identification of specimens. It is imperative that blood collection tubes be properly and clearly marked with pencil or indelible ink (to avoid smudging of the identifying marks). The collection tube must be positively matched with the identifying number of the animal being sampled. Obviously, proper identification of samples must continue throughout processing and analysis until a final value is reported.

Influence of venipuncture site is discussed in Chapter 18. With respect to the effects of venipuncture on serum chemistry values, any influences are probably due in most instances to the degree of tissue trauma, hemolysis, or physical restraint of the animal associated with certain methods rather than to any significant differences in the blood itself.

Chemical restraint agents may alter the blood levels of some analytes and care must be taken in selecting an appropriate agent. Some anesthetics impair mitochondrial respiration, reduce gluconeogenesis and oxygen consumption, and inhibit the activity of enzymes (Bartosek and Guaitani, 1982). Others are capable of inducing hyperuricemia and hyperglycemia (Scott and Trick, 1982). The effects of any particular chemical agent on clinical chemistry analytes should be evaluated thoroughly prior to its adoption as part of a standard bleeding procedure. Ideally, the agent should be evaluated in each species, strain, and sex of animal in which it is to be used.

Diurnal or circadian rhythms are daily fluctuations in certain physiological parameters that, in turn, cause altered levels of some blood analytes (Winkel, et al., 1975). Diurnal variations in enzyme activity are relatively independent of temperature, light, or handling (Bartosek and Guaitani, 1982). If serial collections are required, the best way to compensate for diurnal variation is to conduct sample collections over as short a period of time as possible and at the same time of day.

Whether the animals are fasted or not prior to blood collection affects the level of several analytes. For example, in rats, serum creatinine, lactate dehydrogenase, glucose, corticosterone, and magnesium are altered following an overnight fast (D. C. Villeneuve, unpublished data). Although the degree of change may not be physiologically important, they must be considered when interpreting results of a study. If animals are to be fasted, one must be certain that all animals scheduled for bleeding have their food withheld. It is not acceptable to fast only a portion of the animals because this introduces additional interanimal variation. Fasting of animals prior to blood collection, though not absolutely essential, is recommended in most cases.

The order in which samples are collection and analyzed may influence results. In order to eliminate systematic bias between dose groups, blood should be taken from animals in different dose groups and preferably from different sexes on a random basis. The order in which samples are analyzed should parallel the collection order because systematic bias can also occur during analysis.

The quality of the blood specimen received will directly affect the levels of many analytes. Hemolysis, lipemia, and hyperbilirubinemia affect the actual or measured level of several analytes depending on degree and the methodology used (Glick, et al., 1986); the SOP for each method should list these effects, if any. Rough handling of samples may cause hemolysis and release erythrocyte constituents into the serum. For instance, with serum hemoglobin levels of 1,500 mg/L, lactate dehydrogenase activity may be elevated fivefold (Chin et al., 1979). Normal serum has a straw-yellow color, and a reddish appearance (hemolysis) is indicative of hemoglobin release from erythrocytes. The degree of hemolysis is usually estimated subjectively and must be recorded on the sample collection sheet and in the final report. Lipemia, excess lipid in the blood, and hyperbilirubinemia, excess bilirubin in the blood (also called icterus), are not due to improper sample collection but result from pathological or physiological processes. Lipemia gives serum a milky opalescence and hyperbilirubinemia gives serum a more intense yellow color. The presence of either must be recorded on the sample collection sheet and in the final report.

Several other factors, such as changes in methodology, delays in sample processing, excessive exposure to intensive light, or high or low temperatures and humidity, may affect the measured levels of analytes. Changes in methodology or instrumentation are usually due to failure of equipment used in the primary technique, which necessitates use of a backup procedure. When backup methods are employed, they must be clearly noted in the raw data and accompanied by a full written explanation. Different technicians given the same specimen may generate slightly different results for some analytes, especially if the method used is manual (or not highly automated). This problem can be minimized if one technician is assigned to perform the same analyses for any given study. Delays in sample processing may result in changes of certain analytes. For example, the activity of many enzymes will decrease over time, the degree depending on the particular enzyme and the temperature at which the sample is stored. If delays are necessary, careful consideration must be given to the effects of temperature on the analytes to be measured. High temperatures may inactivate enzymes or hasten denaturation of other serum constituents. Exposure of serum to light will cause a breakdown of bilirubin in the sample, thus decreasing its measured level. Ambient temperature and humidity will affect sample evaporation rates causing variable, but detectable, increases in concentration of many analytes over time. This can be minimized if the sample tubes are covered.

Many drugs and chemicals are known to interfere with the measurement of analytes in human serum (Young, et al., 1975); however, little information is available regarding animal serum. (Use of drugs for the purpose of animal treatment and/or other chemicals for purposes other than those described in the protocol is contraindicated for many toxicology tests). The effects referred to are not those due to toxicological or pathological actions of a compound but rather to direct interference of a compound either with the analyte itself or with the reactions of an analytical system. One example would be the effect of cephalozin on aminotransferases (Dhami, et al., 1979). Potential interference of a test compound or its metabolites with the measurement of serum analytes should be considered in the design or interpretation of a toxicological study. The route by which a test compound is administered may also affect the levels of serum analytes due to differences in rate of absorption, distribution, and metabolism. Possibility of transient intravascular hemolysis following intravenous dosing should be considered a potential source of interference. The time between dosing and sample collection must be carefully recorded because the effects on some analytes may be transitory.

Urinalysis in combination with serum chemistry is preferred for thorough assessment of kidney function. The principal problem encountered with urine samples is in obtaining an adequate but uncontaminated volume. Contamination with fecal material is often a problem when samples are collected from animals in metabolism cages. Bacterial contamination and overgrowth may occur but can be minimized if collection cups are placed on ice, urine receptacles are emptied periodically, samples are refrigerated, or preservatives are added to the samples. Addition of preservatives is convenient, but the type added must depend on the analytes to be measured. Contamination may also occur if the collection device is improperly cleaned and if detergents or tap water contain substances that interfere or alter the concentration of the analyte to be measured (e.g., residues containing calcium or phosphorus).

Collection of an adequate urine specimen may be difficult for several reasons. All animals in a group will not void urine at the same time. Furthermore, the amount voided is not uniform and is influenced by individual water consumption. Catheterization or cystocentesis of the urinary bladder may be used to avoid contamination, but it is difficult to time either procedure in order to catch animals before they spontaneously void. The method of urine collection should be the same for all animals in a group.

VI. STUDY PROTOCOLS

Establishing, updating, and recording deviations from study protocols are important aspects of conducting a toxicological study and are essential for compliance with good laboratory practices (Organization for Economic Co-operation and Development, 1982; U.S. Environmental Protection Agency, 1985; U.S. Food and Drug Administration, 1985). The clinical chemistry section of a protocol should be documented, understood, and approved by all parties involved (e.g., management, study director, head of laboratory, technicians) prior to the initiation of a study. Several items that one needs to address when documenting the clinical chemistry portion of the study protocol are discussed next.

Clinical chemistry instructions are usually included in the clinical pathology section of protocols along with hematology, coagulation, and urinalysis instructions. All individuals directly connected with performing clinical pathology tests must be familiar with the entire protocol to avoid omission of any test. Apart from being a sound practice, this policy is necessary because all laboratories or individuals do not categorize tests identically. For example, some classify methemoglobin assays as hematology tests, whereas others classify them as part of a "clinical chemistry" profile. Listing tests under the categories (i.e. clinical chemistry, hematology, etc.) used by the laboratory conducting the testing will help avoid omissions but should not be a substitute for requiring staff to be familiar with the entire protocol.

Analytes to be measured should be detailed in the protocol. Acronyms such as BUN or CK should not be used as the sole indentifier of an analyte. Typographical errors often create confusion when, for example, AST is inadvertently written as ALT rather than as aspartate aminotransferase.

The SOP for each test to be performed should be referenced. Those SOPs covering more general laboratory procedures such as data storage, specimen preparation, reporting of values, which are common to all or most tests, usually do not need to be quoted individually. A statement that such procedures must be followed is often sufficient.

The following items must be explicitly addressed in the clinical pathology section of any protocol. The type of specimen to be used must be clearly stated. Serum, plasma, and whole blood are not synonymous, and the type of specimen used does make a difference in how it is handled and in the values obtained. The number and types of samples to be collected and tests to be performed at each bleeding interval must be clearly stated. If samples are required for bioavailability or other nonclinical chemistry tests this should be noted. The frequency with which animals are bled and whether or not the same animals are to be bled each time must be specified. For each bleeding interval, the treatment groups to be sampled should be indicated along with the number of male and female animals sampled per group. When the animals are to be fasted prior to blood collection and for how long need to be stated. The method of blood collection (e.g., via orbital sinus, tail vein, cardiac puncture, etc.) and the approximate amount of blood to be collected should be specified. The time interval between administration of treatment (dosing) and blood collection is important to note. Prioritization of analytes should be explicitly stated if it is anticipated that sample volume may not be sufficient for all tests desired.

Factors indirectly affecting the clinical chemistry portion of the study must be stated in the protocol, although not necessarily in the clinical pathology (or chemistry) section. Obviously, the species of animal being tested must be stated. The breed or strain of animal used is important to note because there are often distinct strain-related differences in the levels of some analytes. Although this may influence interpretation of data, test methodology rarely needs to be changed. Similarly, the age of the animals at the start of the test and, in the case of rodents, range of body weight must be indicated. The method of test compound administration is important to specify because this might alter some analyte values. For example, intravenous injection may conceivably result in slight intravascular hemolysis, which will affect measurement of some analytes. The stress of dosing, if by means other than in the feed, may influence the level of some analytes, depending on the time elapsed between dosing and blood sampling and on the animal species. Depending on the logistics of dosing and blood sampling, arrival of specimens at the laboratory may be delayed or scattered over time, which will affect sample processing or scheduling of analyses. Every effort should be made to collect samples over as short a time period as is practicable to minimize delays in processing. Statistical procedures to be employed in analyzing the data should be outlined in the protocol.

Occasionally, certain aspects of the clinical chemistry portion of a study need to be altered after the study is initiated. Changes that alter the basic structure of the protocol are referred to as deviations from protocol and require a formal protocol amendment. Examples of protocol deviations are addition or deletion of tests from the profile and increases or decreases in the number of animals bled or in the frequency of bleedings. Significant changes in test methodology should also be noted in a protocol amendment. An example would be converting from flame photometric measurement of sodium to an ion-selective electrode method. Use of a backup procedure in the event of instrument failure does not constitute a deviation from protocol. Backup procedures should be specified in the SOP for each test. Documentation of any backup procedure used should be kept with raw data, and a note should appear with the data in the final report. Failure to report a value for a specimen due to insufficient quantity of sample does not constitute a deviation from protocol; the reason for the missing value simply needs to be recorded.

VII. STANDARD OPERATING PROCEDURES

Standard operating procedures or SOPs are an important and useful component in any clinical pathology laboratory and are required for GLP compliance. Concise, well-written, and organized SOPs serve as a reference source for both laboratory technicians and those who interpret the data generated. SOPs should be treated as dynamic documents; that is, they are not unalterable although any changes made must be well documented and formally approved. Any deviation from the SOPs requires written justification and approval. These documents should be readily available to all laboratory personnel and read periodically (at least annually), particularly those SOPs concerning the techniques or procedures that a staff member is responsible for performing. Unauthorized duplication of SOPs should not be permitted, and the number of official copies should be strictly controlled and their source (author, originator, etc.) identified. This is to assure that revisions are distributed to all holders of official copies.

Categorization of SOPs in a clinical pathology (chemistry) laboratory can be done in several ways. For the purposes of this chapter, the designations "technical", "instrument", and "procedural" SOPs are used. Technical SOPs deal with specific procedures, such as the determination of serum glucose, urea nitrogen, calcium, etc. Instrument SOPs deal with the operation of specific instruments such as pH meters, balances, or automated chemistry analyzers; they do not necessarily detail any particular procedure. Procedural SOPs deal with a wide variety of procedures common to many tests, such as data handling and recording, specimen preparation, and laboratory administrative details. The exact categories will depend on the particular institution or laboratory. Alternatively, the various SOPs may simply be assigned a number with no attempt made at classification. Whatever classification system is used, each SOP should be assigned a unique identifying number. Although GLP regulations do not specify that there be SOPs for items such as workplace safety or facility evacuation, other regulatory agencies do and it is best to keep a separate category for such SOPs.

Regardless of categorization, all SOPs should be bound together. Three-ring binders are convenient even if several volumes may be required. A table of contents and a cross-reference table are necessities for most SOP manuals. A list of laboratory personnel, their names, signatures, position/job, and qualifications is a useful addendum to laboratory SOP manuals. A summary of individuals to contact in emergencies, for advice, or for authorization on laboratory problems proves invaluable at times. Work and after-hours telephone numbers should be clearly listed for key (preferably all) laboratory personnel.

Formats for SOPs will probably be unique to each laboratory, and there is no real advantage to interlaboratory standardization of such documents. Once a format(s) has been decided upon for use in any given laboratory, it should be adhered to. This facilitates rapid location of vital information and makes editing of documents easier.

Although the actual format of SOPs is not critical, certain types of information must be included. Technical SOPs should have the following information clearly indicated: title, principle of test, instrumentation, reagents, instructions, reference ranges for each species, methodology comments, backup procedures, interpretation, and references. The title is usually the analyte measured, such as calcium, glucose, or aspartate aminotransferases. The title should be succinct with few or no modifiers such as "rapid" or "enzymatic" cluttering it. If two or more methods for the same analyte are used, separate SOPs should be written with subtitles and SOP identification number used to distinguish them. The more common acronym(s) for an analyte may be inserted in the title but should be offset by parentheses; acronyms alone are not suitable as titles. The principle of the test should be a brief description of the reactions involved; diagrams and scientific formulas are helpful. The name and other identification of the equipment used as well as the settings required for that particular analyte should be listed under instrumentation. Under reagents should be listed the reagents required, how to prepare and store them, the manufacturer(s), and any precautions or warnings regarding handling.

Instructions should describe a method step-by-step: instrument settings, placement of control sera, standards, reagent blanks for each run, procedure to follow if specimen values fall outside the linear range or if control sera results are beyond established limits, and expected values for control sera and standards should be discussed. Backup procedures should cross-reference the SOP for the alternative method to be used in case the primary method fails. Reference ranges for each species should be listed. If in-house values are not available, literature values (preferably derived using the same or similar method) may be listed temporarily; at the very least normal human values should be quoted. Methodology comments may include a list of substances known to interfere with the test (e.g., hemoglobin, specific drugs), potential problems, and a trouble-shooting guide. The interpretation section should consist of a brief description of the test's utility, common causes of increased or decreased values, and any species peculiarities. References should include those cited for any of these categories. Addresses and telephone numbers of the technical services for the reagent and control sera manufacturer(s) may be listed in the references also.

The following information should be included in instrument SOPs: name of instrument, manufacturer/distributor, service representative, operating principle(s), operating instructions, maintenance schedules, trouble-shooting list, backup instrumentation, and references. The instrument name is the trade name and model number (serial numbers may be required at times); general instrument type (e.g., centrifugal analyzer, pH meter, flame photometer) may be included as a subtitle in parenthesis. The manufacturer or distributor of the equipment should be listed along with addresses and telephone numbers of technical service departments and names of individuals to contact for advice or other problems. The service representative's name, address, and telephone number should be clearly indicated. The operating principle(s) of the instrument should be discussed, including how it presents, stores, processes, and/or transmits data. Operating instructions should include a step-by-step description of initial setup and daily start-up/shutdown procedures. Calibration, description of instrument controls, and reference to operator maintenance procedures also should be listed under operating instructions. The maintenance schedule should list how, when, and by whom daily and periodic maintenance checks should be performed. A place for recording maintenance and repair procedures is usually kept in a separate log. A trouble-shooting list is a useful item for any instrument SOP. Backup instrumentation or procedures to be used in the event of equipment failure should be indicated with references to the appropriate SOPs. Location of references for equipment such as operation manuals or manufacturer technical bulletins should also be listed.

Procedural SOPs cover a variety of circumstances that will vary among laboratories. In all procedural SOPs, the title should be concise and the purpose of the SOP should be described succinctly at the beginning. There are several fundamental laboratory functions for which procedural SOPs should be generated. Sample collection needs to be standardized with descriptions of sampling technique, anesthetics, or restraint methods employed; types of collection tubes used; and regimens of specimen handling, labeling and recording. Sample preparation procedures such as centrifugation, transference to storage containers, overnight and prolonged storage, and description of specimen quality and volume are required. Systems for recording, storage, and transfer of data need to be described and verified, especially with respect to proofing and approving data prior to final release. The recording, filing, and inspection of control sera and interlaboratory survey program results must be defined. Criteria for deciding if control sera results are unacceptable should be spelled out (i.e., defining when an analytical system is considered "out of control") and remedial actions specified.

VIII. QUALITY ASSURANCE

Assuring the quality of clinical chemistry data generated by the laboratory is a dynamic and continuous process. Preparing and adhering to well-organized SOPs and proper training of personnel helps to maintain quality; however, proving that systems are working properly requires the use of system checks or quality assurance. This is accomplished by the daily use of control sera, participation in interlaboratory survey programs, proper equipment maintenance logs, and through audits by internal or external quality assurance units.

The SOP for each test should include the use of control sera. Control sera are commercially prepared solutions that mimic the composition of serum. The purpose of control sera is to provide a stable sample that can be repeatedly analyzed over a period of months, thus allowing the between-run and day-to-day consistency of the analytical system to be monitored. At least two control sera should be employed, one containing relatively "normal" concentrations of analytes and the other containing "abnormal" concentrations. For tighter control of an analytical method, three control sera are used: normal, low abnormal, and high abnormal. Control sera, abnormal and normal, are analyzed with every batch of specimens. Usually they are placed at the beginning and end of the run and after every 10 to 20 specimens during the run depending on the type of instrumentation, the stability of the technique, and the desired degree of control. Data generated should be displayed and recorded such that the control sera values are clearly identified within each run, including when they were run relative to the other specimens. The interpretation of control sera data is described in many other texts and articles [e.g., see Westgard and Klee (1986) for a more complete discussion].

For most clinical chemistry analytes, it is not essential, although it may be theoretically more correct, to use a species-specific control serum, that is, one derived from the same animal species as the samples being tested. Commercial control sera are usually sufficient. Indeed, these are frequently prepared with material from several animal species such as cattle and pigs. Species-specific control sera are not commercially available and would, therefore, have to be prepared by each laboratory. For certain analytes or procedures, such as isoenzyme electrophoresis of lactate dehydrogenase or creatine kinase, it is technically better to assay a species-specific control serum; however, this is not always feasible either from a technical or economic standpoint. Commercially prepared controls of human origin may have to suffice.

In the United States, there are a number of interlaboratory comparison (or survey) programs currently available, an example being the one administered by the College of American Pathologists (CAP). These programs amount to a type of peer review and allow a laboratory to judge its performance in measuring a particular analyte with that of other laboratories. To obtain usable comparative data, the same specimen must be analyzed by each laboratory participating in the program. This requires that a large batch of specimen be prepared, with an aliquot being sent to each laboratory participating in the program. Usually, at least two (often three) specimens are sent, each having a different amount of the various analytes. These specimens are treated as unknowns by the recipient laboratories and analyzed in a routine manner. Results from all participating laboratories are collated by the center administering the program. For each analyte, the average value reported by all laboratories (or those using only the same methodology) is assumed to be the "true" value. Individual laboratories gauge their performance by determining how much they vary from the "true" value. Significant variance from the "true" value implies that the laboratory may have a problem with that test procedure, and it should be promptly evaluated.

It is important to make certain that all equipment used for testing is functioning correctly and calibrated according to specifications. Water baths and other equipment used to control temperature during an assay must be checked to ensure that temperature settings are accurate and stable. Refrigerators used to store specimens or reagents must be monitored at least daily to assure maintenance of proper temperatures. Spectrophotometers should be calibrated with known instrument performance standards, and periodic checks should be made with these same standards. Maintenance and repairs to equipment should be recorded in permanent log books.

IX. DATA HANDLING

A crucial aspect to any toxicological study is data handling or record keeping. If there is no systematized, reliable way to record, store, and recover data during a study, correct interpretation of the results is impossible. Although GLP regulations are not specific about the way data is to be recorded and stored, there are general provisions for the handling of data (Organization for Economic Co-operation and Development, 1982; U.S. Environmental Protection Agency, 1985; U.S. Food and Drug Administration 1985). All data must be recorded directly, promptly, and legibly in ink. Data should be dated on the day of entry; any subsequent changes or corrections should not obscure the original entry. When an entry is altered, the reason should be indicated next to the mark then signed and dated by the individual making the change. If the data is stored on computers, similar rules apply. No change can be made that will obscure the original entry, and if changes are made, proper documentation must accompany it. With computerized data, it is advisable to have an automatic audit trail generated beyond the very initial stages of data entry. Although this becomes cumbersome and requires more programming and additional memory requirements, it is probably the surest way of recording changes.

Several specific items regarding the recording of clinical chemistry data need to be emphasized. The order in which animals were bled needs to be clearly documented. This "bleeding order" should dictate the order in which samples are analyzed. Original (raw) data should be presented prior to its collation into treatment groups. Interspersed among the original data should be results from standards, blanks, and control sera; these results must be clearly identified to avoid mistaking them for data on test specimens. Other essential information to be recorded with the data are date and time of blood sampling and analysis, test code (what analyte was measured), instrument used, person collecting the blood, analyst performing the test, supervisor approval of data, identification number and sex of each animal, treatment each animal received (i.e., its dose group), and technical comments on sample quality (e.g., hemolyzed, normal).

Most comments regarding data recording and documentation refer to the original or "raw" data. After having been checked, approved, initialed, and dated, raw data are then ready for transmission to another source for collation, statistical analysis, and generation of final tables or graphs. Graphs and tables are not considered raw data although they must accurately reproduce the raw data. The distinction between raw and nonraw data is not always easy to make, and the specifics will vary among laboratories depending on procedures. It is important for each laboratory to define its raw data because it is at this level that all changes or comments must be made. Guidelines for determining what are raw data should refer to the definition in the good laboratory practice codes regulated by the U.S. government (U.S. Environmental Protection Agency, 1985; U.S. Food and Drug Administration, 1985). "*Raw data* means any laboratory worksheets, records, memoranda, notes, or exact copies thereof that are the result of original observations and activities of a nonclinical laboratory study and are necessary for the reconstruction and evaluation of the report of that study."

References

Alper, C. A. (1974). Plasma protein measurements as a diagnostic aid. *N. Eng. J. Med.* **291**, 287–290.

Badylak, S. F., and Van Vleet, J. F. (1981a). Sequential morphologic and clinicopathologic alterations in dogs with experimentally induced glucocorticoid hepatopathy. *Am. J. Vet. Res.* **42**, 1310–1318.

Badylak, S. F., and Van Vleet, J. F. (1981b). Alterations of prothrombin time and activated partial thromboplastin time in dogs with hepatic disease. *Am. J. Vet. Res.* **42**, 2053–2056.

Bartosek, I., and Guaitani, A. (1982). Biochemical and enzymatic control of animal quality. *In* "Animals in Toxicological Research" (I. Bartosek, A. Guaitani, and E. Pacei, eds.), pp. 103–114. New York: Raven Press.

Bovee, K. C., and Joyce, T. (1979). Evaluation of glomerular function: 24 hour creatinine clearance in dogs. *J. Am. Vet. Med. Assoc.* **174,** 488–491.

Boyd, J. W. (1983). The mechanisms relating to increases in plasma enzymes and isoenzymes in diseases of animals. *Vet. Clin. Pathol.* **12,** 9–24.

Buck, W. B., Osweiler, G. D., and Van Gelder, G. A. (1976). "Clinical and Diagnostic Veterinary Toxicology," 2nd ed. Dubuque, Iowa: Kendall/Hunt.

Center, S. A., Bunch, S. E., Baldwin, B. H., Hornbuckle, W. E., and Tennant, B. C. (1983). Sulfobromophthalein and indocyanine green clearances in the dog. *Am. J. Vet. Res.* **44,** 722–726.

Chin, B. Y., Tyler, T. R., and Kosbelt, S. J. (1979). The interfering effects of hemolyzed blood on rat serum chemistry. *Toxicol. Pathol.* **7,** 19–21.

Cornelius, C. E. (1980). Liver function. *In* "Clinical Biochemistry of Domestic Animals," (Kaneko, J. J. ed.), 3rd ed., pp. 201–257. New York: Academic Press.

Davidson, C. S., Leevy, C. M., and Chamberlayne, E. C., eds. (1979). "Guidelines for Detection of Hepatotoxicity Due to Drugs and Chemicals", (NIH Publ. No. 79–313) Washington, DC: U.S. Department of Health, Education and Welfare.

Dhami, M. S., Drangova, R., Farkas, R., Balazz, T., and Feuer, G. (1979). Decreased aminotransferase activity of serum and various tissues in the rat after cefazolin treatment. *Clin. Chem.* **25,** 1263–1266.

Dooley, J. F. (1984a). The role of alanine aminotransferase for assessing hepatotoxicity in laboratory animals. *Lab. Anim.* **13,** 20–23.

Dooley, J. F. (1984b). Sorbitol dehydrogenase and its use in toxicology testing in lab animals. *Lab. Anim.* **13,** 20–21.

Ewing, G. O., Suter, P. F., and Bailey, C. S. (1974). Hepatic insufficiency associated with congenital anomalies of the portal vein in dogs. *J. Am. Ann. Hosp. Assoc.* **10,** 463–476.

Friedel, R., and Mattenheimer, H. (1970). Release of metabolic enzymes from platelets during blood clotting of man, dog, rabbit and rat. *Clin. Chim. Acta* **30,** 37–46.

Glick, M. R., Ryder, K. W., and Jackson, S. A. (1986). Graphical comparison and interferences in clinical chemistry instrumentation. *Clin. Chem.* **32,** 470–475.

Hoe, C. M., and Harvey, D. G. (1961). An investigation into liver function tests in dogs, Part I — Serum transaminases. *J. Sm. Anim. Pract.* **2,** 22–31.

Jones, J. D., and Burnett, P. C. (1972). Implication of creatinine and gut flora in the uremic syndrome: Induction of "creatinase" in colon contents of the rat by dietary creatinine. *Clin. Chem.* **18,** 280–284.

Kaplan, M., and Righetti, A. (1970). Induction of rat liver alkaline phosphatase. The mechanism of serum elevation in obstruction. *J. Clin. Invest.* **49,** 508–516.

Killingsworth, L. M. (1981). "The Role of High Resolution Electrophoresis in the Clinical Evaluation of Protein Status." Freehold, New Jersey: Worthington Diagnostics.

Korsrud, G. O., Grice, H. C., Kuiper-Goodman, T., Knipfel, J. E., and McLaughlan, J. M. (1973). Sensitivity of several serum enzymes for detection of liver damage in rats. *Toxicol. Appl. Pharmacol.* **26,** 299–313.

Laird, C. W. (1977). Clinical pathology: Blood chemistry. *In* "Handbook of Laboratory Animal Science" (E. C. Melby and N. H. Altman, eds.), pp. 347–432. Cleveland: CRC Press.

Leonard, T. B., Neptun, D. A., and Popp, J. A. (1984). Serum gamma gluamyl transferase as a specific indicator of bile duct lesions in the rat liver. *Am. J. Pathol.* **116,** 262–269.

Maclin, E., and Young, D. S. (1986). Automation in the clinical laboratory. *In* "Textbook of Clinical Chemistry" (N. W. Tietz, ed.), pp. 236–283. Philadelphia: Saunders.

Mitruka, B. M., and Rawnsley, H. M. (1981). "Clinical Biochemical and Hematological Reference Values in Normal Experimental Animals and Normal Humans," 2nd ed. New York: Masson Publishing.

Organization for Economic Cooperation and Development (1981). "Guidelines for Testing of Chemicals. Good Laboratory Practice." Paris: Organization for Economic Co-operation and Development.

Organization for Economic Co-operation and Development (1982). "Good Laboratory Practice in the Testing of Chemicals." Paris: Organization for Economic Co-operation and Development.

Osborne, C. A., Low, D. G., and Finco, D. R. (1972). "Canine and Feline Urology." Philadelphia: Saunders.

Polzin, D. J., Osborne, C. A., Stevens, J. B., and Hayden, D. W. (1983). Serum amylase and lipase activities in dogs with primary renal failure. *Am. J. Vet. Res.* **44,** 404–410.

Prasse, K. W., Bjorling, D. E., Holmes, R. A., and Cornelius, L. M. (1983). Indocyanine green clearance and ammonia tolerance in partially hepatectomized and hepatic devascularized anesthetized dogs. *Am. J. Vet. Res.* **44,** 2320–2323.

Rogers, W. A. (1976). Source of serum alkaline phosphatase in clinically normal and diseased dogs: A clinical study. *J. Am. Vet. Med. Assoc.* **168,** 934–937.

Scott, F. W., and Trick, K. D. (1982). Variation of rat serum biochemical parameters following decapitation or anesthesia with ether, halothane, or Innovar-Vet: Rapid Innovar-vet-induced hyperuricemia and hyperglycemia. *Metabolism* **31,** 514–519.

U.S. Food and Drug Administration (1985). "Good Laboratory Practice for Nonclinical Laboratory Studies," (Code of Federal Regulations (CFR), Title 21), pp. 215–229. Washington, DC: U.S. Food and Drug Administration.

U.S. Environmental Protection Agency (1985). "Good Laboratory Practice Standards," (Code of Federal Regulations (CFR), Title 40), pp. 255–268. Washington, DC: U.S. Environmental Protection Agency.

Van Vleet, J. F., and Alberts, J. O. (1968). Evaluation of liver function tests and liver biopsy in experimental carbon tetrachloride intoxication and extrahepatic bile duct obstruction in the dog. *Am. J. Vet. Res.* **29,** 2119–2131.

Werner, M. (1982). "CRC Handbook of Clinical Chemistry," Vol. I, pp. 341–358, 477–487. Boca Raton, Florida: CRC Press.

Westgard, J. O., and Klee, G. G. (1986). Quality assurance. *In* "Textbook of Clinical Chemistry" (N. W. Tietz, ed.), pp. 424–458. Philadelphia: Saunders.

White, J. V., Olivier, B. N., Reimann, K., and Johnson, C. (1984). Use of protein-to-creatinine ratio in a single urine specimen for quantitative estimation of canine proteinuria. *J. Am. Vet. Med. Assoc.* **185,** 882–885.

Winkel, P., Statland, B. E., and Bokeland, H. (1975). The effects of time of venipuncture on variation of serum constituents. *Am. J. Clin. Pathol.* **64,** 433–447.

Woo, J., and Cannon, D. C. (1984). Metabolic intermediates and inorganic ions. In "Clinical Diagnosis and Management by Laboratory Methods" (J. B. Henry, ed.), pp. 133–164. Philadelphia: Saunders.

Young, D. S., Pestaner, L. C., and Gibberman, V. (1975). Effects of drugs on clinical laboratory tests. *Clin. Chem.* **21,** 1D–423D.

20
Selected Issues in Toxicological Pathology

M. D. Clarke
Toxicology Evaluation Division
Bureau of Chemical Safety
Food Directorate
Health Protection Branch
Health and Welfare Canada
Ottawa, Ontario

K. R. Reuhl
Neurotoxicology Laboratories
Department of Pharmacology and Toxicology
College of Pharmacy
Rutgers University
Piscataway, New Jersey

H. C. Grice
CANTOX, Inc.
Nepean, Ontario

I. Introduction

II. Preparation of Histological Sections
    A. Thoroughness of Necropsy
    B. The Problem of Autolysis
    C. Choice of Fixative and Fixation Methods
    D. Blocking and Sectioning Conventions

III. Difficulties of Interpretation in Histopathology
    A. Number of Sections per Organ/Tissue
    B. "Blind" Slide Evaluation
    C. Grading of Neoplastic and Nonneoplastic Lesions
    D. Problems of Appropriate Diagnosis of Proliferative Lesions: The "Stop" Experiment
    E. Remote Effects of Neoplasms: Paraneoplastic and Related Conditions

IV. Pathology Data Format

V. Special Techniques

Handbook of
In Vivo Toxicity Testing

I. INTRODUCTION

Since the formative days of systematic toxicological testing for hazard evaluation, histopathology findings have served as a central reference point. Pathological changes in cells or tissues of test animals have usually been taken to be the best reflection of a compound's toxicity and its potential hazard to humans. The pathologist is specifically trained to identify and interpret morphological alterations and their functional correlates. Consequently, the pathologist is a central figure in any toxicological testing program. Accuracy of the pathological diagnoses and clarity of the pathology report may well determine the usefulness and, indeed, sometimes the validity of the entire study. The pathologist forms the link between the in-life data and all the pathology data, including gross and microscopic findings and clinical pathology. Thus, the pathologist is in the best position to make a valid and coherent assessment of the data.

It is a common misconception of some scientists requiring pathology services that the pathologist need be concerned only with the morphological findings and not with the study design or daily conduct and animal health monitoring. Most pathologists have had the lamentable experience of receiving live animals for necropsy (or worse, bottles of fixed tissues) with little warning and less history. Some study directors may disingenuously consider this a "blind" evaluation, the constituents of which and under what circumstances it may be appropriate are discussed in Section II, B.

Fortunately, such experiences are becoming less frequent. In most present day studies, the pathologist is a full team member throughout all stages of the study. During the design of the experiment, the pathologist provides direction regarding the appropriate experimental outline and conduct to meet the study objectives. If the experiment is to be interdisciplinary, including, for example, detailed behavioral assessment, the pathologist helps identify any potential confounding aspects of the design. During the in-life portion of the study, the pathologist will evaluate clinical data and provide periodic advice to the study director. At the end of the study, the pathologist is directly responsible for accurate and expeditious reporting and interpretation of the histopathology data.

Development of appropriate experimental protocols and proper data analysis are complex problems. Some issues surrounding different study objectives, design protocols, and data interpretation in toxicological pathology, especially pertinent to chronic studies, are discussed in this chapter. Controversial or problematic considerations are illustrated by specific examples from regulatory toxicology. In addition, new methods for the assessment of pathology findings in toxicological research are discussed.

II. PREPARATION OF HISTOLOGICAL SECTIONS

A. Thoroughness of Necropsy

The reliability of incidence figures for lesions, be they "spontaneous" or induced, depends in large part on the thoroughness of the necropsy. An incomplete or hastily performed necropsy will frequently result in subtle (and occasionally not so subtle) lesions going unnoticed. When lesions are occult, the likelihood of missing one may be high. Small cutaneous and subcutaneous lesions may be missed unless the skin is carefully examined and the animal is thoroughly palpated. Detection of lesions in several tissues of rats and mice (skin, subcutaneous tissue, intestinal tract, connective tissue, mammary gland, nasal mucosa, skeleton) depend much more on exhaustive gross and dissecting microscopic inspection than they do on standard or conventional histological sectioning in the absence of grossly evident lesions (Frith *et al.*, 1979; Kulwich *et al.*, 1980; Ward and Reznik, 1983). Small skeletal lesions in particular may be missed. Very few protocols call for radiographic examination of the skeleton, and many do not call for gross examination of long bones or joints. Complete removal of soft tissues to expose the skeleton is usually impractical, but exposure of long bones and joints should be included in the necropsy protocol. In this respect, the pathologist should pay careful attention to clinical findings, such as altered mobility, that might point to affected bones or joints. If clinical examination suggests a possible toxic effect, then appropriate radiographic studies and detailed examination of the suspect tissue should be undertaken.

Clearly, the best way to prevent lesion oversight, with consequent biasing of results, is to undertake a necropsy that includes a thorough gross examination prior to the preparation of lesions for microscopic assessment.

B. The Problem of Autolysis

When clinical examination of animals is rigorously and conscientiously conducted and when criteria for euthanasia are established and adhered to, problems associated with autolysis are minimized (see Chapter 17). If there is seen to be no imminent likelihood of any deaths at the time of late afternoon inspection, then few animals should be lost to advanced autolysis. Unfortunately, cannibalism in mice housed in groups cannot be prevented to quite the same degree, but the incidence can probably be lowered to some extent by careful surveillance.

Even in the best managed studies, however, autolysis will be present in some tissues. This does not mean that the tissues are useless, although the information obtained from them will have to be qualified, depending on the severity of the histological change. Greaves and Faccini (1984) have suggested some guidelines for diagnosis under conditions of autolysis:

1. Autolysed mass: noted grossly; cannot be classified as inflammatory, hyperplastic, neoplastic
2. Autolysed tumors: mass noted grossly; can be distinguished as neoplastic but no further characterization possible (beyond perhaps crude stromal/parenchymal distinction)
3. Partial autolysis: can be diagnosed (precisely) even in the face of some autolysis

Additional factors that should be taken into account concern those tissues that tend to be resistant to autolysis and those that are labile. Tumors of epithelial origin, for example, may still be diagnosable at a stage of autolysis in which lymphomas and other processes (e.g., those requiring histological perception of fine nuclear and cytoplasmic detail) cannot be confidentially distinguished from one another.

C. Choice of Fixatives and Fixation Methods

Proper fixation is a crucial step in the preparation of tissues for microscopic examination. The requirements of the study determine the type of fixative and manner of fixation to be used.

Alternate fixatives are available that combine adequate preservation both for standard light microscopy (LM) and transmission electron microscopy (TEM; McDowell, 1978). However, no fixative is perfect for all applications, and it is the responsibility of the pathologist to foresee competing needs and objectives.

The problem of tissue size becomes particularly acute when samples are taken for both LM and TEM. Optimally, samples for TEM should be taken from perfusion-fixed organs. In most situations requiring TEM, the entire animal is perfused with fixative. However, this may be economically impractical due to the high cost of TEM fixatives, the body size of the species used, and the potentially large number of animals. It must be stressed that properly performed electron microscopy is highly intolerant of poor sample handling. Carelessness will often make the TEM exercise a waste of effort and resources.

Other circumstances requiring special fixation methods frequently arise. For example, preparation of the lungs may require inflation fixation via the trachea. Techniques are readily available (Paget and Thomson, 1979) for the special fixation of various organs and should be consulted prior to initiation of a study.

D. Blocking and Sectioning Conventions

Standardized procedures for blocking and sectioning of tissues are essential for proper assessment. For each animal, tissues should be trimmed and blocked in a reproducible manner, with the same combination of tissues embedded together for each animal. Embedding of tissues in random combinations complicates sectioning, compounds the difficulties of the primary pathologist, and tests the patience of the regulatory evaluator who must not only read the pathology report but occasionally reanalyze the microscopic slides. This is important because of the increasing involvement of regulatory pathologists in slide review. Standard tissue-embedding procedures should be established at the outset of the study and consistently followed.

III. DIFFICULTIES OF INTERPRETATION IN HISTOPATHOLOGY

A. Number of Sections per Organ/Tissue

The extent of the histological examination is crucial to data interpretation. There have been a number of instances in which the regulatory fate of a compound has depended to some extent on the finding of additional tumors following upon recutting of additional sections from previously examined tissues. This situation occurred with the food colors FD & C blue no. 2 and green no. 3, additional gliomas of brain having been found in both instances (Moch, 1986). In the food color FD & C yellow no. 6, proliferative lesions of renal tubular epithelium were the pivotal issue.

Much the same issue has arisen in cases in which it was necessary to compare the concurrent study tumor incidence values with historical control values in the same strain and within the same laboratory. This was the situation in the National Toxicology Program (NTP) chronic inhalation study of propylene oxide on rats and mice (NTP, 1985).

> In inhalation studies, where examination of turbinates is required, recent studies include three sections and older studies only one. . . . Historical data should be used with caution. . . . The chance of detecting microscopic (nasal cavity) tumors . . . were increased because three sections of turbinate were examined from each control and exposed rat. . . . Much of the NTP historical data on nasal tumors is based on a single section of turbinate.

Even without changes in the nature and/or extent of the postmortem examination for a given tissue, historical control comparisons can become more difficult purely because of a significant change in the general understanding of the biology and anatomy of the tissue in question. In the case of nasal tumors in rats, for instance, the nature and extent of the various nasal cavity epithelia in the rat have been thoroughly documented only in the last several years (Gross et al., 1982; Montiero-Riviere and Popp, 1984; Popp and Martin, 1984; Popp and Montiero-Riviere, 1985). Such a change can reasonably be expected to affect the description and interpretation of nasal tumors in rats in the published literature, even without methodological changes.

In the reporting of chronic bioassay results, provisions should be made for comparison of concurrent incidence figures with figures obtained in other laboratories that used slightly differing procedures. This may require a more exhaustive documentation of the numbers and orientation of the standard tissue sections for the study. At present, even the most rudimentary points of a postmortem procedure are frequently overlooked in the drawing of historical comparisons, the result being that bias is frequently introduced. This is a problem not only with extensive tissues requiring careful gross examination (e.g., intestines, mammary gland) but is particularly the case with paired organs, one or both of which may have yielded a histological section. The difficulty is most acute with those small paired organs (adrenal medulla and parathyroid gland) for which homogeneous and reproducible sectioning represents a technical challenge.

The frequency of proliferative changes in the adrenal medulla of rats has produced interpretive difficulties in regulatory toxicology. There has been at least one attempt (Thompson et al., 1981a) to provide statistical methods for comparing animals of differing examination adequacy (i.e., unilateral examination with negative finding, bilateral examination with negative finding, unilateral examination with positive finding, etc.). Clearly, for any particular lesion, the extent of examination must be known both for animals of apparently positive status and for those of apparently negative status. An exception to this, one often cited in bioassay reports, is the category of tissues for which the extent of gross examination, rather than the number of histological sections, defines whether or not an animal is represented in lesion incidence figures. This category generally consists of skin, subcutaneous connective tissue, mammary gland, and intestinal tract. Skeleton and skeletal muscle, although seldom mentioned, are implicitly understood to be part of this group also.

Fortunately, there has been a pronounced tendency for strongly carcinogenic chemicals to manifest their effects in the most susceptible individual animals before they reach 18 months of age (Grice and Burek, 1984). This trend somewhat assures that early scheduled or unscheduled deaths will indicate which tissues should receive particularly careful scrutiny in subsequent unscheduled deaths and in the terminal sacrifice of the bioassay.

Any added complexity of the study due to more explicit reporting of methodology can likely be handled with relatively minor modifications to existing data audit and analysis programs. Some have anticipated that one major proprietary toxicological computer program can eventually reach a half million lines of programming. It is difficult to imagine such vast compilation and analytical capacity not being able to clarify some of the more vexing report ambiguities. The ultimate consumer of the bioassay report is the regulatory evaluator. Sound and timely interpretation of the bioassay data depends on the format and contents of the report; even those studies that are very well executed can often be poorly represented on the printed page. There are several sources of ambiguity frequently encountered by regulatory evaluators in chronic toxicity/oncogenicity study reports. In further sections of this chapter, these problems are outlined along with practical suggestions for their resolution. To a large degree, improvements can be made with very little increased cost.

B. "Blind" Slide Evaluation

For much of the history of toxicological pathology, a running debate over practices in the reading of slides has been conducted between toxicological pathologists and those (chiefly pharmacologists and statisticians) who are uneasy about the "subjective" nature of morphological diagnosis. At various times, this debate has been carried on in toxicological journals (Fears and Schneiderman, 1974; Fears and Douglas, 1978; Weinberger, 1979 and Prasse et al., 1986).

The proponents of "blind" slide reading have cited that no knowledge of a treatment group involved prevents bias, however unconscious, on the part of pathologists. Although many regard blind reading to be appropriate in particular circumstances (Prasse et al., 1986), the concern for possible diagnostic bias resulting from blind readings is to a degree understandable given the pathologist's historical problems in uncovering the appropriate diagnosis (discussed briefly in Sections III, C and III, D).

There has never been, however, any justification for separating particular tissues from the histories and ancillary data of the animals from which the tissues were taken. In order to separate real effects from "noise" and to correctly assign cause and effect with a myriad of lesions in a wide variety of organs, the pathologist must have the opportunity to assemble a complete medical history on the animal whose slides are under examination. This is, for the most part, easily accomplished with most computer systems today (see Section IV). The issue is quite separate from the debate over a pathologist's knowledge of a treatment group; an otherwise very complete medical record can contain everything but treatment group assignment. It is worth mentioning only because there can be no justification for depriving the pathologist of such information as body weight and food consumption data, clinical history and palpation findings, organ weights, hematology and clinical chemistry data, microbiological status (i.e., serology and culture), and gross necropsy findings.

Opponents of blind evaluation have argued that pathologists would respond to such unwelcome constraints by widening the scope of "normal" in order to minimize the likelihood of false positive findings. This does appear quite possible.

A case can be made, however, for the occasional blind reading (i.e., without knowledge of treatment groups) of slides in the context of a very difficult and precisely defined diagnostic issue. Such a case might involve difficult grade-step assignment, for example. Prasse *et al.*, (1986) have suggested that pathologists should evaluate slides without knowledge of the treatment group in three basic situations:

1. Evaluation of defined and particular endpoints (i.e., semiquantitative evaluation)
2. Evaluation of very subtle putative treatment-associated lesions
3. Peer review evaluation

Others (Fears and Schneiderman, 1974) have suggested identification of some (but not all) control treatment groups but no test groups. All these proposals have some merit as long as the blind evaluation is always conducted with full knowledge of the animal's history and ancillary data (minus treatment assignment). Blind evaluation should never be the first and/or only approach to a particular bioassay.

C. Grading of Neoplastic and Nonneoplastic Lesions

There has been, as Salsburg (1986) pointed out, comparatively little work done on the development and sequence of those lesions that comprise the major age-associated disease complexes in aging rodents. The tendency, particularly in proprietary bioassays done for regulatory purposes, has been to tabulate certain lesions in a positive-negative fashion although the lesions in themselves may constitute only small parts of large overall disease syndromes. These lesions are then inappropriately considered as entities that stand alone and unconnected to other lesions to which they are in fact, causally related. These causally related lesions can be present in several different organ systems, as in the case of renal secondary hyperparathyroidism in rats.

The regulatory evaluator, therefore, often sees an abridged version of the qualitative and (especially) quantitative spectrum of lesions seen and noted by the study pathologists. However innocently constructed by the study pathologists, this quantitative simplification has the effect of making binary distinctions of what are more accurately seen as differences of degree. This is often evident as the stated "presence" or "absence" of lesions present in many (and occasionally all) animals to varying degrees (e.g., amyloidosis in mice, chronic progressive nephropathy in rats).

To help circumvent this problem, it is highly desirable for the study report to clarify the basis for diagnostic decision making. In simplest form, this amounts to a glossary with definitions of "present" and "absent" for different lesions or (preferably) with descriptions of grade-step ("ordinal ranking") morphology (Hartung and Durkin, 1986). In such cases, the data currently indicate that some animals have the lesions of interest whereas others do not. As Salsburg (1986) has stated:

> Although a full necropsy on an animal includes a great deal of information that can be used in determining the toxic profile of a treatment, most statistical procedures now in use reduce that information to a single yes or no answer for each animal, and the statistical analysis deals only with the numbers of animals with specific lesions. This "destruction of information" reduces the ability of statistical analysis to answer the more important questions of toxicology.

It is surely inappropriate for the data and subsequent analysis to be based on the assumption that (particularly for the major age-related nonneoplastic lesions) an animal either has it (all) or does not have it (none). This assumption serves only to obscure the quantitative criteria actually employed (however inexactly) by the study pathologists. In most instances, grade-step definitions are much more in keeping with the biological nature of the process and are as easily subjected to statistical analysis:

> Using counts of animals with lesions as the only data, it is impossible to determine no-effect or minimum toxic effect doses. . . . This author believes (that) we are better off abandoning the use of hypothesis tests entirely and concentrating on developing continuous measures of toxicity. When the statistical analysis demands that the pathologist make an absolute determination of whether [the] lesion is there or not, the resulting P values may be influenced more by the pathologist's morning meal than by the sophisticated statistical adjustments that were run on the data (Salsburg, 1986).

Although this statement is radically different from the traditional view in toxicology, the problems associated with binary decision making (null hypothesis, etc.) are nevertheless long overdue for reassessment.

D. Problems of Appropriate Diagnosis of Proliferative Lesions: The "Stop" Experiment

Since anatomical pathology of rodents (in particular of rodents in carcinogenicity bioassays) is in its relative infancy compared to anatomical pathology of humans and some other species, diagnostic terminology has been borrowed from elsewhere and applied to studies involving rodents. To a certain extent, this has been historically inevitable and useful in facilitating communication among investigators of different backgrounds. For lack of information on behavior of lesions, particularly of treatment-associated ones, it has often been necessary to infer behavior of some rodent lesions from the morphological features of the primary lesion alone. That is, malignancy of rat or mouse tumors has often been diagnosed in the absence of evidence of invasion or metastasis. Diagnostic terminology of rodent tumors reflects situations in which an epithelial proliferation apparently induced by treatment has been called a carcinoma because it bore a resemblance to those lesions that behave as carcinomas in other species, not because there was any evidence from within the bioassay itself indicating that the lesion behaved as a malignant epithelial neoplasm.

The controversy surrounding terminology of rodent (especially mouse) hepatocellular tumors is a perfect illustration (Nutrition Foundation, 1983). Particularly in some of the earlier work in chemical carcinogenesis, researchers were cautious enough about terminology to undertake transplantation studies of chemically induced tumorlike lesions in order to assess their ability to grow autonomously (Stewart et al., 1959). It appears that both "spontaneous" and induced neoplasms in rodents are somewhat less liable to malignant behavior than the accepted terminology implicitly predicts. For the most part, however, this has not prevented many investigators from applying the terms carcinoma or sarcoma to these lesions.

What might otherwise remain an arcane laboratory controversy among rodent pathology specialists becomes an issue in the regulatory domain when such "carcinomas" or "sarcomas" are observed at scheduled sacrifice necropsies following uninterrupted treatment, and with a clear statistical relationship to treatment. The cautious regulator tends to deal with these lesions as malignant neoplasms on the basis of morphology alone, generally in the absence of specific behavioral information. However, there exists the possibility that the chemical agent tested may be judged as more oncogenic than is appropriate. This difficulty arises, at least in part, because of the conventional practice of keeping rodents on chronic treatment only until a day or two before sacrifice. If the classical definitions of neoplasia are taken as paramount, it must be clear that such a short time of withdrawal from the "stimuli that evoked the change" (Willis, 1948) is not sufficient to enable a treatment-related lesion that looks like a neoplasm to be diagnosed as a neoplasm because of its persistence, and not simply as a hyperplastic lesion dependent on continued treatment for its maintenance and growth. For example, the ability of forestomach lesions induced by butylated hydroxyanisole (BHA) in rodents to disappear or to persist after cessation of BHA treatment, depending on the duration of treatment, has been a pivotal issue in the controversy about the carcinogenic potential of BHA (Altmann *et al.*, 1986). Nevertheless, there is probably a threshold of extreme anaplasia, rapid growth with high mitotic rate, high incidence of lethal metastasis, etc., beyond which it is clear that the tumor is malignant. Most toxicological pathologists would agree, however, that most rodent tumors do not express such characteristics.

It may be argued that the ultimate behavior of a lesion is more important in the human context because anatomical pathology is largely directed toward prognosis and treatment; in the rodent context, it is directed toward etiology. However, given the number of lesions in humans that mimic neoplasia, even malignant neoplasia, without posing commensurate threat to the individual's life, it is reasonable to seek evidence that shows chemically induced lesions in rodents to resemble life-threatening lesions in other species; at least the autonomy of these lesions from their inciting stimuli should be evident before the lesions are labeled (Shubik, 1984; Furuya *et al.*, 1984).

There are a number of investigators (Bannasch *et al.*, 1974; Treip, 1983; Altmann *et al.*, 1986) who have utilized the so-called "stop experiment" to test the behavioral autonomy of the chemically induced lesion. Generally, this experiment entails the use of parallel treated groups, one of which is continued on treatment until terminal sacrifice while the other is withdrawn from treatment several months or more prior to sacrifice. The incidence and morphology of the chemically induced lesions can then be compared among treated subgroups. Thus, when apparent posttreatment regression has occurred with a class of treatment-associated lesions, such a comparison prevents inappropriate diagnosis. The development of nuclear magnetic resonance imaging of rodent viscera will enable autonomy assessment by stop treatment of all test animal groups, not just of those in satellite dose groups.

E. Remote Effects of Neoplasms: Paraneoplastic and Related Conditions

It is generally recognized that the geriatric test rodent (reflecting a large investment) offers a great source of information on long-term toxic effects. It is not generally recognized that, coincident with the increase in information on toxic effects (or their absence), there has been a decay in the value of some other aspects of this information. This is because geriatric animals very often become encumbered with disease processes that can markedly alter the manner in which they respond to the test chemical. If the disease process (either treatment associated or spontaneous) has no precise human counterpart, the difficulty is compounded further.

These difficulties often result in a conservative interpretation of in-life and postmortem data. The concern about geriatric disease has been reviewed elsewhere (Grice and Burek, 1984). Paraneoplastic and related effects have received much less attention but are potentially important in the interpretation of chronic toxicity data.

Chronic toxicity/carcinogenicity protocols, generally those that involve rats, specify that blood, serum, and urine samples be taken at various intervals. The animals' body and organ weights are important measures, sometimes defining such parameters as the maximum tolerated dose (MTD) and the no-observable-effect level. These measures are often looked to for providing additional information (the "chronic toxicity" aspect) above and beyond that obtained by complete necropsy and for involving endpoints other than the presence or absence of various neoplasms and preneoplastic lesions.

What has tended to be overlooked in this exercise is the spectrum of effects that aging, particularly in the development of tumors at what some call "epidemic" levels (Roe, 1981; 1983), has on the originally homogenous samples of weight- and age-matched animals. There is a case to be made that the development of the many "spontaneous" diseases, particularly tumors, in aged rodents has the effect of subtly dividing the various dose groups into subgroups, each characterized by the systemic effects of a particular tumor or set of tumors.

Some of these effects likely fall into the category of "paraneoplastic syndromes", a generic term used for the many systemic effects resulting from ectopic synthesis of hormones or hormone-like agents by tumor cells (Hall, 1974; Minna and Bunn, 1982). These effects have been thoroughly documented in human cancer patients, in whom the principal target tissues of ectopic synthesis include bone and bone marrow, endocrine organs, central and peripheral nervous systems, gastrointestinal tract, and skin (Minna and Bunn, 1982).

The well-known mouse granulocytic leukemoid reaction (Bateman, 1951; Lan et al., 1981; Thomas et al., 1985) can, in some instances, appear to be a consequence of a distant neoplasm; it can also be the result of infection or trauma. Mammary adenocarcinomas in rats occasionally produce very large quantities of alkaline phosphatase, which is detectable in serum.

The complex effects of tumors on immune function in rodents, particularly on the various T-cell subsets (Greene et al., 1977), also are likely mediated in part by tumor-secreted factors active at sites distant from the tumor itself. Accelerated thymic atrophy was a consequence of transplantation of some cell lines from mammary adenocarcinomas in mice (Thomas et al., 1985), as was hypercalcemia, a well-known paraneoplastic effect in humans and domestic animals (Meuten, 1986). Cancer cachexia and an associated variety of complex metabolic disturbances, such as depressed protein synthesis (Svaninger et al., 1983) and deranged adipose tissue lipogenesis/lipolysis (Thompson et al., 1981b) in tumor-bearing mice, may be the result of mediators secreted by the tumor or by adjacent stimulated macrophages (Beutler and Cerami, 1986). This mechanism can reasonably be expected to exert an effect on body weight and might have a particularly marked influence on the relative weight of organs that are otherwise uninvolved with or distant from the tumor itself.

There is also a category of tumor effects on the host that, although perhaps not the result of ectopic synthesis, can nevertheless complicate interpretation of the bioassay. It has been suggested that the natural killer cell-like activity of large granular lymphocyte (LGL) leukemia cells in F344 rats may influence other disease processes (notably tumor incidence) because leukemia-enhanced "natural immunity" depletes incipient tumor cell clones (Ward, 1982; Ward and Reynolds, 1983). There has been an observed negative relationship between the presence of lymphocytic and hepatocellular neoplasia in F344 rats from the National Toxicology Program bioassay series. Although in some sense perhaps only an exaggeration of a normal secretory function, it is well known that up to one third of the adenohypophyseal tumors in rats secrete mammotropin (prolactin) in sufficient quantities to produce inappropriate lactation, galactocoeles, and increased incidence of mammary neoplasia (Young and Hallowes, 1973).

Although thinly documented in the published literature (Liebelt et al., 1974), at least in comparison to the situation in humans and domestic animals, paraneoplastic syndromes and related effects in rats and mice seem to be capable of interfering with some aspects of interpretation, particularly in the sensitive measurements of body and organ weights and in hematology and serum chemistry. In one study of hematological and clinical chemistry parameters in chronic bioassays with rats (Weil, 1982), it was found that significant skewness, kurtosis, and deviation from normality were present. It may be that effects such as these are at least in part the result of tumor-imposed heterogeneity within treated groups. It is notable in this regard that chronic rodent bioassay reports seldom cite particular animals as having been omitted from statistical treatment of continuous variables because they had tumors. This failure to reject outliers occasionally produces inappropriate statistics, even in such obvious cases as erythrocyte indices for animals with bleeding feet or bleeding ulcerated mammary tumors. Likewise, when an animal's health status is compromised by advanced neoplastic disease, caution must be exercised in interpretation of chronic toxicity finding.

Progress in toxicological pathology will eventually result in identification of those tumors likely to produce paraneoplastic effects. At a still indistinct point in the life of test animals, the increasing value of information on the animals' long-term exposure to a test substance begins to be offset by a diminishing "signal-to-noise" ratio as they become encumbered with the burden of particular geriatric lesions (Grice and Burek, 1984). This effect is probably felt much more in the chronic toxicity aspect of interpretation, although at least one phenomenon, the possible effect of LGL leukemia in F344 rats on incidence of other tumors, complicates the oncogenicity aspect of data analysis.

IV. PATHOLOGY DATA FORMAT

Regulatory evaluators are accustomed to seeing individual animal data from long-term rodent bioassays arranged on a parameter-collated basis. That is, all continuous measures are grouped by sex and treatment group and by date, with means and variances at the bottom of columns. Graphs and tables are often presented for continuous variable measurements like body weight and food consumption. Such formats enable the evaluator to readily grasp the comparisons among animals within each sex and treatment group and among all sex and treatment groups for particular measures or observations. Even tabulation of anatomical pathology data most often resembles the parameter-aggregated continuous measure data in that all findings for a particular organ are collected often with individual animal identification numbers as well as with group incidence fractions.

Although it may be relatively easy to find which animals had a particular lesion (certainly an indispensable part of the submission documentation) with this type of format, it is extremely difficult to put together the entire clinical picture on a particular animal (the "medical history" mentioned in Section III, B of this chapter). In other words, it is very easy to answer the question "Which animals had lesion X?"; it is prohibitively time-consuming to answer the question "Which lesions or symptoms did animal #3684 have?" especially if one is referring to the entire history of the particular animal.

Individual animal medical histories, if available in bioassay reports, facilitate analysis of several study aspects presently very difficult to address for several reasons.

1. They provide a means of evaluating the adequacy of histopathological follow-up of gross lesions seen at necropsy and/or masses palpated during life.

2. They provide for a rough assessment of major causes of death within the study, even if such determinations are not explicitly done by the study pathologist(s).

3. They enable the evaluator to measure possible causal relationships between various lesions in particular animals (e.g., functional adenohypophyseal tumors and mammary changes in rats).

4. They allow estimation of the extent of negative findings in histologically examined tissues, especially in paired organs (e.g., Were both kidneys routinely examined? How many animals with a renal tumor have a normal contralateral kidney? Was the extent of renal examination uniform between dose group?).

5. They provide a validation overview of the adequacy of diagnosis and the appropriateness of overall conclusions to which evaluators have random access. This is particularly important because it is very difficult to do an overall validity check on reports that have only parameter-collated data. Regulatory agencies spend a large portion of the time reviewing and analyzing bioassay data that are collated by parameters.

6. They underscore the synonymous nature of many diagnostic terms used in anatomical pathology data. For those who are relatively unfamiliar with disease terminology in general and rodent pathology in particular, this is a problem that has led to needless misunderstanding between regulatory agencies and sponsors with their contract laboratories.

A useful adjunct to the medical histories form of data organization is the lesion glossary. Glossaries can be satisfactorily included in sections in which the major lesions are described (with appropriate literature citations) and the terminology and grade steps for selected diseases are established.

Much of the difficulty arising from regulatory review of chronic bioassays can be avoided if diagnostic terminology is explicit from the beginning. Regulatory review and decision making can be greatly enhanced by routine availability of a glossary of major lesions as well as by animal-by-animal aggregated data along with traditional parameter-collated formats.

V. SPECIAL TECHNIQUES

The paraffin-embedded, hematoxylin-eosin stained tissue section is the standard technique for histopathological assessment. This method, standardized by almost a century of use, is reproducible, relatively inexpensive, and provides the trained pathologist sufficient morphological information to permit accurate interpretation of pathological lesions in most instances. It is highly unlikely that paraffin sections will be replaced by other techniques for routine tissue examination in the foreseeable future.

Recent developments in biology and microelectronics have spawned a new generation of investigative tools that are of increasing value to the pathologist in toxicological research. Of these emerging technologies, immunocytochemistry is potentially the most important. Cytological techniques have already been used in the diagnosis of tumors and hold great promise for experimental pathology. Electron microscopy (particularly when combined with microanalytical capabilities) and stereology, although not new techniques, are finding expanded applications as a result of microcomputers. Nuclear magnetic resonance (NMR), both as a biochemical instrument and as an imaging tool, is a powerful instrument that can greatly enhance longitudinal studies of tumor development. Other diagnostic imaging techniques, such as computerized tomography (CT) and position emission tomography, are unlikely to find wide application in toxicological research because of their expense.

The first transmission electron microscope (TEM) was developed by Ernst Ruska and his co-workers in Germany during the early 1930s, and electron microscopes were sold in Germany by Siemens in 1939. Major advances in biological applications of TEM followed the development of appropriate embedding media and specialized microtomes for cutting ultrathin sections in the 1950s. In the subsequent three decades, TEM has made major contributions to our understanding of cytology and cell biology. Pathologists have found TEM to aid in studies of pathological mechanisms of disease and in clinical diagnosis.

TEM is most effective and valuable when applied to narrowly defined questions. Consequently, TEM is frequently used in research pathology to elucidate mechanisms of disease and in clinical practice to aid in the diagnosis of tumors or classification of glomerular disease. With the great resolution of TEM, pathologists can evaluate structural changes within cells and thereby document cellular response to xenobiotics or changes in intracellular homeostasis. When a pathologist is confronted with a tumor of uncertain histogenesis or unusual tissue response, TEM can be profitably used to examine these phenomena.

Because of the time and equipment requirements for proper electron microscopy, it is inappropriate as a screening tool, particularly in large toxicological testing schedules. In such circumstances, TEM is used only in response to a specific finding. A routine carcinogenicity assay, for example, may involve hundreds of animals, and many tissue changes may be seen. It is logistically and economically impossible to examine all the animals.

In an attempt to minimize the subjectivity of pathological evaluation, quantitative techniques have been developed to provide reproducible measurements of tissues, cells, and organelles that are amenable to statistical analysis. These techniques, based on well-validated mathematical principles (Weibel et al., 1966; Weibel, 1973; Rohr et al., 1976), are collectively termed morphometry. The volume, surface, and number of structures within a sample may be calculated morphometrically. Stereology is defined as the calculation of three-dimensional structures from two dimensional measures and is best thought of as a component of morphometry. A simple morphometric analysis may be used to determine the depth of invasion of a tumor, as is used in staging melanoma in humans. At a more sophisticated level, it is possible to determine the area and volume fractions of a particular organelle in a cell or the prevalence of a particular cell type in a tissue.

The growing application of morphometry in all areas of structural biology has resulted in an increased number of morphometric hardware and software morphometry packages. These systems have enormously facilitated the labor-intensive task of morphometric data gathering and analysis. However, it must be reiterated that the conduct of morphometric studies should be considered early in the design stages of the study.

References

Altmann, H-J., Grunow, W., Mohr, U., Richter-Reichhelm, H. B., and Wester, P. W. (1986). Effects of BHA and related phenols on the forestomach of rats. *Food Chem. Toxicol.* **24**, 1183–1188.

Bannasch, P., Schacht, U., and Storch, E. (1974). Morphogenese und Mikromorphologie epithelialer Nierentumoren bei Nitrosomorpholin-vergifteten Ratten. I. Induktion und Histologie der Tumoren. *Z. Krebsforsch.* **81**, 311–331.

Bateman, J. C. (1951). Leukemoid reactions to transplanted mouse tumors. *J. Natl. Cancer Inst. (US)* **11**, 671–687.

Beutler, B., and Cerami, A. (1986). Cachectin and tumour necrosis factor as two sides of the same biological coin. *Nature* **320**, 584–588.

Coolidge, B. J., and Howard, R. M. (1979). *"Animal Histology Procedures"* (N.I.H. Publ. No. 80-275). Washington, DC: National Cancer Institute.

Fears, T., and Douglas, J. (1978). Suggested procedures for reducing the pathology workload in a carcinogen bioassay program, Part II: Incorporating blind pathology techniques and analysis for animals with tumors. *J. Environ. Pathol. Toxicol.* **1**, 211–222.

Fears, T. R., and Schneiderman, M. A. (1974). Pathologic evaluation and the blind technique. *Science* **183**, 1144–1145.

Frith, C. H., and Boothe, A. D. (1979). Correlations between gross and microscopic lesions in carcinogenic studies in mice. *J. Environ. Pathol. Toxicol.* **3**, 139–153.

Furuya, K., Maeura, Y., and Williams, G. M. (1984). Abnormalities in liver iron accumulation during N-2-fluorenylacetamide hepatocarcinogenesis that are dependent or independent of continued carcinogen action. *Toxicol. Pathol.* **12**, 136–142.

Greaves, P., and Faccini, J. M. (1984). "Rat Histopathology. A Glossary for Use in Toxicity and Carcinogenicity Studies." Amsterdam: Elsevier.

Greene, M. I., Fujimoto, S., and Sehon, A. H. (1977). Regulation of the immune response to tumor antigens. I. Immunosuppressor cells in tumor-bearing hosts. *J. Immunol.* **116**, 791–799.

Grice, H. C., and Burek, J. D. (1984). The selection of doses in chronic toxicity/carcinogenicity studies. Age-associated (geriatric) pathology: Its impact on long-term toxicity studies. *In* "Current Issues in Toxicology." New York: Springer-Verlag.

Gross, E. A., Swenberg, J. A., Fields, S., and Popp, J. A. (1982). Comparative morphometry of the nasal cavity in rats and mice. *J. Anat.* **135**, 83–88.

Hall, T. C. (1974). Ectopic synthesis and paraneoplastic syndromes. *Cancer Res.* **34**, 2088–2091.

Hartung, R., and Durkin, P. R. (1986). Ranking the severity of toxic effects: potential applications to risk assessment. *Comments Toxicol.* **1**, 49–63.

Humanson, G. L. (1962). "Animal Tissue Techniques." San Francisco: W. H. Freeman.

Hyat, M. A. (1974). "Principles and Techniques of Electron Microscopy Vol. 1: Biological Applications." New York: Van Nostrand-Reinhold.

Kulwich, B. A., Hardisty, J. F., Gilmore, C. E., and Ward, J. M. (1980). Correlation between gross observations of tumors and neoplasms diagnosed microscopically in carcinogenesis bioassays in rats. *J. Environ. Pathol. Toxicol.* **3**, 281–287.

Lan, S., Rettura, G., Levenson, S. M., and Seifter, E. (1981). Granulopoiesis associated with the C3HBA tumor in mice. *J. Natl. Cancer Inst. (US)* **67**, 1135–1138.

Liebelt, R. A., Gehring, G., Delmonte, L., Schuster, G., and Liebelt, A. G. (1974). Paraneoplastic syndromes in experimental animal model systems. *Ann. N.Y. Acad. Sci.* **230**, 547–564.

Lillie, R. D. (1972). "Histopathologic Technic and Practical Histochemistry," 3rd ed. New York: McGraw-Hill.

Luna, L. G. (ed.) (1968). "Manual of Histologic Staining Methods of the Armed Forces Institute of Pathology," 3rd ed. New York: McGraw-Hill.

E. M. McDowell, (1978). Fixation and processing *In* "Diagnostic Electron Micropsy," (B. F. Trump, and R. T. Jones, eds.), Vol. 1, pp. 113–189. New York: Wiley.

Meuten, D. J. (1986). Hypercalcemia of malignancy in man and animals. *Comp. Pathol. Bull.* **18 (3)**, 1–2.

Minna, J. D., and Bunn, P. A., Jr. (1982). Paraneoplastic syndromes *In* "Cancer: Principles and Practice of Oncology" (V. T. DeVita Jr., S. Hellman, and S. A. Rosenberg, eds.), pp. 1476–1517. Philadelphia: Lippincott.

Moch, R. W. (1989). Re-evaluation of pathology data in the regulatory decision process. In press.

Monteiro-Riviere, N. A., and Popp, J. A. (1984). Ultrastructural characterization of the nasal respiratory epithelium in the rat. Am. J. Anat. 169, 31–43.

National Toxicology Program (1985). (Tech. Rep. Ser. No. 267). Washington, DC: U.S. Department of Health and Human Services.

Nutrition Foundation (1983). "The Relevance of Mouse Liver Hepatoma to Human Carcinogenesis Risk: A Report of the International Expert Advisory Committee to the Nutrition Foundation." Washington, DC: Nutrition Foundation.

Paget, G. E., and Thompson, R. (1979). "Standard Operating Procedures in Pathology." Baltimore: University Park Press.

Pearse, A. G. E. (1960). "Histochemistry: Theoretical and Applied," 2nd ed. Boston: Little, Brown.

Popp, J. A., and Martin, J. T. (1984). Surface topography and distribution of cell types in the rat nasal respiratory epithelium: Scanning electron microscopic observations. Am. J. Anat. 169, 425–436.

Popp, J. A., and Montiero-Riviere, N. A. (1985). Macroscopic, microscopic, and ultrastructural anatomy of the nasal cavity, rat. In "Monographs on Pathology of Laboratory Animals: Respiratory System" (T. C. Jones, U. Mohr, and R. D. Hunt, eds.), pp. 3–10. New York: Springer-Verlag.

Prasse, K., Hilderbrandt, P., Dodd, D., Goodman, D., Leader, R., Ferrell, J., Squire, R., Hardistry, J., Newberne, J., Burek, J., De Paoli, A., Boorman, G., Bendele, R., Payne, B., Ward, J., Todd, G., Webster, H., Piper, R., and Patterson, R. (1986). "Blind" microscopic evaluation. Toxicol. Appl. Pharmacol. 83, 184–185.

Roe, F. J. C. (1981). Are nutritionists worried about the epidemic of tumors in laboratory animals? Proc. Nutr. Soc. 40, 57–65.

Roe, F. J. C. (1983). Testing for carcinogenicity and the problem of pseudocarcinogenicity. Nature 303, 657–658.

Rohr, H., Oberholzer, M., Bartsch, G., and Keller, M. (1976). Morphometry in experimental pathology: methods, baseline data and application. Int. Rev. Exp. Pathol. 15, 233–234.

Salsburg, D. S. (1986). "Statistics for Toxicologists." New York: Marcel Dekker.

Shubik, P. (1984). Progression and promotion. J. Natl. Cancer Inst. (US) 73, 1005–1011.

Stewart, H. L., Snell, K. C., Dunham, L. J., and Schleyen, S. M. (1959). "Atlas of Tumor Pathology Section XII Fascicle 40: Transplantable and Transmissible Tumors of Animals." Washington, DC: Armed Forces Institute of Pathology.

Svaninger, G., Bennegard, D., Ekman, L., Ternell, M., and Lundholm, K. (1983). Lack of evidence for elevated breakdown rate of skeletal muscles in weight-losing, tumor bearing mice. J. Natl. Cancer Inst. (US) 71, 341–346.

Thomas, E., Smith, D. C., Lee, M. Y., and Rosse, C. (1985). Induction of granulocytic hyperplasia, thymic atrophy, and hypercalcemia by a selected subpopulation of a murine mammary adenocarcinoma. Cancer Res. 45, 5840–5844.

Thompson, S. W., Rac, V. S., Semonick, D. E., Antonchak, B., Spaet, R. H., and Schellhammer, L. E. (1981a). "The Adrenal Medulla of Rats." Springfield, Illinois: Thomas.

Thompson, M. P., Koons, J. E., Tan, E. T. H., and Grigor, M. R. (1981b). Modified lipoprotein lipase activities, rates of lipogenesis, and lipolysis as factors leading to lipid depletion in C57BL mice bearing the preputial gland tumor ESR-586. *Cancer Res.* **46,** 3228–3232.

Treip, C. S. (1983). The regression of oestradiol-induced pituitary tumors in the rat. *J. Pathol.* **141,** 29–40.

Ward, J. M. (1982). Background variations of tumor incidence in rodent populations. *In* "Safety Evaluation and Regulation of Chemicals." (F. Homburger, ed.), pp. 210–216. Basel: Karger.

Ward, J. M., and Reynolds, C. W. (1983). Large granular lymphocyte leukemia: A heterogeneous lymphocytic leukemia in F344 rats. *Am. J. Pathol.* **111,** 1–10.

Ward, J. M., and Reznik, G. (1983). Refinements of rodent pathology and the pathologist's contribution to evaluation of carcinogenesis bioassays. *Prog. Exp. Tumor Res.* **26,** 266–291.

Weibel, E. R. (1969). Stereological principles for morphometry in electron microscopic cytology. *Int. Rev. Cytol.* **26,** 235.

Weibel, E. R. (1973). Biological applications. *In* "Principles and Techniques of Electron Microscopy" (M. A. Hyat, ed.), Vol. 3, pp. 237–296. Princeton: Van Nostrand-Reinhold.

Weibel, E. R., Kistler, G. S., and Scherle, W. F. (1966). Practical stereologic cytology. *J. Cell Biol.* **30,** 23–33.

Weinberger, M. (1979). How valuable is blind evaluation in histopathologic examinations in conjunction with animal toxicity studies. *Toxicol. Pathol.* **7,** 14–17.

Weil, C. S. (1982). Statistical analysis and normality of selected hematologic and clinical chemistry measurements used in toxicologic studies. *Arch. Toxicol. (Suppl.)* **5,** 237–253.

Willis, R. A. (1948). "Pathology of Tumors." London: Butterworths.

Young, S., and Hallowes, R. C. (1973). Tumors of the mammary gland. *In* "Pathology of Tumors in Laboratory Animals Volume I-Tumors of the Rat-Part 1," (V. S. Turusor, ed.), pp. 31–73. Lyon: International Agency for Research on Cancer.

21
Computer Applications in Toxicological Research

D. R. Krewski
Health Protection Branch
Health and Welfare Canada
Ottawa, Ontario

P. L. Carr
Health Protection Branch
Health and Welfare Canada
Ottawa, Ontario

R. Anderson
Health Protection Branch
Health and Welfare Canada
Ottawa, Ontario

S. G. Gilbert
Health Protection Branch
Health and Welfare Canada
Ottawa, Ontario

I. Introduction

II. Basic Computer Concepts
   A. Computer Hardware
   B. Computer Software
   C. Data Communications
   D. Computer Graphics

III. Toxicology Data Systems
   A. Systems Specifications
   B. Commercial Toxicology Data Management Systems

IV. Other Applications of Computers in Toxicological Research

V. Summary and Conclusions

Handbook of
In Vivo Toxicity Testing

I. INTRODUCTION

Since the first generation of modern computing equipment emerged in the 1940s, virtually no segment of society has remained untouched by electronic information systems. In addition to traditional business and scientific applications, computers today are being used for instrumentation, process control, on-line data acquisition, and information storage and retrieval. The advent of personal computers has also led to the development of integrated office automation systems complete with word processing, scheduling, electronic filing, and electronic mail capabilities.

Computers have been used in toxicological research for many years. Historically, data were transcribed from laboratory records, encoded into the computer, and subjected to statistical analysis. However, the nature of toxicological research has changed markedly in recent years, and the traditional role of the computer has changed to keep pace with the new demands being placed upon informatics technology. Today, computers are being used in protocol design, data acquisition, data management, and data analysis.

Laboratory instrumentation has become increasingly sophisticated. Digitizers allow for direct transfer of analytical results from instruments to computerized storage media. Automated data acquisition systems log experimental data on an ongoing basis, providing up-to-date information on dosing regimens, body weights, and clinical status of experimental subjects during the course of a toxicological study. These systems greatly reduce the number of transcription and coding errors and facilitate editing of anomalous results. Data transfer no longer requires extensive manual intervention, thus freeing human resources for other activities.

Computerization in toxicological research has raised concerns regarding the integrity and security of data. It appears that data can be easily modified on a computer file without exhibiting any trace of being altered, thereby compromising the validity of the experimental data. However, data acquisition and storage systems are now designed with multilevel passwords known only to a very few individuals on the research team, possibly only the study director. This limits the number of people with the ability to alter data and hence enhances data security. It is also possible to record the date and an appropriate identifier at any time data is changed.

Increased computerization in experimental research prompted the U.S. Food and Drug Administration (FDA; 1976) to develop standards for computer technology in nonclinical laboratory studies as a component of their good laboratory practice regulations (GLPs). These regulations have become the standard for conducting nonclinical laboratory studies intended for submission to regulatory agencies in the Western world. Informational systems developed to support nonclinical research must meet GLP standards to ensure quality control in the areas of data collection, data storage and reporting, and data retrieval and audit (Konvicka *et al.*, 1977).

In this chapter, we attempt to elucidate the role of the computer in toxicological research. In Section II, the basic concepts required to understand computing in toxicology are discussed including hardware, software, data communications, and computer graphics. General purpose computer systems for the management of toxicological data are reviewed in Section III. Specialized applications of the computer in toxicological research are presented in Section IV.

II. BASIC COMPUTER CONCEPTS

Simply put, a computer is a device capable of performing arithmetical or logical operations by accepting input information relevant to the problem at hand, performing a sequence of predetermined operations on this information, and providing some form of output. A computer system consists of physical devices called hardware and programmed instructions called software. Both hardware and software have undergone considerable development and refinement since the early days of computer applications (Ralson and Reilly, 1983).

A. Computer Hardware

All computers contain the same basic components but differ in the way in which these components are configured. The heart of the computer is the central processing unit (CPU) in which most arithmetical and logical operations are performed. A microprocessor is a CPU built as a tiny semiconductor chip. It contains much of the arithmetic and control logic circuitry necessary to execute computer programs and control the other components of the machine. The chip itself consists of an integrated circuit containing tens of thousands of transistors fabricated on a sliver of silicon less than 5 mm square and 0.5 mm thick. Each transistor is able to make one simple logic decision or store one bit of information. The CPU is triggered by a clock that controls the basic speed at which instructions are executed. Generally speaking, the faster the clock, the faster an operation can be executed. However, the physical characteristics of the CPU and other components of the computer also have an impact on performance.

Associated with the CPU is the main memory. This is a directly accessible area of internal storage used to store the programs and data during execution. External storage devices such as hard disks, floppy diskettes, and computer tapes are not directly addressable by the CPU. Because of this variety in memory storage, information must be "swapped" in and out of main memory during program execution. Memory size is one of the most important limiting factors in the operation of all computers, with the speed of access directly affecting the speed at which a program will execute.

Devices used exclusively for purposes of input or output are called peripherals. Today, peripherals consist mainly of printers, plotters, and mass storage media such as magnetic tapes and disks. Compact disks can permanently store vast amounts of information, but at present are available for read-only applications. Although there exists a clear need for reduction in paper flow, the reliance on paper or hard-copy output does not appear to be diminishing. As confidence builds in the reliability and security of electronic storage and data transfer media, hard-copy printouts may be reduced.

1. Bits, Bytes, and Words

Computer storage is measured in terms of bits, bytes, and words. A bit is the smallest piece of information a computer stores, consisting of one of two possible values: zero or one. The next unit of storage is the byte, which is simply a small number of bits grouped together. One byte, usually made up of eight bits, is often used to represent one alphanumeric character. Characters are determined by the code set used. The American Standard Code for Information Interchange (ASCII) uses seven bits for data and one bit for parity. (This last bit serves as a check that the seven data bits have been correctly transmitted during data processing.) The seven data bits can form a total of 2^7 or 128 combinations of zeros and ones so that 128 different characters can be represented on an eight-bit machine. A word is a group of bytes used for interim storage of alphanumeric data.

The amount of computer storage is commonly measured in bytes with one "K" bytes denoting $2^{10} = 1,024$ bytes. (The notation "K" bytes evolved from the approximation to 1,000 bytes or 1 kilobyte.) Thus, 640K of internal memory denotes $640 \times 1,024 = 655,360$ bytes. External memory is measured in terms of megabytes (MB) or millions of bytes. For example, 20 MB of disc storage on a microcomputer can accommodate $20 \times 2^{20} = 20,571,520$ bytes of information. Computers vary in processing capability depending on the word size (generally 8–64 bits) and the bus size (generally 8–32 bits). A bus represents the channel by which information is passed within the computer, with larger buses having greater capacity for data transfer.

2. Types of Computers

Computers have traditionally been categorized as mainframes, minicomputers, and microcomputers. The term *mainframe* now designates medium and large scale computer systems. Characteristics of a mainframe include the speed at which the CPU executes its instructions (now several million instructions per second or MIPS), its advanced memory techniques, its interface capability with a variety of peripherals, and its ability to support multiple users performing many different tasks simultaneously.

Minicomputers are essentially scaled-down versions of mainframes that, although less powerful in terms of speed and storage capacity, offer many features of their larger counterparts at less cost. Traditionally, the minicomputer could support fewer users but was considered to be more efficient for on-line engineering or scientific applications.

The microcomputer is a small but complete computer system usually constructed on a single circuit board containing not only the CPU but also the main memory for storing programs and data during execution. Microcomputers are easily able to support well-defined applications such as instrument control and data acquisition. Some general purpose packages such as spreadsheets and word processing programs also run on microcomputers. Several high level programming languages such as BASIC and FORTRAN have also been adapted from larger systems to microcomputers.

Although the differentiation between these types of computers was quite clear in the past, recent technological advances have muddied the distinction among computer types to the point where it is difficult to distinguish among them. At the upper end of the spectrum are the so-called supercomputers that are much faster than the typical mainframe. They are capable of executing exceedingly large numbers of instructions per second and have vast storage capacity. The term supermini is often used to describe a minicomputer manufactured by a traditional mini company; however, it has processing and storage capabilities approaching those of a conventional mainframe. Similarly, the supermicro is a microcomputer capable of supporting a number of users and having processing power approaching that of a minicomputer.

Blurring of the traditional boundaries among types of computers may be attributed in part to two facts: the cost of hardware (or at least the price/performance ratio) has been falling rapidly in recent years, and software applications are becoming less and less machine dependent. As a result, each type of computer is finding a place in the market based not so much on its size and processing capacity, but on the type of application it can support.

B. Computer Software

1. Computer Languages

The so-called first-generation languages used to program computers were machine languages, expressed in terms of the basic internal representation of a computer program as it resides in memory. Because there were no compilers or interpreters to translate higher level languages into this basic form, computers were programmed directly with binary notation.

Second-generation languages were developed around the time virtual memory came into use. These were called symbolic assembler languages. The advantage of assembler languages was that the short mnemonic codes used for specific instructions allowed programmers to converse with the computer more easily while still making efficient use of the machine's limited capacity. Unfortunately, both first- and second-generation languages are totally dependent on the engineering and technological design of the computer on which they run.

Third-generation languages did not come into use until the early 1960s. These were called high level languages and allowed the programmer to represent the equivalent of multiple assembler language instructions in a sentence-like structure or statement. In addition to ease of programming, third-generation languages also represented the first step in gaining independence from the specific machine on which programs were developed. Thus, a program written in a high level language could theoretically be run on many computers with the same general architecture. Some languages like FORTRAN and ALGOL were developed for scientific work, whereas others like COBOL were written for commercial applications. Still others like PL/1 were intended for both purposes. Although third-generation languages have moved a step closer to the real language of the user, they still require relatively large numbers of instruction statements to complete an application. Designed to be used by programming professionals, these languages can also be difficult to debug and time-consuming to maintain.

In response to these problems, fourth-generation languages (4GLs) have emerged in recent years. These languages are typically easier to learn, simpler to use, and can drastically reduce the time required for program development (Martin, 1984). More specifically, 4GLs have been created to respond to meet the following needs: to make the language user-friendly so that end users can solve their own problems, to generate bug-free code from high level statements of programming requirements, to speed up the applications development process and minimize debugging and testing, and to create applications that are easy and quick to change, thereby reducing maintenance costs.

Although the use of fourth-generation languages is growing steadily, they are not without problems. Standards for the production of these languages have not yet evolved. As a result, the capabilities of languages differ appreciably. Some perform many functions, others only a few (Martin, 1985). Some are good for programmers and not users, or vice versa. Another concern with 4GLs is the considerable computer processing power required. Because of their greater generality and flexibility, 4GL applications are often less efficient than those developed in a third-generation language. These problems notwithstanding, 4GLs offer tremendous productivity improvements in comparison with more traditional methods, as well as opportunity for greater user involvement in program development.

Fifth-generation languages involve the use of artificial intelligence in knowledge-based systems, in expert systems, and in processing of human language (Martin, 1985). Fifth-generation systems encode complex knowledge, allowing the user to draw inferences from it. Just as a database includes data, a knowledge base contains data and rules that are exploited in knowledge-based and expert systems. In some cases, fifth-generation systems are used to perform tasks such as understanding speech that, although complex, seem trivial to humans. In other highly specialized areas of knowledge, the fast processing of inferences that are not intuitive to humans, such as decision making in a complex environment, gives such systems an appearance of intelligence.

In order to produce an effective knowledge-based machine, tremendous amounts of quickly accessible data storage is required. Because many inferences can generally be processed simultaneously, parallel processing has become an important feature of modern computer architecture. With parallel processing, instructions or groups of instructions are broken down and processed simultaneously on separate processors. This allows many more instructions to be executed in a given period of time, so that complex decisions can be reached more quickly.

2. Database Management Systems

A database is a set of interrelated data elements in an information processing system required to meet the needs of the end user (Martin, 1983). The introduction of database systems into an organization can have an impact on two areas. First, the database necessitates a change in management thinking and requires a commitment to regard information as a valuable resource that must be protected and maintained. Second, it requires a change in the way applications are developed, such that data will be more readily available to end users.

Prior to the development of database technology, data elements were traditionally stored in sequential files (Wiederhold, 1983, pp. 86–110). Although sequential file systems are adequate for applications that remain static, they are subject to several limitations. First, there is a certain level of redundancy in that the same data elements may be stored in several different places. Second, sequential file systems are somewhat inflexible in that they cannot easily respond to a request that data be grouped in a different way. And third, data in sequential files are not as quickly accessible as data in random access files.

A database system provides a means of structuring data so as to avoid these problems and to provide a way for applications to grow and change as needs change. The actual structure of the database will depend on the type of data relationships and the way it will be used (Wiederhold, 1983, pp. 346–377). The three types of database structures currently in use are hierarchical, network, and relational.

A hierarchical database has the structure of a tree, with a group of master records called parents and a group of subordinates called children (Mills *et al.*, 1986). One parent can have several children but a child can have only one parent. To access a child, the computer is directed through the parent. A network database allows a many-to-many relationship in which the master can have several subordinates and the subordinate can have several masters, with pointers used to identify individual records. A relational database provides still more flexibility because it does not use pointers. A series of tablelike structures are used in a relational database to define a relationship. This means that elements need not be defined at initial design. If a new relationship is required, a new table defining the relationship is built.

The tool that allows the proper use and management of the database is called a database management system (DBMS). The DBMS provides the facility to set up a new database and to define the data elements along with their relationships to other elements. This is done using a data dictionary. Most DBMSs also have a query language facility that is self-contained and nonprocedural to allow information to be retrieved from the database.

3. Applications Life Cycle

The development of a new computer system is a complex undertaking requiring a degree of planning and attention to detail that is often unappreciated by users unfamiliar with systems development. Traditional computer applications go through what is commonly called the applications life cycle (Treasury Board of Canada, 1978). This cycle can be broken down into six distinct phases, with the amount of time spent in each phase depending on the size and type of application. Failure to respect this process is almost certain to result in serious problems or even system failure.

a. Initiation Phase

In the initiation phase, the user must clearly describe the problem or application in general terms and obtain a commitment from management to initiate the development. The project manager should then identify the user's requirements; the human resources needed; the organizational, operational, and financial constraints; and the benefits of the proposed system to the organization. For small applications, these three tasks may be carried out very quickly and with little formal review. For larger systems, this phase may, in conjunction with the feasibility phase, encompass a large portion of the systems development lifecycle.

b. Feasibility Phase

The objective of a feasibility phase is to determine the most appropriate solution to the problem at hand. Organizational compatibility, economic justification, and technical considerations must be taken into account. The end product should be a recommendation for the implementation of the proposed solution to the problem. This phase should be conducted by a team consisting of the project leader, technical specialists, and significant representation from the user community. Once the feasibility study has been completed, a managerial decision must be made as to whether or not to accept the recommendations as stated and proceed with the next phase.

c. Design Phase

At this stage, a formal description of functions to be performed is prepared, along with a detailed system design that can be used as the basis for further development. In particular, data flow diagrams and pseudocode can be used to describe the details of the design. In addition to the design specifications, the documentation should include information on important constraints, changes to previous documents, and hardware and personnel resources to be allocated to the project. Consideration should also be given to potential failure modes and treatment of specific error conditions.

d. Implementation Phase

This phase includes the creation of all forms, manuals, and computer programs. System testing takes place and operations personnel are trained. As discussed later, the implementation and design phases can sometimes be combined with fourth-generation software packages.

System documentation is prepared in the implementation phase and should include four components. The *systems manual* should describe all computer programs in computer terminology. If the system is to be developed with standard programming languages, the *program specifications* should describe the individual programs and have logical diagrams where necessary. The *users' manual* provides detailed instructions about how to use the system. In the event that the system involves computer operations personnel, a *production manual* describing their involvement should be written.

e. Installation Phase

The transition from developmental to operational status occurs in the installation phase. In some applications, it is advisable to go through a preinstallation phase, commonly called beta-testing, in which the system is further tested under a wide variety of possible operational conditions. If the system is a replacement for an existing system, it may be necessary to run the new system in parallel with the existing system to ensure a smooth transfer from the old to the new. All documentation should be completed by this stage, and system approval should be given by authorized personnel.

f. Postinstallation Phase

The last phase of the life cycle involves ongoing maintenance and regular review activities required to keep the system operating smoothly. This will facilitate assessment of the system's performance in relation to the original design objectives as well as the operational criteria used to gauge system efficiency. Updates to the system may be required as operational experience accumulates.

4. 4GLs and Prototyping

In contrast to the traditional systems life cycle, fourth-generation languages can significantly reduce the time and cost required for systems development using a technique called prototyping. Prototyping is a general technique widely used in many scientific and engineering applications. For example, before a final commitment is made to build a new plant or factory, a prototype of the components is used to determine the feasibility of the structure. 4GLs allow the same to be done with information systems.

Complex information systems need to be prototyped because they are very difficult to define fully on paper in advance of systems development. There is much to be learned from experimental operation, and many useful modifications to the original specifications may become apparent with hands-on experience. Changes after the system has been designed and delivered are far more difficult and costly to implement.

In practice, the systems analyst works with an end user who knows the requirements of the new system to create a subset of required screens, reports, and dialogue for database queries. With a model of the dialogue on a terminal, the user is shown how to run the prototype and is left to test it over a period of time. The prototype is then modified as the user gains experience with the system.

Once the user is satisfied with the prototype, computer programmers can begin to build the final operational system. In general, the overall time required to develop a system with prototyping is shorter than the traditional systems life-cycle method. This, coupled with a higher level of user satisfaction and the reduced chance of misunderstandings between analyst and user, has resulted in increased use of prototypes in recent years.

C. Data Communications

In order to interact with the computer, some type of data communications technology is needed. For example, a terminal or microcomputer-based workstation may be connected to a host mainframe. One device connected to one processor represents a very simple type of communications network. Add several terminals talking to several computers and the network becomes much more complicated.

The basic components of a communications network are nodes and links. A node is a processing point within a network. A central computer comprises a host node; a terminal connected to the computer is a terminal node. A link is the physical path that interconnects the nodes and is composed of three components: link interface, telecommunications equipment, and transmission media. The link interface provides the connection between the nodes and the link. Telecommunications equipment such as modems, multiplexors, data services units, and data concentrators are used in the link interface. The transmission media is the element through which the signal is transmitted, including conventional media such as wire cables and more recent innovations such as fiber optics (Silver and Silver, 1986).

A communications network can encompass a large or a small geographic area. In many organizations, much of the communication occurs within a small geographic area, which has resulted in the development of special networks called local area networks (LANs). A LAN is usually confined to a moderate-sized geographic area such as a single building or campus, and is generally used within a single organization.

The LAN is most commonly thought of as interconnecting microcomputers, although this need not be the case (Neilson and Maydell, 1985). A LAN permits the sharing of computer resources, can support a large volume of local traffic, and may act as a common interface between different types of equipment. LANs can be useful in a laboratory environment in which more than one microcomputer is in use and information exchange among nodes in the network is required. A LAN should be carefully thought out and priced before implementation. It is important to consider volume of data to be handled, data to be shared, data transfer rates, connection to other networks, and compatibility with future equipment.

D. Computer Graphics

Computer graphics can be highly effective in presenting research results by providing visual presentations of data trends and comparative analyses among different treatment groups. In recent years, both plotter and storage tube technology have improved dramatically, resulting in much greater flexibility and resolution than was previously available. With graphics output, it is possible to compress an enormous amount of information onto a single screen image. Graphics devices are also becoming more practical for data input. For example, a mouse and digitizer pad can provide a very quick method of entering data into a system.

Many graphics programs available today are in the form of packaged software. Such packages are available for use on a large number of graphics devices. Use of a sophisticated graphic package is comparable to use of a high level language as opposed to use of an assembler language.

There is a current trend in software development to include graphics capabilities in software packages, thereby minimizing the effort required to link data files to graphics routines. Another trend in graphics is image processing and analysis. Equipment is now available to scan, digitize, and store graphic images. This is useful in military and cartographic applications as well as in certain medical applications, but it is very expensive.

III. TOXICOLOGY DATA SYSTEMS

In simplified terms, a typical toxicological study consists of four main phases: protocol generation, data collection, data analysis, and report generation. The data collection phase of a long-term carcinogenicity bioassay can last over two years in which time massive amounts of data will be generated (Gart *et al.*, 1986). Analysis of *in vivo* study data, processing of the pathology specimens, and generation of the final report can require another two years. Because the recording and tabulation of pathology results is time-consuming, attempts have been made to automate this area of the study. Subsequently, some pathology systems have served as the starting point for development of more comprehensive systems. Current commercial systems promise increased staff productivity, decreased time to study report generation, GLP compliance, improved study management, and enhanced data security.

In recent years, a number of general purpose computer systems for the management of toxicological data have been developed for use within the toxicological research laboratory. Four primary factors encouraged the development of computer systems to acquire and process data from toxicological studies. The first is the use of relatively large numbers of animals in toxicological studies, which in turn generates large amounts of data. The volume of data to be acquired is further increased by the monitoring of a number of toxicological indicators for each subject. A second factor is the introduction of good laboratory practice guidelines that mandate more accurate and detailed record keeping (Goeke *et al.*, 1983). The third major factor is the increasing availability of relatively inexpensive computer hardware. All that remained was the development of computer software to accomplish the task.

Software is the most difficult, complex, time-consuming, and costly component in the development of toxicology data systems. The increased sophistication of study protocols and laboratory instrumentation promotes the collection of large amounts of data that ideally will provide more insight into the toxicological properties of the test agent. In terms of computing, the problem then becomes the management and processing of this data into useful information for the experimental toxicologist.

A critical review of the existing toxicology data management systems is not included in this chapter because systems are quickly made obsolete by continual enhancements. In addition, each laboratory has unique requirements that must be defined then compared against the capabilities of the different systems available. Nonetheless, a brief review of some criteria used for selecting a toxicology data system is given followed by a short description of several toxicology data systems currently in use.

A. Systems Specifications

The development or acquisition of a toxicology data system is an important decision because of its impact not only on the conduct of laboratory investigations but also on the functioning of the entire laboratory. Before examining any particular system, one must assess what is wanted from a system. Requirements should be ranked by importance and potential savings arising from computerization.

As a first step in selecting a system, the activities underway in the laboratory should be defined. A diagram, as illustrated in Fig. 1, can be developed to describe the major functional areas involved in the laboratory. These include essential functions relating to activities such as animal husbandry, study conduct, data acquisition, and histopathological diagnosis of toxicological lesions. This particular diagram was developed for one of our own laboratories and will require some modification to meet the particular requirements of other laboratories. Nonetheless, many functions illustrated are general in nature and will be performed in many laboratories.

Once the main functions of the laboratory have been tabulated, each function should be elaborated in greater detail. As illustrated in Fig. 2, the conduct of a study involves a number of activities relating to the acquisition and evaluation of data on an ongoing basis for purposes of monitoring the study's progress. Many of these data acquisition functions have to satisfy GLP requirements. Again, although Fig. 2 typifies the functions of many toxicological research laboratories, the detailed description of activities involved in the conduct of a study have to be tailored to meet the needs of each individual laboratory.

The functional analyses illustrated in Figs. 1 and 2 can serve as a starting point for defining the requirements of a computerized toxicology data management system. These diagrams can be used to develop precise functional specifications for computer systems development, starting

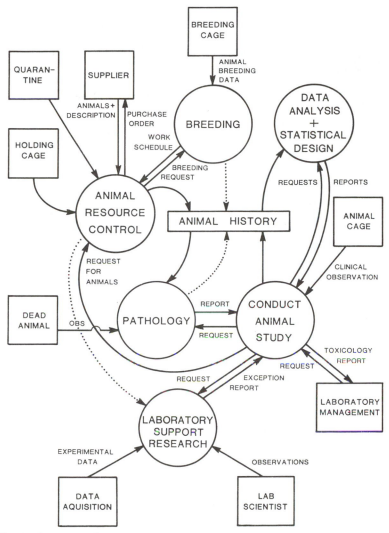

Fig. 1 Representation of a complete toxicology laboratory system. The circles represent major functions that are expanded in subsequent figures. Arrows and lines represent flows of information that must be tracked, input, or produced in reports.

with data flow diagrams that indicate the data-handling needs of the system. Because of this, it is important for functional specifications to be as complete and accurate as possible.

Once the functional requirements of the system have been established, either a system must be developed following the procedures outlined in

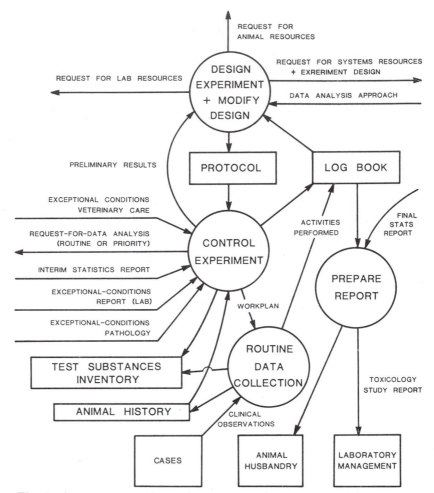

Fig. 2 An expansion of the conduct animal study module from Fig. 1. The circles represent major areas that can be expanded. They are used as major headings for developing functional requirements.

Section II or a commercially available system must be purchased. In the past, many laboratories have chosen to develop their own toxicology data management system (Felsky *et al.,* 1979). This approach can be compared to building your own race car. The race car has the advantage of getting you exactly where you want to go quickly; however, the disadvantages include the skills required to build it and the corresponding maintenance required as the course changes. Developing a toxicology data system is a difficult task that requires time and considerable expertise and should be engineered only with a skilled and experienced computing staff.

An alternative to building your own car is to use public transportation, that is, to acquire a system with fairly general capabilities that has already been developed. Public transportation has the ability to get a large number of people close to their destination but not necessarily precisely where they want to be. The advantages of a commercial system are immediate availability and low maintenance. An established system may also present fewer initial problems than a system developed in house. In addition, expert advice is available from the system's authors when there are problems. Valuable support can also be provided by user groups established to share information among different installations.

Regardless of whether a system is developed in house or purchased outside, there must be good prospects for continued development and support. This is critical because of the high costs associated with maintenance and minor enhancements to an existing system. A major reason for failure of toxicology data systems is poor documentation coupled with loss of key staff familiar with the systems. When this happens, maintenance costs escalate dramatically and maintenance may be virtually impossible because of inadequate documentation. The importance of good documentation by both systems personnel and users cannot be over emphasized. In the future, adequate documentation is sure to become a major thrust of system validation under GLP.

In many ways, the process of selecting a toxicology data system is similar to that of selecting any piece of complex laboratory equipment. In reality, it is more complex because it may represent the purchase of a large computer hardware system or additions to an existing system that may impact on other areas of the organization. An estimate of potential costs and benefits should be developed and the potential impact on other areas of the organization should be considered. Consideration should also be given to staff training and system support. It should be remembered that a toxicology data system is a laboratory tool, and time must be spent in learning how to use it. Thus, the implementation plan should consider coordination of hardware and software, installation of equipment, system validation, and staff training.

B. Commercial Toxicology Data Management Systems

The development of toxicology data management systems has taken two paths, one centralized and one decentralized. In the decentralized approach, the majority of the data acquisition programs are implemented on microcomputers located in the animal rooms or at the pathologist's workbench. This stand-alone approach has the advantage of operational independence but suffers the disadvantage of having the data separated on different computers. To overcome this, systems have been developed to transfer data to a central computer for further processing and storage (Noble, 1984).

In the centralized approach, data is sent directly to one computer. The disadvantage of being dependent on a central computer hardware system has decreased due to the enhanced reliability of computer hardware. Data is conveniently accessible by a large number of users; thus, problems associated with multiple copies of data elements required by many users being on different microcomputers are avoided. In addition, standard well-supported software for data processing and management can be used.

In the remainder of this section, we review five toxicological data management systems. Although systems such as TOXSYS and LABCAT were originally intended for use on independent microcomputers, all systems now have the facility to be linked to a common host computer, thereby combining the features of both centralized and decentralized systems.

a. TOXSYS

Although TOXSYS is no longer being marketed, its early influence on toxicology data systems is still evident. TOXSYS was originally developed by Beckman instruments for chronic toxicity studies. The system was designed around independent workstations (Herrick, 1984). The data collected was then consolidated on a mainframe computer. The workstation used a touchscore approach that allowed quick and accurate data entry. The pathology system in particular was very successful, being capable of both data collection and analysis and some report generation. Reproductive and teratology systems were also developed. Ultimately, the system appeared to have too many software problems and it was abandoned.

b. Toxicology Data Management Systems (TDMS)

One of the first toxicology data systems was developed at the U.S. National Center for Toxicological Research (NCTR). This system uses portable intelligent terminals with a touch screen, balance, and other equipment for data collection. The data is then transmitted to a database residing on a central mainframe for storage and processing. The system is large and complex and was designed primarily for carcinogenicity studies (Cranmer et al., 1978; Konvicka et al., 1978; Lawrence et al., 1979; Firth, 1980; Taylor and Johnson, 1980). One of the great strengths of this system is its capability to store and access large amounts of data.

c. XYBION Path/Tox System

XYBION Medical Systems has developed a successful toxicology data management system. As with most toxicology systems, this one was originally designed to meet the requirements of carcinogenicity studies. The primary feature of the system is a well-developed pathology data system. Reproductive and teratology systems are under development. The system is written in FORTRAN and uses a central microcomputer for data collection and analysis.

d. ARTEMIS Toxicology Data System

ARTEMIS (automatic recording in a toxicology environment and management information system) is a data capture and management system that uses a central minicomputer to collect, store, and process data. ARTEMIS can also be interfaced with front-end microcomputer-based data acquisition systems. It is written in COBOL and uses the commercial database management system INFOS. The system includes data management modules for acute, subchronic, and chronic toxicity tests as well as for teratology and reproductive studies. The system also includes a well-developed and flexible pathology system in which the pathologist can access all study data as individual slides are being examined.

e. LABCAT

LABCAT was initially developed for processing of pathology data on a Apple II microcomputer. It was expanded to include acute and general toxicological studies, genetic toxicology, and a series or more of specialized modules. The system is very flexible and easy to use. The other major advantage is the low start-up cost. The base system can be purchased then gradually expanded. Recently, the system has been moved to the IBM PC environment that takes advantage of the many improvements in hardware speed and disk storage. The system is well suited to a stand-alone environment but may require special arrangements for storage and processing of large studies with multiple sources of data. A newsletter called *LABCAT NEWS* is published, and a users group has been formed. Plans are also being made to provide a common system validation package.

IV. OTHER APPLICATIONS OF COMPUTERS IN TOXICOLOGICAL RESEARCH

Although we focus on integrated data management systems for use in laboratory experiments in the previous section, it should by no means be construed that this represents the only application of computers in toxicological research. Although often part of a more complete toxicology system, separate pathology systems have also been developed (Frith *et al.*, 1977; Naylor, 1978; Faccini and Naylor, 1979; Herrick *et al.*, 1983; Roe and Lee, 1984).

Specialized software has also been developed for a wide variety of other applications in toxicological research, including highly sophisticated tasks such as DNA sequencing (Gingeras, 1983). The DNASIS package, for example, runs on an IBM PC, XT, or AT compatible microcomputer with as little as 512 KB of memory. It can be used efficiently to carry out a number of analyses used in DNA sequencing.

Computer software has also been developed to carry out structure–activity analysis of chemicals (Golberg, 1983). Programs available for carrying out structure–activity analysis include ADAPT (Jurs *et al.*, 1983; Stouch and Jurs, 1985), CASE (Klopman, 1985; Rosenkranz and Klopman, 1988), SIMCA (Dunn and Wold, 1986; Dunn, 1988), and TOPKAT (Enslein *et al.*, 1983a, 1983b, 1987).

In addition to acquisition and analysis of toxicological data, computers are used to store and retrieve summary information on toxicological hazards. For example, the *International Register of Potentially Toxic Chemicals* (IRPTC) was developed by the World Health Organization (WHO) in conjunction with United Nations Environmental Program Governing Council (1984). The purposes of this system are to facilitate access to existing data on the effects of chemicals on humans and the environment and to identify the important gaps in our existing knowledge in this area.

Toxicological information in the scientific literature can be located with computerized bibliographical systems. Such systems offer literature searches yielding results in minutes, which in the past used to take days of manual searching in journals. TOXLINE (Toxicology Information Online), for example, is a bibliographical database containing information on the biochemical, physiological, and toxicological aspects of drugs and chemicals. TOXLINE and the related data bases TOXLIT and TOXLIT65 each contain approximately 700,000 citations and are updated monthly.

Analysis of toxicological data has been expedited through the widespread use of statistical software packages. Program packages are available to carry out most of the classical forms of statistical analysis (McKenzie, 1982; Frances, 1983; Wilson, 1983). The Statistical Package for the Social Sciences (SPSS, 1986) is designed for the user with little statistical background, can be learned very quickly, and provides a broad range of basic statistical procedures. BMDP (Biomedical Computer Programs) is not as easily learned as SPSS but does provide expanded statistical capabilities and the flexibility of a FORTRAN interface (Dixon, 1985). The Statistical Analysis System (SAS, 1985), like BMDP, is more difficult to learn than SPSS but provides a much more extensive battery of statistical analysis procedures.

The major statistical packages were designed initially for use on large scale computers, although most also come in versions that will run on minicomputers. Recently, microcomputer versions offering some of the capabilities of these same packages have also become available (SAS, 1987). At present, however, the microcomputer packages may not provide attractive alternatives to the larger scale systems due to limitations in function, speed, or input/output capabilities, particularly when large volumes of data need to be processed.

In addition to statistical software packages, customized software to carry out specialized analyses is also available. For example, Thomas *et al.* (1977) and Haseman (1984) have described programs developed for the analysis of histopathological data derived from long-term studies in which small rodents are used. Other programs have been developed specifically for use on microcomputers. These include routines for predicting human health risks based on toxicological data (Crump, 1984, 1988; Sielken, 1988) as well as procedures for analysis of mutagenicity data (Myers *et al.*, 1989).

At the leading edge of computer applications in toxicology lies fifth-generation systems or artificial intelligence (Fiksel, 1987a; 1987b; Fiksel and Covello, 1987). In the future, such systems may be used to computerize parts of the decision-making process related to environmental toxicants. Several pioneering projects are currently underway in this area, including the development of a system to evaluate alternative approaches to the management of hazardous substances used in industry (International Institute of Applied Systems Analysis, 1987).

V. SUMMARY AND CONCLUSIONS

In this chapter, we have discussed a number of fundamental informatics concepts. Computers now come in many sizes and have various capabilities and processing power, ranging from microcomputers used for personal computing and data acquisition to large main frames capable of supporting hundreds of users simultaneously.

Today, high level programming languages in which many machine instructions are encompassed in a single statement are available for scientific applications. Increasingly, fourth-generation languages that minimize systems development time and facilitate information retrieval are being used for database applications. Software development has been systematized to the point where new applications proceed through a well-defined life cycle, from the initiation and feasibility phases through systems design and implementation. Prototyping may be considered as an alternative to the traditional systems life cycle when fourth-generation languages are used because of the reduced time for systems development.

Computerized data management systems are becoming widely used in toxicological laboratories for data acquisition, storage, and analysis. These systems serve a wide variety of needs in the research laboratory and offer increased efficiency in data handling, as well as enhanced compliance with GLP. A toxicological data management system may be developed from scratch to meet the specific needs of the laboratory; however, it is often possible to satisfy most requirements through the acquisition of an existing commercial product. Although not necessarily as efficient as a custom designed and developed system, an existing commercial system offers the advantages of a proven system with immediate availability, low maintenance, and vendor support.

The role of the computer in toxicological research will, no doubt, undergo considerable change in the next decade both to keep pace with research demands and to take advantage of advances in computer technology. The growing use of fourth-generation languages will allow the toxicologist easier access to data and provide greater flexibility in analysis of results. Increasingly sophisticated toxicology data management systems will also find widespread application in the automation of toxicological research. Research design will be greatly aided by widespread access to data bases containing pertinent toxicological information, including raw laboratory results. Emerging technologies, such as artificial intelligence, are also likely to be applied in the management of toxicants present in the environment.

Acknowledgments

The authors would like to thank Drs. Alfred Jay and Annette Shipp for their helpful comments on this chapter, and Terry Chernis for her bibliographical assistance.

References

Cranmer, M. F., Lawrence, L. R., Konvincka, A. J., and Herrick, S. S. (1978). NCTR computer systems designed for toxicologic experimentation. I. Overview. *J. Environ. Pathol. Toxicol.* **1**, 701–709.

Crump, K. S. (1984). An improved procedure for low-dose carcinogenic risk assessment from animal data. *J. Environ. Pathol. Toxicol. Oncol.* **5**, 339–348.

Crump, K. S. (1988). "TOX RISK: Toxicology Risk Assessment Program." Washington, DC: ICF/Clement Associates.

Dixon, W. J. (ed.) (1985). "BMDP Statistical Software." Berkeley: University of California Press.

Dunn, W. J. (1988). QSAR approaches to predicting toxicity. *Toxicology Lett.* **43,** 277–283.

Dunn, W. J., and Wold, S. (1986). Use of chemometrics in environmental toxicology and structure-activity relationships. *Trends Anal. Chem.* **15,** 53–56.

Enslein, K., Borgstadt, H. H., Tomb, M. E., Blake, B. W., and Hart, J. B. (1987). A structure-activity prediction model of carcinogenicity based on NCI/NTP assays and food additives. *Toxicol. Ind. Health* **3,** 267–287.

Enslein, K., Lander, T. R., and Strange, J. R. (1983a). Teratogenesis: A statistical structure-activity model. *Teratog. Carcinog. Mutagen.* **3,** 289–309.

Enslein, K., Lander, T. R., Tomb, M. E., and Landis, W. G. (1983b). Mutagenicity (Ames): A structure-activity model. *Teratog. Carcinog. Mutagen.* **3,** 503–513.

Faccini, I. M., and Naylor, D. (1979). Computer analysis and integration of animal pathology data. *Arch. Toxicol. Suppl.* **2,** 517–520.

Felsky, G., Villeneuve, D. C., and Farmer, D. (1979). An interactive toxicological data handling system for a PDP-12 computer. *Comput. Prog. Biomed.* **10,** 75–80.

Fiksel, J. (1987a). Artificial intelligence: software reasons to analyze risk. *Safety and Health* **135,** 64–66.

Fiksel, J. (1987b). Assessment of the risks associated with knowledge system technology. *Comp. Law.* **4,** 7–10.

Fiksel, J., and Covello, V. T. (1987). Knowledge systems, expert systems, and risk communication. *Environ. Profess.* **9,** 144–152.

Francis, I. (1983). A survey of statistical software. *Computational Statistics and Data Analysis* **1,** 17–27.

Frith, C. H. (1980). Automated and computer-assisted pathology support for a large chronic study. *In* "Innovation in Cancer Risk Assessment (ED_{01}) Study" (J. A. Staffa and M. A. Mehlman, eds.), pp. 231–246. Park Forest South, Illinois: Pathotox Publishers.

Frith, C. H., Herrick, S. S., and Konvicka, A. J. (1977). Computer assisted collection and analysis of pathology data. *J. Natl. Cancer Inst. (US)* **58,** 1717–1727.

Gart, J. J., Krewski, D., Lee, P. N., Tarone, R. E., and Wahrendorf, J. (1986). "The Design and Analysis of Long-Term Animal Experiments" (IARC Scientific Publ. No. 79). Lyon: International Agency for Research on Cancer.

Gingeras, T. R. (1983). Computers and DNA sequences: A natural combination. *In* "Statistical Analysis of DNA Sequence Data" (B. S. Weir, ed.), pp. 15–44. New York: Marcel Dekker.

Goeke, J. E., Hoberman, A. M., and Christian, M. S. (1983). Quality assurance validation of computerized toxicological data. *J. Am. Coll. Toxicol.* **3,** 121–124.

Golberg, L. (ed.) (1983). "Structure-Activity Correlation as a Predictive Tool in Toxicology: Fundamentals, Methods, and Applications." New York: Hemisphere Publishing.

Haseman, J. (1984). Statistical issues in the analysis of rodent bioassay data. *Environ. Health Perspect.* **58,** 385–392.

Herrick, S. (1984). Automated data acquisition systems in the 80s and beyond I. Design. *In* "Toxicology Laboratory Design and Management for the 80s and Beyond" (A. S. Tegeris, ed.), pp. 136–142. Basel: Karger.

Herrick, S. S., Davis, C., Donnelley, D. V., Lockhart, T., Marek, L., and Russel, H. (1983). Histopathology automated system. *Drug Inf. J.* **17**, 287–295.

International Institute of Applied Systems Analysis (1987). "Intelligent Decision Support Systems: Hazardous Substances and Industrial Risk." Laxenburg, Austria: International Institute of Applied Systems Analysis.

Jurs, P. C., Hasan, M. N., Henry, D. R., Stouch, T. R., and Whalen-Pedersen, E. K. (1983). Computer-assisted studies of molecular structure and carcinogenic activity. *Fundam. Appl. Toxicol.* **3**, 343–349.

Klopman, G. (1985). Predicting toxicity through a computer automated structure evaluation program. *Environ. Health Perspect.* **61**, 269–274.

Konvicka, A., Herrick, S., and Lawrence, L. (1977). Effect of good laboratory practice (GLP) guidelines on design of automated research support systems. *Drug Inf. J.* **10**, 75–78.

Konvicka, A. J., Robinson, O., and Weiss, K. (1978). NCTR computer systems designed for toxicological experimentation. II. Experiment start-up system. *J. Environ. Pathol. Toxicol.* **1**, 711–719.

Lawrence, L. R., Konvicka, A. J., Ezell, R., Applegate, J., Green, G., and Fernstrom, E. B. (1979). NCTR computer systems designed for toxicologic experimentation IV. Experiment information system. *J. Environ. Pathol. Toxicol.* **2**, 1011–1019.

McKenzie, J. D. (1982). Standards for statistical packages. *In* "Proceedings of the Statistical Computing Section of the Americal Statistical Association," pp. 255–257. Washington, DC: American Statistical Association.

Martin, J. (1983). "Managing the Data Base Environment." Englewood Cliffs, New Jersey: Prentice-Hall.

Martin, J. (1984). "An Information Systems Manifesto." Englewood Cliffs, New Jersey: Prentice-Hall.

Martin, J. (1985). "Fourth Generation Languages." Vol. 1. Englewood Cliffs, New Jersey: Prentice-Hall.

Mills, H. D., Linger, R. C., and Hevner, A. R. (1986). "Principles of Information Systems Analysis and Design." Orlando, Florida: Academic Press.

Myers, L., Adams, N., Kier, L., Rao, T. K., Shah, B., and Williams, L. (1989). Microcomputer software for data management and statistical analyses of the Ames *Salmonella* test. In: "Statistical Methods in Toxicological Research" (D. Krewski and C. A. Franklin, ed.). New York: Gordon & Breach. In press.

Naylor, D. (1978). The computerization of histopathological data in toxicological laboratory studies using SNOP. *Methods Inf. Med.* **17**, 272–279.

Neilson, W. J., and Maydell, U. M. (1985). A survey of current LAN technology and performance. *Inf. Syst. Operat. Res.* **23**, 215–241.

Noble, J. F. (1984). Automated data acquisition systems in the 80s and beyond II. Operation. *In* "Toxicology Laboratory Design and Management for the 80s and Beyond" (A. S. Tegeris, ed.), pp. 143–158. Basel: Karger.

Ralson, A., and Reilly, E. D. (eds.) (1983). "Encyclopedia of Computer Science and Engineering." Toronto: Van Nostrand-Reinhold.

Roe, F. J. C., and Lee, P. N. (1984). "Histopathological Data Recording, Processing, Reporting and Statistical Analysis, using Computer Program ROELEE 84." Available from P. N. Lee, 25 Cedar Road, Sutton, Surrey, U.K., 5M2 5DG.

Rosenkranz, H. S., and Klopman, G. (1988). CASE, the computer-automated structure evaluation system, as an alternative to extensive animal testing. *Toxicol. Ind. Health* **4,** 533–540.

SAS Institute (1985). "SAS Users Guide: Statistics, Version 5 Edition." Cary, North Carolina: SAS Institute.

SAS Institute (1987). "SAS/STAT Guide for Personal Computers, Version 6 Edition." Cary, North Carolina: SAS Institute.

Sielken, R. L. (1988). "GEN.T: A General Tool for Incorporating Cancer Dose-Response Extrapolation Techniques into Quantitative Risk Assessments." Bryan, Texas: Sielken.

Silver, J., and Silver, M. (1986). "Computers and Information Processing." New York: Harper and Row.

Statistical Package for the Social Sciences (1986). "SPSSX User's Guide." Chicago: Statistical Package for the Social Sciences.

Stouch, T. R., and Jurs, P. C. (1985). Computer-assisted studies of molecular structure and genotoxic activity by pattern recognition techniques. *Environ. Health Perspect.* **61,** 329–343.

Taylor, D. W., and Johnson, C. L. (1980). Data systems support for a large, long-term carcinogenic (ED_{01}) study. *In* "Innovation in Cancer Risk Assessment (ED_{01}) Study" (J. A. Staffa and M. A. Mehlman, eds.), pp. 221–230. Park Forest South, Illinois: Pathotox Publishers.

Thomas, D. G., Breslow, N., and Gart, J. (1977). Trend and homogeneity analyses of proportions and life table data. *Comput. Biomed. Res.* **10,** 373–381.

Treasury Board of Canada (1978). EDP: Planning, approvals and development. *In* "Treasury Board Administrative Policy Manual," (Chapter 440.3). Ottawa: Treasury Board of Canada.

United Nations Environment Program (1984). "International Register of Potentially Toxic Chemicals." Geneva: United Nations Environment Program.

U.S. Food and Drug Administration (1976). Nonclinical laboratory studies, good laboratory practice regulation. *Fed. Regist.* **43,** 59986–60020.

Wiederhold, G. (1983). "Database Design" 2nd ed. New York: McGraw-Hill.

Wilson, S. R. (1983). Benchmark data sets for the flexible evaluation of statistical software. *Comput. Stat. Data Anal.* **1,** 29–39.

22
Compliance with Good Laboratory Practice

Douglas L. Arnold
Toxicology Research Division
Bureau of Chemical Safety
Food Directorate
Health Protection Branch
Health and Welfare Canada
Ottawa, Ontario

I. Introduction

II. Responsibilities

III. Quality Assurance Unit

IV. Concluding Comments

I. INTRODUCTION

National regulatory agencies concerned with the safety of foods and food additives, animal feed additives, drugs for human or animal use, cosmetics, medical devices, radiation-emitting devices, pesticides, and biological products require considerable nonclinical laboratory (i.e., toxicological) data if they are to ensure the highest possible degree of public health protection. These agencies lack the facilities to conduct the necessary nonclinical laboratory testing internally. Consequently, via applicable laws and regulations, manufacturers are usually required to generate the data upon which a regulatory agency bases its safety evaluation.

The U.S. Food and Drug Administration (FDA) was the first agency to propose regulations governing the proper conduct of nonclinical laboratory studies (U.S. FDA, 1976). The regulations were published on December 22, 1978, and became effective on June 20, 1979 (U.S. FDA, 1978). These regulations arose as a result of inspections conducted in the nonclinical testing facilities of several pharmaceutical firms and private contract laboratories, and internal review of a toxicological study conducted in FDA's own laboratories (U.S. FDA, 1976). The types of problems found during the various inspections raised serious doubts about the quality and integrity of the data being submitted to FDA for evaluation, interpretation, and eventual extrapolation for purposes of human safety (U.S. FDA, 1976; Halperin, 1978; Lepore, 1979; Reisa, 1979; Van Houweling *et al.*, 1979).

The nature of the good laboratory practice (GLP) regulations are quite general. The reason for this is basically twofold: first, the FDA, like most regulatory agencies, is responsible for regulating a variety of consumer products and/or chemicals; therefore, the regulations apply to nonclinical laboratory data for all regulated items. Second, the regulations are intended to ensure the quality and integrity of the data but not to limit the utilization of informed scientific judgment and/or innovation in the design and conduct of nonclinical testing programs (U.S. FDA, 1976). It is obvious, therefore, that many aspects of the GLP regulations are nothing more than good science. As such, the study protocol will contain the objectives and methods to be followed during its conduct as well as what necessary information and data will be recorded, all in accordance with the applicable standard operating procedures (SOPs). SOPs are a stepwise listing of how each routine or repetitive procedure is to be performed. Compliance with GLP will facilitate the complete reconstruction of a study in the absence of all principal study personnel for the purpose of a study audit or a reevaluation of results in light of future findings.

II. RESPONSIBILITIES

The GLP regulations instituted by the U.S. FDA (1978) and those subsequently developed by the European Chemical Industry Ecology and Toxicology Center (ECETOC; 1979), the Organization for Economic Cooperation and Development (OECD; 1982), and the U.S. Environmental Protection Agency (U.S. EPA; 1983a, 1983b) have placed certain responsibilities on the management of testing facilities (selecting the study director, providing adequate facilities and adequate number of personnel with proper training, approving study protocols, etc.) and on the study director (preparing the study protocol, ensuring compliance with applicable GLP regulations and SOPs, archiving appropriate materials, preparing the study report, etc). The study director also serves as the major focal point for inspections by regulatory agency investigators. Generally speaking, GLP investigators conduct two types of inspections. One is the routine surveillance inspection to ascertain compliance with GLP regulations. If a satisfactory level of compliance is attained, then such inspections continue on a periodic basis, occurring approximately once every two years (James, 1985). If compliance is unsatisfactory, a follow-up inspection may be scheduled within six months. The second type of inspection is a study audit undertaken because the regulatory agency has some reservations about submitted data. In this instance, the inspection team conducts a detailed investigation of the study(ies) in question from the time of conception through the completed final report. Depending on the type of problems revealed by the audit, the regulations allow for legal action to be taken against the study director and/or other nonclinical laboratory testing facility personnel. The regulatory agency may subsequently refuse to accept any data from the study director and/or testing facility (U.S. FDA, 1978). For details on GLP inspection procedures, see James, 1985.

III. QUALITY ASSURANCE UNIT

Although GLP regulations place certain responsibilities on the management of a nonclinical laboratory, they do not require management to monitor ongoing studies or to review final reports to assure that the data are valid. FDA regulations require that "a testing facility shall have a quality assurance unit (QAU) composed of one or more individuals who shall be responsible for monitoring each study to assure management that the facilities, equipment, personnel, methods, practices, records, and controls are in conformance with the regulations" (U.S. FDA, 1978). Members of the QAU report directly to management. They cannot be associated with the planning or conduct of the study(ies) that they inspect so as to maintain their objectivity. In a larger nonclinical laboratory, it is commonplace to have employees whose sole function is QAU activities, whereas in smaller nonclinical laboratories, it may be necessary for an individual who is assisting in the conduct of study A to perform the QAU function on study B if the study director for study B is not involved in the supervision of that individual and the individual is not involved in either the design or conduct of study B. In some laboratories, the QAU auditing team is made up of QA professionals supplemented with toxicologists who have the expertise to attain the goals and objectives for each particular audit, whereas other laboratories use the QAU as a training exercise for new toxicologists (Hoover and Baldwin, 1984).

The QAU ascertains whether the conduct of the study complies with the protocol, whether proper identification of test articles and study data are maintained, and whether SOPs are available at the bench level and are being followed. In addition, the QAU reviews all final reports to verify data accuracy and assures that the final report is substantiated by appropriate data.

In addition to the preceding functions that are required, the QAU can also undertake several other tasks depending on the wishes of management. For example, GLP regulations require that each nonclinical laboratory provide archival facilities for the orderly storage of data and specimens. The QAU may act as the "keeper" of the archives, limiting access to authorized personnel and storing data and specimens in an orderly manner for expeditious retrieval. Baldwin and Hoover (1985) have also suggested that the toxicologist and QA professionals develop a greater "collegial relationship". For example, they have suggested that a future QAU responsibility might be to ascertain whether an organ function test originally devised for humans could be used for other species, particularly in view of potential species differences that may result in erroneous interpretation of results. Although such a proposal may improve the scientific component of nonclinical laboratory studies, it could possibly detract from the QAU's objectivity.

Requirements regarding academic background and previous job experience of QAU members are determined by the management of the nonclinical laboratory. It is this author's opinion that members of the QAU should have sufficient training, knowledge, and experience in toxicology, analytical chemistry, laboratory animal husbandry, statistics, and computer science so that each member can speak knowledgeably about one or more of these disciplines and seek extramural advice in these disciplines when necessary in the performance of their responsibilities.

Compliance with study protocols and SOPs does not mean that these documents are engraved in stone and cannot be changed during the progress of a study. For example, technologies may change, or the purchase of new equipment may result in SOPs being modified or rewritten. Unforeseen circumstances may necessitate changes in anticipated initiation and completion dates. All changes in protocol and significant changes in SOPs are recorded, dated, and approved by management. All data recordings, changes, and modifications are dated by the appropriate personnel; therefore, if it becomes necessary to reconstruct a study, any questions about which procedures were followed and who performed the task can be readily ascertained. It should also be pointed out that various regulatory agencies have modified or have proposed modifications to the GLP regulations that they have found through experience to be burdensome or unnecessary for the attainment of their objectives (U.S. FDA, 1980, 1984; James, 1985).

QAU inspections must be performed at intervals adequate to assure the integrity of the study. Organizations such as ECETOC (1979) and OECD (1982) have indicated that the nature of each nonclinical laboratory study is such that they do not suggest a rigid inspection schedule. The U.S. FDA (1978) and U.S. EPA (1983a, 1983b) regulations specifically require that any study lasting more than six months be inspected by the QAU every three months. Although a fixed time interval may be appropriate to ascertain that the QAU is functioning in a manner to attain its objective, for a multifaceted chronic study that might include a reproductive phase, an immunological and a hormonal evaluation component, etc., periodic inspections should be supplemented with inspections of each new phase of the study as each is initiated. Beyond this basic requirement, the extent, frequency, and depth of each QAU inspection may well be determined in part by the current and previous QAU findings in regard to the laboratory's compliance with GLP regulations.

Each inspection conducted by the QAU should be followed by a written report to management and the study director detailing its observations. If serious deviations are found, then an initial verbal communication from the QAU should precede the written report. Something akin to circumstances that can lead to an invalidation of the study can precipitate a verbal communication prior to the written report. Concurrently, if immediate corrective action is taken to rectify any serious problem found by the QAU, such action should be indicated in the QAU written report. Because the study director has responsibility for the technical conduct of a study, he or she may find it useful to accompany the QAU during its inspections, particularly for a multifaceted study.

Upon completion of a study, a copy or draft of the final report is submitted to the QAU for verification of raw data, methods, and SOPs used during the study. The summary report is substantiated by documented evidence. The documented evidence can consist of raw data, room log book entries, final reports of participating scientists, etc. It is not practical to verify all data summaries contained in the final report or all documented deviations from the study protocol and SOPs; however, a sufficient number must be checked so that the QAU can assure management of the study's validity.

IV. CONCLUDING COMMENTS

The U.S. FDA proposal to introduce GLP regulations was initially viewed by many with a great deal of apprehension. The commercial sector voiced concern about the increased costs of nonclinical laboratory testing while some toxicologists expressed apparent indignation, assuming that their scientific ability and integrity were being questioned. However, it soon became apparent that a large majority of the findings that led to the proposal of GLP regulations generally involved slovenly laboratory and management practices concerning study conduct and control, as well as poor data recording practices. Those few instances in which fraudulent practices were discovered obviously necessitated adequate safeguards and penalties to discourage future recurrences. Following FDA implementation of GLP regulations, and their subsequent adoption by other national regulatory and international agencies, GLP has become an accepted "way of life" in nonclinical laboratories. It probably goes without saying that regulatory agencies now have more confidence in the integrity and validity of the nonclinical laboratory data submitted to them, which should assist them in attaining their various mandates.

It should be added that the use of laboratory animals for nonclinical testing, as well as the disposal of animal wastes, carcasses, and other materials from a toxicological study, requires adherence to other laws and regulations; however, these vary markedly among federal and local jurisdictions and are, therefore, beyond the scope of this text.

Acknowledgments

The author thanks Drs. L. Bradshaw, K. Khera, and P. D. Lepore for their comments and suggestions, and Patsy Matcheskie for her typing assistance.

References

Baldwin, J. K. and Hoover, B. K. (1985). GLP trends today and tomorrow. *J. Am. Coll. Toxicol.* **4,** 305–308.

European Chemical Industry Ecology and Toxicology Center (1979). "Good Laboratory Practice," (Monograph No. 1). Brussels: European Chemical Industry Ecology and Toxicology Center.

Halperin, J. A. (1978). The GLP's: Why we need them; How we'll use them. *J. Parenter. Drug Assoc.* **32,** 57–62.

Hoover, B. K., and Baldwin, J. K. (1984). Meeting the Quality Assurance Challenges of the 1980s: Team auditing by toxicologists and QA professionals. *J. Am. Coll. Toxicol.* **3,** 129–139.

James, G. W. (1985). The FDA's good laboratory practices; inspectional procedures and findings. *In* "Chemical Safety Regulation and Compliance" (F. Hamburger and J. K. Marquis, eds.) pp. 113–118. Basel: S. Karger.

Lepore, P. D. (1979). What is GLP and why? *Proc. 12th Annu. Symp. Soc. Toxicol. Can.* 6–36.

"Good Laboratory Practice in the Testing of Chemicals" Paris: Organization for Economic Co-operation and Development.

Reisa, D. M. (1979). Validation and verification of existing data. *Proc. 12th Annu. Symp. Soc. Toxicol. Can.* 135–142.

U.S. Environmental Protection Agency (1983a). Part III, toxic substances control; Good laboratory practice standards; Final rule. *Fed. Regist.* **48,** 53922–53944.

U.S. Environmental Protection Agency (1983b). Part IV, pesticide programs; Good laboratory practice standards; Final rule. *Fed. Regist.* **48,** 53946–53969.

U.S. Food and Drug Administration (1976). Department of Health, Education and Welfare, nonclinical laboratory studies, proposed regulations for good laboratory practice. *Fed. Regist.* **41,** 51206–51228.

U.S. Food and Drug Administration (1978). Department of Health, Education and Welfare, nonclinical laboratory studies, good laboratory practice regulations. *Fed. Regist.* **43,** 59986–60020.

U.S. Food and Drug Administration (1980). Department of Health, Education and Welfare, good laboratory practice for nonclinical laboratory studies: Amendment of good laboratory practice regulations. *Fed. Regist.* **45,** 24465–24466.

U.S. Food and Drug Administration (1984). Department of Health and Human Services: Good laboratory practice regulations; Proposed rule. *Fed. Regist.* **49,** 43530–43537.

Van Houweling, C. D., Norcross, M. A., and Lepore, P. D. (1979). An overview of good laboratory practices. *Clin. Toxicol.* **15,** 515–526.

23

The Conduct of a Chronic Bioassay and the Use of an Interactive – Integrated Toxicology Data System

Douglas L. Arnold
Peter F. McGuire
Eduardo A. Nera
Toxicology Research Division
Bureau of Chemical Safety
Food Directorate
Health Protection Branch
Health and Welfare Canada
Ottawa, Ontario

I. Introduction
II. Study Protocol
III. The Quarantine Period
IV. Study Initiation: Distribution to Test Groups
V. Housing
VI. Animal Weighing Subsystem
VII. Detailed Clinical Subsystem
VIII. Pathology Subsystem
IX. Host Computer Facility
X. Quality Assurance Unit
XI. Discussion
XII. Future Trends

I. INTRODUCTION

In this chapter, the conduct of a toxicological study is integrated with the requirements of good laboratory practice (GLP) regulations, a computer system to record and process the study data, a health monitoring program, and a disease surveillance and animal quality control program.

II. STUDY PROTOCOL

A protocol is prepared by the study director in consultation with members of the study core team, which include a toxicologist, pathologist, statistician, laboratory animal care specialist, and personnel from other disciplines as necessary (see Chapter 2; Arnold *et al.*, 1978). The protocol must be approved by management. For compliance with GLP, the approved protocol must contain but is not limited to the following:

1. A descriptive title and a statement of the purpose for the study
2. The identification of the test and control compounds by name, chemical abstract number, or code number
3. The name and address of the study sponsor and the facility conducting the study
4. The proposed starting and completion dates
5. The justification for the test system selected
6. The species, strain, substrain, number, body weight range, sex, source of supply, and age of the test animals, where applicable
7. The method of animal identification
8. A description of the experimental design, including the methods to control bias
9. A description and/or identification of the diet used in the study, including the contaminants and their acceptable limits and any other relevant information about the diet
10. The route of test article administration, the vehicle to be used (if any), and the reason for its choice
11. The dosage of the test or control compounds to be administered and the method, frequency, and duration of administration
12. The type and frequency of tests, analyses, and measurements to be made (i.e., body weight determinations, toxicant stability tests, tissue and/or excrement analyses for test chemical and/or its metabolites, etc.)
13. A clear indication of how the various procedures will be undertaken (standard operating procedures)
14. A list of the proposed statistical methods to be used
15. The records to be maintained
16. The date the sponsor approved the protocol and the signature of the study director

For additional comments on the study protocol, consult the regulations of the U.S. Food and Drug Administration (FDA; 1978; 1987), the U.S. Environmental Protection Agency (EPA; 1983a, 1983b), the Organization for Economic Co-operation and Development (OECD; 1982), and the European Chemical Industry Ecology and Toxicology Center (ECETOC; 1979).

Due to the plethora of data collected in conjunction with the conduct of any chronic study, some form of electronic data processing system is required. Commercial vendors have computer hardware and software packages to achieve these needs as well as to satisfy the requirements of GLP. However, many systems are primarily designed for standard tests and often are not flexible enough to deal with some of the complex toxicological studies described in Part V. It is possible to develop software to meet local situations. A series of semi-independent subsystems are described here that are designed to collect specific types of data. These subsystems have many similarities with their commercially available counterparts. To make these independent subsystems as useful as possible, a computer of sufficient capacity to store and integrate all animal room and laboratory data is required. The ability to access such data in a timely manner will improve study management and allow the study director to make well-informed decisions about the study's conduct and direction. One aspect of electronic data gathering that cannot be overlooked is validation of the software. Does the software collect, handle, and store data in the manner desired, or are there unsuspected quirks in the system? For GLP purposes, all electronic data gathering, handling, and storage systems must be validated (Goeke *et al.*, 1984; "The Gold Sheet", 1985; "Food Chemical News", 1986).

After the study protocol is approved, the animals are ordered in accordance with the specifications stated in the protocol. Upon arrival, a copy of the animal requisition form together with the bill of lading are forwarded to the study director and constitute part of the study's raw data. As each animal is removed from its shipping container, its health is evaluated, it is assigned a number for audit trail purposes, and then it is placed in a cage for the quarantine period. When rodents are used, a specific number of randomly selected animals, based on the size of the study population, are killed during the quarantine period for serological, microbiological, and pathological evaluation (Chapter 8; Fox *et al.*, 1979; Balk, 1983).

III. THE QUARANTINE PERIOD

For rodents, the quarantine period preceding the initiation of a study is generally 2 weeks. Based on our past experience with a particular laboratory animal vendor, we find that animals may be quarantined in the test room if the room has been appropriately washed and sanitized after the conclusion of the preceding study. This practice eliminates a number of logistical problems that arise when animals are relocated while minimizing environmental perturbations known to have a significant effect on experimental results (Lane-Petter, 1963; Weihe, 1971). More commonly, confidence in the vendor's quality control program will result in animals being acclimatized for a period of 7 to 10 days prior to study initiation while evaluation of the in-house quality control specimens continues. Ideally, each study is housed in a single room and monitored by the same staff from the start of the quarantine/acclimation period through study termination (Lawrence *et al.*, 1979). Additionally, each study should have its own group of control animals. The practice of pooling control animal data derived from several different studies, wherein the concurrent control group size is often only 10 animals and the test group size is 50 animals, is unacceptable (i.e., the control group size becomes 50 animals by pooling control animal data from five studies).

During the quarantine/acclimation period, all animals are fed the control diet to be used during the test period, and the feed and water are usually supplied *ad libitum*. The quarantine/acclimation period may also provide a brief buffer period to work out unexpected logistic snags as well as to obtain pretest/baseline biological data (i.e., hematology, serum biochemistry, etc.).

For purposes of GLP, shipping documents for feed and bedding are retained as part of the study's raw data. If the feed and/or bedding manufacturers offer a certification program, one should invest in such a service, which is often performed for the manufacturer under contract with an independent laboratory. It is also recommended that periodic reverification by another laboratory be undertaken, particularly for studies in which excessive contamination can jeopardize the study's validity.

IV. STUDY INITIATION: DISTRIBUTION TO TEST GROUPS

Upon completion of the quarantine period and evaluation of the available pretest quality control data, animals are randomly allocated to the experimental groups and randomly assigned their cage positions (see Chapter 7; Fox *et al.*, 1979). To accomplish this, two sets of computer-generated random numbers are used. (These listings form part of the study's raw data.)

An alphanumeric term can be used to identify each cage. The first two characters of the alpha portion of the identification code may be used to indicate the treatment group (A to Z) and sex (M or F), whereas the numeric portion identifies the cage position in a sequential numbering scheme. Additional alphas or digits can be used to specify the month or year when the study was initiated, who the sponsor is, etc. When an animal is assigned to its cage, it is marked or tattooed with its unique identifier. Other test animal groupings that may be incorporated into the study design include:

1. Interim kills: this option is particularly valuable when the progression and onset (latent period) of any toxicological or pathological lesion are studied.
2. Sentinel animals: these animals can be used for latent disease monitoring (Fox *et al.*, 1979; Hamm, 1985; Chapter 8).
3. A group of animals to study recoverability or reversibility: this group can be fed the test substance for some fixed period, at which time a subgroup is killed and the remaining animals are fed control diet for an additional period prior to their being killed (Arnold *et al.*, 1983; Iverson *et al.*, 1985).

If any of these choices are exercised, such animals are predesignated in accordance with the protocol. At this time, it is also necessary to indicate the disposition of each and every animal received from the vendor for purposes of audit accountability. To accomplish this, the software package used for data collection first has to be "initialized". Specifically, the design of the study is "described" to the computer along with the number of test groups, their designation, and the number of animals in each group. The protocol should indicate when animals are to be killed for disease surveillance or for interim kill purposes; depending on the sophistication of the software package, the microprocessor can prompt the operator when one of these predesignated groups is to be utilized. However, if one of the designated animals dies prior to its utilization for disease surveillance or interim kill purposes, no substitution can be allowed. This maintains the integrity of the study design.

Designation of test groups by the use of letters or other "codes" and inclusion of predesignated subgroupings in the study design raise concerns when qualitative or subjective data (i.e., severity of clinical lesions, gradations of an animal's demeanor) are required by the study protocol. Practical attempts to shield treatment and other information about the study population from animal room staff members are often fruitless. To overcome potential and systematic biases, two equally qualified individuals are assigned to acquire subjective data on an alternating basis, or the various subgroupings may be statistically compared to ascertain that they are, in fact, similar. Such comparisons may provide insight into confounding factors among various subgroups (Lagakos and Mosteller, 1981).

V. HOUSING

A study conducted in compliance with GLP requires justification for the test model chosen. However, this exercise will probably have little impact on the usual choice of the rat, the mouse, or occasionally the hamster as the test animals for most toxicological studies, particularly for chronic studies. Regardless of the species chosen, individual housing of test animals is often preferred for statistical and health monitoring purposes (see Chapters 7, 9, and 17).

For chronic rodent studies, one may wish to house animals in plastic shoe box-type cages that can be equipped with filter tops to help minimize the spread of airborne infections. Use of softwood bedding in these cages can interfere with the objectives of some studies due to enzyme induction and/or toxicological components (Fox, 1977; Vlahakis, 1977). However, hardwood bedding should also be monitored for pentachlorophenol (PCP), because wood initially slated for furniture is usually treated with PCP then occasionally "recycled" for hardwood bedding. Cages are changed at least once a week or as frequently as necessary to keep the animals clean and dry and to minimize the accumulation of ammonia fumes (Fox, 1977). From the point of GLP compliance, if applicable protocols or standard operating procedures (SOPs) state that cages, water bottles, and feed cans should be cleaned/sanitized at specified intervals, a room log book to record such events is highly recommended since it provides an inspector with data concerning protocol and SOP compliance.

During the conduct of any chronic study, a significant number of cages become vacant as animals die, are euthanized, or are removed for various reasons. When a sufficient number of cage vacancies are created, economic and resource considerations (Cranmer et al., 1978, Lawrence et al., 1977, 1979) often dictate changes in cage position to eliminate such gaps. Mantel (1980) has suggested that a fixed cage position be maintained throughout the major portion of a chronic study. Some claim that knowing the animal's accurate location throughout a toxicological study will permit adequate analysis of environmental parameters (Lawrence et al., 1979); however, statistical difficulties often arise if consolidation involves fewer racks in fewer rooms (Lawrence et al., 1977).

VI. ANIMAL WEIGHING SUBSYSTEM

The animal weighing subsystem (AWS) is a software package used to systematize data collection. The operator is prompted through the data collection procedures, directly acquiring quantitative data via a scale microprocessor interface and recording qualitative data via a touch screen overlaid on the cathode ray tube (CRT). Unanticipated or infrequent observations may be entered into the system via the microprocessor keyboard and viewed on the screen, which is called the "notebook" or free text screen.

When the AWS is activated, the individual must identify himself or herself before the system will function. Each individual has a unique identification code assigned by the study director, which may be changed periodically to enhance security. The identification code also indicates whether the individual activating the system can enter data or only view data previously entered. Subsequently, the system prompts the individual to enter the study number, to ascertain that the proper diskettes are being accessed, and then the date, which, in the absence of an electronic calendar, allows entrance only to the subsystem subsequent to the date of the previous entry. When all these functions have been performed correctly, the operator is then prompted stepwise through each required/preprogrammed data acquisition operation.

Data pertinent to body weight are obtained by interfacing a scale with the microprocessor. The first step required in this operation is the calibration of the scale when a self-calibrating fully duplex scale is not used. When a self-calibrating scale is used, the microprocessor can be programmed to have the scale calibrate itself before each animal is weighed. With a noncalibrated scale, the system can be programmed to prompt the operator to calibrate the scale with an appropriate series of weights. The program will not proceed unless the calibration is performed and each weight is accurate to within a specified range. When this step is completed, the video screen will display the first animal's identification code and prompt the operator to weigh the animal, its "old" (current week's) feed container, and its "new" (next week's) feed container.

The practice of weighing all test animals in the same weighing vehicle increases the potential for spreading communicable diseases and parasites among the study animals. Lawrence et al. (1979) have recommended weighing each animal in the pretared clean cage that the animal will reside in during the subsequent week, which also means that animal handling is reduced during the cage changing/body weighing procedure. However, unless the animal handler either washes his or her hands or uses a clean set of disposable gloves for each animal, the chance of "passing" disease organisms and parasites still exists. For transferring mice, one can use forceps dipped in alcohol after each animal is handled and move the animals via their tail, but this practice is not advocated because it may result in unnecessary pain to the animal. However, due to the close proximity of test animals, any infectious disease that has established itself in the animal room will likely spread whenever conventional and/or practical methods of animal handling are used.

All body weight data entered into the subsystem are checked against the previous weeks' body weight. Weights that exceed the preprogrammed range for reasonableness are brought to the operator's attention for verification. Because major weight changes during the conduct of a chronic rodent study usually occur during the first few weeks of the test, the preprogrammed range may be larger for this period.

Following acquisition of the first data set by the AWS during the quarantine period, subsequent weekly determinations of body, feed bowl, and/or water bottle weights will result in a greater amount of information being displayed on the CRT. For example, the change in body weight and the amount of feed and/or water consumed during the previous week is displayed for use by the animal technician as part of our health monitoring program (see Chapter 17; Arnold et al., 1977). Rats that have been on test for more than 80 weeks often lose up to 25% of their maximum body weight over a several week period, although their health status is satisfactory. Consequently, the subsystem can be programmed to compare the present week's body weight against the previously recorded maximum body weight value for purposes of health monitoring.

When all required weighings have been performed, the next screen to appear lists approximately 30 terms describing adverse health effects. The individual undertaking this clinical examination (see Chapter 17; Arnold et al., 1977;) may select up to 5 terms to describe any findings. The list also includes terms to indicate when an animal is removed from the test (i.e., for quality control testing, terminal kill or euthanizia) or has died on test. Selection of these terms directs the microprocessor's subsystem not to accept any subsequent entries for this animal. At the next weekly determination of body weight, etc., all adverse health terms recorded during the previous week's clinical examination are displayed on the CRT. Also available in this menu is a term requesting that a detailed clinical examination be performed. When such an examination is required, the request is also recorded (i.e., transferred) to the detailed clinical examination subsystem to be described. During the current superficial clinical examination, the operator may indicate via the touch screen that there are no changes in the terms selected for the previous week's clinical, or other terms may be chosen.

The number of animals dying on test and the number of autolyzed animals serve as good indicators of the effectiveness of a health monitoring program. Animals should remain on test for as long as reasonably possible, providing they do not appear to be moribund or in pain. Killing moribund animals ensures that tissue specimens are useful for pathological evaluation. By applying appropriate criteria (see Chapter 17; Arnold *et al.,* 1977, 1980,) for euthanasia of moribund animals, it is possible to reduce the incidence of animals dying on test during a chronic study to approximately 5% of the initial test population and to reduce the losses due to autolysis to less than 1%.

Before any data gathering session is terminated, the program requires that the newly acquired data be "backed up". The data from the weekly diskettes should be subsequently transferred to a minicomputer for storage on magnetic tapes either in-house or in a host (large) computer facility (HCF). Simple statistical analysis for treatment effects on body weight or feed consumption can be done on a weekly basis. Observations made during the superficial clinical evaluation may be summarized but may only be included in a weekly summary of study data, if the incidence rate of a specific observation is at least 10% in any test group and the observation has been made for two consecutive weeks for the same animal. Such procedures avoid cluttering the summary with possible transient observations.

VII. DETAILED CLINICAL SUBSYSTEM

As its name implies, the detailed clinical subsystem (DCS) involves an extensive examination of a test animal for signs of toxicity and changes in health. The person performing the detailed clinical examination must have sufficient experience with diseases of the test species if observations are to be valid. The DCS is activated and operated in a manner analogous to the AWS. For ease of discussion, this subsystem is described as a stand-alone subsystem. With rodent studies, we have integrated it with the AWS; however, for a study in which larger animals are used, the two subsystems are independent. For example, when monkeys are used, feed and water consumption and menstrual cycle status (i.e., bleeding or not) are determined daily in addition to a visual clinical examination. Consequently, minor variations in subsystem programming can be tailored to study needs.

Following activation of the system, the initial screen contains a summary of the clinical finding(s) from the AWS, the animal's number, and the animal's body weight and feed consumption for the previous week. The DCS will then prompt the operator to perform specific functions, such as determining the animal's present body and feed-can weight. The program can then prompt the operator to perform a urinary "dip-stick" evaluation (i.e., test for the presence of glucose, ketones, bilirubin, protein, and blood), a visual examination of the animal (i.e., haircoat, excrement, etc.), and/or an external palpation of the animal's visera (see Chapter 17). Each screen contains a header term for the activity to be performed and a list of symptomatic terms. In addition, when cysts or other palpable masses are found, the dimensions and location are recorded. Selection of a clinical term(s) is accomplished by touching the screen at the appropriate location. The microprocessor then inserts an asterisk to indicate the selected term. In subsequent weeks, the previous week's selection of terms are indicated to the left of the term and the current selection to its right. The list of clinical terms displayed on the screen are comprehensible to a layperson, but the data retained on the floppy disk uses SNOMED (Systemized Nomenclature of Medicine; see Côté, 1977; Beckett, 1977; Donnelly, 1977; Gantner, 1977; Percy *et al.,* 1977 for additional information) coding to facilitate correlation of gross pathological findings with histological observations when appropriate. If an incorrect term is selected, provisions to delete data prior to its transfer to the floppy disk do exist. However, once the operator completes the evaluation of an animal and the data is written on the disk, no data in the animal's file can subsequently be changed via the touch screen or keyboard. When data correction is necessary, the operator must initiate a written request to the study director indicating the reason for the requested change. If the study director approves the request, the change can be executed either on the floppy disk prior to its transmission to the host computer facility (HCF) or by the HCF. The original observation and requested change are retained as part of the study's raw data.

Detailed clinicals may be performed on a scheduled, periodic basis when each animal is examined; or only specific animals may be examined. For example, during the weekly body weight determination and clinical examination, one of the terms available is a "request" to have a detailed clinical examination performed. This information is then transferred from the AWS to the DCS. The DCS indicates to the operator which animals require a detailed examination. Once the AWS data or personal examination of the test animals have been reviewed, additional animals can be added to the list of animals that the DCS subsystem has prompted for examination. At the beginning of a chronic study, detailed clinical examinations need be scheduled only monthly if dosages are properly selected. However, as the animals get older and the incidences of toxicological signs (particularly those having a pathological origin) and geriatric diseases increase, there will be a greater requirement for detailed clinical examinations. Animals whose health has deteriorated to the point at which daily monitoring of body weight and water and feed consumption is required are placed in a separate bank of cages and possibly may undergo frequent detailed examinations. These cages are designated as the intensive observation unit (IOU; Arnold *et al.*, 1977) and allow for frequent visual observations as a means of minimizing the number of animals dying on test. An animal's stay in the IOU should be of short duration (i.e., usually a week or two), due solely to its deteriorating health; therefore, it would have no impact on the statistical analysis of environmental parameters previously mentioned.

When an animal is to be euthanized, the data contained in its detailed clinical file is available to the pathologist prior to necropsy. The study director can review the data, thereby monitoring the progress of the study. This review may lead to protocol amendments requiring additional clinical tests to evaluate toxicological manifestations.

VIII. PATHOLOGY SUBSYSTEM

The major responsibilities placed on the pathologist for nonclinical laboratory studies are outlined in Chapter 2. The major emphasis in this section pertains to the recording aspects of the histopathological data.

A thorough and accurate assessment of all gross and histopathological lesions is a fundamental requirement for the interpretation and extrapolation of study results. The methods and quality control procedures utilized in the National Cancer Institute's Carcinogenesis Testing Program, as well as related concerns (Ward *et al.*, 1978), should be addressed by all pathologists involved with toxicological studies.

The decision to euthanize any animal is a joint one among a senior animal technician or the animal laboratory veterinarian, the study director, and the pathologist participating in the study. The need to minimize the loss of potential tissue specimens due to autolysis has to be balanced against biasing the survivability data. Therefore, for the euthanasia program to be effective, the criteria for euthanasia must be clearly defined (see Chapter 17) and adherance ensured.

The pathology subsystem (PS) consists of components to record gross observation data during necropsy, significant observations during tissue trimming and sampling, and histopathological data. Data are entered into the microprocessor via a separate routine. The procedure at necropsy allows for entry of body and organ weight data and requires entry of terminal hematological, bacteriological, or other samples taken. A free text entry mode is used to record all significant observations at the time of tissue trimming, selection, and sampling. Because the histopathological evaluation process often requires that lesions be examined several times or by more than one pathologist before a final diagnosis is made, the free text entry will retain all comments in a chronological order. To assist pathologists in the histopathological evaluation process, they are allowed access to review data acquired by the AWS and DCS.

The PS is activated in the same manner as the other subsystems. Following its activation, the operator of the PS is prompted via the CRT to select one of the three available routines (necropsy, tissue selection and sampling, or histopathology). In addition, a query function exists if the operator wishes to view data entered previously. When an animal is to be necroposied, the operator is prompted to identify the animal, then the system verifies that the animal is a member of the study population. Some laboratories often assign a pathology number to each animal as opposed to using the animal's unique identification code. Such a procedure helps to assure that the pathologist's evaluations, both macro and micro, are conducted in an unbiased or "blind" manner; however, it is a somewhat controversial procedure (Weinberger, 1973; Fears and Schneiderman, 1974; Zbinden, 1976; Fears and Douglas, 1978; Prasse et al., 1986; Arnold et al., 1988).

The program will then prompt the operator to identify the entire necropsy team via the keyboard. This requirement is included for GLP purposes so that the number and qualifications of the personnel performing the task can be easily ascertained. Additionally, as pointed out by Frith et al., (1978), the identification of individuals involved in fixing, sampling, and staining tissues, as well as in blocking and monitoring specimens, can be used as a managerial and quality control measure. Next, the system will prompt the operator to indicate an animal's general condition and the method and reason for sacrifice (i.e., was the animal's death a component of the disease surveillance program or a required interim kill, due to poor health, or did the animal die on test).

The pathologist or parapathologist who conducts the necropsy examination may dictate the information to a technical clerk who operates the microprocessor and enters the data. The necropsy component is programmed in a manner similar to the other subsystems in that all functions required by the protocol to be performed during the necropsy are displayed on the CRT. Once the operator indicates that the data entry for that animal is complete, the operator cannot change any data entered unless authorized by the study director. Therefore, to minimize erroneous input, the clerk asks the pathologist to confirm all entries on each screen prior to recording the information on the disk. Some laboratories prefer the pathologists to dictate all findings into a tape recorder for subsequent entry into their data system.

The exact sequence of events during necropsy depends on the requirements in the protocol. For example, if samples of liver or other organs are required for biochemical, enzyme histochemistry, or electron microscopic studies, it is imperative that such samples be obtained as soon as possible after the animal has been exsanguinated. The microprocessor can prompt for each organ that is to be weighed in a fixed sequence. Subsequently, the microprocessor verifies that all samples required by the protocol (i.e., hematology, bacteriology, immunology, biochemistry, analytical chemistry, electron microscopy, etc.) have been obtained. Any missing specimens are brought to the attention of the operator.

When the pathologist wishes to record an observation, a screen listing a topographical index or field can be displayed and the particular organ indicated. The screen with the morphological index can then be displayed and the term(s) that represent appropriate change(s) can be indicated via the touch screen. Edit functions conducted during necropsy ascertain that observations specific to one sex are not entered for an animal of the opposite sex (Kellenbenz *et al.*, 1978). For any changes in paired organs (kidney, testis, adrenals, etc.), the program specifies whether it is a unilateral or bilateral effect. Status reports provide the current number of animals still on test as opposed to the number of animals that have been necropsied; any discrepancies are indicated (Henry and Johnson, 1979).

Most laboratories do not ascertain organ weights for euthanized, moribund animals being necropsied during a chronic study because of the small sample size and the confounding factor of time when data are statistically analyzed. If organ weights are deemed necessary, they can best be handled through the use of serial or terminal kills, which minimize the effect of tumorigenic processes and the consequences of the animal's morbidity (i.e., dehydration/starvation) on organ weights. The microprocessor, in accordance with the applicable SOP, indicates which organs and in what sequence they are to be weighed. A member of the necropsy team prepares the organs for weighing by trimming off any extraneous tissue (i.e. fat, connective tissue, etc.) and placing each on the scale that has been interfaced with the microprocessor.

When the necropsy is completed, all unexamined/unselected components of the carcass are often discarded. For a rodent study, it is suggested that the remaining carcass be retained for a finite period until an initial histopathological examination has been undertaken.

After necropsy, tissues are sampled prior to being processed for histology. Tissue sampling in our laboratory is usually conducted by the pathologist; the microprocessor operator may be either the pathologist or a technical clerk. After activating the PS, the pathologist can elicit from the PS program which animal's tissues require sampling. The pathologist can then review the necropsy findings and add any significant observations made during tissue sectioning via the touch screen. In addition, terms not available in the listing can be added via the keyboard. Once the pathologist has no further data to enter and has indicated to the PS that all tissues listed on the microprocessor's CRT have been sampled, no additional terms can be added or changed without approval of the study director.

The histopathological evaluation of tissues and organs is the only major procedure that cannot be performed with the assistance of system prompts. For this evaluation, the operator first selects a particular organ or tissue from the list provided on the CRT screen. The list contains all tissues and organs required by the protocol or any for which an evaluation has not been completed. For the selected organ or tissue, the system displays all possible SNOMED terms so that lesions can be classify in conformance with the SNOMED system of classification. Additionally, descriptive terminology or other "notes" and pertinent information from the evaluation can be manually entered into the system via the keyboard.

Our quality control program for the PS requires that an entry be made for each animal tissue and organ stipulated in the study protocol. Any omissions can be listed when the pathologist commands the program to proceed from one animal to the next. In appropriate situations, the entry may indicate that the tissue was examined but no remarkable lesions were observed; or the tissue was not available with an explanation as to why the tissue could not be evaluated adequately (i.e., due to autolysis, improper processing, etc.).

IX. HOST COMPUTER FACILITY

The host computer facility (HCF) refers to an internal or external computer facility that has a number of responsibilities including storing/banking of all electronic raw data during the conduct of a study, preparing periodic data summaries, and performing many other data manipulation exercises. Other functions can include performing authorized changes to the data base and preparing necessary software to verify whether data sent by modem was received intact.

As previously described, data are initially recorded on floppy disks by microprocessors. These data may be accumulated on hard disk or magnetic tape then sent to the HCF or sent directly from floppy disks to the HCF via a telephone modem.

The HCF may provide the means necessary for a statistical analysis of the data under the direction of the study statistician. Many statistical analysis procedures are available from commercial sources, but unique experimental situations may require the adaptation of statistical procedures for the analysis of biological data not previously considered (Arnold and Bickis, 1980; Arnold et al., 1983).

The HCF retains electronically acquired data until a final study report is generated and accepted by management or the sponsor. All tapes or records are then returned to the study director for archive storage in compliance with GLP.

X. QUALITY ASSURANCE UNIT

"A testing facility shall have a quality assurance unit composed of one or more individuals who shall be responsible for monitoring each study to assure management that the facilities, equipment, personnel, methods, practices, records, and controls are in conformance with the regulations in this part" (U.S. FDA, 1978). As indicated, the quality assurance unit (QAU) oversees the conduct of a GLP study at the bench or animal room level for management.

The staff of the QAU audits data to ascertain whether the computer system is handling all functions in the manner intended. QA personnel can check for errors in the following ways:

1. They can determine who entered the data into the system.
2. They can evaluate check procedures for data reasonableness.
3. They can determine how data is stored, what kinds of report are generated, and who has access to stored data and/or reports generated.
4. They can determine how data are manipulated for report purposes; that is, data statistically evaluated; are programs available for testing the accuracy of the data handling system to ascertain that it functioned as desired?
5. They can determine the status and adequacy of the systems documentation.
6. They can determine how errors of input or possibly errors of software origin are assessed and corrected.
7. They can evaluate security procedures.

"Any significant problems which are likely to affect study integrity found during the course of an inspection [by the QAU] shall be brought to the attention of the study director and management immediately" (U.S. EPA, 1978). Solving problems as soon as possible is necessary both to maintain good scientific practices and to curb costs resulting from slovenly practices. Consequently, the QAU staff can best perform their function if they are highly trained members who act as managements' eyes and ears while they assist the study director by pointing out any inappropriate procedures before these become problems. For more information on the QAU, see Chapter 22.

XI. DISCUSSION

The necessity of acquiring and storing data in an "error-free" manner is paramount for good science and compliance with GLP. There is an obvious need for computer systems to accomplish these requirements in a nonclinical laboratory setting. Many benefits can be derived from the use of a computer system: enhanced study management and acquisition of validated data are two. Computers allow one to obtain study status reports on a daily basis. Being able to review data immediately after they are collected assists the study director in detecting unexpected trends or findings, such as a greater than expected toxicity, an unusual clinical sign or pathological lesion, or a change in spontaneous tumor latency periods. Armed with this timely information, a study director, in consultation with the appropriate participating scientists, can amend an experimental protocol to accommodate such contingencies without dramatically altering or prematurely terminating the experiment. He or she also can initiate additional procedures in a timely manner to investigate such unexpected observations.

Areas in which experimental design and interpretation might be improved by the timely access to study data includes:

1. Choice of study subpopulations: some researchers intentionally select the most homogenous subset of animals from the potential test population for monitoring selected blood and urine parameters (Bare *et al.,* 1978), whereas others monitor their study animals via longitudinal periodic monitoring (Stavric, 1980). Nonrandom selection of test animals or study subgroups for monitoring will, in most cases, unnecessarily bias the data.
2. Effect of cage position on experimental observations (Lagakos and Mosteller, 1980; Mantel, 1980).
3. Usefulness of the interim kill for detecting early pathological changes or for differentiating toxic effects from those caused by aging.

XII. FUTURE TRENDS

In recent years, more and more data, such as that collected in the hematological (see Chapter 18), clinical chemistry (see Chapter 19), or immunological laboratory (see Chapter 16), are electronically captured at the source. However, getting these instruments to communicate with a computer handling data often depends on the resourcefulness of in-house personnel to develop interfaces for such equipment. Recording animal room temperatures and humidity, controlling and recording animal room light cycles, monitoring cage washing machines by recording water temperatures and halting operations whenever the minimal water temperature is not achieved, and prompting diet preparers to weigh out X grams of each component are recent extensions of this technology. To reduce data gaps regarding fundamental aspects of experimental design and conduct that were previously mentioned, computers handling toxicological data should contain data management software that can allow examination of data in novel ways. Statistical software packages to prepare graphs and other visual aids for data evaluation are soon to be the norm and should improve study protocols, study conduct, and data evaluation, interpretation, and extrapolation.

Acknowledgments

The authors wish to thank Drs. J. J. Berky, P. D. Lepore, D. W. Taylor, and Mr. D. Legault for their comments, Mr. A. Peterkin for his assistance in preparing the chapter, and Ms. Patsy Matcheskie for her typing assistance.

References

Arnold, D. L., and Bickis, M. G. (1980). The effect of sodium saccharin on several urinary constituents of the rat and the statistical evaluation thereof. "Proceedings, Saccharin Working Group of the Toxicology Forum, Given Institute of Pathology, Aspen, Colorado", pp. 71–86. Washington, DC: International Life Sciences Institute.

Arnold, D. L., Charbonneau, S. M., Zawidzka, Z. Z., and Grice, H. C. (1977). Monitoring animal health during chronic toxicity studies. *J. Environ. Pathol. Toxicol.* **1**, 227–239.

Arnold, D. L., Farber, E., and Krewski, D. (1988). Carcinogenicity testing: Histopathology and the blind method. *Comments Toxicol.* **2**, 67–80.

Arnold, D. L., Fox, J. G., Thibert, P., and Grice, H. C. (1978). Toxicology studies. I. Support personnel. *Food Cosmet. Toxicol.* **16**, 479–484.

Arnold, D. L., Krewski, D. R., Junkins, D. B., McGuire, P. F., Moodie, C. A., and Munro, I. C. (1983). Reversibility of ethylenethiourea-induced thyroid lesions. *Toxicol. Appl. Pharmacol.* **67**, 264–273.

Arnold, D. L., Moodie, C. A., Grice, H. C., Charbonneau, S. M., Stavric, B., Collins, B. T., McGuire, P. F., Zawidzka, Z. Z., and Munro, I. C. (1980). Long-term toxicity of ortho-toluenesulfonamide and sodium saccharin in the rat. *Toxicol. Appl. Pharmacol.* **52**, 113–152.

Balk, M. W. (1983). Overview of the state of the art in health monitoring. *In* "The Importance of Laboratory Animal Genetics, Health, and the Environment in Biomedical Research" (E. C. Melby, Jr., and M. W. Balk, eds.) pp. 3–23. New York: Academic Press.

Bare, J. J., Janakiraman, T., Phillips, B. M., Platt, R. D., and Whitesell, J. H., Jr. (1978). A computer system and statistical methodology for the analysis of blood and urine chemistry data in laboratory animals. *Drug Inf. J.* **12**, 141–147.

Beckett, R. S. (1977). History of coding nomenclature in a general hospital medical records department. *Pathologist* **31**, 395–401.

Côté, R. A. (1977). The SNOP-SNOMED concept: Evolution towards a common medical nomenclature and classification. *Pathologist* **31**, 383–389.

Cranmer, M. F., Lawrence, L. R., Konvicka, A. J., and Herrick, S. S. (1978). NCTR computer systems designed for toxicologic experimentation. I. Overview. *J. Environ. Pathol. Toxicol.* **1**, 701–709.

Donnelly, W. H. (1977). Application of SNOMED to state-wide data banks. *Pathologist* **31**, 404–407.

European Chemical Industry Ecology & Toxicologic Center (1979). "Good Laboratory Practice" (Monogr. No. 1). Brussels, Belgium: European Chemical Industry Ecology & Toxicology Center.

Food Chemical News (1986). FDA inspections to cover GLP software validation. *Food Chem. News* **28**, 20–24.

Fears, T. R., and Douglas, J. F. (1978). Suggested procedures for reducing the pathology workload in a carcinogen bioassay program, Part II: Incorporation blind pathology techniques and analysis for animals with tumors. *J. Environ. Pathol. Toxicol.* **1**, 211–222.

Fears, T. R., and Schneiderman, M. A. (1974). Pathologic evaluation and the blind technique. *Science* **183**, 1144–1145.

Fox, J. G. (1977). Clinical assessment of laboratory rodents on long term bioassay studies. *J. Environ. Pathol. Toxicol.* **1**, 199–226.

Fox, J. G., Thibert, P., Arnold, D. L., Krewski, D. R., and Grice, H. C. (1979). Toxicology studies. II. The laboratory animal. *Food Cosmet. Toxicol.* **17**, 661–675.

Frith, C. H., Zamie, J., and Herrick, S. S. (1978). Computer assisted quality control program in a large pathology laboratory. *Bull. Soc. Pharmacol. Environ. Pathol.* **6**, 20–25.

Gantner, G. E. (1977). History of coding. *Pathologist* **31**, 390–394.

Goeke, J. E., Hoberman, A. M., and Christian, M. S. (1984). Quality assurance validation of computerized toxicology data. *J. Am. Coll. Toxicol.* **3**, 121–124.

The Gold Sheet (1985). Computer documentation. *Gold Sheet* **19**, 1–4.

Hamm, T. E., Jr. (1985). Design of a long-term animal bioassay for carcinogenicity. *In* "Handbook of Carcinogen Testing" H. A. Milman and E. K. Weisburger, eds.), pp. 252–281. Park Ridge, New Jersey: Noyes Publication.

Henry, R. L., and Johnson, C. R. (1979). Pathology data quality assurance and data retrieval at the National Center for Toxicological Research. *J. Environ. Pathol. Toxicol.* **3**, 169–178.

Kellenbenz, A., Mosher, A. H., Teal, T. W., and Crocco, R. M. (1978). An interactive pathology/toxicology computer system. *Drug Inf. J.* **12**, 174–180.

Iverson, F., Lok, E., Nera, E., Karpinski, K., and Clayson, D. B. (1985). A 13-week feeding study of butylated hydroxyanisole: The subsequent regression of the induced lesions in male Fischer 344 rat forestomach epithelium. *Toxicology* **35**, 1–11.

Legakos, S., and Mosteller, F. (1981). A care study of statistics in the regulatory process: The FD&C Red No. 40 experiments. *J. Natl. Cancer Inst. (US)* **66**, 197–212.

Lane-Petter, W. (1963). The physical environment of rats and mice. *In* "Animals for Research: Principles of Breeding and Management" (W. Lane-Petter, ed.), pp. 1–20. New York: Academic Press.

Lawrence, L. R., Konvicka, A. J., Ezell, R., Appleget, J., Green, G., Fernstron, E. B., and Johnson, C. R. (1979). NCTR computer systems designed for toxicologic experimentation. IV. Experiment information system. *J. Environ. Pathol. Toxicol.* **2**, 1011–1019.

Lawrence, L. R., Konvicka, A. J., and Herrick, S. S. (1977). Information systems as utilized by the National Center for Toxicological Research. *Drug Inf. J.* **11**, 104–108.

Mantel, N. (1980). Assessing laboratory evidence for neoplastic activity. *Biometrics* **361**, 381–399.

Organization for Economic Co-operation and Development (1982). "Good Laboratory Practice in the Testing of Chemicals; Final Report of the Group of Experts on Good Laboratory Practice." Paris: Organization for Economic Co-operation and Development.

Percy, C., Henson, D., Thomas, L. B., and Graepel, P. (1977). International classification of diseases for oncology (ICD-O). *Pathologist* **31**, 402–403.

Prasse, K., Hilderbrandt, P., Dodd, D., Goodman, D., Leader, R., Ferrell, J., Squire, R., Hardisty, J., Newberne, J., Hilderbrandt, P., Burek, J., De Paoli, A., Boorman, G., Bendele, R., Payne, B., Ward, J., Todd, G., Webster, H., Piper, R., and Patterson, R. (1986). Letter to the editor. *Toxicol. Appl. Pharmacol.* **83**, 184–185.

Stavric, B. (1980). The effect of saccharin upon urinary and serum protein in mature rats. "Proceedings, Saccharin Working Group of the Toxicology Forum, Aspen, Colorado," pp. 86–93. Washington, DC: International Life Sciences Institute.

U.S. Environmental Protection Agency (1983a). Toxic substances control; Good laboratory practice standards; Final rule. *Fed. Regist.* **48**, 53922–53944.

U.S. Environmental Protection Agency (1983b). Pesticide programs; Good laboratory practice standards; Final rule. *Fed. Regist.* **48**, 53946–53969.

U.S. Food and Drug Administration (1978). Nonclinical laboratory studies, good laboratory practice regulations. *Fed. Regist.* **43**, 59986–60020.

U.S. Food and Drug Administration (1987). Good laboratory practice regulations, final rule. *Fed. Regist.* **51**, 33768–33782.

Vlahakis, G. (1977). Brief communication: Possible carcinogenic effects of cedar shavings in bedding of C3H-A^{v}y fB mice. *J. Natl. Cancer Inst. (US)* **58**, 149–150.

Ward, J. M., Goodman, D. G., Griesemer, R. A., Hardisty, J. F., Schueler, R. L., Squire, R. A., and Strandberg, J. D. (1978). Quality assurance for pathology in rodent carcinogenesis tests. *J. Environ. Pathol. Toxicol.* **2**, 371–378.

Weihe, W. H. (1971). The significance of the physical environment for the health and state of adaptation of laboratory animals. *In* "Defining the Laboratory Animal," pp. 353–378. Washington, DC: National Academy of Sciences.

Weinberger, M. A. (1973). The blind technique. *Science* **181**, 219–220.

Zbinden, G. (ed.) (1976). *Progress In Toxicology: Special Topics* **2**, 14–15. Berlin: Springer-Verlag.

Part VII
Data Analysis and Evaluation

24
Statistical Analysis

M. J. Goddard
Environmental Health Directorate
Health Protection Branch
Health and Welfare Canada
Ottawa, Canada

R. T. Burnett
Environmental Health Directorate
Health Protection Branch
Health and Welfare Canada
Ottawa, Canada

B. T. Collins
Canadian Wildlife Service
Environment Canada
Ottawa, Canada

D. J. Murdoch
Department of Statistics and Actuarial Science
University of Waterloo
Waterloo, Canada

I. Introduction
II. Analysis of a Single Continuous Variable
    A. Comparison of a Treatment with a Control Diet
    B. Analysis of Several Unrelated Treatment Groups
    C. Analysis of a Graded Set of Diets
    D. More Complex Designs
III. Analysis of Growth Curve Data
    A. Multivariate Linear Models
    B. Biologically Motivated Nonlinear Models
    C. Nonparametric and Robust Methods
IV. Categorical Data
V. Statistical Analysis of Survival Data
    A. The Model
    B. Parametric Methods
    C. Nonparametric Methods

Handbook of
In Vivo Toxicity Testing

611

I. INTRODUCTION

The nature of data produced and experimental designs employed by *in vivo* toxicity tests is extremely varied. As a result, an experimenter must have some familiarity with the broad spectrum of statistical techniques used in this field. Given this wide spectrum of methodology that is possibly of interest and the intricate nature of much of this material, it is not reasonable to expect a statistician, let alone a toxicologist, to be fully aware of the assumptions, techniques, and pitfalls of all the different methods. Special situations require specialized statistical, as well as toxicological, expertise.

It is, therefore, impossible to treat the subject of statistical methodology comprehensively in one chapter. As a result, our prime purposes in this chapter are to indicate the range of analyses available, to provide the investigator with a means to identify the statistical problem faced, and to indicate where further material can be sought. Occasionally, it is feasible to provide a few detailed instructions. In most cases, however, the investigator is encouraged to seek professional statistical advice. Another of our aims herein is to provide the investigator with a basis for understanding some ideas underlying the advice given. Other works presenting an overview of statistics in toxicological studies include Gad and Weil (1982, 1986) and Salsburg (1986).

There are five substantive sections that follow. Each attempts to provide advice on a specific type of data. The subsections are not unrelated; similar comments and approaches may be discussed in different sections. Where this occurs, the context specific for the problem at hand is emphasized.

After an investigator has decided on the objectives and toxicological procedures for a study, he or she must think about the form of analysis even before initiating the study. The decision as to which method will be used depends on many things, and statisticians often broadly categorize methods by the nature of the "response" variate of interest. In the next few paragraphs, we attempt to describe this broad categorization and indicate how the remainder of this chapter is organized based on this. It is worth noting that this discussion is meant to be instructive rather than exhaustive.

In many toxicological experiments, the main objective involves the measurement of one important variable. Often, a test is made to see if this is related to other variables. A primary distinction is whether this "response" variable is "continuous" or "discrete". Time-to-tumor development and body weight are examples of continuous variates, whereas "clear"/"red"/"blue" and "presence"/"absence" of a tumor are discrete responses.

Continuous variates are considered first, with further distinction made between those that have limits and those that do not. Some distributions allow for negative values (for example, a weight difference, which can be negative, zero, or positive). Other distributions are used for variates that are not negative (for example, the time to tumor). A large body of statistical methodology has developed for normally distributed continuous variables, and this is often described under an umbrella title as the analysis of variance (ANOVA). Recently, there has been considerable interest in the study of "survival" data, particularly in the time to tumor development or time to animal death. Although these methods are also applicable when time is not the variable of interest, the experimenter usually is drawn to this area because time is of prime concern. The decision as to which continuous distribution is appropriate is not simple. Even after the clearly inappropriate distributions are eliminated, several feasible alternatives may exist, and the final choice may require a study of complicated mathematical properties of data and distributions.

There are several categories of discrete-type data. The simplest case is the "binary" in which only one of two possible outcomes occurs. Tumor absence or presence is one example. When there are three or more discrete outcomes, one must determine whether there is an order to the outcomes or not. An example of an ordered discrete variable is the graded size of a tumor in an animal, with possible outcomes being 0, +, ++, or +++, where 0 is less than +, which itself is less than ++ ("less" referring to the size of the tumor mass). An unordered variate might be a type of tumor (e.g., bladder, liver, or pulmonary) that is not graded as "worse" or "better" than the other.

The following sections present material categorized by the nature of the response variate. If it is a continuous variate, then the traditional analysis of variance, described in Section II, may be of major interest. One particular form of traditional analysis is used when "growth curve" analyses are involved. Usually, there will be a sequence of observations on many individuals, with each individual being observed several times. The various attitudes and approaches to this form of analysis are discussed in Section III. The analysis of discrete or "categorical" data is discussed in Section IV. If a continuous variate is the time to a certain event, usually a more complicated methodology is appropriate, and this is discussed in Section V. Section VI is devoted to the analysis of pathological data. One particular type of study in which the analysis of categorical and survival data is combined is presented in this section. Some comments pertaining to the relevance of all response variates and analyses are found in the last section.

II. ANALYSIS OF A SINGLE CONTINUOUS VARIABLE

In this section, we describe procedures for the analysis of a single continuous variable. Some examples of this type of data from toxicological studies are (1) body weight and hematological parameters at a fixed point of time and (2) residue levels and organ weights at the time of death. To give some specificity to the presentation, we consider the analysis of body weight at a fixed age and assume the simplest experiment is of interest with two groups of animals, one fed a control and one fed a diet containing the test substance ("treated" diet).

A. Comparison of a Treatment with a Control Diet

The basic goal of the study is to determine if the treated diet has an effect on body weight. For each diet group, the observed body weights have a distribution over a range of values that reflect the differences among individuals. With statistical analysis, we can assess whether the distribution of the body weights varies among the diets rather than whether the individual body weights differ. For example, if the treated diet reduced body weight gain, then an animal on the treated diet would be smaller than one on the control diet in general; but it could be that some of the largest animals on the treated diet were heavier than some of the smallest animals fed the control diet, that is, the ranges of the two distributions could overlap.

Statistical hypothesis testing is based on assessing whether or not a particular outcome is likely to have occurred when the null hypothesis is true. Under the null hypothesis we assume that the difference in diets has no effect on body weight and the observed distributions are essentially identical. Under the alternative hypothesis, we assume that the distribution of weights under the diets differ. In performing a statistical test, we can either reject or not reject the null hypothesis. Rejecting the null hypothesis when it is true is called a type I error, whereas not rejecting it when it is false is called a type II error. The standard statistical practice is to choose an allowable level for the type I error (usually 5%), called the level of significance for the test. The type II error is more difficult to control because it depends on the magnitude of the difference between the diets. It is usually controlled in the experimental design by the selection of an adequate sample size (Chapter 8).

Because the animals have been allocated at random, the extent to which the distributions can be expected to differ can be assessed. There are two basic types of procedures: parametric and nonparametric analysis. In a parametric analysis, it is assumed that the underlying distribution has some specific form characterized by parameters; for example, the normal distribution has two parameters, the mean and the variance. A hypothesis test can be constructed from a mathematical analysis of the distribution. In a nonparametric analysis, no assumption about the form of the distribution is made and the hypothesis is tested with procedures that are valid for any underlying distribution. In general, a nonparametric analysis is less powerful than a parametric analysis when the assumptions of the parametric analysis are true. Some statisticians feel that the loss of efficiency is small compared to the advantage of not imposing dubious assumptions.

In the classical parametric analysis of the simple two-diet experiment, it is assumed that the weights have a normal distribution. Under this assumption, all information in each sample is summarized by the sample means and variances. Assume that there are n_1 control and n_2 treated animals. Let y_{ij} denote the weight of the jth animal fed diet i (i $= 1$ control, i $= 2$ treated). The sample means $(\bar{y}_i)$ and variances (s_i^2) are defined by

$$\bar{y}_i = \frac{1}{n_i} \sum_{j=1}^{n_i} y_{ij} \tag{1}$$

and

$$s_i^2 = \frac{1}{(n_i - 1)} \sum_{j=1}^{n_i} (y_{ij} - \bar{y}_i)^2. \tag{2}$$

The sample mean and variance are estimates of the population mean (μ_i) and variance (σ_i^2). The variance is further assumed to be identical across all groups, hence the two variance estimates can be pooled:

$$s^2 = \frac{(n_1 - 1)\, s_1^2 + (n_2 - 1)\, s_2^2}{n_1 + n_2 - 2}. \tag{3}$$

The hypothesis that the means of the two distributions are identical is then tested with a t test:

$$t^* = \frac{\bar{y}_1 - \bar{y}_2}{\left[\left(\dfrac{1}{n_1} + \dfrac{1}{n_2}\right)s^2\right]^{1/2}}, \tag{4}$$

which is compared against the critical value of a t distribution with $n_1 + n_2 - 2$ degrees of freedom. (Degrees of freedom is the only parameter of the t distribution and is a measure of the amount of information used in the estimate of the variance.)

The assumptions made in this analysis are not trivial and should be evaluated to ensure that the analysis is appropriate. The assumption of normality can be assessed with graphic procedures (Chambers *et al.*, 1983) or with a G test for goodness of fit (Sokal and Rohlf, 1981). The assumption of equality of variances can be assessed with the Bartlett–Box F test (Sokal and Rohlf, 1981).

If the assumptions are violated, then it may be possible to transform the data to achieve homogeneity of variance or to make the distribution of the observations more like the normal distribution. Logarithmic transformations are often used when residue levels are analyzed. Once a data set has been transformed, it must be remembered that the analysis has been done on a different variable. Reexpressing the results for the original variable in the original scale must be done carefully. For example, the antilog of the mean on a log scale is not the same as the estimate of the mean on the original scale. There is a wide range of possible transformations, the best known system being that of Box and Cox (1964).

Plotting of data can be useful to aid in selecting a suitable transformation or to reveal irregularities in the data. Examination of the plots may reveal outliers (discordant observations) that should be examined closely. It may be reasonable to set these values aside and analyze the remaining data, or it may be decided to include them in the analysis. Outliers may be the most interesting points in the data set (American Society for Testing Materials, 1987).

If the assumption of normality seems appropriate but the variances are not equal, then approximate tests similar in form to the t test are available (Dunnett, 1980). If the assumption that the data are described by the normal distribution does not seem appropriate, then a nonparametric analysis of the data can be done with the Mann–Whitney U test (Gibbons, 1985). In this procedure, the number of times an observation in the treatment diet is lower than one in the control group is counted. Under the null hypothesis in which the two distributions are identical, the probability of unlikely values of this count can be computed without any assumptions about the form of distribution of the original weights.

B. Analysis of Several Unrelated Treatment Groups

Consider the simple toxicological experiments in which there are I diets and n_i animals are assigned to diet i. In most statistics texts, the diets would be called "treatments" and the design a "one-factor completely randomized" design. Let y_{ij} denote the observed response in animal j $(j = 1, 2 \ldots, n_i)$ given diet i. Then an analysis similar to the one described in Section II,A for the one treatment case can be used. The sample variance can be pooled across all treatment groups to give a more accurate estimate of the common population and individual t tests comparing each treatment to the control:

$$s^2 = \frac{\sum_{i=1}^{I} (n_i - 1) s_i^2}{\sum_{i=1}^{I} (n_i - 1)}. \tag{5}$$

Under such a scheme, several comparisons with the mean can be calculated, each one with the possibility of making a type I error. If each test is done at the 5% level or significance and if there really is no difference between the locations of the distributions, then the overall probability that at least one error will be made (i.e., some difference is falsely declared "significant") is above 5%.

The overall probability of making at least one type I error (i.e., of having a "false positive") is called the experiment-wise error rate (Miller, 1981). There are several techniques for controlling the experiment-wise error rate. If all sample sizes are equal, then several treatments can be compared with a control group using Dunnett's many-to-one t test (Miller, 1981) with the experiment error rate controlled. This test has been extended to allow for unequal sample sizes (Dutt *et al.*, 1976).

If the assumption of equality of variances is not appropriate, tests comparing diet groups that control the experiment-wise error rate are available (Dunnett, 1980). If the assumptions about the normal distribution are not appropriate, nonparametric procedures for the comparison of several diets with the control exist (Hollander and Wolfe, 1973).

C. Analysis of a Graded Set of Diets

One common design for a toxicity study is to give a series of graded diet levels. For such an experiment, comparing each dose to the control is an inefficient use of data. It can generally be assumed that if there is a diet effect, it will exhibit a trend with dose. Let d_i denote the dose given to animals on diet i $(d_1 < d_2 < \ldots < d_I)$. Several tests of monotone trend have been proposed. The simplest one involves testing for a linear trend with dose

$$y_{ij} = \mu + \beta d_i + e_{ij}. \tag{6}$$

A test for dose response can be made by testing whether β, the slope of the line, equals zero. This can be done using standard regression methodology (Daniel and Wood, 1981; Draper and Smith, 1981) except that the estimate of variance within the pooled group is used to assess the significance of the estimate of trend instead of the residual sum of squares from the regression.

In this analysis, the linear dose–response curve is viewed only as a means to construct a test for trend with dose. It will provide a valid test even if the functional form of the dose–response curve is different. The test, however, will be most powerful if the correct form of the dose–response equation is used. The regression can be done against other variables such as $\log(d_i)$ or $\exp(d_i)$ if the rate of change with dose decreases or increases with increasing dose. An alternative approach to testing for trend is based on isotonic regression (Williams, 1971; Barlow *et al.*, 1972; Williams, 1972) in which a functional form for the trend is not assumed.

If the assumption of equal variances in each diet group is not true, an alternative test for monotone trend is available (Roth, 1983). A nonparametric test of trend with dose can be done using Jonckheere's test (Hollander and Wolfe, 1973).

D. More Complex Designs

The previous techniques allow an analysis of the most elementary toxicological experiments, but there are many more complex designs available. More complex designs are created when the researcher tries to examine the effect of a combination of treatments or uses a more sophisticated randomization scheme. Four of the most important concepts to understand are: blocking, nesting, interaction, and covariables.

Both blocking and nesting are descriptions of more complex randomization schemes. In the previous designs, it was assumed that each animal was assigned randomly and independently to the diet groups. The assignment of animals, however, may not always follow this ideal. When animals are naturally divided into groups, this grouping may be exploited to improve the precision with which treatment differences are estimated, or it may introduce a substantial degradation of the precision. Groups may be defined through natural classification (e.g., animals from the same litter) or through artificial means, such as sorting the animals into weight classes. Division of animals into groups allows the variance among animals to be partitioned within the group and among the group variance. If the classification scheme is not arbitrary, then the animals within a group will tend to be similar and the variance within a group will be small compared to the variance among the groups.

1. Blocking

If there are I animals in each group and one animal from each group is assigned to each diet, then the groups become a blocking factor in the experiment, and they are called blocks. The advantage of this method of randomization is that the animals on each diet are balanced in terms of the blocking factor; therefore, the differences among diets do not involve the variance among blocks. The precision of the estimates of differences among diets depends only on the variance within blocks. Hence, the blocking factor is chosen because the variance within a block is as small as possible. The simplest case of this design, when there is one treatment and one control group, is analyzed with the paired t test. Even when there are several treatments, the analysis is quite straightforward (Sokal and Rohlf, 1981) as long as each diet has exactly one observation in each block. When some measurements are not available, the experiment is called an incomplete block design, and analysis can become substantially more difficult depending on the pattern of the missing observations.

2. Nesting

If all animals within a group are assigned to the same treatment, the experimental design is said to be nested. For example, in a two-generation study, the F_1 animals might be assigned to the same diet as their parents. The correct statistical analysis of such a design is based on the randomization unit, which is the litter. The "sample size" for the experiment is the number of litters, not the number of animals. Analysis of the results must take into account the variance among and within litters as well as the number of animals in each litter (Jensh, *et al.* 1970; Healy, 1972; Brunden and Kemp, 1980).

3. Interaction

It is often important to examine the effect of a diet in combination with another diet or to examine its effect on different groups of animals (e.g., different sexes, age classes, or weight classes). In these situations, the similarity of the response for one factor (diet) at the different levels of the second factor (diet or group) is of interest. If the response of the first factor varies depending on the level of the second, then these two factors are said to "interact". A description of the effect of each factor must take into account the level of the other.

If the interaction is negligible, the effects of each factor are similar at all levels of the other factor and can be summarized without reference to the other. If the interaction is deemed significant, the effects of each factor can be analysed separately at each level of the other factor. For example, if there is an interaction between diet and sex, then the effect of diet can be studied separately for each sex. The calculation of test statistics and the interpretation of main effects in the presence of interaction are complex (Searle, et al., 1980; Schmoyer, 1984). Several computer packages, such as SAS (SAS Institute, 1985), SPSS (SPSS, 1983), and BMDP (Dixon, 1983) present such analyses. These packages use different algorithms to partition the analysis of variance table and can lead to different significance tests (Speed, et al., 1978; Jennings and Ward, 1982).

4. Covariables

Covariables are variables used to improve the analysis of the main variable under study. A study in which several techniques for the analysis of organ weight were compared using the covariable "final body weight" (Shirley, 1977). In an analysis of covariance, the related variable (e.g., final body weight) is introduced into the analysis so that any differences among the diets in the covariable are removed (Sokal and Rohlf, 1981). This may serve to reduce the estimate of error from that in an analysis of variance and, hence, improve the power of the comparisons.

III. ANALYSIS OF GROWTH CURVE DATA

In any toxicological experiment involving an observation of laboratory animals over a period of time, longitudinal measurements of the physical characteristics of each animal may be taken. These may include body weight and feed consumption as well as hematological and immunological indicators based on periodic blood samples. What these data have in common is that they are measurable quantities being observed as they change over time. Although commonly referred to as "growth curve data", all the examples noted fall within the general category called "repeated measures".

What follows is a survey of the methods available to the toxicologist or biostatistician for the analysis of growth curve data. In Section III, multivariate linear models, biologically motivated nonlinear models, and nonparametric robust methods are considered, respectively.

A. Multivariate Linear Models

Multivariate linear models have been widely studied, and many standard textbooks (e.g., Morrison, 1976) deal with their analysis. In this section, we show how growth curve problems may be analyzed as multivariate linear models.

A simple model is as follows. Suppose observations are taken on several different characteristics of an animal or on the same characteristic at different times. If we assume that the average response depends only on the treatment, then any model must specify the mean response of each characteristic. It must also specify the multivariate behavior, such as correlations among the deviations from the mean. For example, unusually large sized animals will have unusually large weights and will probably eat more than the norm. If these correlations are ignored, as many studies have shown, disastrous increases in the type I error rate can result (e.g., Boik, 1981; Elashoff, 1981; Schwertman et al., 1981).

An important assumption usually made is that treatment affects the average response, but it does not affect the multivariate correlations. Although some study has been made of the case in which the covariances vary (e.g., Chakravorti, 1974), the constant covariance assumption must be made, in many practical situations because estimation of each covariance matrix requires large amounts of data, which are not available.

With univariate linear models, most effort is concerned with modeling the mean response. With multivariate data, however, there are two distinct series to be modeled: the series of responses across different animals and the series within each animal. For example, one model may predict a linear increase in weight over a short term for each animal, with the rates of increase varying across animals according to dose received. This is an example of the so-called multivariate linear growth curve model of Potthoff and Roy (1964). Analysis of variance techniques may be employed, in which case the procedure is known as generalized multivariate ANOVA, or profile analysis. Multivariate models are particularly sensitive to missing data. Kleinbaum (1973) and Laird and Ware (1982) have developed techniques to deal with these problems.

Even assuming constant covariance may not be enough to guarantee stable covariance estimation. For example, if 10 observations are taken on each animal, a covariance needs to be estimated for every pair: 45 covariances and 10 variances. If fewer than 2 or 3 observations per covariance are available, the estimates will be poor. Thus in practice, the model must be simplified.

Grizzle and Allen's (1969) approach to simplifying the model is to select a few interesting parameters or combinations of parameters and ignore the rest. Box (1950) presented a transformation of the data (namely, taking successive differences) that seemed to make each observation independent so that univariate methods could be applied. Sandland and McGilchrist (1979) used ideas from the analysis of time series to simplify the specification of the covariances.

B. Biologically Motivated Nonlinear Models

The estimates and conclusions available from multivariate linear models are often unsatisfying to the toxicologist because the parameters may have no clear biological meaning and the models often ignore well-known behavior of the animals under study. For example, Daniel (1983) has described the increase in body weight of rats as proceeding in three stages: very rapid growth from birth to 16 weeks, more gradual growth to one year, then very gradual decline.

Several simple models of growth have been proposed that allow for rapid initial growth, followed by slower growth or leveling off of body weight. These include the logistic, the Gompertz, and the von Bertalanffy models (Sandland and McGilchrist, 1979). Many data sets fit one or more of these models very well. However, this may be due more to deficiencies in the data sets than to truth of the models (Kowalski and Guire, 1974). Nevertheless, they are clearly preferable to simple linear models in that each of the parameters has a clear physical meaning, and they roughly predict the correct shape.

To fit data to these models generally requires iterative techniques. Because of limitations in such techniques, it is impractical to fit completely arbitrary covariance matrices, therefore, simplifying assumptions must be made. Often, ordinary least-squares techniques are used to fit the data. Because this is equivalent to the assumption of equal, independent errors, increased type I errors can result.

A simple alternative is to assume that the errors follow a first-order autoregressive "AR(1)" process. In this situation, successive errors have a constant correlation. The correlation may be fitted along with the other parameters in the model by maximum likelihood techniques (e.g., Glasebey, 1979). A more general class of covariance models arising from stochastic differential equations is described by Sandland and McGilchrist (1979).

Another application of a biologically motivated model was made by Daniel (1983). He related the body weight to the rate of food intake in a differential equation involving the known energy content in the food. By fitting this model to different treatment groups in a chronic toxicity study, Daniel was able to separate weight changes due to changes in food consumption from those due to changes in metabolism.

Finding estimates of parameters in nonlinear models generally requires iterative techniques. These are numeric methods in which the parameter value that minimizes a (weighted) sum of squared errors or maximizes the likelihood function can be found. For a discussion of these methods and their limitations, see Daniel and Wood (1981). Well-known computer programs to fit nonlinear models include SAS procedure NLIN (SAS Institute, 1985) and BMDP procedure P3R (Dixon *et al.*, 1983).

C. Nonparametric and Robust Methods

With nonparametric and robust methods, the toxicologist can aim to reduce the dependence of inferences on the normal distribution implicit in the discussions in the preceding sections of this chapter. The necessity for this comes largely from the fact that normal analyses are known to be very sensitive to the effects of outliers — observations with far larger variations from the mean than normally expected. Use of these methods attempts to avoid the arbitrariness inherent in most procedures for removing residuals.

One method to reduce the sensitivity to outliers is to analyze, not the observed values, but the ranks of these values among all those observed. Koch *et al.* (1980) have reviewed methods based on ranks. Many methods developed for multivariate linear models have analogues in methods based on ranks. Pendergast and Broffit (1982) proposed the use of M-estimators for growth curve data. M-estimators substitute an arbitrary loss function for the quadratic loss implicit in the normal theory's sums of squares. They found this to be a robust alternative to standard methods, valid for many multivariate distributions. However, their methods, like most nonparametric methods, require substantial computation.

IV. CATEGORICAL DATA

Until the late 1960s, the analysis of categorical data was held by many to involve the application of specialized tests in specific situations. Since then, a "model-building" approach has grown, and modern methods involve the application of techniques not very different from the traditional regression methods for normally distributed data. In this section, we consider those forms of analysis in which the y variates are categorical. Some of the simplest situations with categorical data (the 2 by 2 table and the 2 by k contingency table) are considered first, because these are the cases most frequently encountered in experimental practice. Sometimes it is prudent to make use of some extra information in an analysis, and the "modeling" approach is invoked, which is briefly discussed next. Lastly, we comment on the availability of computer software to aid in the calculations. The types of designs and analyses involving such data are extremely varied. With the broad scope of such material, only a cursory discussion is presented in this section.

Prior to beginning the analysis of categorical data, the careful investigator should examine the mortality rates of the animals on test. If animals in different dose groups experience different mortalities, not all animals are exposed for the same length of time. If animals on the highest dose die rapidly, they may produce fewer tumors than those groups on the lowest dose, which lived long enough for tumors to develop. The analysis of data influenced by dose-dependent mortality rates is discussed in Sections V and VI. The methods outlined in this section are based on the assumption that mortality rates for different dose groups are similar.

Perhaps the simplest of categorical data structures is the 2 by 2 table as shown in Table I. Even such a simple structure can arise from many sampling schemes. Many statistical approaches are the same for different sampling schemes that yield such data. We consider the most common of such methods next.

In toxicity testing, one is often testing for a difference in proportions. By design, a predetermined number of animals are randomly allocated into two groups: one group serves as a control, whereas the other is exposed to the factor of interest. The variable of interest is the number or proportion of animals in each group exhibiting toxic effects. One is interested in testing the difference in proportions of animals that are diseased (or, more generally, "respond").

When the number of animals under test is not large, then a common analytical technique performed is the "Fisher–Irwin exact test". With this test approach, all possible 2 by 2 tables that might possibly occur for the given number of animals in each group and the total number of affected animals (r, s, m, and n in Table I) are determined. For each

Table I
A 2 by 2 Table

	Diseased	Not diseased	Total
Exposed	a	b	m
Not exposed	c	d	n
Total	r	s	N

table, a probability is calculated and a significance test is formed from the combinatorial probabilities equal to that of the observed configuration and from all those configurations that are more extreme than the observed one. The specifics of the calculations for such a test are described in Armitage (1971).

If the number of observations in a 2 by 2 table is large, an approximate test is readily computed and is sufficiently accurate:

$$X_1^2 = \frac{(ad - bc)^2 N}{mnrs}. \tag{7}$$

If there is no difference between proportions responding in the exposed and control groups (null hypothesis), the distribution of X_1^2 is approximately Chi squared with one degree of freedom. In many cases, equation (7) is modified to allow for a "continuity correction" in order to improve the distributional approximation (Fleiss, 1981).

There is one common misapplication of this method. The data described are considered to have arisen in an unmatched fashion. If, however, some matching is performed (for example, two members of each of many litters are chosen and one is exposed but the other not), then the analysis should take this matching into account. In the case in which only one of each group from each litter is taken (the data are "paired"), another test, using McNemar's statistic (Armitage, 1971), is appropriate. However, if there are more than one of each group (i.e., matched but not necessarily paired), an analysis that allows for such "litter effects" is warranted. Several such methods are under study currently, and the interested investigator is referred to Kupper and Haseman (1978) and Haseman and Kupper (1979) for some ideas. By ignoring possible litter effects in an analysis, one may have too sensitive a statistical test because the measure of variability ignores any extrabinomial variation due to differences among litters. If the variation among litters in the analysis is not considered, there is a chance that a sufficiently large difference in the proportions responding will be deemed "significant" when it should be deemed "not significant".

Many of these methods can be extended to tables with more than two rows. If the exposure factor is quantitative, for example, if several dose levels of the same compound are being studied, then a dose–response relationship may be of interest. When the exposure factor is qualitative, involving, for example, different chemicals, one is usually testing for no evidence of differences between the proportions of animals responding to the different compounds.

Table II presents a typical example involving a dose response. Frequently, one is interested in determining if the proportion of animals that

Table II
A 2 by k Table for a Dose Response

Dose	Diseased	Not diseased	Total
x_1	a_1	b_1	m_1
x_2	a_2	b_2	m_2
$\vdots$	$\vdots$	$\vdots$	$\vdots$
x_k	a_k	b_k	m_k
Total	A	B	M

becomes diseased changes as the dose level of the compound is increased. A statistic widely used in this situation (often referred to as the Cochran–Armitage statistic) is

$$X_2^2 = \frac{M\,(M\Sigma_i a_i x_i - A\Sigma_i m_i x_i)^2}{A(M - A)\{M\Sigma_i m_i x_i - (\Sigma_i m_i x_i)^2\}}. \tag{8}$$

Thoughout this subsection, let Σ_i stand for $\Sigma_{i=1}^k$. If there is no dependency of a_i/m_i on x_i, then the distribution of X_2^2 is approximately Chi squared with one degree of freedom. An exact randomization test for X_2^2 similar to the Fisher–Irwin exact test for a 2 by 2 table is possible for small sample sizes (Thomas et al., 1977).

If one is interested only in testing that the k proportions are homogenous (and no dose response is of interest), then a different test is warranted. The expected number of counts for each cell in Table II is calculated by

$$a_i^* = \frac{m_i}{M}\,A \tag{9}$$

and

$$b_i^* = \frac{m_i}{M}\,B.$$

A test statistic comparing the observed and expected values is calculated by

$$X_3^2 = \Sigma_i \left\{ \frac{(a_i - a_i^*)^2}{a_i} + \frac{(b_i - b_i^*)^2}{b_i} \right\}. \tag{10}$$

The distribution of X_3^2, when the underlying probabilities of becoming diseased for the k rows are similar, is approximated by a Chi-squared distribution with $k - 1$ degrees of freedom.

As with the 2 by 2 table, "exact" or combinatorial probabilities can be determined in the dose–response case. These can require considerable amounts of computation. Because the distribution of X_3^2 involves more than one degree of freedom, exact calculations are not usually considered in this situation.

The examples of analyses for categorical data considered so far involve well-defined situations with very few variables. In more complicated situations, there are special test statistics that can be easily calculated. Maxwell (1961) provides an excellent summary of such methods. However, interest recently is centered on a "modeling" approach to the analysis of categorical data. The direction is moving away from the development of an arsenal of specialized techniques, each for its own particular experimental design, toward the use of general methods along lines similar to those of analysis of variance and multiple regression methodology. With general testing methods, customization of a test to a new situation requires only the development of an appropriate model. For example, we have animals exposed to a special combination of risk factors $(x_1, x_2, \ldots, x_u)$. The model is formed by transforming the proportion and expressing this as a function (usually linear) of risk factors or x variates

$$f(p) = \beta_o + \beta_1 x_1 + \beta_2 x_2 + \ldots + \beta_u x_u, \tag{11}$$

where p is a proportion and $f(p)$ is a suitable transformation. Commonly encountered transformations include the "logit", the "probit", and the "arcsine". Examples of more complicated structures analysed with this approach include the combination of 2 by 2 tables and bioassay problems with complicated experimental designs. Cox (1970) has provided an excellent discussion of this approach.

A related technique involves the modeling of the number of responses (instead of the proportion) with a logarithmic transformation. These "log-linear" models can be applied to count data with more than two groups, such as those displayed in a 3 by 3 table. The methodology is outlined in Everitt (1977) and Bishop et al. (1975). The relation between the log-linear and the transformed proportional approaches is described in the latter reference as well as in Bishop (1969). When there are more than two categories in the "response" variable and there is a natural order in these categories (for example, type 1 is "better" than type 2, which is "better" than type 3), then the log-linear model may not be appropriate. Analysis of such data is only now receiving attention in the literature. A discussion of recent developments in this field of ordered categorical data analysis is presented by McCullagh (1980) and McCullagh and Nelder (1983). When data are matched, modeling is still possible although matters are again more complicated both conceptually and computationally (Breslow and Day, 1980).

It is important to realize that there is not a complete equivalence between traditional regression modeling and categorical data modeling. Much care is warranted in the treatment of interactions for categorical data modeling, and consultation with a qualified statistician is advised.

Simultaneous with the development of general modeling methods in the analysis of categorical data has been the creation of powerful statistical computing packages. The investigator with simple categorical data problems will find SPSS very useful. Where modeling of binomial or unordered categorical data is necessary, the investigator may choose between BMDP (program P4F), SAS (procedures FUNCAT and PROBIT), and ECTA (a log-linear models program). GLIM, a general statistical package by Royal Statistical Society, warrants special mention. This program is flexible and powerful, but it requires the user to become familiar with specific ways of entering data and reading output. Presently, analysis of ordered categorical data is not computerized as extensively as that of simple categorical data; neither is analysis of matched data. There are some isolated programs with a small circle of adherents, such as POLYR for ordered categorical data at the London School of Hygiene and Tropical Medicine and PECAN for matched data analyses (Storer et al., 1983), but few at the general level of SPSS, SAS, or BMDP.

For toxicologists who have a traditional attitude, there is a battery of specific tests (mostly termed Chi squared) for which only a calculator is necessary. See Maxwell (1961) and Snedecor and Cochran (1980) for excellent discussions on this approach. Alternatively, there is a growing field of general linear model methodology that offers considerable flexibility and power at the expense of complicated computations. However, some statistical sophistication is required.

V. STATISTICAL ANALYSIS OF SURVIVAL DATA

The use of time-to-death information in *in vivo* toxicity experiments has become increasingly popular over the last decade, mainly due to significant advances in statistical methodology. Herein, an overview of these techniques is given. In the first subsection, we summarize some well-known methods of "survival analysis" that apply to a wide range of time-to-some-event responses. In the second and third subsections, we focus on the analysis of tumorigenicity studies. The methodology available in this area is extensive and is laden with various approaches and viewpoints. For further details on survival analysis in general, see Kalbfleisch and Prentice (1980). The discussion herein refers primarily to analyses of animal death, but the reader should realize that other outcomes or events may also be considered. In the following discussion, the terms "failure time" and "time to death" are used synonymously.

A. The Model

Consider an experiment in which N animals are placed on test. Each animal is randomly placed in one of K + 1 groups — a control group and K treatment groups. The animals in the treatment groups receive doses $d_1 < d_2 \ldots < d_K$ at regular time intervals and throughout their lifetime (e.g., via their food and/or water). The animals are observed until they die or are sacrificed, possibly at the termination of the experiment. The time of death is recorded along with the cause of death. Animals dying for reasons unrelated to the treatment are said to be censored, and one can assume only that the time of death from treatment effects is greater than the observed death time.

Suppose we wish to examine the relationship between dose and time to death. Further, suppose that as dose increases, the time to death decreases. (This assumption is not necessary for the general model but is used throughout to illustrate the methods.) As time to death decreases, the probability that an animal will survive a certain length of time (called the survival distribution) will also decrease. Another approach is to relate the dose to the probability that a living animal at some time (t) will die immediately after t. This probability (or "hazard") is often interpreted as a rate and is a function of time and dose. At any time t, the ratio of two hazard functions corresponding to the animals receiving two different doses is called the relative risk of one dose to the other (note that the relative risk may also be a function of time). If the relative risk of dose d_1 to dose d_2 is greater than one at time t, then d_1 is more toxic than d_2 in the sense that animals living to time t and receiving dose d_1 tend to have a higher probability of dying shortly after t than animals that received dose d_2. If the relative risk is independent of time (i.e., it is constant), then the corresponding hazard functions are proportional to each other. This model is termed the "proportional hazards" model. Methods are available (Kalbfleisch and Prentice, 1980) in which the proportional hazard model can be used to allow a parametric specification of the relationship between independent variables (such as dose) and survival distribution, hazard function, or relative risk. These techniques mimic the risk-modeling capabilities of analysis of regression and variance (see Section II) when the principle outcome is time to death.

B. Parametric Methods

The model discussed in Section V,A is based on the assumption that the control group has a hazard function of h(t) and the treatment groups a hazard function of dose $e^{\beta d}$ multiplied by the control group hazard. In order to determine the survival distribution [S(t;d)], the hazard h(t) must be specified. If h(t) has an explicit functional form, the hazard is said to be "parametric"; if no form is specified, the hazard is "nonparametric". In this section we deal solely with parametric hazards.

Recall that the hazard h(t) is the rate of dying or "failure" at time t for living animals in the control group. This hazard may range from a complicated function of time involving several parameters to a simple constant. An objective of this type of modeling procedure is to specify a hazard function that provides a large variety of shapes with few parameters.

There are three basic shapes of hazards commonly used in practice: Wiebull, logistic, and bathtub. The Weibull hazard includes monotone increasing or decreasing functions of time or a constant. The logistic hazard permits bell-shaped functions, whereas the bathtub hazard consists of the three shapes, a monotone decreasing near the origin, a constant, then a monotone increasing function at the end of the observation period. The bathtub hazard is most applicable to time to failure of machinery or instruments. The logistic hazard can model situations in which the test substances of interest may be toxic initially; however, if no effects are observed in the short term, then little chance of a detrimental long-term effect exists. The Weibull hazard model is best suited for most *in vivo* toxicity testing. Other models are discussed in Gross and Clarke (1975).

C. Nonparametric Methods

In Section III, we assume a parametric form for the hazard h(t), but often in practice it is not clear which distribution best describes the data. Furthermore, the main interest in an experiment may center on the relationship of the dose to the survival distribution; it may not be as important to determine the exact form of the distribution. Thus, a technique that assumes no functional form for h(t) is desirable.

A popular form of analysis for this situation is the "log-rank test". A description of this method can be found in Peto *et al.* (1977). Closely related to this method is an approach described by Cox (1972), now popularly called the "proportional hazards model" in which the relative risk between any two dose groups is assumed to be constant over time. Although the log-rank form of the test is readily calculated, it is specific only to the K + 1 groups situation. The proportional hazards technique involves more computation but can be extended easily to more general designs.

As with regression analysis, the time-to-event analysis not only allows examination of a dose-response relationship but also incorporates covariate information (such as sex, age, method of exposure, and species). If the combination of all levels for the covariates is assumed to influence the time-to-event development (i.e., an interaction between sex and age), then stratification techniques may be employed. A stratified analysis assumes that the time-to-event distribution is shifted for each stratum, but the dose-response relationship remains the same across strata. The last assumption may also be examined and, if found unreasonable, information may not be combined across strata. In this event, each stratum will have to be analyzed separately.

A final warning merits special mention. The log-rank and proportional hazards models are currently popular, and a growing battery of software is becoming available. The investigator in possession of a data set and looking for an analysis is cautioned to avoid the temptation of believing the results of any such nonparametric analyses without inspecting them critically. As is the case in other areas of statistical analysis, special care is required to verify underlying assumptions first. The main assumption in this case is that of proportional hazards, for which no test is accepted as best. One possible approach is described in Andersen (1982).

VI. ANALYSIS OF PATHOLOGICAL DATA

The primary purpose of a long-term carcinogenicity experiment is to determine if a test substance alters the normal pattern of tumor development in a particular animal species. The basic data obtained from each animal are the times of appearance of any visible tumors, the time of death, the cause of death (if it can be determined), the list of organs examined at necropsy, and the histopathological diagnoses. The goal in the statistical analysis of survival (time to death) and pathological (tumor presence and cause of death) data is to quantify the strength of evidence regarding the carcinogenic potential of the test agent.

The evaluation of a long-term carcinogenicity experiment is complicated by the fact that there is no single biological response that characterizes a carcinogenic effect. Several alterations in the normal pattern of tumor development should be examined, the most important being an increase in age-specific rates of tumor incidence in exposed animals over some portion of the animals' lifetime. Acceleration in tumor development is another response of interest.

There are a number of design and analytical features of animal carcinogenesis experiments that should be considered. A review of these issues is given by Gart *et al.* (1986) and McKnight (1988). Issues such as the analysis and interpretation of nonneoplastic lesions when such lesions are precursors of a neoplasm, adjustment for intercurrent mortality, and combination of information over different sexes and species require careful consideration.

Further complicating the analysis and interpretation of these data is the presence of occult tumors that can be detected only at necropsy. Influence of dose on the time-to-tumor development cannot be examined directly. Analysis of this type of data requires several additional assumptions both by the pathologist and the statistician. The methods of analyses and these assumptions are briefly described in this section.

Note that the analysis of these data is complex and must be undertaken by an interdisciplinary team consisting of pathologists, toxicologists, statisticians, and other scientists. Although the statistical analysis of tumor and survival data is an essential component of the evaluation of carcinogenicity, sole reliance on statistically significant results is not recommended. For example, minor, nonstatistically significant changes in the tumor pattern may provide evidence of carcinogenicity, particularly in the case of rare tumors. On the other hand, a significant tumor increase in only one sex within an organ that has a high naturally occurring tumor rate may not provide convincing evidence of carcinogenicity (Gart *et al.*, 1986). Thus, the evaluation of data from a number of different aspects is required to determine the role of the test substance in the cancer process.

In Section III, we consider the analysis of data that indicate whether or not an event had occurred. In the current context, the events of interest may include the development of a tumor or the death of an animal due to toxic effects. We now consider the analysis of data that not only show whether or not an event occurred but also include the time until such an event occurs. Ignoring time-to-event data may give misleading information.

Consider the BIBRA nitrosamine study (Peto *et al.*, 1984). It was found that 20% of the female rats tested developed uterine neoplasms in the lower dose groups, whereas only 2% showed such neoplasms in the high dose groups. Thus, an analysis based only on the crude percentages of tumor-bearing animals indicates that an increased dosage of nitrosamine would decrease the incidence of uterine neoplasms. This conclusion does not seem reasonable. Upon examination of the time-to-death data, it was concluded that animals were dying from other causes in the high dose groups at a much higher rate than those in the low dose groups. Thus, the animals given the higher dose are not living long enough to develop uterine neoplasms. Consequently, an analysis is required that accounts for the time to death, especially when the survival experience differs markedly between dose groups.

The objective of some long-term rodent tumorigenicity experiments is to determine whether or not the administration of a test substance results in an increase in tumor occurrence among exposed animals as compared to unexposed controls. In a typical experiment, two or more groups of animals are exposed to different doses of an agent under study in addition to the unexposed control groups. Exposure commences shortly after weaning and continues throughout the major portion of the animal's lifespan, thereby lasting about two years.

The tumor status of an individual animal is normally determined at the time of the animal's death. Because many animals can die prior to the end of the study period either from natural mortality or as a result of tumor development, information on tumorigenicity will accrue throughout the course of the experiment. Animals surviving to the end of the experiment are sacrificed and subjected to the same pathological evaluation as those dying prior to termination time.

The statistical analysis of time-to-tumor data obtained from such studies is complicated by several factors (Haseman, 1984; Lagakos and Louis, 1985). First, inferences are often required concerning unobservable quantities such as time to occurrence of occult tumors (Kalbfleisch *et al.*, 1983; McKnight and Crowley, 1984). In this case, the data available for analysis are the ages of the animals at death rather than the actual time at which the tumor reaches some well-defined stage in its development. Second, many animals dying or sacrificed during the course of the experimental period will not be tumor free and are thus "censored" observations (note that we have slightly modified the use of this term from the last section.) Because the survival patterns may well vary among the different experimental groups being compared, it is important that the statistical analysis of the data provide for intercurrent mortality (Gart *et al.*, 1979). A third complication relates to the distinction between lethal ("fatal") tumors and nonlethal ("incidental") tumors (Peto *et al.*, 1980). A proper assessment of tumorigenicity experiments requires that a distinction be made between these two situations, which, in turn, requires that the cause of death be determined (Kodell *et al.*, 1982).

A. A Compartmental Model for Tumorigenesis

Consider the compartmental model for tumorigenesis shown in Fig. 1. This model has been employed by Kalbfleisch *et al.* (1983), McKnight and Crowley (1984), and others. In the figure, T_1 is the time in the tumor-free state, T_2 is the time in the latent tumor state, $T = T_1 + T_2$ is the time to death as a result of tumor occurrence, and U is the time to death due to competing risks.

In many experiments, the only observable times in the experiment are T and U. The time T represents the time to a fatal tumor death, whereas U represents the time to death from natural causes. If a tumor is present at the time of death in an animal that died from natural causes, then the tumor is said to be "incidental". One method of determining whether the test agent causes an increased occurrence of both fatal and incidental tumors in a similar fashion is given by Peto *et al.* (1980) and discussed in the following section.

B. Fatal and Incidental Tumor Test

Consider the following hypothetical experiment in which 100 animals are placed under observation with 50 animals in a control group and 50 in the exposed group. The animals are followed for a two-year period, and any alive at that time are sacrificed. Note that the following statistical methodology allows for multiple dose groups and a dose-response model to be specified along with interim sacrifices. The time to death (in days, for example), the level of dose (control or exposed), and the cause of death (due to tumor, natural causes, or sacrifice) are recorded. For those animals dying either by natural causes (not related to the tumor of interest)

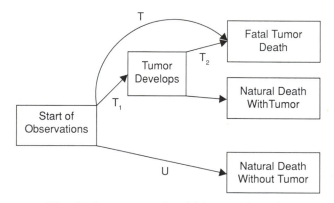

Fig. 1 Compartmental model for tumorigenesis.

or sacrifice, the information regarding tumor presence in also noted. Suppose that 20 animals die because of a fatal tumor throughout the two-year period, 60 animals die naturally, and 20 animals are sacrificed at the termination of the experiment.

Interest centers around determining if animals in the exposed groups are dying sooner (or at a faster rate) from tumors than animals in the control group. Further interest involves whether dose influences the prevalence of nonfatal or incidental tumors. That is, is the probability of a living animal in the exposed group dying from natural causes but also having a tumor greater than the corresponding probability for animals in the control group? It is assumed that the same relationship holds between dose and rate of dying due to fatal tumors and between dose and prevalence of incidental tumors. The test statistic used to answer this question comprises two components: a fatal tumor statistic and an incidental tumor statistic. Calculation of fatal tumor statistics requires, at each of the 20 failure times, the number of animals alive just prior to the fatal tumor death time in each dose group. Note that methods are available to incorporate death times that occur simultaneously, but for simplicity those are not discussed in this chapter (see Peto *et al.*, 1980). Information on all 20 times is combined to form the fatal tumor test statistic (denoted by T_F). A test statistic $Z_F = T_F V_F^{-\frac{1}{2}}$, where V_F is the variance of T_F, may be used to examine the evidence of a relationship between the dose and the fatal tumor death process. For a large number of animals on tests (e.g., 50 animals per dose group), Z_F may be approximated by a standard normal variate.

When an animal dies from natural causes or is sacrificed, and a tumor is found, the tumor is said to be incidental. Because the time-to-tumor development is not known, the methods described in Section V cannot be used to determine if the test substance causes an increased prevalence of incidental tumors. The following is one method suggested by Peto *et al.* (1980) to examine the problem.

Consider only those animals that die from natural causes or are sacrificed. Suppose that time is partitioned into M intervals. (The National Toxicology Program of the U.S. Department of Health and Human Services sometimes uses four intervals for the natural deaths in a standard 2-year experiment: 0–52 weeks, 53–78 weeks, 79–92 weeks, and 93–102 weeks.) The necessary data for the interval are the number of naturally dying animals in the interval and the number with a tumor for each dose group. Similar information is needed to incorporate the terminal sacrifice, which may be thought of as an interval from the termination date of the study (e.g., 2 years) to infinity.

Information over the M intervals is combined to form a statistic T_I

along with a variance V_I. The test statistic $Z_I = T_I V_I^{-\frac{1}{2}}$ may be used to examine whether dose is related to the prevalence of incidental tumors. Again Z_I approximates a standard normal variate if the number of animals in each interval is large.

To examine simultaneously whether dose is related to both the rate of fatal tumor and the prevalence of incidental tumors, the statistic $Z = (T_F + T_I)(V_F + V_I)^{-\frac{1}{2}}$ has been proposed. The test statistic Z, called the "IARC" test, may be approximated by a standard normal variate. When both tests are combined, there is scope for a loss of sensitivity (if one effect is large and the other not) or possibly for an erroneous result (if the effects are large and in opposite directions such that no apparent effect results when they are combined). This should not be surprising. In attempting to summarize two facets of an experiment with one statistic, the investigator may lose some information, therefore, he or she should guard against a serious loss.

The statistical properties of the IARC test are only now being investigated. Although the calculations are simple, it is worth noting that the combination of results in Z involves many underlying assumptions. Two facets of this are considered next. The first involves the realm of theoretical statistics. A test statistic along with its distribution is often selected to perform best against certain possible alternatives. For example, Z_F, based on a Mantel–Haenszel-type test, is most powerful against data arising from an Weibull distribution. That is to say, if the times of occurrence of fatal tumors follow this type of distribution, then Z_F is the most powerful way to test if there is a dose relationship. For incidental tumors, however, Z_I is most powerful for the logistic distribution. Thus, there is a built-in dichotomy in the two tests, and interest now lies in examining how robust these statistics are in other situations and how coherent tests might be formed. Second, the combination of numerators and denominators to obtain Z is only one of several approaches. In choosing to use Z, one implicitly assumes that the specific dose relationship is the same for both types of tumors and that the evidence for both is the same. Possibly one may wish to test if the largest amount of evidence for a dose relationship is significant, or one may not wish to assume that both dose relationships are similar before testing for existence. In this latter case, one should use $Z_F^2 + Z_I^2$ and note that this should follow a Chi-squared density with two degrees of freedom.

In summary, the most common approach to the analysis of pathological data is swinging from the analysis of qualitative (tumor, no tumor) data to the analysis of survival data in order to correct for the possible effects of intercurrent mortality. Carcinogenicity assays are now also evolving to test for more than fatal tumors. At present, the IARC test (Peto *et al.*, 1980) is in vogue. The purpose of this section has been to outline the basis of this.

VII. CONCLUSION

In the preceding sections, we have dealt with material specific to analyses of different types of responses. There are some aspects of the statistical treatment of toxicological data that are common to all analyses discussed, and an investigator should be familiar with them. Most methods described involve the study of very few variable simultaneously. It is important, however, to be alert to possible errors in the unconsidered invocation of Ockham's razor. Omission of an important mitigating factor will prove to be a serious scientific weakness often reflected in an overly simplistic approach in data analysis. Such factors that may influence a relationship under study are sometimes referred to as "confounding factors". It behoves the investigator to take care in the selection of which factors should be considered as "confounders" It often falls to the statistician to decide how to deal with such problems.

Currently, there are different schools of thought on the optimal method of dealing with confounding factors. When possible, allowance for such effects should be considered at the design stage of an experiment. For statistical methods with considerable flexibility in modeling, such as the proportional hazards survival model or log-linear models for categorical data, one way to "adjust" for the effects of a confounding factor is to include the factor in the model along with the main variables of interest. Alternatively, for discrete confounding factors, one can subdivide a data set into subsets according to values of the confounding factor, perform the appropriate analysis within each subset, and combine the separate results for an overall result. Continuous confounding factors can be rendered discrete by grouping like values. The subclasses are referred to "strata", and the whole process is referred to as "stratification".

Failure to take into account the effect of an important confounding factor can lead to seriously misleading results. There is the possibility of considerable bias entering calculations of estimates or test statistics. As well, by allowing for extra factors, one may remove an additional source of variation. This will lead to more precise estimates and tests, and data are used more efficiently. However, consideration of factors that do not influence a relationship of interest can sometimes lead to inefficiency. The majority of the discussion has been focused on unstratified forms of analyses. In many cases, proper incorporation of auxiliary information requires only a minimal elaboration of standard methods.

In order to encompass a wide area of statistical applications, we have presented material that provides general and flexible methods succinctly. In most cases, we have used assumptions that we hope lend clarity to the methodology presented. We are concerned with conveying the underlying statistical idea in the analyses of different types of data; at times, this involves overly simplified examples.

The methods discussed involve either the estimation of parameters or the testing of hypotheses. It is often thought that the goal in statistical treatment of data is to provide an estimated value or a significance level (a "p value"). This is usually insufficient. A proper statistical estimation includes consideration of the uncertainty of the estimate. (The same arithmetical average can be obtained from a sample of 2 and a sample of 2,000, but the precisions are different.) Significance levels, too, are usually best understood in the context of "statistical power". For example, a test of the different between two means may not indicate significance at the traditional 5% level, and one may be inclined to ask how large the difference would have to be for the significance level to go below 5%. It is important to distinguish clearly differences that are biologically meaningful from those that are not when test results are statistically significant (or insignificant). Such considerations require considerable experience and knowledge of the toxicological context as well as the statistical sophistication. Often, this is best resolved by a collaborative effort.

The range of statistical techniques that someone involved with *in vivo* toxicity testing might encounter is very large. There is no way to do justice to so wide a field in one chapter. Our objectives have been to help the prospective client of statistical services to determine the area of statistical methods that he or she may require, to discuss the underlying ideas, and to indicate which articles, books, and software packages may be of use. For the most part, we recommend that the investigator seek professional statistical advice in order to increase the chances of a valid and efficient design and appropriate data analysis.

References

American Society for Testing Materials (1987). Standard recommended practice for dealing with outlying observations. Designation E178-80 *In* "Book of ASTM Standards," Vol. 14.02, pp. 140–165. Washington, DC: American Society for Testing and Materials.

Andersen, P. K. (1982). Testing goodness of fit of Cox's regression and life model. *Biometrics* **38,** 67–77.

Armitage, P. (1971). "Statistical Methods in Medical Research." Oxford: Blackwell Scientific Publications.

Barlow, R. E., Bartholomew, D. J., Bremner, J. M., and Brunk, J. D. (1972). "Statistical Inference under Order Restrictions." New York: Wiley.

Bishop, Y. M. M. (1969). Full contingency tables, logits and split contigency tables. *Biometrics* **25,** 383–399.

Bishop, Y. M. M., Fienberg, S. E., and Holland, P. W. (1975). "Discrete Multivariate Analysis." Cambridge, Massachusetts: MIT Press.

Boik, R. J. (1981). *A priori* tests in repeated measures designs: Effects of nonsphericity. *Psychometrika* **46,** 241–255.

Box, G. E. P. (1950). Problems in the analysis of growth and wear curves. *Biometrics* **6,** 362–389.

Box, G. E. P., and Cox, D. R. (1964). An analysis of transformations (with discussion). *J. R. Statist. Soc. Ser. B* **26,** 211–252.

Breslow, N. E., and Day, N. E. (1980). "Statistical Methods in Cancer Research," Vol. 1, The analysis of case-control studies (IARC Sci. Publ. No. 32). Lyon: International Agency for Research on Cancer.

Brunden, M. N., and Kemp, P. L. (1980). Animal litters as experimental units — a generalization and implementation on SAS. *36th Annu. Conf. Appl. Statist. Newark.*

Chambers, J. M., Cleveland, W. S., Kleiner B., and Tukey, P. A. (1983). "Graphical Methods for Data Analysis." Monterey, California: Wadsworth.

Chakravorti, S. R. (1974). On some tests of growth curve model under Behrens-Fisher situation. *J. Multivariate Anal.* **4,** 31–51.

Cox, D. R. (1970). "The Analysis of Binary Data." London: Chapman and Hall.

Cox, D. R. (1972). Regression models and life tables. *J. R. Statist. Soc. Ser. B* **34,** 187–220.

Daniel, D. L. (1983). The analysis of bodyweight data. *R. Statist. Soc. (March 17, 1983).*

Daniel, C., and Wood, F. (1981). "Fitting Equations to Data," 2nd ed. New York: Wiley.

Dixon, W. J., ed. (1983). "BMDP Statistical Software." Berkeley: University of California Press.

Draper, N. R., and Smith, M. (1981). "Applied Regression Analysis," 2nd ed. New York: Wiley.

Dunnett, C. W. (1980). Pairwise multiple comparisons in the unequal variance case. *J. Am. Statist. Assoc.* **75,** 796–800.

Dutt, J. E., Mattes, K. D., Soms, A. P., and Tao, L. C. (1976). An approximation to the maximum modulus distribution of the trivariate T with a comparison to the exact values. *Biometrics* **32,** 465–469.

Elashoff, J. D. (1981). Repeated measures bioassay with correlated errors and heterogenous variances: A Monte Carlo study. *Biometrics* **37,** 475–482.

Everitt, B. S. (1977). "The Analysis of Contingency Tables." London: Chapman and Hall.

Fleiss, J. L. (1981). "Statistical Methods for Rates and Proportions." New York: Wiley.

Gad, S. C., and Weil, C. S. (1982). Statistics for toxicologists. *In* "Principles and Methods in Toxicology" (A. W. Hayes, ed.), pp. 273–320. New York: Raven Press.

Gad, S. C., and Weil, C. S. (1986). "Statistics and Experimental Design for Toxicologists." Caldwell, New Jersey: Telford Press.

Gart, J., Chu, K., and Tarone, R. E. (1979). Statistical issues in interpretation of chronic bioassay tests for tumorigenicity. *J. Nat. Cancer Inst. (US)* **62,** 957–974.

Gart, J. J., Krewski, D., Lee, P. N., Tarone, R. E., and Wahrendorf, J. (1986). "Statistical Methods in Cancer Research," Vol. III, The design analysis of long term animal experiments. (IARC Sci. Publ. No. 79). Lyon: International Agency for Research on Cancer.

Gibbons, J. D. (1985). "Nonparametric Statistical Inference," 2nd ed. New York: Marcel Dekker.

Glaseby, C. D. (1979). Correlated residuals in non-linear regression applied to growth data. *Appl. Statist.* **28**, 251–259.

Grizzle, J. E., and Allen, D. M. (1969). Analysis of growth and dose response curves. *Biometrics* **25**, 357–381.

Gross, A., and Clark, V. A. (1975). "Survival Distributions: Reliability Applications in the Biomedical Sciences." New York: Wiley.

Haseman, J. K. (1984). "Statistical issues in the analysis of rodent bioassay data," (Tech. Rep.) Research Triangle Park, North Carolina: Biometry and Risk Assessment Program, National Institute of Environmental Health Sciences.

Haseman, J. K., and Kupper, L. L. (1979). Analysis of dichotomous response data from certain toxicological experiments. *Biometrics* **35**, 281–293.

Healy, M. J. R. (1972). Animal litters as experimental units. *Appl. Statist.* **21**, 155–159.

Hollander, M., and Wolfe, D. A. (1973). "Non-parametric Statistical Methods." New York: Wiley.

Jennings, E., and Ward, J. H. (1982). Hypothesis testing in the case of the missing cell. *Am. Statistician* **36**, 25–27.

Jensh, R. P., Brent, R. L., and Barr, M. (1970). The litter effect as a variable in teratogenic studies of the albino rat. *Am. J. Anat.* **128**, 185–192.

Kalbfleisch, J. D., and Prentice, R. L. (1980). "The Statistical Analysis of Failure Time Data." New York: Wiley.

Kalbfleisch, J. D., Krewski, D. R., and Van Ryzin, J. (1983). Dose-response models for time-to-response toxicity data. *Can. J. Statist.* **11**, 25–49.

Kleinbaum, D. G. (1973). A generalization of the growth curve model which allows missing data. *J. Multivariate Anal.* **3**, 117–124.

Koch, G. G., Amara, I. A., Stokes, M. E., and Gillings, D. B. (1980). Some views on parametric and non-parametric analysis for repeated measurements and selected bibliography. *Int. Statist. Rev.* **48**, 249–265.

Kodell, R. L., Farmer, J. W., Gaylor, D. W., and Cameron, A. M. (1982). Influence on cause-of-death assignment on time-to-tumor analyses in animal carcinogenesis studies. *J. Nat. Cancer Inst. (US)* **69**, 659–64.

Kowalski, C. H., and Guire, K. E. (1974). Longitudinal data analysis. *Growth* **38**, 131–169.

Kupper, L. L., and Haseman, J. K. (1978). The use of a correlated binomial model for the analysis of certain toxicological experiments. *Biometrics* **34**, 69–76.

Lagakos, S. W., and Louis, T. A. (1985). Statistical analysis of rodent tumorigenicity and experiments. *In* "Toxicological Risk Assessment, Vol. 1, Biological and Statistical Criteria" (D. Clayson, D. Krewski, and I. Munro, eds.), pp. 149–163. Boca Raton, Florida: CRC Press.

Laird, N. M., and Ware, J. H. (1982). Random effects models for longitudinal data. *Biometrics* **38**, 963–974.

McCullagh, P. (1980). Regression models for ordinal data. *J. R. Statist. Soc. Ser. B* **42**, 109–142.

McCullagh, P., and Nelder, J. A. (1983). "Generalized Linear Models." London: Chapman and Hall.

McKnight, B. (1988). A guide to the statistical analysis of long-term carcinogenicity assays. *Fundam. Appl. Toxicol.* **10**, 355–364.

McKnight, B., and Crowley, J. (1984). Tests for differences in tumor incidence based on animal carcinogenesis experiments. *J. Am. Statist. Assoc.* **79**, 639–648.

Maxwell, A. E. (1961). "Analyzing Qualitative Data." London: Methuen.

Miller, R. J. (1981). "Simultaneous Statistical Inference," 2nd ed. New York: Springer-Verlag.

Morrison, D. F. (1976). "Multivariate Statistical Methods," 2nd ed. New York: McGraw-Hill.

Pendergast, J. F., and Broffitt, J. D. (1982). "Robust estimation in growth curve models," (Tech. Rep. No. 184). Gainesville: University of Florida.

Peto, R., Pike, M. C., Armitage, P., Breslow, N. F., Cox, D. R., Howard, S. V., Mantel, N., McPherson, K., Peto, J., and Smith, P. G. (1977). Design and analysis of randomized clinical trials requiring prolonged observation of each patient. II. Analysis and examples. *Br. J. Cancer* **35**, 1–39.

Peto, R., Pike, M. C., Day, N. E., Gray, R. G., Lee, P. N., Parish, S., Peto, J., Richards, S., and Wahrendorf, J. (1980). Guidelines for simple, sensitive significance tests for carcinogenic effects in long-term animal experiments. *IARC Monogr. Evol. Carc. Risk Chem. Humans, Annex Suppl.* **2**, 311–426.

Peto, R., Gray, R., Brantom, P., and Grasso, P. (1984). Nitrosamine carcinogenesis in 5120 rodents: Chronic administration of sixteen different concentrations of NDEA, NDMA, NPYR and NPIP in the water of 4440 inbred rats, with parallel studies on NDEA alone of the effect of age starting (3, 6 or 20 weeks) and of species (rats, mice or hamsters). *IARC Sci. Publ.* **57**, 627–655.

Potthoff, R. F., and Roy, S. N. (1964). A generalized multivariate analysis of variance model useful especially for growth curve problems. *Biometrika* **51**, 313–326.

Roth, A. J. (1983). Robust trend tests derived and simulated: Analogs of the Welch and Brown-Forsythe tests. *J. Am. Statist. Assoc.* **78**, 972–980.

SAS Institue (1985). "SAS User's Guide: Statistics." Cary, North Carolina: SAS Institute.

SPSS (1983). "SPSS User's Guide." New York: McGraw-Hill.

Salsburg, D. S. (1986). "Statistics for Toxicologists." New York: Marcel Dekker.

Sandland, R. L., and McGilchrist, C. A. (1979). Stochastic growth curve analysis. *Biometrics* **35**, 255–271.

Schmoyer, R. L. (1984). Everyday application of the cell means model. *Am. Statistician* **38**, 49–52.

Schwertman, N. C., Magrey, J. M., and Fridshal, D. (1981). On the analysis of incomplete growth curve data: A Monte Carlo study of two non-parametric procedures. *Commun. Statist.-Simula. Computa.* **B10**, 51–66.

Searle, S. R., Speed, F. M., and Milliken, G. A. (1980). Population marginal means in the linear model: An alternative to least squares means. *Am. Statistician* **34**, 216–221.

Shirley, E. (1977). The analysis of organ weight data. *Toxicology* **8**, 13–22.

Snedecor, G. W., and Cochran, W. G. (1980). "Statistical Methods," 7th ed. Ames: Iowa State University Press.

Sokal, R. R., and Rohlf, F. J. (1981). "Biometry," 2nd ed. San Francisco: W. H. Freeman.

Speed, F. M., Hocking, R. R., and Hackney, O. P. (1978). Methods of analysis of linear models with unbalanced data. *J. Am. Statist. Assoc.* **73,** 105–112.

Storer, B. E., Wacholder, S., and Breslow, N. E. (1983). Maximum likelihood fitting of general risk models to stratified data. *Appl. Statist.* **32,** 172–181.

Thomas, D. G., Breslow, N. E., and Gart, J. J. (1977). Trend and homogeneity analyses of proportions and life table data. *Comput. Biomed. Res.* **10,** 373–381.

Williams, D. A. (1971). A test for differences between treatment means when several dose levels are compared to a zero dose control. *Biometrics* **28,** 519–531.

Williams, D. A. (1972). The comparison of several dose levels with a zero dose control. *Biometrics* **28,** 519–531.

25
Interpretation and Extrapolation of Toxicological Data

David B. Clayson
Toxicology Research Division
Bureau of Chemical Safety
Food Directorate
Health Protection Branch
Health and Welfare Canada
Ottawa, Ontario

Daniel R. Krewski
Biostatistics and Computer Applications Division
Environmental Health Directorate
Health Protection Branch
Health and Welfare Canada
Ottawa, Ontario

I. INTRODUCTION

In the previous chapters of this text, a wide variety of *in vivo* laboratory tests that may be used to establish the toxic properties of chemical substances are discussed in detail. Identification of potential health hazards through these tests is only the first step toward effective regulation and safe use of chemicals. There remains a need to estimate the level of risk that these agents present to humans under the actual or proposed conditions in which they will be used (risk assessment). Once this risk is estimated, the most appropriate way to regulate these substances (risk management) must be determined.

The process of risk assessment and risk management has been the subject of systematic study in recent years (National Research Council, 1983; Royal Society Study Group, 1983; World Health Organization, 1985; Krewski and Birkwood, 1987). Despite some minor differences in detail, most current frameworks for this process distinguish between hazard identification in which toxic phenomena are qualitatively described and risk estimation in which a more quantitative evaluation of adverse effects is conducted. These two steps together comprise what may be termed toxicological risk assessment. As discussed later in this chapter, a number of approaches used to identify and estimate the potential human risks based on experimental data have been developed.

In contrast to the scientific enterprise of hazard identification and risk estimation, risk management requires consideration of a host of social, economic, and political factors. The potential risks must be weighed against offsetting benefits, and regulatory and nonregulatory options must be considered for the control of risk (Ruckleshaus, 1983; U.S. Department of Health and Human Services, 1985). Inclusion of these extra-scientific factors in the overall management of risk can lead to legitimate differences in the strategies chosen for controlling risk in different circumstances, even in the presence of a common scientific data base. This may occur as a result of different economic or political conditions or as a result of differences in social policy or cultural perspective. Thus, effective risk management requires an appropriate blend of risk assessment, technical feasibility, human intervention, and political support (Starr, 1985).

In this chapter, we discuss the interpretation and extrapolation of toxicological data for purposes of human risk assessment. Fundamental to this is the validation of laboratory data to ensure that it is of sufficient quality to serve as the basis for further evaluation (Part II). Identification of health hazards is discussed in Part III. Current approaches to risk estimation are treated in Part IV. These include the application of safety factors and mathematical models to experimental data in order to establish human safety standards. The assumptions underlying these procedures are enunciated, and the need to consider all available biological data in order to select the most suitable statistical method for handling risk is emphasized.

The issues involved within the broader context of risk management are treated briefly in Part V. As noted previously, this is largely a politically mediated process, balancing actual or perceived health risks against the usefulness of the substance of interest within the prevailing regulatory climate. Some snags, lacunae, and pitfalls in risk assessment are discussed in Part VI. These include scientific uncertainties surrounding the risk assessment process, the possibility of synergistic effects between environmental agents, and the existence of uniquely susceptible population subgroups. Conclusions are presented in Part VII.

II. VALIDATION OF EXPERIMENTAL DATA

Hazard identification and risk estimation are both completely dependent on the quality of available toxicological data. Quality can only be assured through strict attention to detail during each stage of the study, which includes experimental design, choice and care of the animals to be used, detailed monitoring throughout the course of the study, thoroughness of the necropsy and histopathological examinations, and integration of the results for analysis. A weakness at any stage may well compromise the outcome, and the entire experiment may have to be repeated. If not detected, any deficiency may lead to an entirely incorrect perspective of the risk posed by the test agent.

Avoidance of gross errors is best achieved by encouraging the involved scientists from all disciplines to participate fully during the planning stage of the study. For example, early involvement of a biostatistician helps greatly to ensure that adequate numbers of animals are allocated to each study group and that they are randomized properly between these groups to avoid bias. Consideration should also be given to relative doses administered to animals in different treatment groups, to the study duration, to use of appropriate controls, and to other factors dictated by experimental protocol (International Life Sciences Institute, 1984; Bickis and Krewski, 1985; Gart et al., 1986).

Appropriate statistical tests to analyze the significance of all study results are usually necessary at the end of any toxicological study (Gad and Weil, 1984; Chapter 24). However, statistical analysis is completely dependent on the soundness of the data to be analyzed. Inadequate attention to the details of research cannot be corrected by statistical methods. Sloppy work inexorably means tarnished conclusions. Audits of data throughout a study ensure that good laboratory practices (GLPs), introduced by the U.S. Food and Drug Administration (1976) and adopted by other agencies (U.S. Environmental Protection Agency, 1983a, 1983b), will more easily be maintained and inadequate work practices will be curbed. Furthermore, full attention to this code of practice will greatly reduce inadequate attention to toxicological detail.

Much of the responsibility for adherence to GLPs rests with the study director. At minimum, he or she should apply the following criteria to ensure that the toxicological data package is adequate for purposes of analysis and evaluation.

1. Standard operating procedures: the study director should ensure that the data package contains each category of information mentioned in the study protocol and standard operating procedures. For example, lack of a specific item of information on one group of animals may eventually lead to a complete re-analysis of a substantial part of the data, thus wasting statistical resources and unnecessarily frustrating those who may urgently need the final results.

2. Evaluation of anomalous results: the study director should scan all data for discordant results, such as an abnormally heavy tissue at necropsy or an animal that has gained an unusual amount of weight at one point and apparently lost it by the next weighing. In these cases, the original records should be reviewed to ensure that the apparent anomaly is not due to transcriptional errors. Use of computerized data gathering methods will greatly lessen the possibility of such errors.

3. Confirmation of judgmental results: some toxicological data necessarily involves an element of personal judgment. In the case of histopathological diagnoses, for example, the results depend on the individual pathologist's judgment and previous experience with specific lesions. Before presenting data for statistical analysis, the study director should decide whether the data demands a further review by a second or third pathologist because of the presence of unusual lesions or lesions that have been particularly difficult to diagnose.

4. Priority of analyses: in some instances, the study director may identify specific parts of data as priorities for analysis. Such a procedure can be used, for example, if a new product is being developed and knowledge of its mutagenicity, clastogenicity, or carcinogenicity may preclude further highly expensive developmental work.

Once an experiment has been completed and validity of the results ascertained, the process of toxicological risk assessment can begin in earnest. This involves a careful evaluation of all available toxicological data, interpretation of their biological significance, and extrapolation of laboratory findings to the human situation.

III. HAZARD IDENTIFICATION

The toxicologist ostensibly has a number of options that may determine the relevance of experimental results obtained in a surrogate species to the human population. Thus, he or she may choose to use a species in which the absorption, distribution, and metabolism of a test agent resembles that in humans as closely as possible. The chosen species should similarly resemble the human species in its biological behavior; for example, a species that possesses a menstrual cycle may be judged more relevant than one with an estrous cycle in certain investigations. Unfortunately, however, economic and time constraints usually lead the toxicologist to choose inexpensive, short-lived, and easily bred animals for research, which leaves the risk assessor to assume that the results obtained are directly applicable to humans. Even if higher order animals are employed, there is no guarantee that they will react similarly to humans. For example, use of the cynomolgus monkey to study the effects of caffeine on pregnancy (Gilbert *et al.,* 1985) and on the behavioral characteristics of the offspring have produced results of questionable relevance to humans because theophylline is a major metabolite of caffeine in cynomolgus monkeys but not in humans.

In the past, the dilemmas that arose from the use of surrogate species were avoided by the use of two basic assumptions: the surrogate species predicts adequately for humans, and humans are as sensitive to the toxic effects of an agent as are the most sensitive experimental species. A growing understanding of the pharmacokinetic, physiological, and pathological processes involved in disease etiology promises a more rational and a more accurate assessment of the likely human toxicology of an agent. Such an approach requires the integration of the total toxicological data package and a greater feeling for the mechanisms of a particular toxicological effect (see Section IV, D).

The second major concern of the toxicologist is to conduct experiments that either demonstrate a toxic effect or give a reasonable assurance that the toxic effect does not occur (Clayson and Krewski, 1986). This is generally achieved with adequate numbers of test animals and an exaggerated dose, although evaluation of toxic effects induced by high doses is not always straightforward (Section IV, D).

In a carcinogenesis study, for example, it is theoretically possible to demonstrate a positive effect using 5 experimental and 5 control animals provided all the experimental animals and none of the controls develop cancer. Such a limited experiment is, however, quite insufficient to judge whether the agent fails to elicit a carcinogenic response. In the case of agents judged not to be carcinogenic, it is necessary to use more animals, the actual number chosen being a compromise between what can be afforded and what is desirable (Clayson and Krewski, 1986). For example, in carcinogenicity studies, groups of 50 or more male and 50 or more female animals for each dose group including controls are usually considered adequate (Sontag *et al.,* 1976).

Use of exaggerated doses presents problems (Section IV, D). The major concern should be to ensure that high doses do not induce forms of toxicity that do not occur at lower doses and thus obscure the significance of high dose results to the human situation. The solution to this problem again requires careful consideration of all available toxicological evidence. For example, the use of 2% dietary butylated hydroxyanisole (BHA) induces toxic effects and subsequent tumors in the forestomach of rats (Clayson et al., 1986). Neither toxic effects nor forestomach tumors are observed at doses below 0.25% BHA in the diet.

IV. RISK ESTIMATION

The fundamental problem of regulatory toxicology has been defined as the determination of safe levels of human exposure to toxicants present in the environment (Clayson and Krewski, 1986). Despite the fact that absolute safety can never be guaranteed, it is the responsibility of the regulatory toxicologist to determine acceptable levels of human exposure to chemicals present in or added to the overall human environment, including those in air, water, food, and drugs.

For risk assessment purposes, toxic processes may be divided into those that are stochastic and those that are nonstochastic in nature. Stochastic processes such as carcinogenesis result from the random occurrence of one or more biological events in specific individuals. The consequence of this is that the response of a particular individual under specified conditions of exposure cannot be predicted with certainty. On the other hand, nonstochastic events such as enzyme inhibition are more uniform in nature and occur predictably following an animal's exposure to a certain critical level of the toxicant under study. Different approaches to risk assessment are usually employed for these two categories of response.

A. Safety Factors and Thresholds

Nonstochastic effects usually exhibit a threshold level below which the toxic effect may not occur. Because the precise identification of a population threshold is a difficult proposition (Schneiderman et al., 1979), it has become common practice to identify an experimental dose level at which no adverse effects are apparent. Recognizing that the absence of any observed toxic effects in a small sample of homogeneous experimental animals does not guarantee zero risk, this dose has been termed the no-observed effect level (NOEL).

With nonstochastic toxic effects, the usual procedure is to apply a safety or uncertainty factor to the NOEL and assume that the derived level will be safe for humans (Dourson and Stara, 1983). The magnitude of the safety factor involves a number of considerations including the quality and extent of available experimental data, the uncertainty in the data itself, the nature and severity of the health effects induced, the possibility of differential sensitivity among population subgroups, and the potential for differences between the test species used and humans. A larger safety factor may sometimes be applied to the lowest-observed effect level (LOEL) in the absence of a NOEL in the study or studies at hand. Each of the relevant factors may be allocated a value of 5 or 10, or another value if deemed appropriate, and the product of these components is adopted as the overall safety factor. In many cases, a safety factor of $10 \times 10 = 100$ is used, with the first factor of 10 allowing for human variability in response and the second for the use of a surrogate species. This use of safety factors represents a prudent approach to risk assessment. In special cases, very low safety factors may be acceptable. For example, the cardiac drug digitoxin is considered to be so important in the control of cardiac disease that a safety factor (therapeutic index) of 2 may be used.

Safety factors are seldom used to assess the effects of toxic agents that lead to stochastic processes because it is not possible to define a no-effect level with any degree of confidence. Nevertheless, it has been suggested that a safety factor of the order of 5,000 might be used with some carcinogens based on a minimal response to the agent in a standard bioassay (Weil, 1972; Truhaut, 1979, 1980). This approach has not been widely adopted for carcinogens, but use of a suitable safety factor may be appropriate if carcinogenic effects can be clearly demonstrated to depend on the previous occurrence of nonstochastic toxic effects (Clayson, 1987).

B. Linear Extrapolation and Virtual Safety

The threshold assumption has been called into question for certain delayed, irreversible toxic effects occurring as a result of genotoxic or initiating events. Thus, stochastic processes are used to describe the actions of many chemical carcinogens and mutagens. Because these substances are often tested at high dose levels in animals, alternative methods are required to assess risks associated with human exposure to lower doses. These methods are more recent and more controversial than the use of safety factors. Nonetheless, practical evaluations should comprise three separate stages: a detailed consideration of whether the results of the animal test are likely to be applicable to humans (Clayson, 1987); an attempt to estimate the differences in response between humans and the surrogate animal species (Rall *et al.*, 1987); and a mathematical approach to dose extrapolation from the high doses usually given to animals to the expected human exposure levels (Krewski *et al.*, 1986).

Because any nonzero dose may be associated with some degree of risk in the absence of a population threshold, complete safety can only be assured through the complete elimination of exposure. This may be impractical with chemicals that are ubiquitous in the environment or deemed necessary in view of significant offsetting benefits.

As a way out of this dilemma, Mantel and Bryan (1961) have proposed a concept of virtual safety in which the zero risk principle is abandoned in favor of a negligible or *de minimis* risk philosophy. More precisely, Mantel and Bryan have defined a virtually safe dose (VSD) as one that limits risk to some suitably low level. A lifetime risk of 1 in 100 million or 10^{-8} was suggested as a negligible risk by these authors, although recent trends have been toward use of a value on the order of 10^{-6} (U.S. Environmental Protection Agency, 1980). Although the selection of an acceptable level of risk is clearly a societal rather than a scientific decision, there is some evidence that voluntary risks of 1 in 1 million are largely ignored (Royal Society Study Group, 1983).

Because the occurrence of a single lesion in a group of 50 test animals corresponds to an additional 20,000 cases in a population of 1 million, risks in the order of 10^{-6} cannot be estimated with practically feasible numbers of experimental animals. Safety assessment of chemicals relies on procedures analogous to the overstress tests used to assess the reliability of manufactured items. It is necessary to extrapolate downward from the "accelerated" doses used in the laboratory. To perform this extrapolation, Mantel and Bryan originally relied on a probit model with a shallower slope than had been observed experimentally to perform this extrapolation.

Since that time, many other models have been developed by various investigators (Brown and Koziol, 1983; Krewski *et al.*, 1983). Most are sufficiently flexible to provide a good fit to the experimental data and appear to have at least some biological basis. However, it is now well known that different models can lead to markedly different results upon extrapolation to low risk levels, leaving the regulator in a dilemma as to which result to believe. This task is made no less difficult by the fact that statistical goodness-of-fit tests have little chance of distinguishing between two plausible models at the experimental dose levels (Crump, 1984). The undefined nature of many disease processes presents further complications that can be addressed only through mechanistic studies designed to elucidate disease etiology.

Such model dependency has produced a tendency toward conservatism in risk extrapolation. In many cases, it is assumed that the worst case may be embodied in the hypotheses of low dose linearity in which the risk is presumed to be directly proportional to the level of exposure in the low dose region (Crump et al., 1976; Hoel et al., 1983; Murdoch et al., 1987). Thus, statistical procedures for linear extrapolation have been advocated by many investigators (Crump, 1984; Krewski et al., 1983) and endorsed by certain regulatory authorities (U.S. Environmental Protection Agency, 1980; World Health Organization, 1984). Although these procedures are likely to be reasonably accurate when the so-called linear hypothesis holds, the method can be quite conservative if the dose–response curve approaches zero at a sublinear rate (Krewski et al., 1983).

By way of comparison with the safety factor approach, linear extrapolation to a target risk of 10^{-6} might be comparable to an uncertainty factor of up to 50,000 fold (Krewski et al., 1984). This can be further increased if an additional adjustment for species difference is considered appropriate or desirable according to scientifically based methodology. Despite its apparent stringency, linear extrapolation has been used in a number of instances, including the determination of Canadian federal guidelines for trace levels of carcinogenic contaminants in drinking water (Somers, 1983, 1984). This same approach has been used by the World Health Organization (1984) for establishing the objectives of quality drinking water.

C. Transspecies Extrapolation

Satisfactory techniques for quantitative transspecies extrapolation presently do not exist (Clayson, 1983). Therefore, the regulator has usually assumed that humans are at least as sensitive to a stochastic effect such as carcinogenesis as is the most sensitive experimental species (Clayson, 1985a). However, the price paid for this assumption is overestimation of the risk presented by some carcinogens to the human population. For example, Booth et al. (1981) have presented evidence that the human liver may be considerably less sensitive to the carcinogenic effects of aflatoxin B_1 than is the rat liver.

This area of biologically based risk assessment has until recently been largely neglected because the possible mechanisms involved in carcinogenesis have not been considered. Efforts to estimate potency (Clayson, 1983; Gold et al., 1984) indicate substantial interspecies differences with some but not all carcinogens (National Academy of Sciences, 1981).

One area that may offer promise for improvement in the manner in which risk estimates are translated from one species to another is the use of pharmacokinetic modeling (Anderson *et al.,* 1987; Krewski *et al.,* 1987; Menzel, 1987). By constructing physiological models to describe the metabolism of a substance and the concentration of the reactive metabolite at the target tissue, the researcher may be better able to predict tissue concentrations in humans if the relevant metabolites can be identified and the appropriate model parameters can be determined (Fiserova-Bergerova, 1983). Although representing a potentially useful technique for improving the risk assessment process, this approach cannot be applied in those cases in which the reactive metabolites are too unstable to permit their measurement *in vivo.*

D. Biological Risk Assessment

Hazard identification and statistical studies of risk alone are inadequate for the full determination of the risk that a particular chemical may pose to humans. There is a need to determine whether the biological consequences of the experimental conditions, including the species and strain of test animal, the degree of dose exaggeration, and the length of the test, render data unsuitable for extrapolation to particular human populations. Such a process may be termed biological risk assessment (Clayson, 1987).

Toxicological studies of carcinogenic effects are generally conducted at or near the maximum dose levels that animals will survive without deteriorating in overall condition or losing more than 10% of their body weight. Maximum dose levels ensure that negative results will not be superseded by positive results obtained at a higher dose level. However, there has recently been growing concern about use of such high doses because they may in themselves present difficulties in evaluating the likelihood of similar effects from lower doses.

In teratological and reproductive studies, Khera (1984, 1985, 1987a, 1987b) has pointed out that those levels of test agent that induce toxic signs in the mothers may lead to fetal wastage and to deformities in the offspring that show a constant pattern dependent on the species used rather than on the individual test agent. The relevance of such results for humans or animals exposed to much lower doses is thus questionable. Such a dilemma was clearly demonstrated by teratogenicity tests of the trichothecene (Vomitoxin; Khera *et al.,* 1982).

Haseman (1985) pointed out that the test agents used in 18 of 31 feeding bioassays conducted by the U.S. National Toxicology Program were identified as carcinogens solely as a result of feeding at the maximum tolerated dose (MTD). Because the MTD is relatively loosely defined as the maximum dose that does not affect the clinical condition of the animal nor lead to more than a 10% reduction in body weight (Munro, 1977), there can be little confidence that none of the chemicals to which Haseman (1985) has referred was associated with toxicity related to carcinogenesis; all were therefore of limited human relevance. This issue is addressed by the U.S. Environmental Protection Agency in its *Proposed Guidelines for Carcinogen Risk Assessment* (1984).

> "Positive studies at levels above the MTD should be fully reviewed to ensure that the responses are not due to factors which do not operate at exposure levels below the MTD. Evidence indicating that high dose testing produces tumor responses by indirect mechanisms that may be unrelated to effects at lower doses should be dealt with on an individual basis."

This represents a considerable step forward in deciding the relevance of animal experiments to humans. However, it is still difficult to understand why this approach should not be valid at doses below the MTD if the critical toxic event is not acutely life threatening and is specific to the tissue in which tumors are induced. Recent work on the mechanism of induction of forestomach tumors in rats by tert-butylated hydroxyanisole (BHA) is an example. It appears that high levels of this agent induce cellular proliferation in the forestomach epithelium, which is related to tumor formation. Because this proliferation also occurs at levels below the MTD, the possibility of tumor occurrence at these lower doses cannot be dismissed. However, this proliferative stimulus appears to show a NOEL well above human exposure levels, thereby casting uncertainty on the relevance of the animal results to humans (Ito *et al.*, 1982, 1983; Nera *et al.*, 1984; Iverson *et al.*, 1985; Rodriques *et al.*, 1986).

A further complication in the interpretation of animal carcinogenicity studies arises in the use of untreated animals that naturally develop a moderate to high incidence of tumors in specific tissues (Tarone *et al.*, 1981). These tumors in control animals are very likely to be accompanied by initiated cells that, for one reason or another, do not develop into tumors in the lifetime of the test animal (Clayson *et al.*, 1983). A change in the tissue environment induced by high doses of a test agent may enable more of these initiated cells to develop into cancers. This supports the suggestion that the agent is a carcinogen. If human tissues do not contain similar initiated cells, such a test agent is most unlikely to be effective in humans. That is, in assays such as those in which male B6C3F1 mice developed a high incidence of tumors in liver tissue even when untreated (Tarone *et al.*, 1981), it is difficult to decide whether the inducing agent is a true carcinogen or simply an enhancing agent acting through cytotoxicity and subsequent cellular regeneration or in other ways (Clayson, 1987). The importance of this observation can be seen in Soderman's (1982) database analysis, which shows that of 811 chemicals that have been adequately tested for carcinogenicity, 120 produced an increase in liver cell carcinomas in mice. Moreover, in 25 to 30 examples, this tumor was the only lesion to suggest that the chemical was carcinogenic.

The instability of these relatively high yields of tumors in control animals presents a further problem. These tumors are sensitive to the laboratory environment in which the study is conducted (Tarone et al., 1981). Thus, any use of historical controls to increase confidence in the validity of a particular result must take into account any between study variation, which may be present as a result of such differences (Tarone, 1982; Yanagawa and Hoel, 1985; Krewski et al., 1988).

The problems raised by background tumors have been recognized in the test for lung adenoma in StA mice (Shimkin and Stoner, 1975; Maronpot et al., 1986). This test is seldom used because the incidence of induced tumors were unstable. Similarly, the inadequacy of the bladder implantation technique became apparent when it was demonstrated clearly that implantation of paraffin pellets without a test chemical led to bladder carcinoma in 50% of the test animals in a lifetime mouse study (Jull, 1951, 1979; Clayson, 1979).

V. RISK MANAGEMENT

Identification of a specific hazard and estimation of the risk that an agent might pose represents only the first steps toward effective control of that hazard. The subsequent management of risk is largely a politically based process that depends on balancing society's perception of the risks involved, the usefulness or desirability of the agent, and the current regulatory climate.

In many cases, the public tends to view risk in a pragmatic manner: as much attention is often paid to the perceived benefits as to the magnitude of the risk. In the area of life-style, for example, individual decisions are possible. Many members of the public choose to ignore the adverse effects of cigarette smoking despite the overwhelming evidence that this activity is associated with a high level of mortality, involving perhaps 30% of all cancer deaths (Krewski, 1985), 30% of all cases of coronary heart disease (U.S. Surgeon General, 1983), and 85% of all cases of chronic obstructive lung disease (U.S. Surgeon General, 1984). In contrast, the public clearly shows great concern over the possibility that marginally toxic chemicals may find their way into the general environment or food supply (Roberts, 1981).

Most nations enact separate laws to control food, water, air, occupational settings, and use of drugs. With multiple legislation, both differing public perceptions of risk and differing needs for regulation in specific areas can be considered. The severity of regulation may differ among nations, as exemplified by the Delaney amendment to the U.S. Food and Drug Act (U.S. Food and Drug Act, 1958) that makes it illegal to add known human or animal carcinogens to food intended for human consumption in the United States. Other Western nations do not have similar restrictions but rely on a more general and possibly more effective prohibition against the addition of substances to the food supply that may be injurious to health. Similarly, regulators in different countries may differ in their opinion as to what constitutes an unacceptable hazard. The list of food dyes permitted in various countries, for example, demonstrates a wide divergence of opinion among nations. Such disparity is a barrier to the harmonization of international trade in processed foodstuffs; however, the hazard and level of risk associated with these substances is, in all probability, minimal. The risk management strategies selected in different countries also demonstrate how governments judge and manage scientific uncertainty and respond to local political and cultural pressures.

Although the community as a whole looks for a risk-free environment, individuals fiercely maintain their right to decide what risks they are prepared to accept, whether they be cigarette smoking, motorcycle racing, or Russian roulette. Consequently, progress in rationalizing the process of risk management has been slow. Risk-benefit analysis has been widely discussed as a means of rationalizing the regulatory approach (Krewski, 1987). However, it presents two major difficulties. First, it is often difficult to assess risks and benefits in identical units in order to permit logical comparisons. Who, for example, is able to place a dollar value on the development of the perfect cola beverage from the community's viewpoint? Second, although the introduction of a new agent or process may present an overall benefit to the community at large, the risk is often borne by a group of individuals other than those who garner the benefits. For example, although a new industrial process may present a hazard to the workers involved, the owners reap most of the primary benefit.

Such considerations make the application of risk-benefit analyses difficult except in certain relatively simple cases. For example, the use of a highly toxic drug may be entirely appropriate to control an otherwise debilitating or fatal disease. The individual patient is thereby given a chance to survive a potential calamity. Through informed consent, he or she expresses a willingness to accept the risk in view of the possible benefit. Use of a highly toxic drug, however, places the onus on attending physicians to avoid subjecting less severely ill patients to unjustified risks associated with that particular form of therapy.

Regardless of the manner in which decisions are ultimately made, the scientific data base on which risk assessment is based forms a critical component of the overall process. Thus, the most useful contribution that a toxicologist can make to the process of risk management is to present information that is as accurate as possible on the toxicology of the chemical agent in question. This will require careful attention to all aspects of the design, conduct, and evaluation of individual studies as described in the previous chapters of this book.

VI. UNCERTAINTIES IN RISK ASSESSMENT

Toxicology is currently relied on to protect the general population from hazards inherent in various components of the environment. Although identification of hazards in laboratory animals may be defined in terms of relatively rigid approaches and experimental protocols, interpretation of their significance in terms of risk assessment and risk management presents many problems.

A number of major uncertainties that range from transspecies extrapolation and high to low dose extrapolation to human heterozygosity have been discussed in this chapter. These problems can be effectively solved only through an increased knowledge of the mechanisms of the toxic processes under consideration (Clayson, 1987). Such mechanistic studies will, for example, make it possible to determine whether a process observed in one species is likely to occur in another species. Eventually, it will be possible to calculate the likely magnitude of response in the human species. Mechanistic considerations should no longer be regarded as irrelevant to regulatory toxicology, and should increasingly play a greater role in the toxicologist's decision with respect to which toxic effects manifest in animals are relevant to the human population.

Perhaps the biggest problem facing toxicology risk assessment is the fact that, while experimental animals are exposed to just one compound, humans are, in contrast, exposed to large numbers of different agents. Single-chemical toxicity studies thus have intrinsically limited applicability to humans. However, the testing of a vast number of individual agents jointly is impossible. It has been estimated that about 60,000 chemicals at any one time are produced and used in industry and commerce. An even greater number of chemicals probably occurs naturally as components of foodstuffs, as air or water pollutants, or from other sources. There are not enough trained personnel or adequate laboratory resources for each of these chemicals to be examined in isolation. The opportunity to study chemicals systematically in pairs or in larger aggregates, each of which might require a number of different ratios of the individual components for adequate testing (Clayson, 1985b), is quite beyond available resources now or in the foreseeable future.

There are at present few examples of synergism between agents in humans. Excluding drug interactions in the pharmaceutical area, the most prominent is the enhancing effect of cigarette smoking on the incidence of lung cancer induced by inhalation of asbestos fibers (Selikoff and Lee, 1976). In animals, there is more information. Carcinogenesis promotion (Berenblum and Shubik, 1947a, 1947b, 1949; Pitot and Sirica, 1980) represents perhaps the best documented example of synergism between two agents with seemingly different properties. Enzyme induction often represents a diminution in the effectiveness of a carcinogen's action by another agent (Richardson et al., 1952; Conney et al., 1956; Wattenberg, 1978). However, this represents only a small fraction of the knowledge that needs to be acquired on agent-agent interactions if accurate risk assessment is to be achieved.

A further series of problems arises from individuals within the human population who possess genetic abnormalities or personal idiosyncrasies. Xeroderma pigmentosum is an example of a genetic abnormality; some individuals with this condition are unable to remove ultraviolet light-induced thymine dimers and other lesions from their DNA. Consequently, they are often extremely prone to sunlight-induced skin lesions ranging from erythema to cancer (Setlow et al., 1977). Individual susceptibility also includes those humans who develop asthmatic symptoms when exposed to specific substances. With some substances, such idiosyncratic responses may be readily noticeable in the population and may lead to serious consequences, including death, in some individuals. Sulfur dioxide, for example, has led to severe bronchial asthma and death. Use of sulfur dioxide has, therefore, been prohibited and regulated in certain situations in which alternatives have been identified. With substances that appear to induce less serious consequences in fewer individuals and with those that occur naturally in certain important components of the food supply, less restrictive action may be considered appropriate. Adequate protection may sometimes be afforded if an attending clinician helps an individual understand those factors that contribute to his or her personal discomfort. Situations in which the offending agent is present may also be identified through component and additive labeling of specific products.

VII. SUMMARY AND CONCLUSIONS

The previous chapters of this book have focused on a wide variety of *in vivo* toxicological tests that may be used to evaluate the potential risks associated with specific toxicants present in the human environment. To ensure that the scientific data base on which toxicological risk assessment is based is as reliable and complete as possible, it is important that individual tests be conducted to the strictest experimental standards. This requires proper experimental design and analysis, careful adherence to standard operating procedures called for under GLP, evaluation of any anomalous results by the study director, and confirmation of judgmental results (such as in the histopathological diagnosis of difficult lesions).

Once toxicological data have been assembled, it is necessary to determine whether or not the substance under investigation demonstrates a hazard to humans. The critical elements of hazard identification include the selection of the most appropriate laboratory tests for safety evaluation and the determination of whether test outcomes are positive or negative. Subsequent quantitative analyses may then be used to arrive at estimates of risk and to establish acceptable levels of human exposure to substances added to or present in the environment. In this regard, application of a suitable safety factor for the dose shown to induce no adverse effects in animals has traditionally been employed to arrive at acceptable human exposures. Although this approach may be appropriate for non-stochastic effects likely to demonstrate a threshold, linear extrapolation to low doses may be more appropriate with stochastic effects for which a population threshold may not exist. In either case, use of these methods should be accompanied by careful consideration of the biological consequences of the experimental conditions, such as secondary high-dose toxic phenomena.

These approaches to toxicological risk assessment ultimately form the basis for effective risk management. Despite the scientific uncertainty surrounding risk assessment, careful interpretation and evaluation of the toxicological data at hand can lead to sound regulatory decisions concerning risk. Toxicology has progressed substantially since the last century when the main preoccupation was detecting and controlling sand in sugar or arsenic oxide in flour. There are still many problems to be solved before toxicological science becomes a precise way to prevent human exposure to excessive levels of potentially deleterious agents. It is clear that sound toxicological data gathering combined with a deep understanding of the problems in the use of that data to protect human health will be needed. Failure to recognize the problems that face the community in applying the results of toxicological data can be as disastrous as no toxicology at all.

Acknowledgments

The authors thank Douglas L. Arnold, Patricia Birkwood, Diane Kirkpatrick, David Clegg, and Don Wigle for their helpful comments and Judy Graham for her bibliographical assistance.

References

Andersen, M. E., Clewel, H. J., Gargas, M. L., Smith, F. A., and Reitz, R. H. (1987). Physiologically-based pharmacokinetics and the risk assessment process for methylene chloride. *Toxicol. Appl. Pharmacol.* **87**, 185–205.

Berenblum, I., and Shubik, P. (1947a). The role of croton oil applications, associated with a single painting of a carcinogen, in tumour induction of the mouse's skin. *Br. J. Cancer* **1**, 379–382.

Berenblum, I., and Shubik, P. (1947b). A new, quantitative approach to the study of the stages of chemical carcinogenesis in the mouse's skin. *Br. J. Cancer* **1**, 383–391.

Berenblum, I., and Shubik, P. (1949). The persistence of latent tumour cells induced in the mouse's skin by a single application of 9,10-dimethyl-1:2-benzanthracene. *Br. J. Cancer* **3**, 384–386.

Bickis, M., and Krewski, D. (1985). Statistical design and analysis of the long-term carcinogenicity bioassay. *In* "Toxicological Risk Assessment, Vol. I, Biological and Statistical Criteria" (D. B. Clayson, D. Krewski, and I. Munro, eds.), pp. 125–147. Boca Raton, Florida: CRC Press.

Booth, S. C., Bosenberg, H., Garner, R. C., Hertzog, P. J., and Norpoth, K. (1981). The activation of aflatoxin-Bl in liver slices and in bacterial mutagenicity assays using livers from different species including man. *Carcinogenesis* **2**, 1063–1068.

Brown, C. C., and Koziol, J. A. (1983). Statistical aspects of the estimation of human risk from suspected environmental carcinogens. *SIAM Rev.* **25**, 151–181.

Brown, K. G., and Hoel, D. G. (1983). Modelling time-to-tumour data: Analysis of the ED_{01} study. *Fundam. Appl. Toxicol.* **3**, 458–469.

Clayson, D. B. (1979). Guest Editorial: Bladder cancer in rats and mice: Possibility of artifacts. *Natl. Cancer Inst. Monogr.* **52**, 519–524.

Clayson, D. B. (1983). Trans-species and trans-tissue extrapolation of carcinogenicity assays. *In* "Organ and Species Specificity in Chemical Carcinogenesis" (R. Langenbach, S. Nesnow, and J. R. Rice, eds.), pp. 637–651. New York: Plenum.

Clayson, D. B. (1985a). Problems in interspecies extrapolation. *In* "Toxicological Risk Assessment, Volume 1: Biological and Statistical Criteria" (D. Clayson, D. Krewski, and I. Munro, eds.), pp. 105–122. Boca Raton, Florida: CRC Press.

Clayson, D. B. (1985b). Dose relationship in experimental carcinogenesis: dependence on multiple factors including biotransformation. *Toxicol. Pathol.* **13**, 119–127.

Clayson, D. B. (1987). The need for biological risk assessment in reaching decisions about carcinogens. *Mutat. Res.* **185**, 243–269.

Clayson, D. B., Iverson, F., Nera, E., Lok, E., Rogers, C., Rodrigues, C., Page, D., and Karpinski, K. (1986). Histopathological and radioautographical studies on the forestomach of F344 rats treated with butylated hydroxyanisole. *Food Chem. Toxicol.* **24,** 1171–1182.

Clayson, D. B., and Krewski, D. (1986). The concept of negativity in experimental carcinogenesis. *Mutat. Res.* **167,** 233–240.

Clayson, D. B., Krewski, D., and Munro, I. C. (1983). The power and interpretation of the carcinogenicity bioassay. *Regul. Toxicol. Pharmacol.* **3,** 329–348.

Conney, A. H., Miller, E. C., and Miller, J. A. (1956). The metabolism of methylated aminoazo dyes. V. Evidence for induction of enzyme synthesis in the rat by 3-methylcholanthrene. *Cancer Res.* **16,** 450–459.

Crump, K. S., Hoel, D. G., Langley, C. H., and Peto, R. (1976). Fundamental carcinogenic processes and their implications for low dose risk assessment. *Cancer Res.* **36,** 2973–2979.

Crump, K. S. (1984). An improved procedure for low-dose carcinogenic risk assessment from animal data. *J. Environ. Pathol. Toxicol. Oncol.* **5,** 339–348.

Dourson, M. L., and Stara, J. F. (1983). Regulatory history and experimental support of uncertainty (safety) factors. *Regul. Toxicol. Pharmacol.* **3,** 224–238.

Fiserova-Bergerova, V. (ed.) (1983). "Modelling of Inhalation Exposure to Vapors: Uptake, Distribution and Elimination." Boca Raton, Florida: CRC Press.

Gad, S. C., and Weil, C. S. (1984). Statistics for toxicologists. *In* "Principles and Methods of Toxicology" (A. W. Hayes, ed.), pp. 273–320. New York: Raven Press.

Gart, J. J., Krewski, D., Lee, P. N., Tarone, R. E., and Wahrendorf, J. (1986). "Statistical Methods in Cancer Research, Vol. III: The Design and Analysis of Long-Term Animal Experiments." Lyon: International Agency for Research on Cancer.

Gilbert, S. G., Stavric, B., Klassen, R. D., and Rice, D. C. (1985). Fate of chronically consumed caffeine in the monkey (Macaca fascicularis). *Fundam. Appl. Toxicol.* **5,** 578–587.

Gold, L. G., Sawyer, C. B., Magaw, R., Backman, G. M., de Veciana, M., Levinson, R., Hooper, N. K., Havendor, W. R., Bernstein, L., Peto, R., Pike, M. C., and Ames, B. N. (1984). A carcinogenic potency database of the standardized results of animal bioassays. *Environ. Health Perspect.* **58,** 9–319.

Haseman, J. K. (1985). Issues in carcinogenicity testing: Dose selection. *Fundam. Appl. Toxicol.* **5,** 66–78.

Hoel, D. G., Kaplan, N. L., and Anderson, M. W. (1983). Implication of nonlinear kinetics on risk estimation in carcinogenesis. *Science* **219,** 1032–1037.

International Life Sciences Institute (1984). Interpretation of extrapolation of chemical and. biological carcinogenicity data to establish human safety standards. *In* "Current Issues in Toxicology" (H. C. Grice, ed.), pp. 1–152. New York: Springer-Verlag.

Ito, N., Fukushima, S., Hagiwara, A., Shibata, M., and Ogiso, T. (1983). Carcinogenicity of butylated hydroxyanisole in F344 rats. *J. Natl. Cancer Inst. (US)* **70,** 343–352.

Ito, N., Hagiwasa, A., Shibata, M., Ogiso, T., and Fukushima, S. (1982). Induction of squamous cell carcinoma in the forestomach of F344 rats treated with butylated hydroxyanisole. *Gann* **73,** 332–334.

Iverson, F., Lok, E., Nera, E., Karpinski, K., and Clayson, D. B. (1985). A 13 week feeding study of butylated hydroxyanisole: the subsequent regression of the induced lesions in male Fischer 344 rat forestomach epithelium. *Toxicology* **35,** 1–11.

Jull, J. W. (1951). The induction of tumours of the bladder epithelium in mice by the direct application of a carcinogen. *Br. J. Cancer* **5,** 328–330.

Jull, J. W. (1979). The effect of time on the incidence of carcinomas obtained by the implantation of paraffin wax pellets into mouse bladder. *Cancer Lett.* **6,** 21–25.

Khera, K. S. (1984). Maternal toxicity—A possible cause for fetal malformations in mice. *Teratology* **29,** 411–416.

Khera, K. S. (1985). Maternal toxicity: A possible etiological factor in embryo–fetal deaths and fetal malformations of rodent-rabbit species. *Teratology* **31,** 129–153.

Khera, K. S. (1987a). Maternal toxicity of drugs and metabolic disorders—A possible etiologic factor in the intrauterine death and congenital malformation: A critique on human data. *CRC Crit. Rev. Toxicol.* **17,** 345–375.

Khera, K. S. (1987b). Maternal toxicity in humans and animals: Effects on fetal development and criteria for detection. *Teratog. Carcinog. Mutagen.* **7,** 287–295.

Khera, K. S., Whalen, C., Angers, G., Vesonder, R. F., and Kuiper-Goodman, T. (1982). Embryotoxicity of 4-deoxynivalenol (vomitoxin) in mice. *Bull. Environ. Contam. Toxicol.* **29,** 487–491.

Krewski, D. (1985). Cancer prevention: A historical perspective. *Risk Abstr.* **2,** 139–145.

Krewski, D. (1987). Risk and risk management: Issues and approaches. *In* "Environmental Health Risks: Assessment and Management" (R. S. McColl, ed.), pp. 29–51. Waterloo: University of Waterloo Press.

Krewski, D., and Birkwood, P. (1987). Risk assessment and risk management. *Risk Abstr.,* in press.

Krewski, D., Brown, C., and Murdoch, D. (1984). Determining "safe" levels of exposure: Safety factors or mathematical models? *Fundam. Appl. Toxicol.* **4,** S383–S394.

Krewski, D., Crump, K. S., Gaylor, D. W., Howe, R., Portier, C., Salsburg, D., Sielkon, R. L., and Van Ryzin, J. (1983). A comparison of statistical methods for low dose extrapolation using time to tumor data. *Fundam. Appl. Toxicol.* **3,** 140–160.

Krewski, D., Murdoch, D., and Dewanji, A. (1986). Statistical modeling and extrapolation of carcinogenesis data. *In* "Modern Statistical Methods in Chronic Disease Epidemiology" (S. H. Moolgavkar and R. L. Prentice, eds.), pp. 259–282. New York: Wiley-Interscience.

Krewski, D., Murdoch, D., and Withey, J. (1987). The application of pharmacokinetic data in carcinogenic risk assessment. *In* "Pharmacokinetics and Risk Assessment: Drinking Water and Health," Vol. 8, pp. 441–468. Washington, DC: National Academy Press.

Krewski, D., Smythe, R. T., Dewanji, A., and Colin, D. (1988). Statistical tests with historical controls. *In* "Carcinogenicity: The Design, Analysis and Interpretation of Long-Term Animal Studies" (H. C. Grice and J. L. Ciminera, eds.), pp. 23–38. New York: Springer-Verlag.

Mantel, N., and Bryan, W. R. (1961). "Safety" testing of carcinogenic agents. *J. Natl. Cancer Inst. (US)* **27,** 455–470.

Maronpot, R. R., Shimkin, M. B., Witschi, H. P., Smith, L. H., and Cline, J. M. (1986). Strain A mouse pulmonary tumor test results for chemicals previously tested in the National Cancer Institute Carcinogenicity tests. *J. Natl. Cancer Inst. (US)* **76,** 1101–1112.

Menzel, D. (1987). Physiological pharmacokinetic modeling. *Environ. Sci. Technol.* **21,** 944–950.

Munro, I. C. (1977). Considerations in chronic toxicity testing: the chemical, the dose, the design. *J. Environ. Pathol. Toxicol.* **1**, 183–197.

Murdoch, D. J., Krewski, D., and Crump, K. S. (1987). Mathematical models of carcinogenesis. *In* "Cancer Modelling" (J. R. Thompson & B. W. Brown, eds.). New York: Marcel Dekker. In press.

National Academy of Sciences (1981). "The Health Effects of Nitrate, Nitrite and N-Nitroso compounds: Part 1 of a 2 Part Study by the Committee on Nitrite and Alternative Curing Agents in Food," pp. 9-47–9-48. Washington, DC: National Academy Press.

National Research Council, Committee on the Institutional Means for the Assessment of Risks to Public Health (1983). "Risk Assessment in the Federal Government: Managing the Process." Washington, DC: National Academy Press.

Nera, E. A., Lok, E., Iverson, F., Ormsby, E., Karpinski, K. F., and Clayson, D. B. (1984). Short-term pathological and proliferative effects of butylated hydroxyanisole and other phenolic antioxidants in the Forestomach of Fischer 344 rats. *Toxicology* **32**, 197–213.

Pitot, H. C., and Sirica, A. E. (1980). The stages of initiation and promotion in hepatocarcinogenesis. *Biochim. Biophys. Acta* **605**, 191–215.

Rall, D., Hogan, M. D., Huff, J. E., Schwetz, B. A., and Tennant, R. W. (1987). Alternatives to using human experience in assessing health risks. *Annu. Rev. Public Health* **8**, 355–385.

Richardson, H. L., Stier, A. R., and Borsos-Nachtnebel, E. (1952). Liver tumor inhibition and adrenal histologic responses in rats to which 3'-methyl-4-dimethylaminoazo-benzene and 20-methylcholanthrene were simultaneously administered. *Cancer Res.* **12**, 356–361.

Roberts, H. (ed.) (1981). "Food Safety." New York: Wiley-Interscience.

Rodrigues, C., Lok, E., Nera, E., Iverson, F., Page, D., Karpinski, K., and Clayson, D. B. (1986). Short-term effects of various phenols and acids on the Fischer 344 male rats forestomach epithelium. *Toxicology* **38**, 103–117.

Royal Society Study Group (1983). "Risk Assessment: A Study Group Report." London: Royal Society.

Ruckelshaus, W. D. (1983). Science, risk and public policy. *Science* **221**, 1026–1028.

Schneiderman, M. A., Decouflé, P., and Brown, C. C. (1979). Thresholds for environmental cancer: Biologic and statistical considerations. *Ann. N.Y. Acad. Sci.* **329**, 92–130.

Selikoff, L. J., and Lee, D. H. K. (1978). "Asbestos and Disease." New York: Academic Press.

Setlow, R. B., Ahmed, F. E., and Grist, E. (1977). Xeroderma pigmentosum: damage to DNA is involved in carcinogenesis. *In* "Origins of Human Cancer" (H. H. Hiatt, J. D. Watson, and J. A. Winsten, eds), Vol. B, pp. 889–902. Cold Spring Harbor, New York: Cold Spring Harbor Laboratory.

Shimkin, M. B., and Stoner, C. D. (1975). Lung tumors in mice: Application to carcinogenesis bioassay. *Adv. Cancer Res.* **21**, 1–58.

Soderman, J. V. (1982). "CRC Handbook of Identified Carcinogens and Noncarcinogens: Carcinogenicity-Mutagenicity Data Base." Boca Raton, Florida. CRC Press.

Somers, E. (1983). Environmental health risk management in Canada. *Regul. Toxicol. Pharmacol.* **3**, 75–81.

Somers, E. (1984). Risk estimation for environmental chemicals as a basis for decision making. *Regul. Toxicol. Pharmacol.* **4**, 99–106.

Sontag, J. M., Page, N. P., and Saffiotti, U. (1976). Guidelines for carcinogen bioassay in small rodents. (Tech. Rep. NCI-CG-TR-1). Washington, DC: U.S. Department of Health, Education and Welfare.

Starr, C. (1985). Risk management, assessment and acceptability. *Risk Anal.* **5,** 97–102.

Tarone, R. E. (1982). The use of historical control information in testing for a trend in proportions. *Biometrics* **38,** 215–220.

Tarone, R. E., Chu, K. C., and Ward, J. M. (1981). Variability in the rates of some common naturally-occurring tumors in Fischer 344 rats and (C57BL/6N × C3H/HEN)F$_1$ (B6C3F1) mice. *J. Natl. Cancer Inst. (US)* **66,** 1175–1181.

Truhaut, R. (1979). An overview of the problem of thresholds for chemical carcinogens. *In* "Carcinogenic Risks/Strategies for Intervention" (W. Davis & C. Rosenfeld, eds.), pp. 191–202. (IARC Sci. Publ. No. 25). Lyon: International Agency for Research on Cancer.

Truhaut, R. (1980). The problem of thresholds for chemical carcinogens — Its importance in industrial hygiene, especially in the field of permissible limits for occupational exposure. *Am. Ind. Hyg. Assoc. J.* **41,** 685–692.

U.S. Department of Health and Human Services, Committee to Coordinate Environmental and Related Programs (1985). "Risk Assessment and Risk Management of Toxic Substances." Washington, DC: Department of Health and Human Services.

U.S. Environmental Protection Agency (1980). Water quality criteria documents; availability. *Fed. Regist.* **45,** 79318–79379.

U.S. Environmental Protection Agency (1983a). Toxic substance control; good laboratory practice standards; final rule. *Fed. Regist.* **48,** 53922–53944.

U.S. Environmental Protection Agency (1983b). Pesticide programs; good laboratory practice standards; final rule. *Fed. Regist.* **48,** 53948–53969.

U.S. Environmental Protection Agency (1984). "Proposed Guidelines for Carcinogenic Risk Assessment." Washington, DC: U.S. Environmental Protection Agency.

U.S. Food and Drug Act (1958). Public Law 85–929. 85th Congress. H.R. 13254, September 6.

U.S. Food and Drug Administration (1976). Department of Health, Education and Welfare, Food and Drug Administration, nonclinical laboratories studies, proposed regulations for good laboratory practice. *Fed. Regist.,* 51206–51228.

U.S. Surgeon General (1983). "The Health Consequences of Smoking: Cardiovascular Disease." Washington, DC: U.S. Government Printing Office.

U.S. Surgeon General (1984). "The Health Consequences of Smoking: Chronic Obstructive Lung Disease." Washington, DC: U.S. Government Printing Office.

Wattenberg, L. W. (1978). Inhibition of chemical carcinogenesis. *J. Natl. Cancer Inst. (US)* **60,** 11–18.

Weil, C. S. (1972). Statistics versus safety factors and scientific judgement in the evaluation of safety for man. *Toxicol. Appl. Pharmacol.* **21,** 454–463.

World Health Organization (1984). "Guidelines for Drinking Water Quality, Vol. I, Recommendations." Geneva: World Health Organization.

World Health Organization (1985). "Risk Management in Chemical Safety" (ICP/CEH 506/m01 56881). Geneva: World Health Organization, European Regional Program on Chemical Safety.

Yanagawa, T., and Hoel, D. G. (1985). Use of historical controls for animal experiments. *Environ. Health Perspect.* **63,** 217–224.

Index